PLEASE TAKE GOOD CARE OF THIS BOOK

DATE OF RETURN
UNLESS RECALLED BY LIBRARY

Current Clinical Pathology

Antonio Giordano, MD, PhD
Temple University
Philadelphia
United States

Series Editor

Alfonso Baldi • Paola Pasquali
Enrico P. Spugnini
Editors

Skin Cancer

A Practical Approach

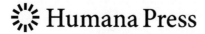 Humana Press

Editors
Alfonso Baldi
Department of Environmental
Biological and Pharmaceutical Sciences
and Technologies
Second University of Naples
Naples
Italy

Enrico P. Spugnini, DVM, PhD
S.A.F.U. Department
Regina Elena Cancer Institute
Rome
Italy

Paola Pasquali
Department of Dermatology
Pius Hospital De Valls
Tarragona
Spain

ISBN 978-1-4614-7356-5   ISBN 978-1-4614-7357-2   (eBook)
DOI 10.1007/978-1-4614-7357-2
Springer New York Heidelberg Dordrecht London

Library of Congress Control Number: 2013945181

Printed on acid-free paper

Humana Press is a brand of Springer
Springer is part of Springer Science+Business Media (www.springer.com)

Contents

Contributors

Yasser A. Alqubaisy, MD Department of Dermatology and Cutaneous Surgery, University of Miami Leonard M. Miller School of Medicine, Miami, FL, USA

Peter E. Andersen DTU Fotonik – Department of Photonics Engineering, Technical University of Denmark, Roskilde, Denmark

Anna Maria Anniciello Pathology Unit, National Institute of Tumours Fondazione "G. Pascale", Naples, Italy

Federica Arginelli Department of Dermatology, University of Modena and Reggio Emilia, Modena, Italy

Enrico Baldessari Plastic Surgery, Casa di Cura Addominale EUR, Rome, Italy

Fondazione Futura-onlus, Rome, Italy

Alfonso Baldi Department of Environmental, Biological and Pharmaceutical Sciences and Technologies, Second University of Naples, Naples, Italy

Fondazione Futura-onlus, Rome, Italy

Feliciano Baldi Department of Biochemistry, Section Pathology, Second University of Naples, Naples, Italy

Christina Banzhaf Department of Dermatology, Faculty of Health Sciences, Roskilde Hospital, University of Copenhagen, Roskilde, Denmark

Raymond Barnhill Department of Pathology and Laboratory Medicine, David Geffen School of Medicine at UCLA, and Jonsson Comprehensive Cancer Center, Los Angeles, CA, USA

Alexander Bianchi Department of Biochemistry, Section of Pathology, Second University of Naples, Naples, Italy

Stefano Bizzi Advanced Computer Systems (ACS), Rome, Italy

Emanuela Bonoldi Pathology Unit, Hospital A. Manzoni, Lecco, Italy

Gerardo Botti Pathology Unit, National Institute of Tumours Fondazione "G. Pascale", Naples, Italy

Beniamino Brunetti, MD Plastic and Reconstructive Surgery Unit,
Campus Bio-Medico of Rome University, Rome, Italy

Piergiacomo Calzavara-Pinton, MD Department of Dermatology,
University of Brescia, Brescia, Italy

Elia Camacho Department of Dermatology, Pius Hospital De Valls,
Valls, Spain

Stefano Campa Plastic and Reconstructive Surgery Unit,
Campus Bio-Medico of Rome University, Rome, Italy

Emilia Caputo Department of Genetics and Biophysics,
Institute of Genetics and Biophysics, Naples, Italy

Michele Caraglia, MD, PhD Department of Biochemistry and Biophysics,
Second University of Naples, Naples, Italy

Sonal Choudhary, MD Department of Dermatology and Cutaneous
Surgery, University of Miami Leonard M. Miller School of Medicine,
Miami, FL, USA

Claudio Clemente Department of Pathology and Cytopathology,
San Pio X Hospital, Milan, Italy

Department of Pathology and Cytopathology, IRCCS Policlinico
San Donato, San Donato Group, San Donato Milanese, Milan, Italy

Alistair Cochran Departments of Pathology, Laboratory Medicine
and Surgery, David Geffen School of Medicine at UCLA, and Jonsson
Comprehensive Cancer Center, Los Angeles, CA, USA

Francesco Cognetti, MD Division of Medical Oncology "A",
Medical Oncology Department, National Cancer Institute Regina Elena,
Rome, Italy

Stefania Crispi, PhD Institute of Genetics and Biophysics, I.G.B.,
A.Buzzati-Traverso, CNR, Naples, Italy

Alfredo D'Avino Department of Biochemistry, Section of Pathology,
Second University of Naples, Naples, Italy

Maria De Falco Department of Biology, Section of Evolutionary and
Comparative Biology, University of Naples "Federico II", Naples, Italy

Antonio De Luca, PhD Department of Mental and Physical Health and
Preventive Medicine, Section of Human Anatomy, Second University of
Naples, Naples, Italy

Michele De Nuntiis Plastic Surgery, Casa di Cura Addominale EUR,
Rome, Italy

Fondazione Futura-onlus, Rome, Italy

Emanuele Dragonetti Futura-onlus, Rome, Italy

Maria Elena Errico Pathology Unit, Paediatric Hospital Santobono-
Pausilipon, Naples, Italy

Katherine M. Ferris, BA Department of Dermatology and Cutaneous Surgery, University of Miami Hospital, Miami, FL, USA

Angeles Fortuño-Mar, MD, PhD, MBA Eldine Patologia Laboratory, Valls, Tarragona, Spain

Renato Franco Pathology Unit, National Institute of Tumours Fondazione "G. Pascale", Naples, Italy

Anna Maria Frezza Medical Oncology, University Campus Bio-Medico, Rome, Italy

Riccardo Garcea Plastic Surgery, Casa di Cura Addominale EUR, Viale Africa, Rome, Italy

Joan Ramon Garcés, MD Department of Dermatology, Universitat Autònoma de Barcelona, Hospital de la Santa Creu i Sant Pau, Barcelona, Spain

Umberto Gianelli Department of Pathophysiology and Transplantation, University if Milan, Milano, Italy

Salvador Gonzalez Dermatology Service, Ramon y Cajal Hospital, Alcalá University, Madrid, Spain

Faculty of Dermatology Service, Memorial Sloan-Kettering Cancer Center, New York, NY, USA

Ira Gordon, DVM Department of Radiation Oncology Branch, National Cancer Institute, Bethesda, MD, USA

Anna Grimaldi Department of Biochemistry and Biophysics, Second University of Naples, Naples, Italy

Gregor B.E. Jemec Department of Dermatology, Faculty of Health Sciences, Roskilde Hospital, University of Copenhagen, Roskilde, Denmark

Barbara E. Kitchell, DVM, PhD, DACVIM Department of Small Animal Clinical Sciences, Center for Comparative Oncology, Veterinary Medicine Center, Michigan State University, East Lansing, MI, USA

Aleksandar L. Krunic, MD, PhD, FAAD, FACMS Department of Dermatology, University of Illinois at Chicago, Chicago, IL, USA

Department of Dermatology, Northwestern University Feinberg School of Medicine, River Forest, IL, USA

Susanne Lange-Asschenfeldt Department of Dermatology, Charité – Universitätsmedizin, Berlin, Germany

Stephan Lautenschlager, PhD Dermatologisches Ambulatorium Stadtspital Triemli, Zurich, Switzerland

Outpatient Clinic of Dermatology, Triemli Hospital, Zurich, Switzerland

Angela Lombardi Department of Biochemistry and Biophysics, Second University of Naples, Naples, Italy

Miguel Alejandro López Dermatologic Surgery and Cutaneous Oncology
Section, Department of Dermatology, Hospital Militar "Dr. Carlos Arvelo",
Caracas, Venezuela

Amalia Luce Department of Biochemistry and Biophysics,
Second University of Naples, Naples, Italy

Joseph Malvehy Dermatology Department & CIBER-ER, Melanoma Unit,
Hospital Clínic, Barcelona, Spain

Marco Manfredini Department of Dermatology (ACS), University of
Modena and Reggio Emilia, Skin Center, Modena, Italy

Mario Manganaro Advanced Computer Systems, Rome, Italy

Ashfaq A. Marghoob Hauppauge Dermatology Section, Memorial
Sloan-Kettering Skin Cancer Center Hauppauge, Long Island, NY, USA

Federica Zito Marino Pathology Unit, National Institute of Tumours
Fondazione "G. Pascale", Naples, Italy

Sebastian Marschall DTU Fotonik – Department of Photonics
Engineering, Technical University of Denmark, Roskilde, Denmark

Michael P. McLeod, MS Department of Dermatology and Cutaneous
Surgery, University of Miami Leonard M. Miller School of Medicine,
Miami, FL, USA

Martin C. Mihm Jr. Pathology and Dermatology Department,
Harvard Medical School, Boston, MA, USA

Melanoma Program, Department of Dermatology, Brigham and Women's
Hospital, Boston, MA, USA

Melanoma Program, Dana Farber and Brigham and Women's Cancer
Center, Boston, MA, USA

Mette Mogensen, MD, PhD Department of Dermatology, Faculty of
Health Sciences, Roskilde Hospital, University of Copenhagen, Roskilde,
Denmark

Department of Dermatology, Bispebjerg Hospital, University of
Copenhagen, Copenhagen, Denmark

Eduardo K. Moioli Section of Dermatology, University of Chicago,
Chicago, IL, USA

Raffaele Murace Futura-onlus, Rome, Italy

Paola Muti Juravinski Hospital and Cancer Centre, Hamilton, ON, Canada

Department of Oncology, McMaster University, Hamilton, ON, Canada

Giovanni Francesco Nicoletti Dipartimento di Scienze Ortopediche,
Traumatologiche, Riabilitative e Plastico-Ricostruttive, Second University
of Naples, Naples, Italy

Keyvan Nouri, MD Department of Dermatology and Cutaneous Surgery, University of Miami Leonard M. Miller School of Medicine, Miami, FL, USA

Department of Dermatology, Sylvester Comprehensive Cancer Center/ University of Miami Hospital and Clinics, Miami, FL, USA

Carmen Nuzzo Division of Medical Oncology "A", Medical Oncology Department, National Cancer Institute Regina Elena, Rome, Italy

Pablo Luis Ortiz-Romero, MD, PhD Department of Dermatology, Instituto de investigación i +12, hospital 12 de Octubre, Facultad de Medicina. Universidad Complutense, Madrid, Spain

Giuseppe Palmieri, MD Department of Cancer Genetics, Institute of Biomolecular Chemistry, National Research Council (CNR), Sassari, Italy

Evangelia Papadavid Department of Dermatology, Athens University Medical School, Attikon University Hospital and Andreas Syggros Cutaneous Lymphoma Clinic, Athens, Greece

Paola Pasquali Department of Dermatology, Pius Hospital De Valls, Cambrils, Tarragona, Spain

Paolo Persichetti Plastic and Reconstructive Surgery Unit, Campus Bio-Medico University of Rome, Rome, Italy

Maria Simona Pino Division of Medical Oncology "A", Medical Oncology Department, National Cancer Institute Regina Elena, Rome, Italy

Michele M. Pisano Department of Molecular, Cellular and Craniofacial Biology, University of Louisville Birth Defects Center, Louisville, KY, USA

Susana Puig, MD, PhD Melanoma Unit, Dermatology Department, Hospital Clínic, Barcelona, Spain

Maria Teresa Rossi Department of Dermatology, University of Brescia, Brescia, Italy

Paulo Vilar-Saavedra Center for Comparative Oncology, Veterinary Medicine Center, Michigan State University, East Lansing, MI, USA

Raffaella Sala Department of Dermatology, University of Brescia, Brescia, Italy

Virginia Sanchez Dermatology Service, CEU University, Madrid, Spain

Daniele Santini Medical Oncology, University Campus Bio-Medico, Rome, Italy

Peter Sarantopoulos Department of Pathology and Laboratory Medicine, David Geffen School of Medicine at UCLA, and Jonsson Comprehensive Cancer Center, Los Angeles, CA, USA

Alessandra Scarabello Istituto Dermatologico San Gallicano, Rome, Italy

Alon Scope, MD Department of Dermatology, Sheba Medical Center, Ramat Gan, Ganey Tikva, Israel

Stefania Seidenari Department of Dermatology, University of Modena and Reggio Emilia, Skin Center, Modena, Italy

Enrico P. Spugnini, DVM, PhD S.A.F.U. Department, Regina Elena Cancer Institute, Rome, Italy

Stefania Tenna Plastic and Reconstructive Surgery Unit, Campus Bio-Medico of Rome University, Rome, Italy

Lotte Themstrup Department of Dermatology, Faculty of Health Sciences, Roskilde Hospital, University of Copenhagen, Roskilde, Denmark

Giuseppe Tonini Medical Oncology, University Campus Bio-Medico, Rome, Italy

Martina Ulrich Department of Dermatology, Charité – Universitätsmedizin, Berlin, Germany

Job Paul van der Heijden, MSc Department of Dermatology, Academic Medical Center, University of Amsterdam, Amsterdam, The Netherlands

Bruno Vincenzi Medical Oncology, University Campus Bio-Medico, Rome, Italy

Leonard Witkamp, MD, PhD KSYOS TeleMedical Center, Amstelveen, The Netherlands

Ximena Wortsman, MD Department of Radiology and Dermatology, Faculty of Medicine, Institute for Diagnostic Imaging and Research of the Skin and Soft Tissues, Clinica Servet, University of Chile, Providencia, Santiago, Chile

Maria De Falco, Michele M. Pisano,
and Antonio De Luca

Key Points

- Skin embryology: the embryology of the both epidermis and dermis is described.
- Epidermal development: the development of the epidermis beginning the third week of fetal life and its regulation is treated.
- Skin structure: the structure and the ultrastructure of adult skin are detailed.

Introduction

Skin Structure

The integumentary system is formed by skin and several skin appendages (glands, hair, nails, and teeth) [1]. The skin is the largest organ in the body

M. De Falco
Department of Biology,
Section of Evolutionary and Comparative Biology,
University of Naples "Federico II",
Naples, Italy

M.M. Pisano
Department of Molecular,
Cellular and Craniofacial Biology,
University of Louisville Birth Defects Center,
Louisville, KY, USA

A. De Luca, PhD (✉)
Department of Mental and Physical Health and
Preventive Medicine, Section of Human Anatomy,
Second University of Naples,
Via L. Armanni 5, Naples, 80138, Italy
e-mail: antonio.deluca@unina2.it

(in adults it weighs from 3 to 5 kg) and represents both its border and its intermediary with environment [1, 2]. The skin covers the whole outer surface of the body, including the wall of the outer auditory canal (meatus). It proceeds with the mucosae of the alimentary canal and respiratory and urinary-genital ways [3]. Its total thickness varies from 1.5 to 4.0 mm [3]. Human skin is formed by two distinct layers: the outer epidermis, a stratified pavement epithelium, and the underlying dermis consisting of connective tissue, principally dense at interlaced bundles (Fig. 1.1).

The two skin layers are interconnected with each other through epidermal-dermal junctions. These are undulating in section and formed by ridges of the epidermis, known as rete ridges, that project into the dermis. The junction provides mechanical support for the epidermis and acts as a partial barrier against exchange of cells and large molecules. Below the dermis, there is a fatty layer, the panniculus adiposus, usually designated as "subcutaneous." This is separated from the rest of the body by a vestigial layer of striated muscle, the panniculus carnosus [4].

There are two main kinds of human skin. Glabrous skin (non-hairy skin), covering the palms and soles, is grooved on its surface by continuously alternating ridges and sulci. It is characterized by a thick epidermis divided into several layers, including a compact stratum corneum; by the presence of encapsulated sense organs within the dermis; and by a lack of hair follicles and sebaceous glands. On the contrary, hair-bearing

Fig. 1.1 Histological section of human skin. The human skin is composed by a superficial upper layer, the epidermis covering a deeper layer, the dermis. Inside the dermis, numerous glands (*arrows*), blood vessels (*bv*), and hair follicles (*hf*) are evident. Below the dermis is visible the subcutaneous fat (*stars*). Mallory trichromic stain. Original magnification 2.5×

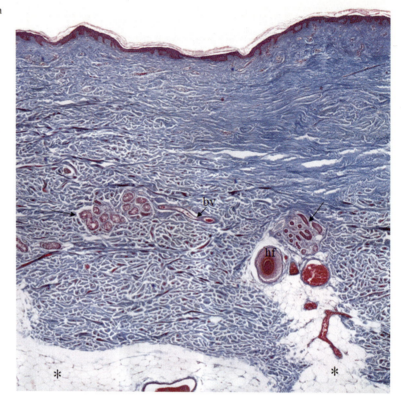

skin has both hair follicles and sebaceous glands but lacks encapsulated sense organs [4].

The integumentary system has not only principally protection functions but also thermoregulation, respiration, and perception functions [1]. The skin is the first line of defense against environmental (mechanical, chemical, osmotic, thermal) insults and microbial infection, as well as water and electrolyte loss [2, 3]. It confronts these attacks by undergoing continual self-renewal to repair damaged tissue and replace old cells [5]. Stem cells are located in the adult hair follicle, sebaceous glands, and in the basal layer of the interfollicular epidermis [5, 6]; they have the function to maintain tissue homeostasis, regenerating hair and repairing the epidermis after injury [5].

Embryology of the Skin

The skin develops by the juxtaposition of two embryological elements: the prospective epidermis, which originates from a surface area of the early gastrula, and the prospective mesoderm, which is brought into contact with the inner surface of the epidermis during gastrulation [4, 7, 8].

The epidermis originates almost completely from the covering ectoderm, and only few cells (melanocytes and Langerhans' cells) migrate from other areas. On the contrary, the dermis develops from two different mesenchymal areas; the larger part arises from somatopleure (lateral mesoderm) and the smaller part arises from somites (paraxial mesoderm) [1]. Both components of the skin should be considered as donors and receptors of information. Morphogenesis of the skin depends on a careful and constant dialogue between them [9]. Before skin morphogenesis, several cell interactions take place, in order to specify first the formation of dermal progenitors [10, 11] and second their densification inside the sub-ectodermal space [9]. These two first steps lead to the formation of the embryonic skin, formed by an upper epidermis overlying a dense dermis. The next step is the initiation and organization of regular repetitive appendage primordia. Finally, the final step is the organogenesis of the epidermal primordia (placode) in a complete, mature appendage [9].

Development of the Epidermis

After gastrulation, the embryo surface emerges as a single layer of neuroectoderm, which will ultimately specify the nervous system and the skin epithelium [5]. The covering ectoderm develops from epiblast during the third week of fetal life and represents the ectoderm that does not differentiate in nervous tissue. During the fourth week,

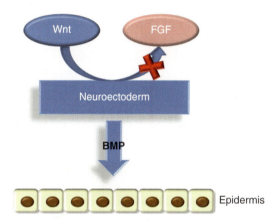

Fig. 1.2 The epidermis formation. Wnt signaling blocks FGF activity on the neuroectoderm that can express BMP proteins so developing the epidermis

the covering ectoderm separates from neural tube and closes on nervous system, forming a continuous coating on embryo surface. At the crossroads of this decision is Wnt signaling, which blocks the ability of ectoderm to respond to fibroblast growth factors (FGFs) [5]. In the absence of FGF signaling, the cells express bone morphogenetic proteins (BMPs) and become fated to develop into epidermis [5] (Fig. 1.2). Initially, the covering ectoderm is composed by a single layer of undifferentiated, cuboidal, and glycogen-filled cells [4, 12] (Fig. 1.3a). At this early stage, cell proliferation is the dominant process [13]. At the end of the fourth week, the epidermis forms a second layer that lies outer and originates simple squamous epithelium called periderm, a purely embryonic structure, which is unique to primates [4] (Fig. 1.3b). Its cells flatten, cornify, and eventually spread to several times the diameter of the deeper cells. The inner, basal layer includes stem cells and represents the germinal layer (stratum germinativum) of epidermis, whereas the periderm establishes the protection barrier on contact with amniotic fluid [1].

Between 8 and 11 weeks, the germinal layer actively proliferates and originates a third

Fig. 1.3 Development of the epidermis. (**a**) The covering ectoderm is formed by a single layer of cuboidal, undifferentiated cells; (**b**) the epidermis is composed by a second superficial layer called periderm; (**c**) the germinal basal layer originates a third middle layer, the intermediate layer, whose cells are characterized by the presence of microvillus projections at the surface of the periderm; (**d**) during the fifth month, the intermediate layer proliferates, forming one or more other layers. The periderm cells form numerous blebs and get away in the amniotic fluid (See more details in the text)

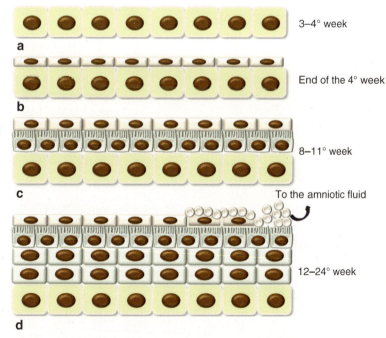

middle layer, the intermediate layer (Fig. 1.3c). Development of this layer is associated with asymmetric cell division of embryonic basal keratinocytes [14–16]. Glycogen is abundant in all layers, and a few microvillous projections occur at the surface of the periderm. The surface cells are flat and polygonal [4, 17]. These three layers persist about a month and then the epidermis later on evolves. During the fifth month (12–16 weeks), there are one or more intermediate layers (Fig. 1.3d). These cells contain mitochondria, Golgi complexes, and a few tonofilaments, as well as abundant glycogen both within and between cells. Microvilli become much more numerous [4]. From this stage onward, dome-shaped blebs start to project from the centers of the periderm cells. At first, the blebs are simple, but later their surface becomes dimpled and infolded [4]. The periderm gets away, and in some weeks (by 24 weeks), it is removed in the amniotic fluid, forming, together with shed lanugo, sebum, and other materials, the vernix caseosa [4]. The periderm may be no more than a protective coating for the fetus before keratinization of the epidermis. On the other hand, features such as the abundant microvilli, raised blebs, coated- and smooth-membrane vesicles, and increasing cell size suggest that it may have an important function such as the uptake of carbohydrate from the amniotic fluid [4, 17].

In the same time, like basal keratinocytes, intermediate cells undergo proliferation and/or differentiation. The loss of their proliferative capacity is associated with the maturation of intermediate cells into spinous cells [14, 16, 18]. The basal layer together with the spinous layer forms the Malpighian layer [19]. The spinous layer cells undergo further maturation to form the granular layer (stratum granulosum) and the outer cornified layer (stratum corneum) [1, 18].

In the epidermis of the hand and foot, among granular and cornified layers, a thin additional layer, called bright (glossy) layer (stratum lucidum) for its refraction property, lies. This layer is formed by cells containing the fluid eleidin that replaces the granules. All the epidermis layers are formed by cells called keratinocytes because they contain keratin by 14 weeks [4].

The germinal layer continuously produces cells that differentiate in keratinocytes, move toward the upper layers, degenerate, and finally are eliminated in the environment. During this migration among layers, keratinocytes pass through several maturation phases and their structural transformations originate morphological differences. Hemidesmosomal and desmosomal proteins are already detectable in the basal keratinocytes at 10 weeks [4].

Epidermal cells must undergo growth arrest before they can initiate a differentiation program [13]. Moreover, the morphological changes that are a hallmark of epidermal stratification are associated with changes in the expression of keratin differentiation markers [16, 20]. In fact, during normal epidermal development, commitment to the epidermal lineage involves the repression of the non-epidermal keratin pair K8/K18 [16, 21] and the induction of the epidermal keratin pair K5/K14 [6, 16, 22, 23]. Keratinocytes belonging to the spinous layer are big and polyhedric cells, synthesizing high quantity of keratin and keratohyalin, the two specific proteins of the epidermis. In the granular layer, these proteins are organized in two several types of subcellular aggregates: keratohyalin granules and keratin bundles. Some derivatives of keratohyalins, particularly the filaggrin, used to tightly join cells together, are first detectable at 15 weeks [4]. Moreover, cells forming the layer just beneath the periderm become to express loricrin [13, 23–25]. Specifically, keratohyalin granules appear at 21 weeks in the uppermost layer [4]. The initiation of terminal differentiation results in the induction of K1 and K10 expression in the newly formed suprabasal keratinocytes [18, 26, 27]. In addition, cornified envelope proteins, which are rich in glutamine and lysine residues, are synthesized and deposited under the plasma membrane of the granular cells [5]. When the cells become permeabilized to calcium, they activate transglutaminase, generating γ-glutamyl-ε-lysine cross-links to create an indestructible proteinaceous sac to hold the keratin macrofibrils (including various keratins, involucrin, loricrin, and filaggrin) [5, 13]. In the higher part of granular layer, the cells start to show the first signs of terminal differentiation and degeneration: flattening cell form, destruction of cellular organelles, dense chromatin granules, and breaking of the nuclear envelope. When the cells pass into the cornified layer, they completely degenerate, lose nuclei, and assume the shape of flattening sacs full of keratin, forming 15–30 layers of dead cells. Terminal differentiation is a slow process that requires many newly synthesized proteins in all layers of the epidermis [13].

The plane of union between epidermis and dermis is smooth until early in the fourth month when epidermal thickenings grow down into the dermis of the palm and sole. About 2 months later, corresponding elevations first appear on the skin surface. These epidermal ridges complete their permanent, individual patterns in the second half of fetal life [28].

The Regulation of Epidermal Development

The process during which the unspecified surface ectoderm adopts an epidermal fate is defined as epidermal specification [16].

Generally, keratinocytes take about 4 weeks to pass from the germinal layer to the outside of the body, and the epidermis structure depends on both their proliferation rate and differentiation processes. The fine balance among proliferation and differentiation is regulated by a complex system of interaction between many growth factors (Table 1.1). Some of these stimulate keratinocyte proliferation (epidermal growth factor, fibroblast growth factor, transforming growth factor-α, insulin, and interleukins), whereas others inhibit it (transforming growth factor-β1 and transforming growth factor-β2, interferons, and tumor growth factor) [1]. These pathways may be variably activated, both spatially and temporally, leading to a diverse series of transcribed genes [4].

TGF-α is made by the basal cells and stimulates their own division. If the TGF-α gene is linked to a promoter for keratin 14 (one of the major skin proteins expressed in the basal cells) and inserted into the mouse pronucleus, the resulting transgenic mice activate the TGF-α

Table 1.1 Main growth factors involved in proliferation and differentiation of keratinocytes

Proliferative	Anti-proliferative
EGF	TGFβ1
FGF	TGFβ2
TGF-α	Interferons
Insulin	Tumor growth factor
Interleukins	NF-κB
KGF	

gene in their skin cells and cannot downregulate it. The result is a mouse with scaly skin, stunted hair growth, and an enormous surplus of keratinized epidermis over its single layer of basal layer [19, 29].

Another growth factor needed for epidermal development is keratinocyte growth factor (KGF), a paracrine factor produced by the fibroblasts of the underlying dermis. KGF is received by the basal cells of the epidermis and probably regulates their proliferation. If the gene encoding KGF is fused with keratin 14 promoter, the KGF becomes an autocrine factor in the transgenic mice. These mice have a thickened epidermis, baggy skin, too many basal cells, and no hair follicles, not even whisker follicles [19, 30].

Many studies have demonstrated that the dermis provides the initial signals required for epidermal specification [16]. In vertebrates, the acquisition of the epidermal fate is associated with the induction of p63 expression, which is the first transcription factor to be specified for the epidermal lineage [16, 31–36]. It has been demonstrated that mice that are deficient for *p63* gene function have truncated or absent limbs, poorly developed skin, and die shortly after birth, presumably due to dehydration [13, 37, 38]. p63 is involved in the development of the embryonic basal layer (Fig. 1.4a). In the epidermis, at least six p63 isoforms are expressed, which fall into two categories: those that encode proteins with an amino-terminal transactivation domain (TA isoforms) and those that encode proteins that lack this domain (ΔN isoforms) [13]. Among the TA or ΔN isoforms, alternative splicing gives rise to three different carboxyl termini that are associated with the designations of α,

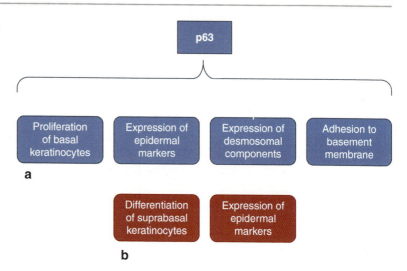

Fig. 1.4 Roles of p63 in the development of the epidermis. (**a**) p63 is involved in several processes important for the formation of the embryonic basal layer; (**b**) p63 isoforms also control terminal differentiation of keratinocytes (See more details in the text)

β, and γ [13, 39]. Regulation by p63 involves an intricate interplay between various p63 isoforms [13, 20]. Specifically, TAp63 isoforms are detected prior to the commitment to stratify and strongly localize to the nucleus, indicating that they may be required to initiate the epithelial stratification program in the developing embryo [13]. Particularly, the TAp63α isoform induces expression of AP-2γ, a transcription factor implicated in the regulation of K5 and K14 expression during epidermal morphogenesis [6, 16, 23, 36, 40–43]. Other than K14 expression, the epidermal fate is also associated to the expression of desmosomal components, important for cell-cell adhesion within the epidermis [18, 44] (Fig. 1.4a). One desmosomal component directly involved by p63 in the embryonic basal layer is Perp [6, 16, 45]. Moreover p63 is important for regulating the adhesion of keratinocytes to the basement membrane which is mediated by integrins, a family of transmembrane receptors for the basement membrane protein laminin [6, 46]. Specifically, it has been demonstrated that p63 induces expression of several integrin subunits, such as integrin α3 [6, 47, 48]. Furthermore, p63 controls basement membrane formation by directly inducing the expression of the basement membrane component Fras1 [6, 18].

The basal layer other producing keratinocytes that undergo terminal differentiation provides the epidermis with mechanical stability and barrier

function (Fig. 1.4b). To this purpose, some keratinocytes terminally differentiated are ultimately sloughed off, whereas other cells which can continuously supply terminally differentiating keratinocytes must be maintained for the life of the organism [16]. In order to prevent premature terminal differentiation, basal keratinocytes must repress the expression of genes that initiate this process and, at the same time, must induce and maintain the expression of genes required for proliferation and K5/K14 expression [16]. It has been demonstrated that ΔNp63α can directly induce K14 expression, and it is probably involved in maintenance of K14 expression in keratinocytes [16, 43, 49]. Moreover, ΔNp63α is able to maintain keratinocyte proliferation by directly inhibiting the expression of two genes induced during epidermal terminal differentiation: p21$^{WAF/Cip1}$, a member of the cyclin-dependent kinase inhibitor (CKI) family [13, 50], and 14-3-3σ, a member of 14-3-3 family of intracellular signaling proteins [13, 16, 51–57]. ΔNp63α binds directly to the p21$^{WAF/Cip1}$ and 14-3-3σ promoters [55], so inhibiting their transcription and then favoring epidermal cell proliferation [13]. In addition, ΔNp63α inhibits p21 expression by preventing Notch signaling, an upstream regulator of p21 in the epidermis [16, 57–59]. Moreover, it has been hypothesized that Notch signaling is involved not only in growth arrest but also in cornification [13]. In fact, it has been demonstrated that addition of JAG-1 to human keratinocytes lift cultures resulted in Notch activation; strong induction of loricrin, involucrin, and peroxisome proliferator-activated receptor-γ (PPARγ); and cornified envelope formation [13, 60] other than in enhanced levels of nuclear NF-κB [13, 61]. Furthermore, p63 also represses two cell cycle inhibitors Ink4a and Arf [6, 62] as well as induces the expression of genes required for cell cycle progression, including ADA and FASN [6, 55, 62–66]. Ink4a regulates cell cycle arrest by blocking phosphorylation of Rb family members, thereby maintaining them in their anti-proliferative states [20, 67]. On the other hand, it has been demonstrated that p63 is able to directly repress the expression of genes required for cell cycle progression including cyclin B2 and cdc2 [6, 16, 68]. This apparent controversy may be explained by supposing that p63 functions to maintain proliferation in early transit amplifying (TA) cells, whereas it acts inducing cell cycle exit in mature TA cells [6, 16]. In fact, it has been demonstrated that p63 directly induces p57^{Kip2}, a cyclin-dependent kinase inhibitor, in order to allow cell cycle exit and undergo terminal differentiation [6, 69, 70]. Specifically, whereas TAp63 isoforms inhibit terminal differentiation [36], ΔNp63 isoforms are first expressed after the single-layered epidermis has committed to stratification [13]. In vivo studies using transgenic mice suggest that one function of ΔNp63α during early epidermal morphogenesis is to counterbalance the effects of TAp63-induced inhibition of differentiation, allowing cells to respond to terminal differentiation program [13, 36]. ΔNp63α may block TAp63 isoforms directly, via a dominant-negative action of TAp63 [13]. As reported for p63 and Notch, another molecule involved in the switch from proliferation to growth arrest is NF-κB [13, 71]. In normal epidermis, NF-κB proteins localize in the cytoplasm of basal cells and then in the nuclei of suprabasal cells [13, 71]. Particularly, it has been shown that NF-κB in association with selective induction of p21$^{WAF/Cip1}$ induces growth arrest [13, 72]. As p63, also NF-κB acts by downregulating molecules that promote cell proliferation [13]. Specifically,

during epidermal development, NF-κB functions by opposing the proliferative activity of TNFR1/JNK [13].

In humans, the earliest morphological sign of stratification during epidermal development is the formation of the intermediate cell layer [14, 16, 73]. The intermediate keratinocytes, which proliferate and express K1, populate the first suprabasal layer of the embryonic epidermis [14–16, 18]. ΔNp63α is the only transcription factor known to be required for the formation of the intermediate layer [16]. In fact, ΔNp63α synergizes with Notch to induce K1 expression [16, 57].

At the same time, it has been shown that ΔNp63α expression is reduced to approximately 25 % in suprabasal keratinocytes with respect to its high expression in basal keratinocytes [6, 74]. Its rapid downregulation in suprabasal keratinocytes is mediated by several processes: first, ΔNp63α transcripts are degraded by micro RNA-203 [6, 75, 76] which is expressed only in suprabasal keratinocytes [6, 75–77]; second, ΔNp63α protein is also actively degraded in suprabasal keratinocytes through the proteosomal pathways by the E3 ubiquitin ligase Itch and p14^{Arf} [6, 78, 79].

The intermediate cell layer exists only transiently, since intermediate cells are replaced by postmitotic keratinocytes that form spinous layer during later developmental stages [14, 16]. Histological analysis has demonstrated that intermediate cells mature directly into spinous cells [16, 18, 73]. Despite ΔNp63α active degradation in suprabasal cell layers, the remaining protein is sufficient to control important aspects of keratinocytes differentiation and particularly seems to be involved also in this process. In fact, ΔNp63α critical target gene is IKKα [18], a previously identified regulator of epidermal, skeletal, and craniofacial morphogenesis [16, 80–82] which is a critical mediator of cell cycle exit during keratinocyte differentiation [6, 18, 83]. Intriguingly, the failure of intermediate cells to mature into spinous cells, lacking IKKα, also resulted in the aborted development of epithelial appendages and limbs [16, 84].

An important trigger of epidermal terminal differentiation is an increase in extracellular Ca^{2+}

concentration, which is involved in regulating the formation of the spinous layer, granular layer, and epidermal barrier [16]. A Ca^{2+} gradient is first established in utero, and in mature epidermis, an increasing gradient of extracellular Ca^{2+} is present from basal to the cornified layers [16, 85–87]. Specifically, protein kinase C (PKC) is activated during keratinocyte differentiation [16, 88]. During terminal differentiation, PKC proteins appear to function specifically in the transition from spinous to granular cells, by contributing to downregulate K1 and K10 expression [16, 89], a process that is associated with the transition from spinous to granular cells [27, 90]. In addition, PKC activation induces expression of loricrin, filaggrin, and transglutaminase, markers of granular keratinocytes [16, 89, 91].

The final step in epidermal stratification involves the formation of the epidermal barrier [16]. The best-studied transcription factor involved in the regulation of epidermal barrier formation is Klf4 which is expressed in the upper spinous and granular layers [16, 92, 93]. Another transcription factor implicated in this process is Grhl3/Get1 [94, 95] which downregulates many genes involved in lipid synthesis and metabolism [16]. Finally, it has been demonstrated that $\Delta Np63\alpha$ is also important for the formation of the epidermal barrier by inducing at least two genes required for barrier formation: Claudin 1 and Alox12 [6, 96, 97]. Moreover, several in vivo and in vitro studies indicated that PPAR activators accelerate differentiation and cornification in fetal and adult epidermis [98–101]. It has been demonstrated that Notch signaling may be involved also in these processes. In fact, Notch may function upstream of PPARs to induce terminal differentiation [13]. Moreover, Notch also induces the caspase 3 in order to promote terminal differentiation during embryonic development of epidermis [13].

Dermis Development

The dermis is the skin layer under the epidermis. It arises from mesenchymal cells that come in part by somatopleure and, in lower size, by dermatomes. In the face and in wide regions of the neck, instead, the dermis arises from cells that migrate from neural crest of the skull [1]. Initially, dermis cells form several junctions between their cytoplasmic extensions and originate the *primordial dermis*, characterized by high cell density and by aqueous extracellular matrix, rich in glycogen and hyaluronic acid [1]. This primordial dermis changes into the *mature* or *definitive dermis*, during the third month, when a great part of its mesenchymal cells differentiate in fibroblasts, which secrete a fibrous extracellular matrix, formed by collagen fibers (especially collagen I and IV) and by elastic fibers [1]. This change gives dermis both a high resistance and notable resilience, allowing it to carry out one of its main functions: to give a physical stable support to the epidermis, essential to establish an effective protective barrier [1]. Other than to provide physical support, the dermis nourishes the epidermis, which is not vascularized. This function is allowed by the development of dense network of blood vessels in the stroma of the dermis [1]. Always during the third month, the surface that divides the dermis from the epidermis loses its primordial flatten shape and becomes highly wavy by the formation of crests and depressions that form very complicate drawing (dermatoglyphics). These waves originate both by epidermis ridges and by dermis eversions (dermal papillae). Interdigitations between ridges and papillae markedly increase adhesion of the epidermis to the dermis, especially in areas exposed to high mechanical efforts [1]. The first visible lines on the skin appear at the end of the third month in the hands and feet (forming fingerprints), and after several weeks, they cover the whole body surface, with drawing that varies from one side to the other [1]. From the fifth month, each region of the skin is marked by a specific network of lines and keeps this configuration also if it is transplanted elsewhere [1]. Formation of dermal papillae divide the dermis in two layers. An upper layer, close to the epidermis, is called papillary layer. It is a thin sheet that maintains many features of the looser connective tissue which forms the primordial dermis [1]. The deeper layer, instead, is much more thick and is called reticular layer, since here the collagen fibers assume an arrangement at weave, or at a reticulum (network), that characterizes the compact connective tissue [1]. The reticular layer of the dermis, in its turn, is close to the hypoderm, or subcutaneous layer, the region which is addressed to become the main fatty storage of the body. Other than by the formation of connective fibers and blood vessels, the dermis development is characterized by appearance, in its stroma, of tactile receptors (Meissner, Pacinian, and Ruffini corpuscles), nerve endings (free or encapsulated), and skin adnexa (hairs and glands) [1].

Structure and Ultrastructure of Adult Epidermis

The epidermis is a complex, terminally differentiated, stratified squamous epithelium formed by one basal and several suprabasal layers of keratinocytes, which provides barrier functions to the skin [2]. The epidermis can be divided into four distinct layers: stratum basale or stratum germinativum, stratum spinosum, stratum granulosum, and stratum corneum [4] (Fig. 1.5). In palmoplantar skin, there is an additional zone, also electron lucent, the stratum lucidum between the granulosum and corneum [4]. Each epidermal layer contains keratinocytes at various stages of differentiation and proliferative potential [2, 102].

The stratum basale is a continuous layer directly in contact with a basement membrane. It is generally described as only one cell thick, but may be two to three cells thick in glabrous skin and hyperproliferative epidermis. The basal cells are small and cuboidal and have large nuclei that vary from euchromatic (in stem cells and in young keratinocytes) to eterochromatic (in older keratinocytes), dense cytoplasm containing many free polyribosomes, mitochondria, dense tonofilament bundles [4], included actin microfilaments and keratin filament bundles, and melanin granules [3]. Moreover, basal keratinocytes specifically express K5 and K14 [103]. The basal cells are linked to basement membrane through hemidesmosomes. Almost always, basal surfaces of basal cells are many pleated, interacting with basement membrane projections [3]. The basal layer is composed by dividing cells that give rise to several upper layers where keratinocytes progressively differentiate [4]. Close to the basal layer, the epibasal keratinocytes enlarge to form the spinous/prickle cell layer or stratum spinosum. This stratum contains more mature keratinocytes, disposed in more layers and closely packed. These cells show interacting surfaces through projections and indentations and

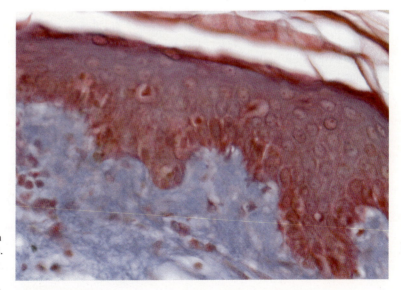

Fig. 1.5 Histological section of the mature adult epidermis. Mallory's trichrome stain. Original magnification 40×

are interconnected with each other through desmosomes. In their cytoplasm, there are many abundant keratin bundles integrated with desmosomes. This feature allows a strong cohesion to the epidermis and a high strength to traction [3]. The suprabasal layer (spinous) cells express K1 and K10 [103]. The cytoplasm of the cells of the stratum spinosum show moderately euchromatic nuclei, with large nucleoli, numerous polyribosomes, and typical vacuoles containing melanin granules (melanosomes) [3]. The melanin comes from melanocytes of the epidermis. Melanin granules are more numerous in the deeper part of stratum spinosum and progressively are degraded by keratinocytes, so that they lack in the superficial part of the stratum [3]. The stratum spinosum is succeeded by the stratum granulosum or granular layer, so called for the presence of the intracellular granules of keratohyalin inside keratinocytes cytoplasm [4]. At high magnification, the dense mass of keratohyalin granules from human epidermis has a particulate substructure, with particles of irregular shape on average 2 nm length and occurring randomly in rows or lattices [4, 104]. The granular cells also contain a highly phosphorylated protein, rich in histidine, called basic profilaggrin [3]. The cytoplasm of the cells of the upper, spinous layer and granular cell layer also contains smaller lamellated granules averaging 100–300 nm in size, which are known as lamellar granules or bodies, membrane-coating granules, or Odland bodies [4, 105]. These are numerous within the uppermost cells of the spinous layer and migrate toward the periphery of the cells as they enter the granular cell layer. They discharge their lipid components into the intercellular space, playing important roles in barrier function and intercellular cohesion within the stratum corneum [4]. The granular cells contain pyknotic nuclei and show degenerated organelles [3]. Granular cells also express and produce filaggrin, loricrin, and transglutaminase 3 (TG3) [103, 106].

In the palmoplantar region, the cells forming the stratum lucidum are still nucleated and may be referred to as "transitional" cells [4]. The outermost layer of epidermis is the stratum corneum where cells, now called corneocytes, have lost nuclei and cytoplasmic organelles. The cells become flattened and the keratin filaments align into disulphide cross-linked macrofibers, under the influence of filaggrin, the protein component of the keratohyalin granule, responsible for keratin filament aggregation [107]. The corneocyte has a highly insoluble cornified envelope within the plasma membrane, formed by cross-linking of the soluble protein precursor, involucrin [108], following the action of a specific epidermis transglutaminase also synthesized in the high stratum spinosum [109]. The process of desquamation involves degradation of the lamellated lipid in the intercellular spaces and loss of the residual intercellular desmosomal interconnections. The corneocytes which protect the viable cell layers are continually shed from the skin surface, and the rate of production of cells in the basal layer must match the rate of loss from the surface to produce the normal skin thickness, although increased rates of loss and cell division occur in pathological states [4].

Within the epidermis, there are several other cell populations, namely, melanocytes, which donate pigment to the keratinocytes; Langerhans' cells, which have immunological functions; and Merkel cells [4].

Structure and Ultrastructure of Adult Dermis

The dermis is composed of dense connective tissue at interlaced bundles formed by cells scattered in a supporting matrix (Fig. 1.6). The dermis consists of the following: (a) retiform interlacement of collagen fiber bundles, with a varying amount of elastic fibers; (b) a matrix containing proteoglycans, fibronectin, and other typical element of the matrix; (c) blood vessels; (d) lymphatic vessels; and (e) nerve endings. The matrix is constituted by proteins and polysaccharides linked to each other to compose macromolecules that provide a remarkable capacity for retaining water [4]. Inside the matrix, there are two kinds of protein fibers: collagen, the major constituent of the dermis, which has great tensile strength, and elastin, which makes up only a small proportion of the

Fig. 1.6 Histological section of the adult dermis. Mallory trichromic stain. Original magnification 20×

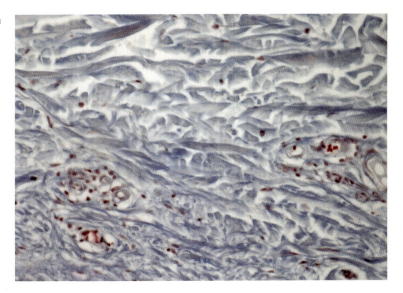

bulk [4]. The cellular components of the dermis include fibroblasts, mast cells, macrophages, and monocytes. Unlike epidermis, the dermis has a very rich blood supply, even if vessels do not the pass through epidermal-dermal junction [4].

The dermis confers a considerable resistance and resilience to the cutis thanks to a large amount and spatial arrangement of its collagen and elastin fibers. Moreover, for the presence of blood and lymphatic vessels, nerves and defensive cells, the dermis is essential for the epidermis survival and for many functions of the cutis [3].

The mature dermis can be divided in two distinct layers: a superficial thin papillary layer and a deeper reticular layer. The papillary layer, close to basal membrane, contains rich blood vessel networks and nerve endings. It is specialized in furnishing a mechanical anchorage and in allowing a physiological metabolism to the overlooking epidermis. In the superficial part, it is characterized by numerous papillae which have round peak and that interact with epidermal ridges [3]. Each papilla contains thin bundles, densely interlaced, of fine collagen fibers of types I and III and some elastic fibers and microfibers, many of those tight to basement membrane of the epidermis. Inside the papilla, there is also a blood capillary ansa, and in the thick, hairless cutis, there are often the Meissner's

corpuscles [3]. The papillae can vary their morphology depending on anatomic region. For example, in the thin cutis of regions at low sensibility and subjected to slight mechanical solicitations, the papillae are sparse and many are small. On the contrary, in the thick cutis of the hands and feet, the papillae are more bulky, densely thickened, and disposed to form curved parallel lines that conform with epidermal ridges [3]. The reticular layer is fused with deeper part of papillary layer. It contains bundles of collagen fibers, prevalently of type I, that are more thick than papillary layer bundles. Bundles inside both dermal layers intermingle with each to other to form a hardy, but deforming, tridimensional network also containing elastic fibers.

Glossary

Dermis Is the skin layer under the epidermis. It is a dense connective tissue which functions as a mechanical device for the attachment of the epidermis and for its nourishing. It contains collagen and elastic fibers, glands, hair follicles and blood vessels. The mature dermis can be divided in two distinct layers: a superficial thin papillary layer and a deeper reticular layer.

Epidermis A stratified pavement epithelium that forms the outermost layer of the skin. It is interconnected with the dermis, the below connective tissue and functions as the first barrier between the organism and the environment. The epidermis can be divided into four distinct layers: stratum basale or stratum germinativum, stratum spinosum, stratum granulosum, and stratum corneum.

Keratinocytes The cells that form all the epidermis layers at various stages of differentiation and proliferative potential. They contain several types of keratins. The basal keratinocytes specifically express K5 and K14.

References

1. Barbieri M, Carinci P. L'apparato tegumentario. In: Barbieri M, Carinci P, editors. Embriologia. 2nd ed. Milano: Casa Editrice Ambrosiana; 1997. p. 422–7.
2. Ivanova IA, D'Souza SJA, Dagnino L. Signalling in the epidermis: the E2f cell cycle regulatory pathway in epidermal morphogenesis, re generation and transformation. Int J Biol Sci. 2005;1:87–95.
3. Williams PL, Warwick R, Dyson M, et al. L'apparato tegumentario. In: Amprino R, editor. Anatomia del Gray. 3rd ed. Bologna: Zanichelli; 1993. p. 66–75.
4. McGrath JA, Eady RAJ, Pope FM. Anatomy and organization of human skin. In: Bums T, Breathnach S, Cox N, Griffiths C, editors. Rook's textbook of dermatology. 7th ed. Hoboken: Blackwell Science Ltd; 2004. p. 45–128.
5. Fuchs E. Scratching the surface of skin development. Nature. 2007;445:834–42.
6. Koster MI. p63 in skin development and ectodermal dysplasias. J Invest Dermatol. 2010;130:2352–8.
7. Ebling FJ. Hormonal control and methods of measuring sebaceous gland activity. J Invest Dermatol 1974;62:161–71.
8. Sengel P. Morphogenesis of skin. Cambridge: Cambridge University Press; 1976.
9. Olivera-Martinez I, Thelu J, Dhouailly D. Molecular mechanisms controlling dorsal dermis generation from the somatic dermomyotome. Int J Dev Biol. 2004;48:93–101.
10. Fliniaux I, Viallet JP, Dhouailly D. Ventral vs. dorsal chick dermal progenitor specification. Int J Dev Biol. 2004;48:103–6.
11. Olivera-Martinez I, Viallet JP, Michon F, et al. The different steps of skin formation in vertebrates. Int J Dev Biol. 2004;48:107–15.
12. Holbrook KA, Hoff MS. Structure of the developing human embryo and fetal skin. Semin Dermatol. 1984;3:185–202.
13. Mack J, Anand S, Maytin EV. Proliferation and cornification during development of the mammalian epidermis. Birth Defects Res. 2005;75:314–29.
14. Smart IH. Variation in the plane of cell cleavage during the process of stratification in the mouse epidermis. Br J Dermatol. 1970;82:276–82.
15. Lechler T, Fuchs E. Asymmetric cell divisions promote stratification and differentiation of mammalian skin. Nature. 2005;437:275–80.
16. Koster MI, Roop DR. Mechanisms regulating epithelial stratification. Annu Rev Cell Dev Biol. 2007;23:93–113.
17. Holbrook KA, Odland GF. The fine structure of developing human epidermis: light, scanning and transmission electron microscopy of the periderm. J Invest Dermatol. 1975;65:16–38.
18. Koster MI, Dai D, Marinari B, et al. p63 induces key target genes required for epidermal morphogenesis. Proc Natl Acad Sci U S A. 2007;104:3255–60.
19. Gilbert SF. The epidermis and the origin of cutaneous structures. In: Gilbert SF, editor. Developmental biology. 7th ed. Sunderland: Sinauer Associates Inc., Publishers; 2003. p. 416–8.
20. Koster MI, Roop DR. The role of p63 in development and differentiation of the epidermis. J Dermatol Sci. 2004;34:3–9.
21. Moll R, Franke WW, Schiller DL, et al. The catalog of human cytokeratins: patterns of expression in normal epithelial, tumors and cultured cells. Cell. 1982;31:11–24.
22. Jackson B, Tilli CL, Hardman M, et al. Late cornified envelope family in differentiating epithelia – response to calcium and UV irradiation. J Invest Dermatol. 2005;124:1062–70.
23. Byrne C, Tainsky M, Fuchs E. Programming gene expression in developing epidermis. Development. 1994;120:2369–83.
24. Mehrel T, Hohl D, Rothnagel JA, et al. Identification of a major keratinocytes cell envelope protein, loricrin. Cell. 1990;61:1103–12.
25. Yoneda K, Steinert PM. Overexpression of human loricrin in transgenic mice produces a normal phenotype. Proc Natl Acad Sci U S A. 1993;90:10754–8.
26. Fuchs E, Green H. Changes in keratin gene expression during terminal differentiation of the keratinocytes. Cell. 1980;19:1033–42.
27. Bickenbach JR, Greer JM, Bundman DS, et al. Loricrin expression is coordinated with other epidermal proteins and the appearance of lipid lamellar granules in development. J Invest Dermatol. 1995;104:405–10.
28. Brainerd Arey L. The integumentary system. In: Developmental anatomy. A textbook and laboratory manual of embryology. 7th ed. Philadelphia/London: WB Saunders Company; 1974. p. 439–41.
29. Vassar R, Fuchs E. Transgenic mice provide new insights into the role of TGF-alpha during epidermal development and differentiation. Genes Dev. 1991;5:714–27.

30. Guo L, Yu QC, Fuchs E. Targeting expression of keratinocyte growth factor to keratinocytes elicits striking changes in epithelial differentiation in transgenic mice. EMBO J. 1993;12:973–86.
31. Lu P, Barad M, Vize PD. Xenopus p63 expression in early ectoderm and neuroectoderm. Mech Dev. 2001;102:275–8.
32. Yasue A, Tao H, Moriyama K, et al. Cloning and expression of the chick p63 gene. Mech Dev. 2001;100:105–8.
33. Bakkers J, Hild M, Kramer C, et al. Zebrafish ΔNp63 is a direct target of Bmp signaling and encodes a transcriptional repressor blocking neural specification in the ventral ectoderm. Dev Cell. 2002;2:617–27.
34. Lee H, Kimelman D. A dominant-negative form of p63 is required for epidermal proliferation in zebrafish. Dev Cell. 2002;2:607–16.
35. Green H, Easley K, Iuchi S. Marker succession during the development of keratinocytes from cultured human embryonic stem cells. Proc Natl Acad Sci U S A. 2003;100:15625–30.
36. Koster MI, Kim S, Mills AA, et al. p63 is the molecular switch for initiation of an epithelial stratification program. Genes Dev. 2004;18:126–31.
37. Mills AA, Zheng B, Wang XJ, et al. p63 is a p53 homologue required for limb and epidermal morphogenesis. Nature. 1999;398:708–13.
38. Yang A, Schweitzer R, Sun D, et al. p63 is essential for regenerative proliferation in limb, craniofacial and epithelial development. Nature. 1999;398:714–8.
39. Yang A, Kaghad M, Wang Y, et al. p63, a p53 homolog at 3q27-29, encodes multiple products with transactivating, death-inducing, and dominant-negative activities. Mol Cell. 1998;2:305–16.
40. Leask A, Byrne C, Fuchs E. Transcription factor AP2 and its role in epidermal-specific gene expression. Proc Natl Acad Sci U S A. 1991;88:7948–52.
41. Sinha S, Degenstein L, Copenhaver C, et al. Defining the regulatory factors required for epidermal gene expression. Mol Cell Biol. 2000;20:2543–55.
42. Kaufman CK, Sinha S, Bolotin D, et al. Dissection of a complex enhancer element: maintenance of keratinocytes specificity but loss of differentiation specificity. Mol Cell Biol. 2002;22:4293–308.
43. Romano RA, Birkaya B, Sinha S. A functional enhancer of keratin K14 is a direct transcriptional target of ΔNp63. J Invest Dermatol. 2007;127:1175–86.
44. Cheng X, Koch PJ. In vivo function of desmosomes. J Dermatol. 2004;31:171–87.
45. Ihrie RA, MArques MR, Nguyen BT, et al. Perp is a p63-regulated gene essential for epithelial integrity. Cell. 2005;120:843–56.
46. Larsen M, Artym VV, Green JA, et al. The matrix reorganized: extracellular matrix remodeling and integrin signaling. Curr Opin Cell Biol. 2006;18:463–71.
47. Kurata S, Okuyama T, Osada M, et al. p51/p63 controls subunit alpha3 of the major epidermis integrin

anchoring the stem cells to the niche. J Biol Chem. 2004;279:50069–77.
48. Carrol DK, Carrol JS, Leong CO, et al. p63 regulates an adhesion program and cell survival in epithelial cells. Nat Cell Biol. 2006;8:551–61.
49. Candi E, Rufini A, Terrinoni A, et al. Differential roles of p63 isoforms in epidermal development: selective genetic complementation in p63 null mice. Cell Death Differ. 2006;13:1037–47.
50. Vermeulen K, Van Bockstaele DR, Berneman ZN. The cell cycle: a review of regulation, deregulation and therapeutic targets in cancer. Cell Prolif. 2003;36:131–49.
51. Dellambra E, Patrone M, Sparatore B, et al. Stratifin, a keratinocyte specific 14-3-3 protein, harbors a pleckstrin homology (PH) domain and enhances protein kinase C activity. J Cell Sci. 1995;108:3569–79.
52. Dellambra E, Golisano O, Bondanza S, et al. Downregulation of 14-3-3σ prevents clonal evolution and leads to immortalization of primary human keratinocytes. J Cell Biol. 2000;149:1117–30.
53. Missero C, Calautti E, Eckner R, et al. Involvement of the cell-cycle inhibitor Cip1/WAF1 and the E1A-associated p300 protein in terminal differentiation. Proc Natl Acad Sci U S A. 1995;92:5451–5.
54. Pellegrini G, Dellambra E, Golisano O, et al. p63 identifies keratinocyte stem cells. Proc Natl Acad Sci U S A. 2001;98:3156–61.
55. Westfall MD, Mays DJ, Sniezek JC, et al. The ΔNp63α phosphoprotein binds the p21 and 14-3-3σ promoters in vivo and has transcriptional repressor activity that is reduced by Hay-Wells syndrome-derived mutations. Mol Cell Biol. 2003;23:2264–76.
56. Mhawech P. 14-3-3 proteins – an update. Cell Res. 2005;15:228–36.
57. Nguyen BC, Lefort K, Mandinova A, et al. Cross-regulation between Notch and p63 in keratinocyte commitment to differentiation. Genes Dev. 2006;20:1028–42.
58. Rangarajan A, Talora C, Okuyama R, et al. Notch signaling is a direct determinant of keratinocyte growth arrest and entry into differentiation. EMBO J. 2001;20:3427–36.
59. Baldi A, De Falco M, De Luca L, et al. Characterization of tissue specific expression of Notch-1 in human tissues. Biol Cell. 2004;96:303–11.
60. Nickoloff BJ, Qin JZ, Chaturvedi V, et al. Jagged-1 mediated activation of Notch signaling induces complete maturation of human keratinocytes through NF-κB and PPargamma. Cell Death Differ. 2002;9:842–55.
61. Guan E, Wang J, Laborda J, et al. T cell leukemia-associated human Notch/trans location-associated Notch homologue has I kappa B-like activity and physically interacts with nuclear factor-kappa B proteins in T cells. J Exp Med. 1996;183:2025–32.
62. Su X, Cho MS, Gi YJ, et al. Rescue of key features of the p63-null epithelial phenotype by inactivation of Ink4a and Arf. EMBO J. 2009;28:1904–15.

63. D'Erchia AM, Tullo A, Lefkimmiatis K, et al. The fatty acid synthase gene is a conserved p53 family target from worm to human. Cell Cycle. 2006;5:750–8.

64. Sbisa E, Mastropasqua G, Lefkimmiatis K, et al. Connecting p63 to cellular proliferation: the example of the adenosine deaminase target gene. Cell Cycle. 2006;5:205–12.

65. Truong AB, Kretz M, Ridky TW, et al. p63 regulates proliferation and differentiation of developmentally mature keratinocytes. Genes Dev. 2006;20:3185–97.

66. Lefkimmiatis K, Caratozzolo MF, Merlo P, et al. p73 and p63 sustain cellular growth by transcriptional activation of cell cycle progression genes. Cancer Res. 2009;69:8563–71.

67. Classon M, Dyson N. p107 and p130: versatile proteins with interesting pockets. Exp Cell Res. 2001;264:135–47.

68. Testoni B, Mantovani R. Mechanisms of transcriptional repression of cell-cycle G2/M promoters by p63. Nucleic Acids Res. 2006;34:928–38.

69. Martinez LA, Chen Y, Fischer SM, et al. Coordinated changes in cell cycle machinery occur during keratinocyte terminal differentiation. Oncogene. 1999;18: 397–406.

70. Beretta C, Chiarelli A, Testoni B, et al. Regulation of the cyclin-dependent kinase inhibitor p57Kip2 expression by p63. Cell Cycle. 2005;4:1625–31.

71. Seitz CS, Lin Q, Deng H, et al. Alterations in NF-kappaB function in transgenic epithelial tissue demonstrate a growth inhibitory role for NF-kappa B. Proc Natl Acad Sci U S A. 1998;95:2307–12.

72. Seitz CS, Deng H, Hinata K, et al. Nuclear factor kappaB subunits induce epithelial cell growth arrest. Cancer Res. 2000;60:4085–92.

73. Weiss LW, Zelickson AS. Embryology of the epidermis: ultrastructural aspects. II. Period of differentiation in the mouse with mammalian comparisons. Acta Derm Venereol. 1975;55:321–9.

74. King KE, Ponnamperuma RM, Gerdes MJ, et al. Unique domain functions of p63 isotypes that differentially regulate distinct aspects of epidermal homeostasis. Carcinogenesis. 2006;27:53–63.

75. Yi R, Poy MN, Stoffel M, et al. A skin microRNA promotes differentiation by repressing 'stemness'. Nature. 2008;452:225–9.

76. Lena AM, Shalom-Feuerstein R, di Val Cervo PR, et al. miR-203 represses 'stemness' by re pressing [Delta]Np63. Cell Death Differ. 2008;15:1187–95.

77. Sonkoly E, Wei T, Janson PC, et al. MicroRNAs: novel regulators involved in the pathogenesis of Psoriasis? PLoS One. 2007;2:e610.

78. Rossi M, Aqeilan RI, Neale M, et al. The E3 ubiquitin ligase Itch controls the protein stability of p63. Proc Natl Acad Sci U S A. 2006;103:12753–8.

79. Vivo M, Di CA, Fortugno P, et al. Downregulation of DeltaNp63alpha in keratinocytes by p14ARF-mediated SUMO-conjugation and degradation. Cell Cycle. 2003;8:3537–43.

80. Hu Y, Baud V, Delhase M, et al. Abnormal morphogenesis but intact IKK activation in mice lacking the IKKα subunit of IκB kinase. Science. 1999;284: 316–20.

81. Li Q, Lu Q, Estepa G, et al. Identification of 14-3-3σ mutation causing cutaneous abnormality in repeated-epilation mutant mouse. Proc Natl Acad Sci U S A. 1999;102:15977–82.

82. Takeda K, Takeuchi O, Tsujimura T, et al. Limb and skin abnormalities in mice lacking IKKα. Science. 1999;284:313–6.

83. Marinari B, Ballaro C, Koster MI, et al. IKK[alpha] is a p63 transcriptional target involved in the pathogenesis of ectodermal dysplasias. J Invest Dermatol. 2008;129:60–9.

84. Sil AK, Maeda S, Sano Y, et al. IκB kinase-α acts in the epidermis to control skeletal and craniofacial morphogenesis. Nature. 2004;428:660–4.

85. Menon GK, Grayson S, Elias PM. Ionic calcium reservoirs in mammalian epidermis: ultrastructural localization by ion-capture cytochemistry. J Invest Dermatol. 1985;84:508–12.

86. Menon GK, Elias PM, Lee SH, et al. Localization of calcium in murine epidermis following disruption and repair of the permeability barrier. Cell Tissue Res. 1992;270:503–12.

87. Elias PM, Nau P, Hanley K, et al. Formation of the epidermal calcium gradient coincides with key milestones of barrier ontogenesis in the rodent. J Invest Dermatol. 1998;110:399–404.

88. Lee E, Yuspa SH. Changes in inositol phosphate metabolism are associated with terminal differentiation and neoplasia in mouse keratinocytes. Carcinogenesis. 1991;12:1651–8.

89. Dlugosz AA, Yuspa SH. Coordinate changes in gene expression which mark the spinous to granular cell transition in epidermis are regulated by protein kinase C. J Cell Biol. 1993;120:217–25.

90. Yuspa SH, Kilkenny AE, Steinert PM, et al. Expression of murine epidermal differentiation markers is tightly regulated by restricted extracellular calcium concentrations in vitro. J Cell Biol. 1989;109:1207–17.

91. Dlugosz AA, Yuspa SH. Protein kinase C regulates keratinocyte transglutaminase (TGK) gene expression in cultured primary mouse epidermal keratinocytes induced to terminally differentiate by calcium. J Invest Dermatol. 1994;102:409–14.

92. Garrett-Sinha LA, Eberspaecher H, Seldin MF, et al. A gene for a novel zinc-finger protein expressed in differentiated epithelial cells and transiently in certain mesenchymal cells. J Biol Chem. 1996;271: 31384–90.

93. Segre JA, Bauer C, Fuchs E. Klf4 is a transcription factor required for establishing the barrier function of the skin. Nat Genet. 1999;22:356–60.

94. Ting SB, Caddy J, Hislop N, et al. A homolog of Drosophila grainy head is essential for epidermal integrity in mice. Science. 2005;308:411–3.

95. Yu Z, Lin KK, Bhandari A, et al. The Grainyhead-like epithelial transactivator Get-1/Grhl3 regulates epidermal terminal differentiation and interacts functionally with LMO4. Dev Biol. 2006;299:122–36.

96. Lopardo T, Lo IN, Marinari B, et al. Claudin-1 is a p63 target gene with a crucial role in epithelial development. PLoS One. 2008;3:e2715.

97. Kim S, Choi IF, Quante JR, et al. p63 directly induces expression of Alox12, a regulator of epidermal barrier formation. Exp Dermatol. 2009; 18:1016–21.

98. Hanley K, Komuves LG, Bass NM, et al. Fetal epidermal differentiation and barrier development in vivo is accelerated by nuclear hormone receptor activators. J Invest Dermatol. 1999;113: 788–95.

99. Hanley K, Jiang Y, He SS, et al. Keratinocyte differentiation is stimulated by activators of the nuclear hormone receptor PPARalpha. J Invest Dermatol. 1998;110:368–75.

100. Kim DJ, Bility MT, Billin AN, et al. PPARbeta/delta selectively induces differentiation and inhibits cell proliferation. Cell Death Differ. 2006;13:53–60.

101. Komuves LG, Hanley K, Lefebvre AM, et al. Stimulation of PPARalpha promotes epidermal keratinocyte differentiation in vivo. J Invest Dermatol. 2000;115:353–60.

102. Fuchs E, Byrne C. The epidermis: rising to the surface. Curr Opin Genet Dev. 1994;4:725–36.

103. Aberdam D, Candi E, Knight RA, et al. miRNAs, 'stemness' and skin. Trends Biochem Sci. 2008; 33:583–91.

104. Lavker RM, Matoltsy AG. Substructure of keratohyalin granules of the epidermis as revealed by high resolution electron microscopy. J Ultrastruct Res. 1971;35:575–81.

105. Odland GF. Structure of the skin. In: Goldsmith LA, editor. Physiology, biochemistry and molecular biology of the skin. New York: Oxford University Press; 1991. p. 3–62.

106. Candi E, Schmidt R, Melino G. The cornified envelope: a model of cell death in the skin. Nat Rev Mol Cell Biol. 2005;6:328–40.

107. Lynley AM, Dale BA. The characterization of human epidermal filaggrin, a histidine-rich keratin filament-aggregating protein. Biochim Biophys Acta. 1983; 744:28–35.

108. Rice RH, Green H. The cornified envelope of terminally differentiated human epidermal keratinocytes consists of cross-linked protein. Cell. 1977;11:417–22.

109. Buxman MM, Wuepper KD. Cellular localization of epidermal trans-glutaminase: a histochemical and immunochemical study. J Histochem Cytochem. 1978;26:340–8.

Epidemiology and Prevention of Cutaneous Tumors

Alessandra Scarabello and Paola Muti

Key Points

- The ISTAT 2010 data report that skin tumors account for 11 % of all tumors.
- Squamoous cell carcinomas account for about 20 % of all nonmelanoma skin cancers (NMSC) and about 75 % of NNSC mortality.
- Merkel cell carcinoma presents an incidence increase by about 8 % annually and a mortality of more than 30 % at 2 years.
- UV radiation represents the major risk factor for development of melanoma and nonmelanoma tumors. Other risks factors are radiodermatitis, burns, ulcers, scars, chronic diseases, immunosuppression and genetic diseases with a disturbance of pigmentation and/or the reparative DNS system.
- There are two different types of melanomas (MM) with clinical and biological characteristics that ascribe substantially to two different etiopathogenic mechanisms: the most common (de novo of from a pre existing nevus) develops as a MM in situ with horizontal growth and only later a vertical growth; a second type (de novo) with a rapid vertical growth and an aggressive biological behavior.
- For the first type of MM (with superficial diffusion), risk factors have been identified. Public education and awareness raising campaigns have been organized with the aim of reducing the incidence.
- There has been improvement in early diagnosis with the aid of the noninvasive diagnostic methodologies.

A. Scarabello
Istituto Dermatologico San Gallicano, Rome, Italy

P. Muti (✉)
Juravinski Hospital and Cancer Centre,
711 Concession Street, 1st Floor, 60 (G) Wing,
Room 125, Hamilton, ON L8V 1C3, Canada

Department of Oncology, McMaster University,
Hamilton, ON, Canada
e-mail: muti@mcmaster.ca

Introduction

Skin cancer is the most common type of neoplasia in the world, with a preponderance in the Caucasian population and a higher incidence in areas with a greater solar exposure: it accounts for 35–45 % of all cancers among Caucasians [1], 4–5 % among Hispanics, 2–4 % among Asians, and 1–2 % in the black population [2].

Among whites the incidence has shown an increasing trend in the last 30 years, with a greater stability observable instead in the colored populations [1] thanks to the photoprotection provided by the greater quantity of melanin [3] and the different structures of the melanosomes [4]. Precise information concerning the real incidence and/or mortality of cutaneous tumors is difficult to collect, except for the melanomas, in that generally cutaneous carcinomas are not registered in national tumor registers and are rarely a cause of death. However, we should not underestimate these carcinomas as they represent nonetheless a pathology in rapid increase everywhere and one which is often rather disabling. It also appears at times as an occupational pathology in professions with a chronic and/or increased exposure to ultraviolet radiation. The high incidence of this pathology also makes it one of the major health costs in terms of diagnosis, therapy, and follow-up in the area of oncological pathology.

Nonmelanoma Cutaneous Tumors

Epidemiology

Nonmelanoma cutaneous tumors are the most common malignant neoplasias in the USA, with more than two million new cases every year [5] and in Europe [6]. Among these carcinomas, we must include basal cell carcinomas and squamous cell carcinomas, by a long way the two most frequent nonmelanoma cutaneous tumors. There are also other cutaneous tumors, less frequent, such as adnexal tumors (these are as important as cutaneous "spies" of systemic pathologies as, e.g., sebaceous adenoma is for Muir-Torre syndrome, a multiple oncological disease), neuroendocrine cutaneous carcinomas (Merkel cell carcinomas), dermatofibrosarcomas protuberans (Darier-Ferrand tumors), and the B and T cutaneous lymphomas.

Basal cell carcinomas (BCC) and the squamous cell carcinomas (SCC) are the most common forms of cutaneous tumors. The incidence of BCC varies according to gender and geographical latitude: 175–1073 cases for every 100,000 men of the Caucasian race and 124–415 cases for every 100,000 Caucasian women; SCC shows an incidence of 63–214 cases for every 100,000 Caucasian men and 22–50 cases for every 100,000 Caucasian women. We can say that SCC, which accounts for about 20 % of all nonmelanoma cutaneous tumors, can sometimes be a cause of death (about 75 % of deaths due to nonmelanoma cutaneous tumors), usually in very elderly and not well-cared patients [7].

Merkel cell carcinoma, an aggressive tumor at an advanced age – beyond the sixth decade – with a slight preponderance among males, shows an incidence in the USA of three cases per million inhabitants, with an increasing trend of about 8 % annually during the last 20 years. It has a mortality of about 30 % at 2 years and an average survival at diagnosis, often made at a metastatic stage of the disease, of 6–8 months [8]. The incidence of this neoplasia shows a more than elevenfold increase in patients affected by AIDS, obviously also with a lowering of the average age – more than 50 % of subjects have an age of less than 50 – and a fivefold increase in patients in immunosuppressive therapy after an organ transplant: immunodeficiency plays a fundamental role in the development of this neoplasia [9]. Patients with light phototypes show a greater incidence compared to those with dark phototypes, and the most frequent onset sites are the photo-exposed areas. Often other photo-related cutaneous tumors – synchronous and metachronous – present in an affected patient. Ultraviolet radiation therefore represents a factor promoting the onset of this neoplasia, the etiopathogenetic mechanism of which is not yet completely clear [10]. An important role seems to have been revealed in viral infections: the viral genome is found in 80 % of cases of Merkel cell carcinomas [11]. Patients with such tumors show also an increased risk of multiple myeloma-type hematological neoplasias, non-Hodgkin lymphomas, and chronic lymphocytic leukemia [12].

The ISTAT 2010 data report that skin cancers account for 11 % of all tumors, with an increasing trend, registering 6,000 new cases every year, with an incidence of 12 new cases for every 1,000 inhabitants, with a basal cell carcinoma/squamous cell carcinoma relationship of 10:1. In the 5-year

Table 2.1 Record of cases at the "Celio" military hospital in Rome in the 5-year period 2006–2010

Cutaneous tumors			
Nonmelanomas	312	Melanomas	86
Basal cell carcinomas	282	Superficial spreading melanoma	84
Squamous cell carcinomas	26	Nodular melanoma	2
Cutaneous lymphomas	2		
Merkel cell carcinomas	1		
Kaposi's sarcoma	1		

period 2006–2010 at the "Celio" military hospital in Rome, 35,000 examinations and 10,000 video dermatoscopes were carried out: 312 new cases of nonmelanoma cutaneous tumors were discovered – of which 282 were basal cellular carcinomas, 26 squamous cell carcinomas, 2 cutaneous lymphomas, 1 Merkel cell carcinoma, and 1 Kaposi's sarcoma – and 86 new cases of melanomas (Table 2.1) [13].

Risk Factors

In all races UV radiation is the major risk factor for the onset of nonmelanoma cutaneous tumors (BCC and SCC), which appear in fact predominantly in photo-exposed areas, in almost 90 % of cases in the head and neck. Other possible risk factors are radiodermatitis, burns scars, ulcers, chronic infections and immunosuppression, genetic diseases with albinism and xeroderma pigmentosum, or chronic diseases like systemic lupus erythematosus [2].

Melanomas

Epidemiology

In the USA more than 60,000 new cases of melanoma are registered every year, and melanomas represent the sixth most frequent neoplasia in men and the seventh in women [2]; the increase in the incidence of melanomas both in the USA and in Europe is estimated at between 3 and 7 %

annually among the Caucasian population (less among blacks) and represents one of the tumors with the highest mortality rates and at an age more than a decade lower than that of other solid tumors (breast, colon, lung, and prostate cancers) [14]. This increase in incidence is considered to be due to a greater awareness among the population thanks to prevention campaigns and so to a more likely early diagnosis with the result that there is no parallel increase in mortality. A detailed analysis of melanoma cases registered in the 20-year period 1988–2006, subdivided according to thickness (four different groups: <1, 1.01–2, 2.01–4, >4 mm), shows that all four categories record a significant increase in incidence, with a greater increase in cases of thin melanomas in women and of thick melanomas in men [15].

Two principal types of registrable melanomas have been identified with two different etiopathogenetic mechanisms: the most common melanoma, which has a superficial diffusion arising de novo or on a preexisting melanocytic nevus and develops as a melanoma in situ with a subsequent horizontal growth and only in much later phases a vertical growth with a progressive metastatic potential; and a second type of melanoma, arising de novo, which has a rapid vertical growth (Breslow index of thickness at diagnosis >1), an immediately aggressive biological behavior, a high metastatic potential, and an unfavorable prognosis [16], the pathogenetic mechanism of which is not yet well known. Thin melanomas with a slow evolution, instead, seem to be connected to exposure to ultraviolet radiation, both UVA and UVB, with a variable risk factor in terms of accumulated doses of radiation, type of exposure (intermittent or continuous), and sunburn [17]. Additionally, the use of tanning lamps, which became widespread in the 1980s, has caused an increase in the risk of the development of melanoma in relation to the accumulated dose of ultraviolet radiation. In fact, a recent study by the University of Minnesota has revealed an increase in this risk by a factor of 1.74 in subjects who are habitual users of UV tanning lamps compared to nonusers, with a close correlation between the increase in risk and the total dose of

UV radiation (in terms of the total hours of exposure and number of sessions) [18] without overlooking the age of the subjects who are tanning lamp users. In fact, the International Agency for Research on Cancer has considered tanning lamps as carcinogenic – causing all types of cutaneous tumors – highlighting how the risk of developing a melanoma is increased by 75 % in subjects who regularly use tanning lamps up to the age of 30 [19].

It is obvious how the close correlation between environmental UV radiation and the development of melanoma influences directly the incidence in terms of ethnicity and latitude and indirectly the onset sites and the differences between genders [20].

From analyzing the cases of melanomas in relation to solar exposure and latitude, it would seem that intermittent exposure, for the most part recreational, leading with a greater probability to solar burns of various grades, represents an important risk factor at all latitudes. Instead, chronic exposure, for the most part occupational, representing a risk in terms of total doses of radiation absorbed, would seem to have a greater influence on the risk of developing melanomas at low latitudes, considering also the type of skin of the resident populations [21]. In Norway the incidence of melanomas in the last 50 years has shown a notable increase, with a difference of about two to three times between the south and north. The area of the body most seriously affected turns out to be the trunk in both sexes. These data would suggest that at these low altitudes the predominant risk factor is the phototype, which is to be correlated more to recreational solar exposure than to chronic exposure during the entire lifetime. Similar considerations can be made about the rest of Europe, with the only difference that in the south of Europe, there seems to be a difference in the site of onset also with respect to gender: the trunk appears to be the predominant site for men and the legs for women [22].

This same prevalence for the trunk in men and the legs in women in terms of the site of onset of the melanoma is similarly recorded in other parts of the world: Asia, Latin America, the USA, and Canada [20, 23–25].

These observations have suggested that the difference in the onset site of the melanoma between the two sexes can be in some way connected to sexual hormones. It is interesting to note that the melanomas of the trunk frequently present mutations of the BRAF gene, closely associated to a polymorphism of MC1R, the expression of which is modulated by the sexual hormones [26]. It is true that other differences between men and women could explain the difference in the anatomic site of the melanoma: clothing, lifestyle, occupations, solar exposure, and the different degrees of attention to preventive behaviors between the sexes [27]. The different habits of life explain indeed the different incidence of melanomas in the Middle East, where an incidence among men almost two times greater than that of women is recorded, probably because women are more protected by their covering clothing and by their limited presence in the open air, both for work and leisure [28].

A separate category is represented by the colored population of Africa, in which melanomas are extremely rare, for the most part in the acroposthion, and have an unfavorable prognosis, often due to the lateness of diagnosis. The sites most affected are those less rich in protective melanin: the subungual exostoses and the palmoplantar areas. Risk factors additional to the intense doses of UV radiation are immunosuppression (also from HIV), chronic diseases, and genetic diseases, like albinism, in which the protective constitutional conditions are less than those typical of that race [29].

Melanomas of the Mucosas

The melanoma of the mucosa is a rare form of melanoma distinct from the cutaneous form by reason of its biological behavior and pathogenesis. It accounts for 1.3–1.4 % of all melanomas, appears most frequently in colored races, and is located predominantly (up to 50 % of cases) in the head and neck area [30]. It shows an onset at a later age compared to cutaneous melanomas and often, considering that this site is richly vascularized, is already metastatic at the time of diagnosis, with the result that it has a very unfavorable prognosis [31].

The risk factors are to a very limited degree ascribable to UV radiation and recognize instead other mechanisms linked to potential tumor promoters like tobacco. Thirty percent of melanomas of the oral cavity develop on the melanoses, and it is well known that cigarettes cause an increase in the melanocytes [32]. Survival to 5 years varies from 12 to 34 % according to the location of the first lesion and obviously to its thickness at the time of diagnosis [31].

Melanomas at Pediatric Age

Melanomas at pediatric age, understood as the period from the uterus to the age of 21, are rare, but not insignificant, and are however increasing, although with some differences in the various age ranges (congenital/neonatal melanomas 3.8 %, infant melanomas 23 %, adolescent melanomas 73.2 %) [33]. On average the pediatric melanoma represents 1–4 % of all cases of melanoma and 1–3 % of neoplasias at pediatric age [34]. In the last few decades, this incidence has shown an increase of 3 % per year, from 1973 to 2001, with a slight prevalence in females, fortunately with an improvement in survival of 4 % per year [35], possibly thanks to a more widespread primary prevention and a more effective secondary prevention.

In melanomas of the pediatric age, a predominant role seems to be played by genetic conditions of susceptibility with mainly endogenous risk factors, such as the total number of nevi, the presence of congenital nevi of average or large dimensions (transformation risk from 2 to 10 %), a light phototype, and the presence of freckles and burns from solar exposure in childhood [36], the latter an exogenous risk factor but with some predisposition. Other predisposing factors are congenital diseases with an alteration in the reparative capacity of the DNA after UV radiation damage (e.g., xeroderma pigmentosum), which show an increase of 2,000 times in the risk of developing melanomas in pediatric age and immunosuppression conditions (iatrogenic,

infective, and hematological disorders) with an increase in risk of three to six times [34].

Melanomas: Mortality

Despite a significant increase in the incidence of melanomas in the last few decades, a comparable increased trend of mortality has not been registered. The number of deaths due to melanomas appears stable or only slightly increased, and an improvement in survival rates has been universally recorded [37]. Such a divergence would seem to be due principally to an improvement in early diagnosis, thanks to campaigns of primary and secondary prevention, and to the optimization of surgical techniques with the support of a more effective adjuvant therapy [38]. The prognosis of the melanoma is directly proportional to the thickness of the original lesion: in fact, the initial stages of the melanoma are fully manageable surgically with a survival rate at 5 years which reaches 95 %. In contrast, for more advanced forms of the melanoma, with a metastatic condition, the prognosis is unfavorable on account of the aggressive biological behavior of the disease and the poor response to the systemic therapies currently available [39].

From these findings we conclude that early diagnosis is the only effective weapon to reduce the mortality rate of this neoplasia.

Prevention

By prevention we mean the implementation of the most suitable measures to prevent the appearance of something damaging. The prevention of melanomas is therefore realized through "primary prevention," aimed at the identification of risk factors, endogenous and exogenous, and at the containment of these factors and/or their effects, combined with "secondary prevention," aimed at reducing the number of deaths due to melanomas, principally through early diagnosis, given that this seems to be the key factor for the reduction in the mortality of this neoplasia.

Risk Factors

Traditionally, the risk factors identified for melanomas are divided into endogenous and exogenous factors. In the first group we include phototype; the total number of nevi – the risk of the transformation of each single nevus is estimated at around 1 out of 200,000 per year [40] – a variable percentage between 22 and 50 % of diagnosed melanomas show histologically an origin associated with nevi [41] and a specific genetic susceptibility; in the second group we include first and foremost natural and artificial ultraviolet radiation, to which we can then add other risk factors such as socioeconomic condition, habits of behavior, and occupational activity.

Endogenous Risk Factors

The exact pathogenesis of melanomas remains as yet not completely clear, but an important role seems to be ascribable to a polymorphism of certain genes involved in the determination of the color of the skin and hair, in the case of sporadic melanomas, and of certain other genes, in the case of familial melanomas. We can subdivide the endogenous risk factors into two groups: "traditional," among which we include phototype, the total number of nevi above 50, and the presence of atypical nevi and freckles; and "new" risk factors, identified thanks to the development of cellular and molecular investigation techniques, definable in terms of genetic susceptibility to the development of melanomas.

In a variable percentage of the cases of melanomas, in fact, we can find a positive familial anamnesis for the same disease: the prevalence varies from 1.3 % in studies conducted in the north of Europe to almost 16 % in studies conducted in Australia. This confirms that there exists a great variability in the family history of melanomas, probably because environmental risk factors are decisive in terms of the onset of the disease even if on a predisposing phenotypical and genotypical base [42].

It is clear that melanoma originate from the combination of a series of genetic and epigenetic events: for the onset, progression, and metastatic diffusion of the neoplasia, numerous irreversible changes must take place within the genome – mutations, deletions, and an amplification of the target gene – but also a complete series of epigenetic phenomena, that is, modifications in gene expression, without an alteration of the DNA (DNA methylation or histone deacetylation) seem to be decisive [43]. Currently four genes have been identified associated with a condition of susceptibility to genetically determined melanomas: CDKN2A, an oncosuppressor important in the control of the entry of the cell into the cellular cycle, CDK4, ARF, and BRAF [44]. Another three loci seem to be involved: a locus on chromosome 1p22 [45], a locus on chromosome 9q21 [46], and, more recently identified, the locus 20q11.22 [47].

Other susceptibility genes, but with a lower penetrance, involved in the melanogenesis and in particular in the definition of the relationship between the eumelanin and pheomelanin and therefore in the determination of the color of the skin and hair, are MC1R, αMSH, OCA2, ASIP, TYR, and TYRPT1 [48–50]. Such genes, in that they are involved in melanogenesis, are therefore directly and/or indirectly responsible for the determination of another endogenous risk factor, the most important, the phototype. The variability of cutaneous pigmentation depends not only on the dimension, shape, and distribution of the melanosomes in the epidermis but also on the quantity of eumelanin and pheomelanin produced by the melanocytes and their relationship. The incidence of melanoma, in fact, shows a wide variability according to race in terms above all of the color of the skin in that this represents the greater or lesser capacity of the individual to cope with damage due to ultraviolet radiation (UVA and UVB), with a factor of protection 13 times greater for blacks as opposed to whites [51]. In addition, genetic or epigenetic phenomena responsible for alterations in the functions of such genes and their products can contribute to render the skin still more sensitive to UV-induced damage of the DNA and so predispose the subject to the development of melanoma and non-melanoma cutaneous tumors [52].

This supposed genetic susceptibility, which puts blood relations potentially more at risk of developing melanomas compared to the general population, implies in the affected subject a relatively greater risk of developing a secondary melanoma. Unfortunately, these molecular alterations have not to date produced useful data relating to the possible plasma and/or tissue biomarkers of the disease and/or their progression [53].

Exogenous Risk Factors

The direct pathogenetic role of ultraviolet radiation (UV) is by now universally recognized for nonmelanoma cutaneous tumors (BCC and SCC) and strongly probable for cutaneous melanomas. The UV radiation spectrum is subdivided on the basis of wavelength (λ): UVA radiation accounts for about 94 % (λ: 320–400 nm), UVB about 5 % (λ: 280–320 nm), and UVC about 1 % ($\lambda < 280$ nm). The Earth is not at risk from UVC radiation because this is normally absorbed by the ozone layer and therefore does not reach the surface, but, instead, it is extensively affected by the other types, the energy of which is absorbed by the cellular proteins and the DNA, sometimes with mutagenic effects [54].

At the cutaneous level, the UVA penetrates deeply and is not absorbed directly by the DNA of the keratinocytes but can damage the cells through oxidative stress. The UVB radiation, instead, is absorbed by the epidermis and can cause direct damage to the DNA with the formation of dimers, thymine, cytosine, and other potentially carcinogenic photoproducts. Some forms of melanoma, connected to some well-known genetic alterations, could recognize analogous pathogenetic mechanisms at the level of the DNA of the melanocytes [55]. Knowledge of the genetics of the melanocytes and of melanogenesis together with data relating to the interactions of UV radiation with the DNA demonstrates how intense solar exposure with the aggravating factor of burns, even at a young age, can in fact result in the development of melanomas. It has been suggested that two different mechanisms of interaction between UV radiation and melanomas exist that involve different genes: a total of intermittent intense solar exposure would pro-mote the development of melanomas on the trunk (a zone not daily photoexposed) in young patients with numerous nevi; and chronic photo exposure would promote the development of melanoma in photo-damaged areas at an advanced age in subjects with a history of photo-induced cutaneous carcinomas [56].

In the same way as solar radiation, the artificial ultraviolet radiation of tanning lamps increases the risk of the induction of melanoma and in general of cutaneous tumors.

Primary Prevention

Primary prevention has as its objective the reduction of damage due to ultraviolet radiation and therefore focuses on the organization of education campaigns to make the population aware of the need to use sun protection products of a suitable protection factor in accordance with phototype, applied in the correct quantity and with the correct frequency; to wear hats and sunglasses; to take photo-protective supplements; to abstain from direct solar exposure in the midday period to avoid sunburn and to permit the melanocytes to activate themselves in the synthesis of new protective melanin; and to avoid intermittent intense exposure in favor of a gradual progressive and safe solar exposure [57]. In parallel, the use of tanning lamps and tanning beds is discouraged [58].

Secondary Prevention

The objective of secondary prevention is the early diagnosis of the disease that, in the case of melanoma, turns out to be the only potentially successful weapon, bearing in mind the poor response to the therapies currently available.

The first objective of this prevention is certainly the identification of subjects at risk. Potential risk factors include the following: a personal history of melanomas (the risk of secondary melanomas is 5–8 %); a positive familial anamnesis of melanomas (two or more affected family members within the second degree of

Table 2.2 Index of the increase in the risk of developing cutaneous melanomas

Total number of nevi	Increased risk of melanoma (number of times)
11–25	1.6
26–50	4.4
51–100	5.4
>100	9.8
1–5 atypical nevi	3.8
More than 6 atypical nevi	6.3

relationship); the number of nevi (the risk progressively increasing in accordance with the number of nevi – see Table 2.2); the presence and/or history of dysplastic nevi (the risk increasing by 6.3 times for more than 6 atypical/dysplastic nevi); a light skin (risk 4 times); blue eyes and red hair (risk 2 times); a personal history of cutaneous carcinomas (risk 2–3 times); sunburns and excessive sun/UV lamp exposure (risk 2–3 times); males as opposed to females; age (the risk of the development of melanomas increases with age); and new pigmented lesions appearing after 50 years of age [59].

Different strategies have been proposed to improve the early diagnosis of melanomas including campaigns of education of the population for cutaneous self-exploration, the awareness raising of general practitioners about routine examinations of the entire integument also on the occasion of consultations for different reasons, mass screening campaigns, and the development of noninvasive technologies auxiliary to clinical diagnosis. Large-scale statistical investigations have demonstrated the probable utility of mass screening: the data are however insufficient to confirm unequivocally the benefits of such an effort [60–63].

The patient certainly plays a fundamental role in the diagnosis of melanomas: more than 70 % of melanomas are "suspected" by the patient himself/herself or by friends or family members. In recent years, thanks also to better information (in the mass media, newspapers, magazines, etc.), people have shown an improvement in the early recourse to the doctor. Today, the appearance of a mark in evolution or the presence of a change in a nevus, present for some time, is rightly interpreted by the inexpert patient as warning signs. Therefore, the efforts made since the 1980s, the years in which the ABCD criterion was introduced (a useful acronym to remember the warning signs of a cutaneous pigmented lesion: Asymmetry, Border, Color, Dimension) [64], in the education and awareness raising of the population in terms of self-diagnosis, a noninvasive and inexpensive procedure, have been bearing fruit [65, 66]. In the case of nodular melanomas with lesions characteristically with a rapid growth – estimated at around 0.4 mm per month – it is frequently (41 % of times) the patient himself/herself who notices the lesion, but unfortunately at an already advanced stage of development (a thickness >2 mm), with negative repercussions in terms of prognosis [67]. The "evolution" of the cutaneous lesion is therefore very important but it is not included in the ABCD rules, unless the acronym is widened to ABCDE, where the E refers to the tendency of the lesion to Evolve in time [68]. In particular, for nodular lesions with a rapid growth, the acronym EFG has been introduced, respecting better the clinical characteristics of such a melanoma: E for "Elevated," F for "Firm," and G for "Growing" (a compact nodule that grows).

Such diagnostic criteria, useful to the specialist on the occasion of a screening examination, have an easy approach and applicability also on the part of the patient himself/herself and/or his/her family. Detailed educational campaigns, undertaken with the assistance of illustrative photographic images, have increased the awareness and the specificity of self-diagnosis [69].

The most reliable instrument for a certain diagnosis remains however a histological examination, but the cutaneous localization of such a disease, which offers the possibility of the clinical diagnosis of a suspected lesion, permits also the use of noninvasive diagnostic methods to achieve a highly reliable diagnosis. The aim is to achieve a sensitive and specific selection of the lesions to be removed no longer for diagnostic reasons but, on the contrary, for therapeutic reasons. In the last 30 years, an improvement in the early diagnosis of melanomas has been obtained thanks to the introduction of noninvasive

Table 2.3 Comparison of the different diagnostic algorithms available

Algorithm for dermoscopic diagnosis	Sensitivity (%)	Specificity (%)	Diagnostic accuracy (%)
Pattern analysis	85	79	71
ABCD	84	75	76
7-point checklist	78	65	58
Cash	98	68	–
Menzies method	85	85	81

Rigel et al. [72]

methodical investigative instruments, such as dermatoscopy, digital videodermatoscopy (introduced in the 1990s), and confocal microscopy (introduced after 2000). The use of dermatoscopy or epiluminescence microscopy provides a surface visualization of the dermo-epidermic structure and, in particular, of the distribution and architectural organization of the melanocytes, melanin, and capillary vessels in the cutaneous thickness. The quality of the images has been optimized by the use of polarized light to reduce the effects of reflection, refraction, and diffraction of the cutaneous surface. The use of these instruments has allowed an improvement in the sensitivity and specificity of the clinical diagnosis of melanomas from 71 to 91 % [70]. However, despite this improvement we cannot leave out of consideration the training and experience of the operator [71]. With the aim of improving the sensitivity and specificity of the dermoscopic diagnosis, different algorithmic systems have been created applicable in the analysis of the images obtained (pattern analysis, ABCD rules, seven-point checklist, CASH, Menzies method, Table 2.3), all of which have demonstrated a significant utility but absolutely cannot be carried out without human intervention and above all the experience of the observer [73–75].

A good and trained clinical eye remains the best weapon in the identification of suspicious lesions, to be subsequently examined with the methodical instruments available.

Digital dermatoscopy, offering the possibility of a recording of the images of atypical pigmented lesions, allows us to create a kind of map of the integument of a patient with a high risk of melanoma and numerous nevi with the aim of having a point of reference for periodic checks and the subsequent identification of new lesions and/or modifications, even minimal, in preexisting lesions [76]; the realization of detailed photographs can be useful also for the patient for self-examination at home [77].

Due to its technical characteristics, such a method is not applicable in the case of nodular lesions, for which it can offer only an assistance, however useful, in terms of a comparison between the photographic images of the entire cutaneous surface – the map – and the previous periodic checks.

In the last decade a new noninvasive diagnostic technique has been confirmed, confocal microscopy, which allows us to obtain in vivo images of cutaneous lesions at various levels of depth and the entire epidermis and the dermis up to a depth of 400 μm [78]. Specific cytological and architectural patterns are being defined, connected to the histological and histopathological picture, to be used for the correct interpretation of the images obtained from the confocal microscope, without the need to have recourse to a cutaneous biopsy. These would also be useful for the better focalization of the most suspicious areas in the case of large lesions and/or cutaneous/mucous areas which are difficult or delicate to approach by reconstructive surgery, such as the face and the genital areas, to achieve the desired examination [79]. In the diagnosis of cutaneous melanomas, the confocal microscope has demonstrated an average sensitivity of more than 90 % and a specificity of 86 %: this therefore places it, although there are still many limitations in this "young" methodology, in the role of support diagnostic technique to the more established dermatoscopy (sensitivity 83.2 % and specificity 85.8 %) and to the indisputable histopathology [79].

Glossary

Cutaneous carcinomas Malignant neoplasias originating from the keratinocytes

Melanoma A malignant neoplasia deriving from the melanocytes

Melanoma – primary prevention The realization of the most suitable measures to prevent the development of melanoma: the identification of risk factors, endogenous and exogenous, and the containment of these factors and/or their effects.

Melanoma – secondary prevention The realization of the most suitable measures to reduce the number of deaths due to melanomas.

Nevus A benign proliferation with melanocytic origin

Risk factors Any element, endogenous or exogenous, capable of promoting the development of a damaging and fearful event

References

1. Ridky TW. Non-melanoma skin cancer. J Am Acad Dermatol. 2007;57:484–501.
2. Gloster HM, Neal K. Skin cancer in skin color. J Am Acad Dermatol. 2006;55:741–60.
3. Montagna W. The architecture of black and white skin. J Am Acad Dermatol. 1991;24:29–37.
4. Brenner M, Hearing VJ. The protective role of melanin against UV damage in human skin. Photochem Photobiol. 2008;84:539–49.
5. Roger HW, Weinstock MA, Harris AR, et al. Incidence estimate of non-melanoma skin cancer in the United States, 2006. Arch Dermatol. 2010;146:283–7.
6. Karim-Kos HE, De Vries E, Soerjomataram I, et al. Recent trends of cancer in Europe: a combined approach of incidence, survival and mortality for 17 cancer sites since the 1990s. Eur J Cancer. 2008;44:1345–89.
7. Alan M, Ratner D. Cutaneous squamous cell carcinoma. N Engl J Med. 2001;344:975–83. Am Journal of Preventive Medicine 2001;20:47–58.
8. Girschik J, Fritschi L, Threlfall T, Slevin T. Deaths from non-melanoma skin cancer in Western Australia. Cancer Causes Control. 2008;19:879–85.
9. Lanoy E, Dores GM, Madeleine MM, et al. Epidemiology of non-keratinocytic skin cancers among persons with AIDS in the United States. AIDS. 2008;23:385–93.
10. Norval M. The mechanisms and consequences of ultraviolet-induced immunosuppression. Prog Biophys Mol Biol. 2006;92:108–18.
11. Becker JC, Houben R, Ugurel S, et al. MC polyomavirus is frequently present in Merkel cell carcinoma of European patients. J Invest Dermatol. 2009;129:248–50.
12. Howard RA, Dores GM, Curtis RE, et al. Merkel cell carcinoma and multiple primary cancers. Cancer Epidemiol Biomarkers Prev. 2006;15:1545–9.
13. Spagnolo A, Astorino S. Corso di aggiornamento. Roma: Dermatologia militare; 2010.
14. Bevona C, Sorber AJ. Melanoma incidence trends. Dermatol Clin. 2002;20:589–95.
15. Criscione VD, Weinstock MA. Melanoma thickness trends in the United States, 1988–2006. J Invest Dermatol. 2010;130:793–7.
16. Houghton AN, Polsky D. Focus on melanoma. Cancer Cell. 2002;2:275–8.
17. Gandini S, Sera F, Cattaruzza MS, et al. Meta-analysis of risk factors for cutaneous melanoma II. Sun exposure. Eur J Cancer. 2005;41:45–60.
18. Lazovich D, Vogel RI, Berwick M, et al. Indoor tanning and risk of melanoma: a case–control study in highly exposed population. Cancer Epidemiol Biomarkers Prev. 2010;19:1557–68.
19. El Ghissassi F, Baan R, Straif K, et al. Special report. Policy. A review of human carcinogenesis – part d: radiation. Lancet Oncol. 2009;10:751–2.
20. Eide MJ, Weinstock MA. Association of UV index, latitude, and melanoma incidence in non-white populations – US Surveillance, Epidemiology and End Results (SEER) Program, 1992–2001. Arch Dermatol. 2005;141:477–81.
21. Chang YM, Barret JH, Bishop DT, et al. Sun exposure and melanoma risk at different latitudes: a pooled analysis of 5700 cases and 7216 controls. Int J Epidemiol. 2009;38:814–30.
22. Naldi L, Altieri A, Imberbi GL, et al. Sun exposure, phenotypical characteristics, and cutaneous malignant melanoma. An analysis according to different clinico-pathological variants and anatomical locations (Italy). Cancer Causes Control. 2005;16:893–9.
23. Zemelman V, Roa J, Ruiz T, Valenzuela CY. Malignant melanoma in Chile: an unusual distribution of primary sites in men from low socioeconomic strata. Clin Exp Dermatol. 2006;31:335–8.
24. Pruthi DK, Guilfoyle R, Nugent Z, et al. Incidence and anatomic presentation of cutaneous malignant melanoma in central Canada during a 50-year period: 1956–2005. J Am Acad Dermatol. 2009;61:44–50.
25. Uehara S, Kamo R, Harada T, Ishii M. Survival analysis of malignant melanoma in Japan – multivariate analysis of prognostic factors. Osaka City Med J. 2009;55(55):35–52.
26. Perez-Gomez B, Aragones N, Pollan M. Divergent cancer pathways for early onset and late onset cutaneous malignant melanoma, a role for sex-site interaction. Cancer. 2010;115:2499.
27. Whiteman DC, Stickley M, Watt P, Hughes MC, et al. Anatomic site, sun exposure, and risk of cutaneous melanoma. J Clin Oncol. 2006;24:3172–7.
28. Noorbals MT, Kafaie P. Analysis of 15 years of skin cancer in central Iran (Yadz). Dermatol Online J. 2007;13:1.
29. Asuquo ME, Ebughe G. Cutaneous cancer in Calabra, Southern Nigeria. Dermatol Online J. 2009;15:11.
30. McLaughlin CC, Wu XC, Jemal A, et al. Incidence of non-cutaneous melanomas in the U.S. Cancer. 2005;103:1000–7.
31. Manolidis S, Donald PJ. Malignant mucosal melanoma of the head and neck: review of the literature and report of 14 patients. Cancer. 1997;80:1373–6.
32. Axell T, Hedin CA. Epidemiologic study of excessive oral melanin pigmentation with special reference to

the influence of tobacco habits. Scand J Dent Res. 1982;90:434–42.

33. Lange JR, Palis BE, Chang DC, et al. Melanoma in children and teenagers: an analysis of patients from the National Cancer Data Base. J Clin Oncol. 2007;25: 1363–8.

34. Downard CD, Rapkin LB, Gow KW. Melanoma in children and adolescents. Surg Oncol. 2007;16: 215–20.

35. Strouse JJ, Fears TR, Tucker MA, et al. Pediatric melanoma: risk factor and survival analysis of the surveillance, epidemiology and end data base. J Clin Oncol. 2005;23:4735–41.

36. Markovic SN, Erickson LA, Rao RD, et al. Malignant melanoma in the 21st century, part 1: epidemiology, risk factor, screening, prevention, and diagnosis. Mayo Clin Proc. 2007;82:364–80.

37. MacKie RM, Bray C, Vestey J, et al. Melanoma incidence and mortality in Scotland 1979–2003. Br J Cancer. 2007;96:1772–7.

38. Schneider JS, Moore DH, Mendelsohn ML. Screening program reduced melanoma mortality at the Lawrence Livermore National Laboratory, 1984 to 1996. J Am Acad Dermatol. 2008;58:741–9.

39. Balch CM, Buzaid AC, Soong SJ, et al. Final version of the American joint committee on cancer staging system for cutaneous melanoma. J Clin Oncol. 2001;19:3635–48.

40. Tsao H, Bevona C, Goggins W, Quinn T. The transformation rate of moles (melanocytic nevi) into cutaneous melanoma: a population-based estimate. Arch Dermatol. 2003;139:282–8.

41. Bevona C, Goggins W, Quin T, et al. Cutaneous melanoma associated with nevi. Arch Dermatol. 2003;139:1620–4.

42. Olsen CM, Carroll HJ, Whiteman DC. Familial melanoma: a meta-analysis and estimates of attributable fraction. Cancer Epidemiol Biomarkers Prev. 2010;19:65–76.

43. Howell PM, Liu S, Ren S, et al. Epigenetics in human melanoma. Cancer Control. 2009;16:200–18.

44. Pho L, Grossman D, Jeachman SA. Melanoma genetics: a review of genetic factors and clinical phenotypes in familial melanoma. Curr Opin Oncol. 2006;18:173–9.

45. Gillanders E, Juo SH, Holland EA, et al. Localization of novel melanoma susceptibility locus to 1p22. Am J Hum Genet. 2003;73:301–13.

46. Jonsson G, Bendahl PO, Sandberg T, et al. Mapping of novel ocular and cutaneous malignant melanoma susceptibility locus to chromosome 9q21.32. J Natl Cancer Inst. 2005;97:1377–82.

47. Brown KM, MacGregor S, Montgomery GW, et al. Common sequence variants on 20q11.22 confer melanoma susceptibility. Nat Genet. 2008;40:838–40.

48. Gudbjartsson DF, Sulem P, Stacey SN, et al. ASIP and TYR pigmentation variants associated with cutaneous melanoma and basal cell carcinoma. Nat Genet. 2008; 40:886–91.

49. Landi MT, Kanetsky PA, Tsang S, et al. MC1R, ASIP, and DNA repair in sporadic and familial melanoma in a Mediterranean population. J Natl Cancer Inst. 2005; 97:998–1007.

50. Duffy DL, Box NF, Chen W, et al. Interactive effects of MC1R and OCA2 on melanoma risk phenotypes. Hum Mol Genet. 2004;13:447–61.

51. Johnson BL, Moy R, White GM. Ethnic skin: medical and surgical. Toronto: Mosby Publications; 1998.

52. Council ML, Gardner JM, Helms C, et al. Contribution of genetic factors for melanoma susceptibility in sporadic US melanoma patients. Exp Dermatol. 2009;18: 485–7.

53. Gould Rothberg BE, Bracken MB, Rimm DL. Tissue biomarkers for prognosis in cutaneous melanoma: a systematic review and meta-analysis. J Natl Cancer Inst. 2009;101:452–7.

54. Hussein MR. Ultraviolet radiation and skin cancer: molecular mechanism. J Cutan Pathol. 2005;32: 191–205.

55. Setlow RB, Grist E, Thompson K, Woodhead AD. Wavelengths effective in induction of malignant melanoma. Proc Natl Acad Sci U S A. 1993;90:6666–70.

56. Thomas NE, Edmiston SH, Alexander A. Number of naevi and early life ambient UV exposure are associated with B-RAF mutant melanoma. Cancer Epidemiol Biomarkers Prev. 2007;16:991–7.

57. Bouknight P, Bowling A, Kovach FE. Sunscreen use for skin cancer prevention. Am Fam Physician. 2010; 82:989–90.

58. Demko CA, Borawski EA, Ebanne SM, et al. Use of indoor tanning facilities by white adolescents in the United States. Arch Pediatr Adolesc Med. 2003;157: 854–60.

59. Goodson AG, Grossman D. Strategies for early melanoma detection: approaches to the patient with nevi. J Am Acad Dermatol. 2009;60:736–7.

60. U.S. Preventive Services Task Force. Screening for skin cancer: U.S. Preventive Services Task Force recommendation statement. Ann Intern Med. 2009;150:188–93.

61. Wolff T, Tai E, Miller T. Screening for skin cancer: an update of the evidence for the U.S. Preventive Services Task Force. Ann Intern Med. 2009;150:194–8.

62. Vandaele MM, Richert B, Van der Endt JD, et al. Melanoma screening: results of the first one-day campaign in Belgium ("melanoma Monday"). J Eur Acad Dermatol Venereol. 2000;14:470–2.

63. Carli P, De Giorgi V, Giannotti B. Skin cancer day in Italy: method of referral to open access clinics and tumor prevalence in the examined population. Eur J Dermatol. 2003;13:76–9.

64. Rigel DS, Friedman RJ. The rationale of the ABCDs of early melanoma. J Am Acad Dermatol. 1993;29: 1060–1.

65. Friedman RJ, Rigel DS, Kopf AW. Early detection of malignant melanoma: the role of physician examination and self-examination of the skin. CA Cancer J Clin. 1985;35:130–51.

66. Carli P, De Giorni V, Palli D. Self-detected cutaneous melanoma in Italian patients. Clin Exp Dermatol. 2004;29:593–6.

67. Chamberlain AJ, Fritschi L, Kelly JW. Nodular melanoma: patients' perceptions of presenting features and

implications for earlier detection. J Am Acad Dermatol. 2003;48:694–701.

68. Abbasi NR, Shaw HM, Rigel DS, et al. Early diagnosis of cutaneous melanoma: revisiting the ABCD criteria. JAMA. 2004;292:2771–6.

69. Robinson JK, Ortiz S. Use of photographs illustrating ABCDE criteria in skin self-examination. Arch Dermatol. 2009;145:332–3.

70. Vestergaard ME, Macaskill P, Holt PE, Menzies SW. Dermoscopy compared with naked eye examination for the diagnosis of primary melanoma: a meta-analysis of studies performed in a clinical setting. Br J Dermatol. 2008;159:669–76.

71. Piccolo D, Ferrari A, Peris K, et al. Dermoscopic diagnosis by trained clinician vs a clinician with minimal dermoscopy training vs computer-aided diagnosis of 341 pigmented skin lesions: a comparative study. Br J Dermatol. 2002;147: 481–6.

72. Rigel DS, Russak J, Friedman R. The evolution of melanoma diagnosis: 25 years beyond the ABCDs. CA Cancer J Clin. 2010;60:301–16.

73. Henning JS, Dusza SW, Wang SQ, et al. The CASH - color, architecture, symmetry, and homogeneity - algorithm for dermoscopy. J Am Acad Dermatol. 2007;56:45–52.

74. Dolianitis C, Kelly J, Wolfe R, Simpson P. Comparative performance of 4 dermoscopic algorithms by non experts for the diagnosis of melanocytic lesions. Arch Dermatol. 2005;141:1008–14.

75. Annessi G, Bono R, Sampogna F, et al. Sensitivity, specificity, and diagnostic accuracy of three dermoscopic algorithmic methods in the diagnosis of doubtful melanocytic lesions: the importance of light brown structureless areas in differentiating atypical melanocytic nevi from thin melanoma. J Am Acad Dermatol. 2007;56:759–67.

76. Argenziano G, Mordente I, Ferrara G, et al. Dermoscopic monitoring of melanocytic skin lesions: clinical outcome and patient compliance vary according to follow-up protocols. Br J Dermatol. 2008;159:331–6.

77. Chiu V, Won E, Malik M, Weinstock MA. The use of mole-mapping diagrams to increase skin self-examination accuracy. J Am Acad Dermatol. 2006; 55:245–50.

78. Meyer LE, Otberg N, Sterry W, Lademann J. In vivo confocal scanning laser microscopy: comparison of the reflectance and fluorescence mode by imaging human skin. J Biomed Opt. 2006;11: 44012–6.

79. Brazan AL, Landthaler M, Szeimies RM. In vivo confocal scanning laser microscopy in dermatology. Lasers Med Sci. 2007;22:73–82.

Cutaneous Squamous Cell Carcinoma: Focus on Biochemical and Molecular Characteristics

Michele Caraglia, Giovanni Francesco Nicoletti, Angela Lombardi, Gerardo Botti, and Renato Franco

Key Points

- cSCC is an emerging problem for the world health due to its diffusion and spread in the population.
- The main etiopathogenetic factors of cSCC are the exposure to sun's UV and the infection by HPV.
- The molecular alterations of cSCC reside in the inactivation of the p53 family protein and particularly of p63, mutations in PATCH and INK4a/ARF tumor suppressor genes, the amplification of the expression of the EGFR family proteins, ras-activating mutations, Fas and

Fas ligand depressed expression, and alterations of molecules associated to intra-tumor vessels such as podoplanin.

- cSCC can be grouped in two categories: *sun exposure-related tumors*, such as *preinvasive lesions* (actinic or solar keratoses (AKs), cSCC in situ (Bowen's disease)) and *invasive lesions* (invasive cSCC (cSCCI), clear-cell cSCC, spindle cell (sarcomatoid) cSCC, and cSCC with single cell infiltrates) that derive from preinvasive lesions, and *non-sun exposure-related lesions*, such as de novo cSCC, lymphoepithelioma-like carcinoma of the skin (LELCS), and verrucous carcinoma (VC), not related to solar exposure.
- The treatment of nonadvanced cSCC is radical surgery or other local approaches with radical intention. The treatment of advanced cSCC is based upon the use of conventional chemotherapy agents (i.e., 5 fluorouracil, bleomycin, cisplatin, doxorubicin) that has given varying results.
- Biological agents such as cis-retinoic acid and interferon-α (alone or in combination) have been used in the advanced stage but with limiting effects.
- New emphasis has been given by the target-based agents cetuximab and gefitinib raised against EGFR and used

M. Caraglia, MD, PhD (✉) • A. Lombardi
Department of Biochemistry and Biophysics,
Second University of Naples,
Via S.M. Costantinopoli, 16,
Naples 80138, Italy
e-mail: michele.caraglia@unina2.it

G.F. Nicoletti
Dipartimento di Scienze Ortopediche,
Traumatologiche, Riabilitative e Plastico-Ricostruttive,
Second University of Naples,
Naples, Italy

G. Botti • R. Franco
Pathology Unit,
National Institute of Tumours Fondazione "G. Pascale",
Naples, Italy

A. Baldi et al. (eds.), *Skin Cancer*, Current Clinical Pathology,
DOI 10.1007/978-1-4614-7357-2_3, © Springer Science+Business Media New York 2014

alone or in combination with chemotherapy or radiotherapy.

- Some target-based agents used in the
treatment of other skin tumors such as
melanoma can determine the risk of
occurrence of cSCC. This is the case of
the raf inhibitors that elicit Erk hyperactivation in Ras-mutated cSCC precursor
cells.

- The limited activity of interferon-α in
cSCC can be explained on the basis of
multiple escape mechanisms to the antiproliferative and apoptotic activity of
the cytokine. Several strategies designed
to overcome resistance mechanism are
described. On these bases, new molecular biology-based protocols can be
designed for the treatment of advanced
cSCC.

Introduction

Nonmelanoma skin cancer (NMSC) is the most
common cancer of Caucasians, accounting
approximately for 80 % of basal cell cancer and
20 % cutaneous squamous cell carcinoma
(cSCC) [1]. cSCC is associated with relative
risk of metastasis. Recently a relative increase
of cSCC incidence has been documented, probably attributable to sun exposure, intensifying
UV exposure, and more frequent skin examinations [2].

Histopathological variants show significant
different clinical behavior [3–6]. They recognize
different biological background, and their correct classification is critical for diagnosis and
treatment [7, 8].

Epidemiology

cSCC incidence is not easily determined,
although it is known for its substantial contribution to morbidity and mortality in the elderly
individuals [9, 10].

However, in recent years, there has been a
significant increase in the incidence of this tumor
[11]. In details, it has been recorded in longitudinal studies of both the USA and Canada that
cSCC has grown by 50–200 % over the past
10–30 years [2, 12, 13].

Moreover, the incidence of cSCC increases
proceeding from the poles to the equator, about
twice any decrease of 8–10°, reaching its maximum at the equator [14]. Among whites, cSCC
incidence is 100–150 per 100,000 persons per
year, being ten times more frequent in the group
of persons older than 75 years.

Mortality for cSCC reported in the early 1990s
is of 1 % per year [10] accounting the majority of
NMSC deaths [15] and 20 % of all skin-cancer-
related deaths [16].

Etiological Factor

Many etiological factors have been demonstrated in the pathogenesis of cSCC, including
environmental, genetic, viral, and altered host
immunity (Table 3.1) [17–19]. Exposure to
ultraviolet radiation has been recognized as the
main cause of this type of cancer [20, 21]. In
detail, sunlight ultraviolet B radiation (wavelength: from 290 to 320 nm) seems to play the
most relevant role [22–24] inducing dimerization of thymidine in the p53 tumor suppressor
gene. Therefore, tumor development requires
inability to repair DNA damage [25].
Consequently, cSCC is more common in areas
with high UV exposure [20].

Albinism, *xeroderma pigmentosum*, and *epidermodysplasia verruciformis* are the cutaneous
genetically inherited skin diseases with high propensity of risk for developing cSCC [15, 22, 23].

Immunodepression is related to high incidence
of cSCC, that is up to 64–250-fold greater than
that in the general population [26, 27]. In solid
organ transplant patients, cSCC appears as multiple lesions, with high propensity of recurrence
and metastatization [28]. In these patients, cSCCs
develop within 10 years from organ transplant
[29]. HPV has also been found in cSCC with
higher evidence in immunosuppressed patients

Table 3.1 Risk factors for the development of cutaneous squamous cell carcinoma

Exposure to ultraviolet radiation
Ultraviolet A
Ultraviolet B
Therapy with methoxsalen and ultraviolet A radiation
Exposure to ionizing radiation
Genodermatosis
Oculocutaneous albinism
Xeroderma pigmentosum
Infection with human papillomavirus, especially types 6, 11, 16, and 18
Exposure to chemical carcinogens
Arsenic
Polycyclic aromatic hydrocarbons
Immunosuppression
Organ transplantation
Leukemia and lymphoma
Immunosuppressive medications
Chronically injured or diseased skin
Ulcers
Sinus tracts
Osteomyelitis
Radiation dermatitis
Certain chronic inflammatory disorders, such as dystrophic epidermolysis bullosa
Precursor lesions
Actinic keratoses
Arsenical keratoses
Radiation-induced keratoses
Bowen's disease (squamous cell carcinoma in situ)
Erythroplasia of Queyrat (squamous cell carcinoma in situ of the penis)

[20, 21]. cSCC could also occur in cutaneous sites with scars, sinus tracts, and burns. The latter are more aggressive with an overall metastatic rate of 40 % [16, 21].

Molecular Pathology of cSCC

Different pathways are deregulated in cSCC, dependently from etiological factor.

UV-Driven cSCC

UV radiations are very toxic agents for skin. The wave lengths of absorption depends upon molecular structure, being shorter around 200 nm for conjugated bonds in organic molecules and longer around 300 nm, in the range of solar spectrum, for linear repeats or ring structures. Therefore, DNA containing many ring structures, i.e., bases, and conjugated bonds represents the most relevant absorber of UV in the cell with consequent gene mutations [30]. The effects of UV on human skin can be considered acute or chronic. Between the acute effects, DNA damage is essentially due to the induction of primarily cyclobutane-type pyrimidine dimers and pyrimidine pyrimidone photoproducts [31–33].

Therefore, base modifications occur where a tandem of pyrimidine exists. Radiation induces primarily $C \rightarrow T$ and $CC \rightarrow TT$ transitions that are the hallmark of UV-induced mutagenesis [34]. Subsequently, when DNA polymerase cannot interpret the DNA template, the enzyme inserts A residues by default [35]. In addition, UV induces also cytosine photohydrates, purine photoproducts, and single-strand breaks in the DNA and the production of specific reactive oxygen species (ROS), responsible for the induction of single-strand breaks, DNA–protein cross-links, and altered bases in DNA [36, 37]. Acute UV-induced skin damage is also responsible for the induction of p53 expression through different mechanisms. p53 is a critical protein that causes cell cycle arrest, either favoring the cellular repair pathways to remove DNA damage before DNA synthesis and mitosis [38–40] or promoting apoptosis in cells with excessive DNA damage [41]. p53 protein increases in epidermal cells after exposure to UV radiation, as demonstrated in SKH-hr1 mice [42]. In details, it seems to be induced when DNA damage has characterized by pyrimidine dimers and DNA stands break [42]. In addition, p53 phosphorylation is induced by UV radiation through involvement of the ATM, ATR, and p38, and of the ERK1/2 and JNK-1 mitogen-activated protein (MAP) kinases-dependent pathways [43–46]. Thus, serine residue phosphorylation promotes stabilization of p53 by (1) disrupting the interaction of p53 with Mdm2, (2) enhancing p53 transcriptional activity, and (3) favoring p53 nuclear localization. The final effects of p53 activation are essentially cell cycle arrest followed by DNA repair occurring through two major pathways: non-excision repair (NER) and base excision repair (BER). In details, in NER pathway p53 transactivates the two xeroderma pigmentosum-associated gene products (p48XPE and XPC) and GADD45; [47–49] in BER pathway, p53 plays a role in regulating DNA polymerase, which is directly involved in DNA repair/synthesis [50]. When DNA damage is too deep, activated p53 in damaged skin induces apoptosis, through activation of a wide variety of transcriptional factors related to activation of the apoptosomal complex, such as the Bcl-2 family members Bax, p53-upregulated modulator of apoptosis (PUMA), Noxa, p53-upregulated apoptosis-inducing protein 1 (p53AIP1), and PIGa (galectin-7) [51–53]. Moreover, it has been demonstrated that UVB-induced apoptosis is related also to activation of Fas–Fas ligand, potent activators of pro-caspase 8 cleavage and, at the same time, of the cytochrome c release from mitochondria, followed by activation of the Apaf-1–pro-caspase 9 complex that both induce apoptosis [54]. Finally, UV-induced acute skin damage can also stimulate cell survival mechanisms and induce cell proliferation in the form of cell hyperplasia. In fact, UV triggers proliferation through activation of growth factor receptors such as erbB receptors and cytokine receptors, such as receptors for tumor necrosis factor (TNF) and interleukin-1 (IL1) [55, 56].

Chronic UV irradiation causes p53 mutation and loss of Fas–Fas ligand interaction with consequent apoptosis deregulation.

p53 mutations seem to be an early genetic event in the development of UV-induced skin cancers. In fact it has been described in approximately 53 % of premalignant actinic keratosis (AK) lesions [57]. In addition, 40 % of Bowen's disease carry p53 mutations [58]. Many reports have recorded p53-mutant cell clones in nonneoplastic cells of sun-exposed skin [57–62]. However, p53 mutations in cSCC and in their respective precursors seem to be different from those in nonneoplastic skin areas [61]. This suggests that not all UV-induced p53mutations confer a malignant phenotype to neoplastic cells and that there is a latency from the occurrence of p53 mutation and cancer development. Some in vivo experiments have demonstrated that the occur-

rence of the most critical p53 mutations is recorded from 17 to 80 daily UVB exposures and skin tumors around 80 to 30 weeks later [63, 64]. Analyzing both $C \rightarrow T$ and $CC \rightarrow TT$ transitions in p53 gene, it has been observed that mutations are much earlier, being present at the first week from the beginning of chronic UV irradiation, with higher frequency at 4–8 weeks [65].

Therefore, selective expansion of p53-mutant cells occurs in the context of epidermis, due to both the resistance to UV-induced apoptosis and the proliferative advantage over normal keratinocytes in response to UV irradiation [64, 66, 67] (Fig. 3.1). Regression of a part of precancerous p53-positive clones can be observed after discontinuation from UV irradiation [64, 68] although tumor occurrence is only delayed [69].

p53 Family Protein p63 and cSCC Pathogenesis

The epidermis is continuously regenerated by mitotically active keratinocytes in the inner basal layer which, following detachment from the basement membrane, migrates to the outer cornified layer (terminally differentiated compartment): a process called cornification. The epidermis is continuously renewed by a regulated balance between proliferation and differentiation. The renewal capacity is due to the presence of epidermal stem cells and transient amplifying (TA) cells in the basal layer of the interfollicular epidermis and in the bulge of the hair follicle. The importance of the transcription factor p63 for the formation of the epidermis and other stratified epithelia arises from two lines of evidence. First, p63 is strongly expressed in the innermost basal layer where epithelial cells with high clonogenic and proliferative capacity reside. Second, mice lacking all p63 isoforms have no epidermis or squamous epithelia (prostate, urothelium), probably due to a premature proliferative rundown of the stem and TA cells. Mice knockout for p63 (p63$^{-/-}$) also show lack of epithelial appendages, such as mammary, salivary, and lachrymal glands, hair follicles, and teeth, and have truncated limbs and abnormal craniofacial development. This is most likely

Fig. 3.1 (**a**) UV skin damage-induced apoptosis in functional p53 expressing normal skin; (**b**) Identification of p53-mutated clones in UV-induced cSCC

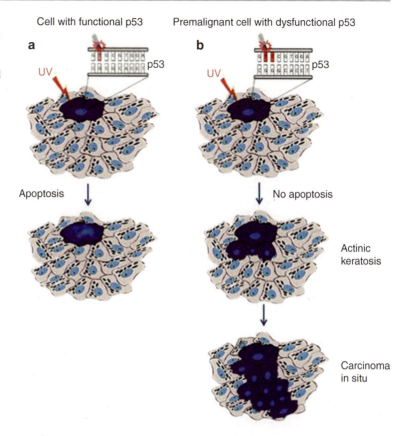

due to failure to maintain or differentiate the apical ectodermal ridge, a structure that is important for coordination of epithelial–mesenchymal interactions and is required for limb outgrowth and palatal and facial structure formation. p63 is expressed from two different promoters that generate two classes of proteins, TAp63, which contains the N-terminal transactivation(TA) domain, and the N-terminal truncated (DNp63) isoform, which lacks the transactivation domain. In addition, alternative splicing at the 3′ end of the transcripts generates three different C-termini: α, β, and γ. However, information about the protein expression levels of splice variants is not currently available due to the lack of isoform-specific antibodies, thus hampering the identification of specific functions.

It is emerging that p63 is involved in tumorigenesis and in controlling chemosensitivity.

The notion that the transcription factor p63 is essential for the formation of the epidermis and other stratified epithelia arises from the fact that mice lacking p63 show profound defects information of the epidermis. Remarkably, genetic mutations of p63 in man are causatively linked to ectodermal dysplastic syndromes. The involvement of p63 in the generation of skin cancer is related to its ability to control apoptosis through both extrinsic and intrinsic pathway. The loss of p63 in cancer can favor the survival of mutated cell clones that in the presence of p63 have not the possibility to develop towards cancer. Moreover, p63 is involved in the control of cell proliferation through the regulation of both the expression and activity of several growth factor receptors. In fact, p63 can affect the fibroblast growth factor receptor 2b (FGFR2b) receptor and its associated signaling, since it has been shown that there is a reduction in keratinocyte proliferation in the epidermis of Fgfr2b$^{-/-}$ embryos. In addition, the proliferative capacity of p63$^{-/-}$ mice keratinocytes could be also reduced as a consequence of increased expression of p21, a direct transcriptional repression target of DNp63. p63 functions as a selective modulator of Notch1-dependent transcription and function and also directly transactivates the Notch ligand, JAGG-1. Thus, a complex cross-talk between Notch and p63 could regulate the balance between keratinocyte self-renewal and differentiation. Moreover, a microarray analysis for p63 target genes, which was then validated in the genetically complemented mice, indicates that the function of p63 in epithelial development is at least in part mediated by IKKα (IκB kinase-α) and GATA-3 [70].

Fas and Fas Ligand

After the initial upregulation of Fas and Fas ligand expression induced by the acute exposure to UV, transcriptional inhibition of Fas ligand expression has been observed after 1 week of continuous UV irradiation in mice, with corresponding decrease in the number of apoptotic cells [65, 71]. Deregulation of Fas–Fas ligand-mediated signaling favors accumulation of p53 mutations, since Fas ligand-deficient mice with prolonged UV irradiation develop more *p53* mutations than wild-type mice [54].

Growth Factor Receptors Belonging to the Superfamily of Erb

The tyrosine kinases human epidermal receptor (HER) family (epidermal growth factor receptor (EGFR), HER-2, HER-3, and HER-4) are transmembrane glycoproteins related to cell proliferation, differentiation, and apoptosis. Altered expression of the HER family is associated with several epithelial tumors such as breast carcinoma and esophageal squamous cell carcinoma. Small studies have also shown altered HER expression in localized squamous cell carcinoma when compared to normal skin. Given the paucity of unresectable or metastatic cSCC, reliable information on the frequency of EGFR expression is limited. One study of 13 metastatic specimens by IHC demonstrated that all had strong membranous expression of EGFR. Another study of locally advanced and nodally metastatic

cutaneous SCC demonstrated EGFR expression above background in only 9 of 21 (43 %) specimens using a quantitative Western blotting technique. Another study using IHC and fluorescence in situ hybridization demonstrated higher levels of EGFR protein expression in cutaneous SCC than in the precursor actinic keratoses and an association between this elevated protein expression and higher EGFR gene copy number. One study, examining the role of EGFR in cSCC arising in the head and neck, demonstrated that primary lesions associated with subsequent metastases were more likely to overexpress EGFR (79 %) than those not associated with subsequent metastases (36 %). Interestingly, metastatic nodal disease exhibited only a 47 % rate of EGFR overexpression; EGFR overexpression in that study was not associated with EGFR gene amplification. Recently, a study on 55 primary tumors and 22 lymph node metastases derived from cSCC of the trunk and extremities has demonstrated that EGFR had no influence on prognosis. It is possible that altered EGFR expression may be associated with local recurrence, which is more frequently life threatening at other sites. HER-2 was negative in all samples and may play little part in CSCC progression as found in squamous cell carcinomas from other sites. High HER-4 expression in lymph node metastases was associated with poor prognosis suggesting a role in progression of cSCC of the trunk and extremities. It is possible that altered HER-4 expression occurs late and is present only in metastases. The altered coexpression of the HER family may play a role (i.e., EGFR/HER-4, HER-3/HER-4, and EGFR/HER-3/HER-4), but the small number of cases in this study meant this could not be analyzed.

Lymphatic Vessel Markers: Podoplanin

Podoplanin, originally detected on the surface of podocytes, belongs to the family of type-1 transmembrane sialomucin-like glycoproteins. Although specific for lymphatic vascular (LV) endothelium, podoplanin is expressed in a wide variety of normal and tumor cells. Podoplanin plays an important role in preventing cellular adhesion and is involved in the regulation of the shape of podocyte foot processes and in the maintenance of glomerular permeability. Moreover, podoplanin is involved in LV formation and does not influence formation of blood vessels.

The expression of podoplanin is induced by the homeobox gene Prox-1, and a specific endogenous receptor was identified on platelets. Immunohistochemical detection of podoplanin/D2-40 in LECs was used in many studies to evaluate the LV microvascular density (LVMD) in peritumoral and tumoral areas and to correlate LVMD with lymph node status and prognosis. Podoplanin significantly increases the detection of lymphovascular invasion in different types of malignant tumors. Podoplanin expression was found in tumor cells of various types of cancer, such as vascular tumors, malignant mesothelioma, tumors of the central nervous system (CNS), germ cell tumors, and squamous cell carcinomas. This expression in tumor cells is useful for pathological diagnosis, and podoplanin seems to be expressed by aggressive tumors, with higher invasive and metastatic potential [72]. Recently, it was demonstrated that podoplanin expression was not associated with the presence of lymph node metastasis, but was a prognosticator of reduced survival indicating a locally aggressive tumor, with survival impact in cSCC. Altered expression of podoplanin is associated with mesothelioma, squamous cell carcinoma of oral mucosa, and germ cell tumors, suggesting that podoplanin may influence invasive and proliferative activity. As cSCC metastases occur preferentially via lymphatic vessels, podoplanin expression may be associated with disease progression. Hyperexpression has been related to undifferentiated skin tumors, but its impact on prognosis and metastasis has not been established. Podoplanin can be suggested as a possible target for the development of novel therapies, and its expression has to be studied in other settings to completely understand its role in cSCC development and progression.

Progression of cSCC

Progression of cSCC is substantially due to activation of proto-oncogenes such as ras and inactivation of tumor suppressor genes such as PTCH or INK4a-ARF. Moreover, epigenetic deregulations have also been described as an important determinant in the progression of cSCC.

Activation of ras Oncogenes

The members of *ras* family, *H-ras, K-ras,* and *N-ras,* encode 21 kDa guanosine triphosphate (GTP)-binding proteins placed on the inner surface of the cell membrane [73]. They are functional in the transduction of signals to the nucleus in order to activate proliferation machinery, when growth factors are activated through intrinsic GTPase. Different human cancers show *ras* mutations in codons 12, 13, and 61 [74] with consequent continuous activation of *ras*-mediated signal transduction. Also human skin cancers contain mutations in all three members of the *ras* family [75].

Activated c-H-*ras* oncogenes derived from UV-exposed cSCC are tumorigenic for NIH 3T3 cells [76]. Therefore, the transfected NIH 3T3 cells induce tumors at the subcutaneous site of injection and spontaneous lung metastases in nude mice [77]. Also *ras* family mutations rely at pyrimidine-rich sequences, suggesting a direct role of UV irradiation [78]. Besides point mutations, deregulation of ras genes could be due to amplification and rearrangement of specific gene sequences [79, 80].

Mutations in PATCH and INK4a/ARF Tumor Suppressor Genes

Mutations in *INK4a/ARF* tumor suppressor gene have been described in a subset of cSCCs. This locus encodes for two independent growth inhibitors: the cyclin-dependent kinase (CDK) inhibitor p16INK4a and the p53 activator p14ARF (mouse p19Arf). p16INK4a inactivates CDK4/6, favoring sequestration of the transcription factor E2F1 by the Rb tumor suppressor protein [81]. p14ARF binds human double-minute protein 2 (HDM2, mouse Mdm2), thereby blocking HDM2-induced translational silencing and degradation of p53 [82]. Also in these cases gene alterations were induced by UV. Recently, in a series of cSCC, all the alterations of the *INK4a/ARF* locus have been analyzed. Point mutations were less common (10 %) and loss of heterozygosity (32.5 %) and promoter hypermethylation of *p16INK4a* and *p14ARF* (36 %) more common [83].

Epigenetic Alterations

Epigenetic alterations described in cancer progression include DNA methylation and histone modifications, the latter consisting in methylation, acetylation, phosphorylation, ubiquitination, and sumoylation, chromatin remodelling and different microRNA profile [84–86]. Gene specific methylation responsible of transcriptional control is described in cSCC development and progression [84–86]. Promoter methylation of FOXE1, a transcriptional factor involved in regulation of many organ development and located on chromosome 9q22, a region frequently lost in cSCC, is highly methylated in cSCC [87]. microRNAs (MiRNAs) appear to play an important role in the epigenetic regulation of cSCC at posttranscriptional level [88]. In fact, a recent study has demonstrated that a distinct microRNA profile is specifically induced by UV radiation [89]. Finally, mitochondrial DNA mutations, affecting displacement loop (D-loop) and other regions, are described in cSCC [90–92].

Human Papillomavirus (HPV) and cSCC

In cSCC carcinogenesis, also HPV infection appears to play an important role significantly reducing p53 expression, particularly in immune-suppressed patients [93]. In details, higher viral load has been recorded in 80 % of cSCC of immunosuppressed organ transplant patients [20], while in immune-competent patients, the frequency of HPV DNA in cSCC varies from only 27 to 70 % depending on detection techniques [23, 29]. On this light, among more than 100 HPV identified subtypes, only the small subgroup of high-risk mucotro-

pic HPV (HPV types 16, 18, 31, 33, 35, and 58) has been demonstrated as responsible of cervical cancer development. In this context E6 gene favors p53 proteosomal degradation with subsequent abolishment of cell cycle arrest or apoptosis.

HPV DNA is often identified in cSCC including more than 40 not high-risk subtypes [94, 95]. The pathogenesis of HPV-induced cSCC is probably different from that observed in cervical cSCC. In fact, low copy of HPV DNA has been found in cSCC, suggesting a possible role for tumor initiation and progression. In details, three mechanisms have been proposed for HPV-induced carcinogenesis: (1) UV radiation-induced immunosuppression that favors HPV infection [96, 97], (2) E6/E7 oncoprotein-related changes in p53 and Rb tumor suppressor gene, and (3) integration of HPV DNA disrupting genomic stability [96]. However, the weak transforming activity of cutaneous HPV in vitro suggests that antiapoptotic activity of E6 protein in cSCC could become relevant only in conjunction with other factors, such as by sunlight (UV) exposure, immunosuppression, and proliferation of epithelium (psoriasis) [95] (Fig. 3.2).

These hypotheses are supported by the evidence that HPV-38, detected in 50 % of skin carcinomas, in 43 % of AK, and in 10 % of nonneoplastic keratinocytes, is responsible of longevity/immortalization of human keratinocytes in vitro [97–99].

Clinicopathological data of HPV-related cSCC show close association with poorly differentiated cancers, lymph nodes metastasis, and late-stage disease, which are related to poor prognosis tumors. HPV status is also characterized by p16 overexpression and low frequency of p53 mutations [100].

Histology

cSCC includes a series of neoplastic disorders with substantial biological differences. They could be grouped in two categories: *sun exposure-related tumors*, such as *preinvasive lesions* (actinic or solar keratoses (AKs), cSCC in situ(Bowen's

Fig. 3.2 Mechanisms of HPV-induced cSCC: Low-risk HPV (**a**) needs cofactors to induce cSCC, differently from high-risk HPV (**b**)

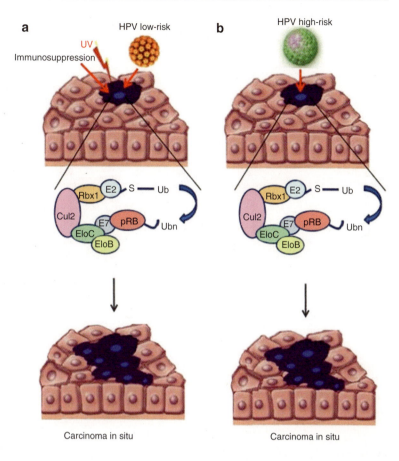

disease)) and *invasive lesions* (invasive cSCC (cSCCI), clear-cell cSCC, spindle cell (sarcomatoid) cSCC, and cSCC with single-cell infiltrates) that derive from preinvasive lesions, and *non-sun exposure-related lesions*, such as de novo cSCC, lymphoepithelioma-like carcinoma of the skin (LELCS), and verrucous carcinoma (VC), not related to solar exposure.

Actinic Keratosis (AK)

It is commonly considered a cSCC precursor lesion. It is related to solar exposure; therefore, it develops in sun-exposed skin areas, including face, neck, dorsal hands, and forearms, upper chest, back, and scalp [4, 5, 15, 101]. Due to its relation to exposure to sun, it generally affects middle-aged or older individuals. It can occur in younger individuals, but always in relation to longtime sun exposure or concomitant sensibility to UV damage, such as immunosuppression [15, 24]. AK spontaneously regresses and evolves to invasive cSCC in only 5–10 % of cases [102]. Different AK variants have been described including hypertrophic, atrophic, acantholytic, pigmented, proliferative, and bowenoid subtypes. Hypertrophic and proliferative variants are associated to a more aggressive biologic behavior [4, 5, 103, 104].

It is characterized by aggregates of atypical, pleomorphic keratinocytes that show nuclear atypia, dyskeratosis, and loss of polarity, extending variously through the epithelium till to cover all the thickness in the bowenoid variant, similar to Bowen's disease [5, 105, 106] (Fig. 3.3a). The profile of dermo-epidermal junction in AKs shows small round epithelial buds protruding slightly into the upper papillary dermis. Solar elastosis in the dermis is always observed.

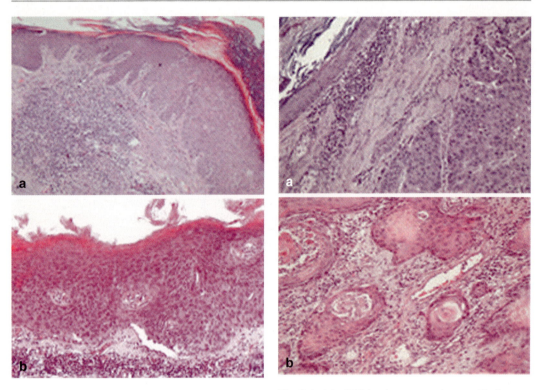

Fig. 3.3 (a) Actinic keratosis, H&E 10×; (b) Bowen's disease, H&E 20×

Fig. 3.4 (a) cSCC in photo-exposed area with the concomitant presence of solar elastosis, H&E 20×; (b) SCC in not photo-exposed area, H&E 20×

Squamous Cell Carcinoma In Situ (cSCCS)/Bowen's Disease

The two definitions are synonymous. Most of them occur in sun-exposed skin areas, such as the head, neck, and hands [107]. Moreover, mucosal surfaces and nail could be frequently involved [108]. Bowen's disease in genital areas is also called *erythroplasia of Queyrat*. Clinical presentation is generally represented by erythematous, scaly patch or plaque [108]. Only 3–5 % of cases progress towards invasive cSCC, and this rate is higher for *erythroplasia of Queyrat* [109]. The invasive cSCC developed from Bowen's disease seems to be more aggressive, since 20 % of these cases develop metastatic disease [110]. Histopathologically, the epidermis is characterized by atypical cells with loss of polarity, high mitotic activity, pleomorphism, and greatly enlarged nuclei through the entire thickness (Fig. 3.3b). Multinucleated cells could be also observed [107]. Atypical cells may involve adjacent follicular epithelium and adnexal structures [5].

Invasive Squamous Cell Carcinoma (cSCCI)

Approximately 97 % of cSCC are associated to AK as a consequence of their strict biological link. Also histological features of cSCC are similar to its precursor but characterized by infiltrative pattern of membrane basement into dermis [3, 111] (Fig. 3.4). Infiltrative dermal component is represented by neoplastic cell nests, often associated to inflammatory infiltrate. cSCCI differentiation is defined by three broad histologic grades, based essentially on nuclear atypia and keratinization (Fig. 3.5a–c). Approximately 0.5 % of metastases has been recorded for well-differentiated tumors, containing cells with slightly enlarged, hyperchromatic nuclei with abundant amounts of cytoplasm [15]. On the contrary, poorly differentiated tumors, containing highly pleomorphic cells with scanty keratin formation, are characterized by much more aggressive clinical behavior [16]. Intermediate differentiated cSCCI share

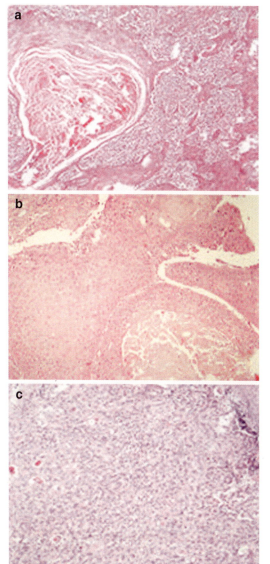

Fig. 3.5 Well-differentiated (**a**), moderately differentiated (**b**), and undifferentiated (**c**) cSCC, H&E 20×

features of both well-differentiated and poorly differentiated tumors.

Clear-Cell cSCC

This rare variant shows neoplastic cells with clear cytoplasm, because of hydropic degeneration of neoplastic cells, and the accumulation of intracellular fluid [112]. Clinically, the lesions as nodules or ulcerated masses are typically present in

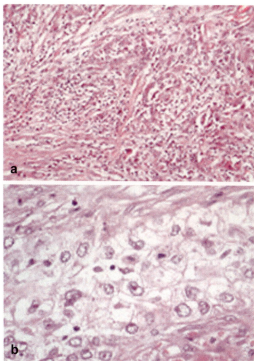

Fig. 3.6 (**a**) Sarcomatoid cSCC, H&E 40×; (**b**) Clear-cell SCC, H&E 40×

sun-exposed surfaces. Histopathologically, three different types have been recognized: (1) keratinizing (type I), (2) nonkeratinizing (type II), and (3) pleomorphic (type III). All three types are characterized by clear cytoplasm without glycogen or mucin, but only trace of lipid, suggesting that clear-cell changes are degenerative [112].

Type I lesions are characterized as sheets or islands of tumor cells with clear, empty-appearing cytoplasm and foci of keratinization. Type II lesions are dermal tumor without keratinizing foci, while type III lesions arise from the epidermis, widely ulcerated, with foci of squamous differentiation, areas of acantholysis, and the presence of dyskeratosis (Fig. 3.6a). Its rarity makes it difficult to distinguish histologic markers of aggressiveness.

Spindle Cell (Sarcomatoid) cSCC

Spindle cell cSCC is a very rare variant of squamous cell carcinoma [113]. It has been observed in sun-exposed areas, but it can develop also in patients with prior exposure to radiation. In the latter case, this variant is considered de novo cSCC and appears to be more aggressive than conventional cSCC [113]. Clinically it is characterized by either bleeding or ulceration. Microscopically spindle cells cSCC is composed by tumoral spindle cells arranged in whorled pattern (Fig. 3.6b). It can be also associated to conventional cSCC and AK [114]. Neoplastic cells can contain also highly pleomorphic giant cells and heterologous elements. The tumor is generally deeply infiltrating, sometimes with the involvement of subcutis, fascia, muscle, and even occasionally bone. High mitotic index is generally present. Immunohistochemical staining is needed, in the absence of conventional cSCC, in order to distinguish it from other spindle cell tumors, such as atypical fibroxanthoma, spindle cell melanoma, or spindle cell sarcoma. Spindle cell cSCC stains, at least focally, high molecular weight cytokeratin and p63 [115].

cSCC with Single-Cell Infiltrates

This is a rare entity, occurring on the face and neck of older individuals. It seems more aggressive than conventional cSCC because it is frequently misdiagnosed [116]. Microscopically, it is formed by loosely arranged neoplastic cells in the dermis, without apparent connection to epidermis or adnexal structures. The diagnosis is very difficult, above all when neoplastic cells are obscured by inflammatory infiltrates. Immunohistochemical staining of neoplastic cells for high molecular weight cytokeratin and p63 allows the recognition of these cells [116].

De Novo cSCC

De novo cSCC generally arises on skin surface previously injured or diseased, particularly long-standing ulcers, burn scars, or osteomyelitis, and also chronic inflammatory conditions such as discoid lupus erythematosus and dystrophic epidermolysis bullosa [117–120]. Marjolin's ulcer refers to cSCC developed in burn scars, first described by Marjolin in 1827 [121]. De novo cSCCs are commonly found on the lower extremities, where burn scars are more prevalent. The time of incidence from the trauma is around 20 to 40 years later [122]. Clinically it is presented as exophytic growths or indurated ulcers. Microscopically, de novo cSCCs are similar to conventional cSCC, with the lack of solar dermis elastosis (Fig. 3.4). It is associated to either ulcers or scars. The epidermis is often atrophic or ulcerated. The incidence of regional lymph node metastasis, particularly for lower extremity lesions, is higher if compared with other cSCC subtypes, reaching as high as 54 % [122]. Its prognosis is very poor, with a 5-year survival rate of only 52–75 % [5].

Verrucous Carcinomas

Verrucous carcinoma (VC) is a relative indolent noninfiltrating tumor, associated with both low-risk (types 6 and 11) and high-risk (types 16 and 18) types of HPV [23]. Four clinicopathological categories based on the involved body skin area are described: oro-aero-digestive VC, ano-urogenital VC, palmoplantar VC (also known as *epithelioma cuniculatum*), and VC found on other sites [123]. Despite this subclassification, all these lesions share similar histological features.

As cutaneous VC concerns, the most frequent category is palmoplantar VC, found on the soles of elderly Caucasian males, but it may also be seen on the toes, the heel, or the dorsum of the foot [124]. They are frequently misdiagnosed as plantar warts, but they finally emerge as bulky exophytic masses. Low-risk HPV types is commonly found in thesetumors [123].

VC lesions found on other cutaneous sites are rarely describes. They are clinically similar to palmoplantar VC, but rarely associated to HPV infections [123].

Microscopically, VC are well-differentiated tumors, with a characteristic endo-exophytic growth pattern, normal stratification of squamous cells, marked acanthosis and papillomatosis, hyperkeratosis with parakeratosis, and a prominent granular layer. Minimal atypia can be also

Fig. 3.7 Verrucous carcinoma, H&E 5×

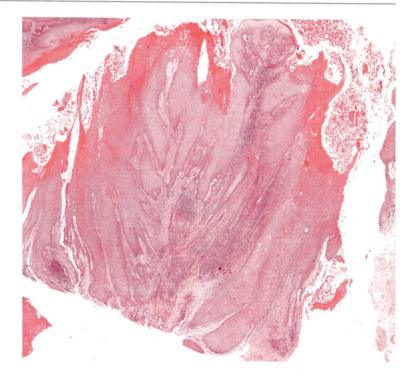

present (Fig. 3.7). Tumoral projections through the dermis descend deeply, and they seem to be responsible of compressive destruction [123].

The distinction between conventional cSCC and VC is very relevant, conventional cSCC being more aggressive. Immunohistochemical staining of bcl-2, Ki-67, and p53 of the lower third of the epidermis in VC and the entire epidermis in cSCC is very useful for the differential diagnosis [125].

Lymphoepithelioma-Like Carcinoma of the Skin

This rare entity occurs in the head and neck of elderly patients. Clinically it is a slowly growing dermal nodule. Histologically it is characterized by syncytial sheets of tumor cells in the mid to deep dermis in an inflammatory background [126]. Only electronic microscopy has demonstrated its squamous origin, due to the presence of desmosomes and tonofilaments [127]. Also in these cases, the diagnosis of neoplastic cells can be difficult, because they are obscured by inflammatory elements. Also in this case, the

immunohistochemical staining of neoplastic cells for epithelial markers, such as cytokeratin and EMA, can facilitate the recognition of neoplastic cells [128].

Therapeutic Approaches Based upon the Targeting of Biological Markers Expressed in cSCC

Treatment of Nonadvanced cSCC

For low-risk, local lesions, the usual treatment is surgical excision, electrodessication and curettage, or cryosurgery. Destructive treatment methods leave no tissue to analyze for marginal control. Nevertheless, using these methods, the 5-year control rate in patients with low-risk primary lesions can be as high as 96 %.

For higher-risk tumors, the primary treatment is surgical excision. The key factor in determining the cure rate is the ability to achieve negative surgical margins. Surgery may be conventional or microscopically controlled, the latter procedure referred to as "Mohs' surgery," after its originator. In this procedure, the targeted lesion is excised and the circumferential margins are assessed microscopically for residual tumor. Margins remaining involved undergo repeated excisions, followed by histological assessment, until negative margins are obtained. Mohs' surgery yields local control rates of 92–100 %, versus 38–87 % for standard surgical excision. Mohs' surgery cure rates decrease as tumor grade increases, with a 45.2 % cure rate for grade 4 cSCC.

Treatment of Advanced cSCC

Chemotherapy

A number of systemic therapies have been used to treat advanced cutaneous SCC, including cytotoxic chemotherapy (cisplatin, 5-fluorouracil [5-FU], bleomycin, and doxorubicin), 13-cis-retinoic acid (13cRA), and immunotherapy (interferon-α 2a [IFN-α]).

A nonrigorous randomized trial comparing bleomycin with other cytotoxic agents (cyclophosphamide, vincristine, methotrexate, and procarbazine) as treatment for 70 patients with SCC, only six of whom had cSCC, showed no statistically significant difference between the two treatment groups [129]. Sadek et al. [130] reported on 14 patients (13 evaluable) from a prospective observational study of patients with advanced cutaneous SCC treated with cisplatin, 5-FU, and bleomycin for 1–4 months. That study resulted in 4 of 13 patients with a complete response (CR) and 7 of 13 with a partial response (PR) [131]. After 1 year, 6 of 13 patients had died from their disease and 6 of 13 had no evidence of disease.

Two case series reported patients achieving a CR with a PR that was achieved in three of seven patients. The median duration of CR was 1 year. Fujisawa et al. [132] reported on two patients achieving a CR after one or two cycles of cisplatin and 5-FU. This therapy seemed to be effective in terms of local control, but was ineffective in preventing metastases.

Guthrie et al. [133] treated three SCC patients with cisplatin and doxorubicin. One patient had a CR for 17 months, one had a PR for 3 months, and one had stable disease (SD). The authors suggested that the combination of cisplatin and doxorubicin had activity in cSCC. A phase II trial by the same group used this regimen in 12 cSCC patients [134]. Interpretation of that trial's results was hampered by the low numbers of enrolled patients and their heterogeneity. Seven patients were treated with chemotherapy alone: two achieved a CR for 4–12 months, two achieved a PR for 3–6 months, and three had no response. Five patients received neoadjuvant chemotherapy followed by surgery or definitive radiation therapy, with two CRs and one PR after induction chemotherapy. The authors concluded that this combination had activity in advanced cutaneous SCC patients and that multimodality therapy was to be preferred over chemotherapy alone.

Wollina et al. [135] used oral capecitabine and s.c. IFN-α in four patients with advanced cutaneous SCC. They reported two patients with CRs and two patients with PRs using this regimen.

Oral 5-FU was administered to 14 patients with advanced cSCC as a single agent [136]. Two patients experienced a PR and seven had SD of varying duration. This report, however, supports the use of fluoropyrimidine-based therapy in advanced cSCC patients, because there may be palliative benefit even with the use of single-agent therapy.

Retinoids and IFN-α in Cutaneous SCC

Retinoids modulate cell differentiation and proliferation; in vitro, some cytokines can act synergistically with retinoids to inhibit cell proliferation and increase apoptosis. Shin et al. [137] assessed the effects of IFN-α, 13cis retinoic acid (13cRA), and cisplatin used to treat unresectable SCC of the skin in a prospective phase II trial. Six of 35 (17 %) patients experienced a CR and 6 of 35 (17 %) had a PR. The response rate of patients with locoregional disease was higher (67 %) than that of patients with metastatic disease (17 %; $P=.007$). They concluded that this combination was useful in treating locally advanced disease, but less so in metastatic disease.

Lippman et al. used 13cRA in combination with IFN-α in a prospective phase II trial enrolling 32 patients with inoperable cSCC. They observed a response in 19 (68 %) of the 28 evaluable patients (7 CRs, 12 PRs). The median duration of response was 5 months. Response rates varied with the extent of disease: 93 % (13 of 14) responded among patients with advanced local disease, 67 % (4 of 6) responded among patients with regional disease, and 25 % (2 of 8) responded among those with distant metastases. This combination appeared to be effective in advanced SCC patients, albeit with greater efficacy in less advanced disease.

Although not focused on treatment of unresectable disease, Brewster and coworkers reported on a phase III trial testing whether adjuvant therapy with 13cRA and IFN-α was effective in preventing recurrences and increasing time to recurrence. Their adjuvant study enrolled 66 patients with "aggressive" SCC. The 66 patients were randomly assigned, following initial surgery, to receive either a combination of 13cRA and IFN-α for 6 months or no systemic adjuvant therapy. Adjuvant radiotherapy was added to the initial treatment plan for tumors with perineural invasion, more than two positive nodes, extracapsular nodal disease, or microscopically positive margins. With a median follow-up of 21.5 months, this systemic treatment did not improve time to recurrence or prevent secondary tumors.

Anti-EGFR Therapy in Cutaneous SCC

Cetuximab, a humanized monoclonal antibody, inhibits EGFR by blocking the extracellular domain of EGFR. This prevents the receptor's ligand from binding and consequent dimerization. One phase II study and two case reports have described its effects in cSCC. In a phase II trial enrolling 36 naïve patients with unresectable or metastatic cutaneous SCC that expressed EGFR [138], 31 patients of 36 enrolled were evaluable for tumor response. The disease control rate (DCR) after 6 weeks of treatment was 69 %, and the overall response rate was 11 %. The mean progression-free survival (PFS) and overall survival (OS) times were 121 days and 246 days, respectively. Among the 31 evaluable patients, development of an acneiform rash did not predict response to treatment, but did predict the mean PFS and OS times. Such drug rashes have been associated with better outcome in other diseases treated with cetuximab, such as SCC of the head and neck.

Randomized trials of cetuximab in metastatic colorectal cancer (mCRC) patients have confirmed the importance of mutational status in the signal transduction apparatus downstream from EGFR, including KRAS and BRAF, and in an immune marker, the Fc antibody receptor [139, 140]. In a subset of 28 patients studied by Maubec and coworkers, mutational status was assessed in exon 2 ($n=28$) and exon 3 ($n=25$) of KRAS and exon 15 ($n=23$) of BRAF kinase. All were found to be wild type. Cutaneous SCC patients possessing the FcγIIa-131 H/H or FcγIIIa-158 V/V variants, associated with better outcome in mCRC patients, had a PFS interval similar to the wild-type 131R and 158 F carriers in the Maubec et al. study [138].

Two case reports of cSCC patients treated with cetuximab have also been published, both achieving CRs [141, 142]. More recently, eight cases of locoregionally advanced or unresectable cSCC treated with either cetuximab alone or cetuximab and radiotherapy and followed up for 23 months were presented. Two patients were treated with cetuximab as single-agent therapy, and four were treated with cetuximab and concomitant radiotherapy. Either cetuximab alone or the combination of cetuximab and radiotherapy can be effective in cSCC, with 6/8 responses, including three CRs and a median OS of 22.5 months. Moreover, the use of cetuximab and radiotherapy according to previously reported modalities seems to be more efficient than single-agent use, with 3 CRs observed in this series. It is noteworthy that most of this study had a very poor prognosis, having received heavy previous surgery and/or radiotherapy for several previous relapses.

Gefitinib inhibits binding to the ATP-binding site of EGFR, rendering it unable to autophosphorylate and activate the receptor. Glisson et al. [143] used gefitinib in a prospective phase II trial, enrolling 18 patients with advanced or recurrent cutaneous SCC. Gefitinib had already been reported to have an 11 % response rate and 53 % control rate in head and neck SCC patients [144]. Four of the 15 evaluable cSCC patients had SD after 4 weeks of treatment.

Erlotinib, much like gefitinib, competitively binds to the ATP-binding site of EGFR. It has been approved for use in non-small cell lung cancer patients who have failed to respond to chemotherapy, and in advanced pancreatic cancer patients, combined with gemcitabine. Read et al. [145] reported results from two patients with unresectable cSCC. One patient achieved a CR after 1 month of treatment and the other achieved a PR after 3 months of treatment. The patient that achieved a CR had a recurrence when the therapy was discontinued.

cSCC Secondary to Raf Kinase Inhibitors

The T→A transversion at position 1799 of BRAF (BRAF V600E) is present in approximately 50 % of patients with metastatic melanoma [146, 147]. Recently, it was also demonstrated that this mutation can be present in about 25 % of the patients affected by hepatocellular carcinoma in which medical treatment with Raf inhibitor have received approval by US and European agencies. BRAF V600E induces constitutive signaling through the MAPK pathway, stimulating cancer cell proliferation and survival [147]. The clinical development of inhibitors of oncogenic BRAF, termed type I BRAF inhibitors, which block the active conformation of the BRAF kinase, has led to a high rate of objective tumor responses and improvement in overall survival, as compared with standard chemotherapy in melanoma [148, 149]. However, nonmelanoma skin cancers – cSCC and keratoacanthomas (KA) – have developed in approximately 15–30 % of patients treated with type I BRAF inhibitors such as vemurafenib and dabrafenib (GSK-2118436) [150, 151].

KA and cSCC most frequently develop within 8–12 weeks of beginning therapy. Similar treatment-related skin neoplasms have been described with the structurally unrelated multikinase inhibitor sorafenib [152, 153]. Sorafenib has been reported to have pan-RAF inhibitory properties [154], although the overall cellular potency of

this compound against RAF proteins is much less pronounced when compared with selective inhibitors [155]. Perhaps not surprisingly, sorafenib-induced skin tumors occur much less frequently and are more delayed in onset [152, 153]. Together, these observations suggest that RAF inhibition may play a direct role in the development of skin tumors.

Recently, four international centers contributed 237 KA or cSCC tumor samples from patients receiving an RAF inhibitor (either vemurafenib or sorafenib; $n = 19$) or immunosuppression therapy ($n = 53$) or tumors that developed spontaneously ($n = 165$). Each sample was profiled for 396 known somatic mutations across 33 cancer-related genes.

Mutations were detected in 16 % of tumors (38 of 237), with five tumors harboring two mutations. Mutations in TP53, CDKN2A, HRAS, KRAS, and PIK3CA were previously described in squamous cell tumors. Mutations in MYC, FGFR3, and VHL were identified for the first time. A higher frequency of activating RAS mutations was found in tumors from patients treated with an RAF inhibitor versus populations treated with a non-RAF inhibitor (21.1 % v 3.2 %; $P = .01$), although overall mutation rates between treatment groups were similar (RAF inhibitor, 21.1 %; immunosuppression, 18.9 %; and spontaneous, 17.6 %; P = not significant). Tumor histology (KA v cSCC), tumor site (head and neck v other), patient age (>70 v <70 years), and sex had no significant impact on mutation rate or type.

In another study, a molecular analysis to identify oncogenic mutations (HRAS, KRAS, NRAS, CDKN2A, and TP53) in the lesions from patients treated with the BRAF inhibitor vemurafenib was performed.

Among 21 tumor samples, 13 had RAS mutations (12 in HRAS). In a validation set of 14 samples, 8 had RAS mutations (4 in HRAS). Thus, 60 % (21 of 35) of the specimens harbored RAS mutations, the most prevalent being the activating HRAS Q61L. Increased proliferation of HRAS Q61L-mutant cell lines exposed to vemurafenib was associated with MAPK-pathway signaling and activation of ERK-mediated transcription. In a mouse model of HRAS Q61L-mediated skin carcinogenesis, the vemurafenib analogue PLX4720 was not an initiator or a promoter of carcinogenesis but accelerated growth of the lesions harboring HRAS mutations, and this growth was blocked by concomitant treatment with a MEK inhibitor.

The paradoxical hyperactivation of MAPK by RAF inhibitors predicts that upstream oncogenic events, either activating mutations in RAS or mutations or amplifications in receptor tyrosine kinases that strongly elevate levels of the RAS–GTP complex in the absence of a BRAF V600E mutation, would potentiate signaling through the MAPK pathway [156, 157]. Some preclinical experimental models have demonstrated that signaling occurred preferentially through CRAF, with RAF inhibitors thought to induce a conformational change in CRAF/BRAF heterodimers or BRAF homodimers that resulted in pathway hyperactivity [158, 159]. The functional studies of the previous report showing HRAS-primed activation of the MAPK pathway in models of SCC treated with BRAF inhibitors provide evidence that the toxicity related to BRAF inhibition may arise from paradoxical MAPK-pathway activation in humans. Recent studies have shown that vemurafenib resistance can be mediated by receptor tyrosine kinases such as the platelet-derived growth factor and insulin-like growth factor 1 receptors [160, 161]. Preexisting amplification of the EGFR gene in the A431 cell-line model also resulted in paradoxical MAPK-pathway signaling in functional assays, although at a lower level than that driven by oncogenic HRAS. These data from in vitro models suggest that similar mutations or amplifications of receptor tyrosine kinases may account for the development of cSCC and KA in the 40 % of samples in which no RAS mutations were found.

The timing of the appearance of these lesions after vemurafenib treatment is decidedly different from that of secondary cancers associated with cytotoxic chemotherapy. In the case of vemurafenib, the lesions tend to appear within the first few weeks after the start of therapy,

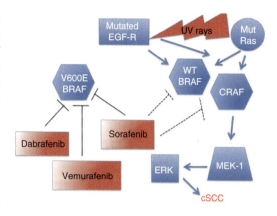

Fig. 3.8 Mechanism of induction of cSCC by raf inhibitors. (*Right part*) UV rays due to solar exposure can induce mutations in ras or EGFR (or other tyrosine kinase receptors) that, in turn, can induce a hyperactivation of MEK and ERK signaling in skin cells. (*Left part*) Specific inhibitors of V600E BRAF (i.e., vemurafenib and dabrafenib) or sorafenib (that at a lesser extent inhibits also CRAF and WT BRAF) induces a hyperactivation of MEK and ERK signaling in ras- or EGFR-mutated cells accelerating the transformation process. This could be due to the formation of functional heterodimers between BRAF and CRAF leading to the activation of the downstream signaling

whereas cancers that are due to the genotoxic effects of chemotherapy develop years after exposure. The specificity of vemurafenib for a limited number of kinases [162, 163], along with the finding that RAS mutations occur frequently in lesions arising preferentially in sun-damaged skin, suggests that vemurafenib may not have direct carcinogenic effects but instead may potentiate preexisting initiating oncogenic events.

In the skin carcinogenesis model, the BRAF inhibitor PLX4720 drove paradoxical activation of the MAPK pathway and proliferation of HRAS Q61L-transformed keratinocytes, with decreased latency and accelerated growth of cSCC and KA. PLX4720 was not itself a true tumor promoter because it could not substitute for TPA. Instead, PLX4720 accelerated the growth of preexisting RAS-mutant lesions. The use of more specific inhibitors or the concomitant inhibition of MEK could be useful strategies in order to counteract this detrimental side effect of Raf inhibitors (for a summary, see Fig. 3.8).

Molecular Strategies for the Sensitization of SCC to Antiproliferative Effects of Anticancer Agents

As described above, type I IFNs and above all IFN-α have been widely used in the therapy of cSCC; however, contrasting data are available about the clinical effectiveness of IFN-α monotherapy in this tumor. In fact, the benefit of IFN-α treatment is limited, and the clinical practice is far from taking in consideration IFN-a as a standard therapy of cSCC. The poor activity of this cytokine in SCC is based upon the presence of multiple mechanisms of tumor resistance that have been widely studied in the recent time.

In detail, alteration of JAK/STAT components of the IFN-α-induced signaling has been indicated as potential resistance mechanism for IFN-α antiproliferative effects. The activated JAK-1 can stimulate STAT-3 that acts as adapter to couple the phosphoinositol-3 kinase (PI3K)-dependent pathway [164]. The p85 regulatory subunit of PI3K, which activates a series of serine kinases, binds to phosphorylated STAT3 and subsequently undergoes tyrosine phosphorylation. Consequently, PI3K is activated and can transduce its signals through Akt activation. Akt apparently promotes cell survival by phosphorylating multiple targets, including the Bcl-2 family member BAD, the apoptosis-inducing enzyme caspase-9, and the Forkhead transcription factor (FKHRL)1 that regulates Fas ligand gene expression. Therefore, IFN-α-induced phosphorylation of STAT-3 can prevent apoptosis and counteracts the antitumor activity promoted by STAT-1 and STAT-2 activation [165]. Another target of the IFN-α-induced Akt activation is NF-kB, which mediates antiapoptotic signals [166]. IFN induces NF-kB activation through a "canonical" and a "noncanonical" pathway. The first pathway is mediated by the IFN-α induction of the ubiquitin cross-reactive protein (ISG 15) and of two ubiquitin-conjugating enzymes (UbcH5 and UbcH8). A molecular target of these enzymes is the inhibitor of kB (IkB) protein, a cytoplasmic protein that binds and inactivates NF-kB. Therefore, IkB degradation activates NF-kB that triggers the transcription of genes involved in the antiapoptotic process. In parallel there is another survival pathway, activated by type I IFNs, called "noncanonical," which involves the linkage of TNF receptor-associated factors (TRAFs) and NF-kB-inducing kinase (NIK) [167, 168].

An additional survival mechanism induced by type I IFNs is the activation of specific protein tyrosine phosphatases (PTP) that dephosphorylate and inactivate STATs and IFN-receptor-associated kinases [169]. In particular, two mammalian SH2-containing cytoplasmic PTPs, Shp-1 and Shp-2, have been implicated in the regulation of IFN signaling. After IFN-α binding, Shp1 is associated to the IFN-α receptor, complexed to Jak1 and Tyk2. In this complex, it exerts a negative feedback by inhibiting the IFN-α-stimulated Jak/STAT pathway. Moreover, Shp2 has a positive effect on the mitogenic stimulation of Erk-1/2 and on the expression of platelet-derived growth factor receptor and, on the other hand, inhibits JNK under cellular stress [168, 169]. Other Jak/STAT pathway inhibitors have been identified, such as the suppressors of cytokine signaling (SOCS) [170]. These proteins contain an SH2-domain and can inhibit Jak, thus playing a negative control on the Jak/STAT signaling. IFN-α can specifically induce SOCS1 and 3 that are candidates for the specific inhibition and turning off the IFN-α-dependent signaling [168, 170].

An interesting and well-studied survival pathway activated in SCCs after IFN-α treatment includes the epidermal growth factor receptor (EGFR) and its downstream targets. Our group has shown that IFN-α, at growth inhibitory concentrations, enhances the expression and signaling activity of EGFR in epidermoid cancer cell lines [171, 172]. Therefore, the enhanced expression and function of EGFR in tumor cells could represent a stress response that is activated to provide an escape mechanism to the growth inhibition induced by IFN-α [171, 173]. In fact, EGF causes a protective response in tumor cells against IFN-α-induced apoptosis that occurs through the triggering of a stress kinase pathway [174]. It is well known that EGF acts through the binding to its specific receptor, EGFR, a transmembrane protein with a cytoplasmic tyrosine kinase domain [175]. The phosphorylation of its intracytoplasmic tail allows the interaction of

EGFR with cytoplasmic factors that can induce Ras activation only when Ras is isoprenylated and, therefore, linked to the inner side of the cell membrane. In fact, the latter event allows its interaction for co-localization with EGFR-associated nucleotide exchange factors that favor GTP:GDP exchange and the subsequent Ras activation. The stimulation of Ras induces the activation of the Ras/Raf/mitogen-activated protein kinase (MAPK) cascade, a main antiapoptotic pathway counteracting the IFN-α-mediated apoptosis [172, 176, 177]. Another important antiapoptotic pathway regulated by EGF and Ras is the signaling via Akt/PKB, an important survival pathway as previously reported [178, 179].

In addition, we recently showed that in H1355 lung SCC, IFN-α increases the expression of the eukaryotic translation elongation factor 1A (eEF-1A) through decrease of its ubiquitination and its possible rescue from proteasome-dependent degradation. This effect seems to be mediated by the phosphorylation of serine and threonine residues in eEF-1A, lacking the site responsible for polyubiquitination. The phosphorylation of eEF-1A could be mediated by C-Raf that is presumably activated by the upregulation of EGFR IFN-α mediated. eEF-1A catalyzes the first step of the protein synthesis elongation cycle and is involved in several cellular processes. In H1355, eEF-1A is an antiapoptotic factor. In fact, the reduction of eEF-1A expression by RNA interference enhances the apoptotic cell death induced by IFN-α in H1355. Therefore, the overexpression of eEF-1A is a further survival pathway activated by type I IFNs [180].

We recently demonstrated [181] that in human SCC KB the adenylate cyclase/cAMP axis could be part of a complex survival response to the apoptosis and growth inhibition activated by IFN-α. Incubation of KB cells with IFN-α (1.000 IU/ml) caused both a reduced activity of adenylate cyclase enzyme and a parallel decrease of intracellular cAMP content. In agreement with these observations, we have found a reduction in the activity of PKA, one of the main targets of cAMP, and in the phosphorylation state of transcription factor cAMP-response-element-binding-protein (CREB), one of the main PKA substrates and reported to be involved in the IFN-α-mediated transcriptional events. Interestingly, the concomitant treatment of KB cells with IFN-α and cAMP reconstituting agent (8-Bromo-cAMP) was able to induce both an increase of the apoptosis onset and the restoration of cAMP levels and PKA activity. On the other hand, the concomitant addition to the cells of IFN-α and of the PKA inhibitor KT5720 caused an antagonism on apoptosis occurrence and potentiated the reduction of PKA activity induced by the cytokine alone. In agreement with its known action on both growth and apoptosis control in many cell types, cAMP can, at least in part, mediate the IFN-α-induced apoptosis in KB cells either via PKA-dependent or independent pathways [182]. In support of this hypothesis, there is the evidence that another PKA activator 8-chloro-cyclic adenosine monophosphate inhibits Erk-1/2 activity in the presence of an increased EGFR expression and activity in KB cells [183]. In these experimental conditions, the growth-promoting activity of EGF was completely abolished when EGF treatment was performed in combination with cAMP reconstituting agent [184].

Future Perspectives to Enhance the Antitumor Activity of Type I IFNs

The understanding of the molecular mechanisms regulating the signal transduction pathway mediated by IFN-α and of the escape mechanisms activated in cancer cells could be useful in the design of new therapeutic strategies able to strengthen the antitumor activity of type I IFNs overcoming survival pathways.

PI3K/Akt pathway represents an IFN-induced escape mechanism modulated by the overactivation of STAT-3 and EGFR. The development of novel compounds able to block this pathway and recently studied in clinical trials opens a new scenario in the treatment of cancer with type I IFNs [184].

Another approach combining proteasome inhibitors (i.e., bortezomib) with type I IFNs requires future investigations. In fact, proteasome inhibitors have shown antitumor activity in both solid and hematological malignancies. These compounds block activation of NF-kB, resulting in increased apoptosis, decreased angiogenic cytokine production, and inhibition of tumor cell adhesion to stroma. Additional mechanisms of action include c-Jun N-terminal kinase activation, effects on growth factor expression, and anti-angiogenic properties [185, 186].

As previously described, the overactivation of the EGFR/Ras/Raf/MAPK pathway is a crucial escape mechanism to the growth inhibition and apoptosis induced by IFN-α. It is advisable to use specific inhibitors of this pathway in order to enhance the antitumor activity of type I IFNs. Gefitinib (Iressa) is an orally active, selective EGFR tyrosine kinase inhibitor that blocks the signal transduction pathways involved in the proliferation and survival of cancer cells. We have shown that the combination of IFN-α with the selective EGFR tyrosine kinase inhibitor gefitinib induces cooperative antitumor effect on human neck squamous cell carcinoma-derived cell lines both in vitro and in vivo [187]. Simultaneous exposure to gefitinib and IFN-α produced synergistic antiproliferative and proapoptotic effects compared with single drug treatment. Furthermore, daily treatment of gefitinib (50 mg/kg p.o.) in combination with IFN-α regimen (50,000 units s.c. three times weekly) induced tumor growth delay and increased survival rate on nude mice carrying human neck squamous cell carcinoma cell-line xenografts. Furthermore, gefitinib suppresses the IFN-α-induced phosphorylation/activation of EGFR and ERK1/2 both in vitro and in vivo showing that it may overcome the previously described mechanisms of the IFN-α-induced EGFR-mediated survival escape [187].

A promising way of interfering with Ras function seems to be the inhibition of farnesyltransferase, the enzyme coupling a 15-carbon isoprenyl group to Ras proteins, by farnesyltransferase inhibitors (FTIs). R115777 is a potent and selective nonpeptidomimetic competitive FTI with antitumor activity that catalyzes the farnesylation of a number of proteins, including the small GTP-binding protein Ras. R115777 has displayed the most interesting activity in hematologic neoplasms with a schedule based on oral administration twice a day for 3 consecutive weeks with a week of rest [188]. We have found a cooperative antitumor effect of IFN-α and R115777 combination both in vitro and in vivo on nude mice xenografted with

KB cells, through the enhancement of apoptosis and antagonism on the IFN-α-induced hyperactivation of Ras and its terminal enzyme Erk [189]. In detail, we have demonstrated that IFN-α increases Raf-1/Bcl-2 interactions. Raf-1, the immediate downstream target of Ras, has been reported to activate bcl-2 through interaction and subsequent phosphorylation on serine-70 of bcl-2 and displacement of bcl-2 from bad. This induces the antiapoptotic activity of bcl-2. All these effects were antagonized by the concomitant treatment of KB cells with R115777 and IFN-α. In fact, the synergistic growth inhibitory and proapoptotic effects produced by the IFN-α/FTI combination involve the inhibition of both Erk and Akt survival pathways acting in these cells in a Ras-dependent fashion [189]. Considering that the overactivation of STAT-3 is another IFN-α-induced escape mechanism, the inhibitory activity of R11577 on STAT-3 phosphorylation and DNA binding could additionally explain the synergistic antitumor activity of FTI and type I IFNs.

Another compound able to block the EGFR downstream pathway is sorafenib, a Raf kinase inhibitor. When the C-Raf kinase activity was blocked by sorafenib, a strong increase of IFN-α-induced apoptosis has been observed [180]. In addition, sorafenib was completely able to block the decrease in ubiquitination of eEF-1A. As previously described, eEF-1A is an antiapoptotic factor whose activity links the protein synthesis machinery to growth factor-elicited survival pathway and represents an important molecular target to improve strategies based on apoptosis induction [180].

We described interesting effects with the use of MAPK inhibitors. PD098059, a specific MEK1 inhibitor, enhanced apoptosis caused by IFN-α [172]. An additional important finding is that PD098059 specifically abrogated the recovery from apoptosis induced by EGF in IFN-α-treated cells [172]. Unfortunately, PD98059 has not been shown to be sufficiently soluble nor sufficiently bioavailable to be conducive to clinical testing. Due to this limitation, PD98059 only has activity in vitro. However, several new MEK inhibitors (PD184352, PD 0325901, and AZD6244) have been examined in early-phase clinical trials with satisfying preliminary results in terms of safety and clinical response (for a summary, see Fig. 3.9) [190].

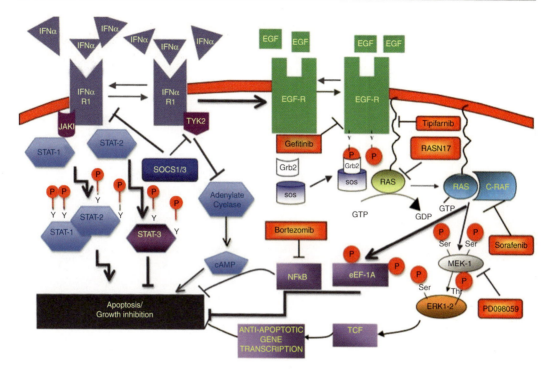

Fig. 3.9 Survival pathways activated by type I interferons. In this figure, both the type I IFN signaling pathway (*on the left*) and the principal tumor resistance mechanisms induced by IFN-α are resumed. After the binding of the receptors with IFN-α, the activated JAK-1 phosphorylates in tyrosine residues STAT-1 and STAT-2 that subsequently form homo/heterodimers that translocate to the nucleus inducing the expression of genes that inhibit proliferation and trigger apoptosis. On the other hand, JAK-1 can also stimulate STAT-3 that acts as adapter to couple the p85 regulatory subunit of PI3K. Consequently, PI3K is activated and can transduce its signals through Akt activation that finally inhibit apoptosis and generate a survival signal. Another survival pathway elicited by IFN-α is NF-κB that also mediates antiapoptotic signals and the proteasome inhibitor bortezomib can potentiate the apoptosis induced by IFN-α. It has been demonstrated that IFN-α activates in SCC cells a pro-survival EGF-dependent pathway through both EGFR overexpression and hyperactivation. EGF binds its specific receptor, EGFR, a transmembrane protein with a cytoplasmic tyrosine kinase domain. The phosphorylation of its intracytoplasmic tail allows the interaction of EGFR with cytoplasmic factors that favor GTP:GDP exchange and the subsequent Ras activation only when Ras is linked to the inner side of the cell membrane and, therefore, isoprenylated (see the *black tail*). The stimulation of Ras induces the activation of the MAPK cascade, a main antiapoptotic pathway counteracting the IFN-α-mediated apoptosis. The use of an EGFR-associated tyrosine kinase inhibitor gefitinib or of a farnesyltransferase inhibitor tipifarnib or of a plasmid encoding for dominant negative Ras RASN17 or of a MEK-1 inhibitor PD098059 can inhibit the EGFR→ras pathway potentiating IFN-α-induced apoptosis. Other two recent escape mechanisms involve the eukaryotic elongation factor-1A and the adenylate cyclase/cAMP axis. eEF-1A catalyzes the first step of the protein synthesis elongation cycle and is involved in several cellular processes through decrease of its ubiquitination and its possible rescue from proteasome-dependent degradation. The phosphorylation of eEF-1A could be mediated by C-Raf that is presumably activated by the upregulation of EGFR IFN-α mediated. This phosphorylation stabilizes eEF-1A expression and increases its levels mediating an antiapoptotic effect. The use of a specific inhibitor of raf kinase activity sorafenib inhibits these effects and potentiates IFN-α-induced apoptosis. The adenylate cyclase/cAMP axis could be part of a complex survival response to the apoptosis and growth inhibition activated by IFN-α. IFN-α caused both a reduced activity of adenylate cyclase enzyme and a parallel decrease of intracellular cAMP content and of its targets PKA. The end result is the reduction in the phosphorylation state of transcription factor CREB, one of the main PKA substrates. The reconstitution of intracellular cAMP potentiates the apoptosis induced by IFN-α. Another Jak/STAT pathway inhibitor is SOCS that contains an SH2-domain and can inhibit Jak, thus playing a negative control role on the Jak/STAT signaling. *EGFR* epidermal growth factor receptor, *MAPK* Ras/Raf/mitogen-activated protein kinase, *eEF-1A* eukaryotic translation elongation factor 1A, *CREB* cAMP-response-element-binding-protein, *PTP* protein tyrosine phosphatases, *SOCS* suppressors of cytokine signaling, *Ser* serine, *Thr* threonine, *Y* tyrosine, → stimulating activity, –| inhibiting activity

Table 3.2 Classification of cutaneous SCC into risk-based categories

Low malignant potential	Intermediate malignant potential	High malignant potential	Indeterminate malignant potential
SCC arising in AK	Acantholytic (adenoid) SCC	Invasive Bowen's disease	Clear-cell SCC
Verrucous and HPV-related SCC	Lymphoepithelioma-like carcinoma (LELCS)	Adenosquamous carcinoma	Signet ring cell SCC
Spindle cell SCC unassociated to UV radiation	Jadassohn tumor with invasion	Malignant proliferating pilar tumor (SCC arising in PPT)	Papillary SCC
Tricholemmal carcinoma		Desmoplastic SCC	Pigmented SCC
		De novo SCC	Follicular SCC
		SCC arising in chronic conditions	SCC arising from adnexal cysts
		Radiation-induced SCC	Squamoid eccrine ductal carcinoma

AK actinic keratosis, *PPT* proliferating pilar tumor, *SCC* squamous cell carcinoma

Prognosis

cSCC are generally characterized by a favorable outcome. However, cSCC histopathological variants share different etiopathogenetic, biological, and clinical features, some of them related to poor prognosis (Table 3.2). The correct recognition of histopathological variant could help to correct prognostic stratification of patients. Besides histological categories, other histological and clinical factors have been demonstrated as particularly useful to predict clinical outcome. Since most cSCC derives from a superficial precursor lesion, its behavior is generally indolent. As previously established, cSCC with single cell infiltrates, with exclusive dermal activity, and de novo cSCC, represent the categories with significant poor prognosis. Among histological factors, (1) tumor size (2) depth of invasion, (3) degree of differentiation, (4) anatomical location, and (5) perineural and (6) perivascular invasion are the most characterized factors that limit the prognosis of these tumors [16]. In particular tumor size and depth of infiltration seems to be the most relevant histological negative prognostic factors. In fact, tumor greater than 2 cm in size are associated to a significant higher risk of metastases and recurrence if compared to cases less than 2 cm [191]. Similarly, a poor outcome has been recorded for tumors exceeding 4 mm in depth or involving both the deeper dermis and the

hypodermis, with a sevenfold increase in the probability of metastases [192, 193]. Moreover, lesions exceeding 8 mm in depth additionally increase the risk of metastases to regional lymph nodes, suggesting prophylactic node dissection as therapeutic strategy [193].

Concerning the degree of histologic differentiation, we have already discussed in this chapter that poorly differentiated tumors particularly from the ear or the lip will be threefold more likely to metastasize if compared to tumors that are well differentiated [16].

Tumors with perineural involvement (PNI), observed in approximately 14 % of all cSCCs show a significant greater risk of local recurrence (23 %) if compared to those without PNI (9 %) [194]. Similarly, invasion of capillary lymphatics is associated to significant incidence of metastases, local recurrence, and disease-related death [194].

The most important clinical features related to the development, recurrence, and metastases seem to be the host immunosuppression, such as the active use of immunosuppressive agents during transplant therapy or infection by HIV [195–198]. All these factors can greatly increase the likelihood of cSCC development, recurrence, and malignant spread. Suppression may be also due to an underlying malignancy. In fact, long-term immunosuppressant use in transplant recipients increases significantly the manifestation of cSCC if compared to general population. Although the risk of metastases of the single lesions of these patients does not seem higher if compared to cSCC of general population, the elevated number of primary lesions has the effect to increase the overall risk of metastases [197, 198]. Finally, the inappropriate treatment, with methodologies different from surgical excision, such as cryotherapy, curettage, electrodesiccation, and radiation, could significantly reduce the curability rate of cSCC, increasing the risk of local recurrences and metastasis [16].

Glossary

13cRA 13-cis-retinoic acid
5-FU 5-fluorouracil
AK Actinic keratosis
AKs Actinic or solar keratoses
BER Base excision repair
CDK Cyclin-dependent kinase
CNS Central nervous system
CR Complete response
CREB cAMP-response-element-binding-protein
cSCC Cutaneous squamous cancer
DCR Disease control rate
D-loop Displacement loop
eEF-1A Eukaryotic translation elongation factor 1A
EGFR Epidermal growth factor receptor
HDM2 Human double-minute protein 2
HER Human epidermal receptor
HPV Human papillomaviruses
IFN-α Interferon alpha
IL1 Interleukin-1
KA Keratoacanthomas
LELCS Lymphoepithelioma-like carcinoma of the skin
LV Lymphatic vascular
LVMD LV microvascular density
MAP Mitogen-activated protein
mCRC Metastatic colorectal cancer
MiRNAs microRNAs
MTAs Molecularly target-based agents
NER Non-excision repair
NMSC Nonmelanoma skin cancer
OS Overall survival
PFS Progression-free survival
PNI Perineural involvement
PR Partial response
PTP Protein tyrosine phosphatases
PUMA p53-upregulated modulator of apoptosis
ROS Reactive specific oxygen species
SOCS Suppressors of cytokine signaling
TA Transient amplifying
TNF Tumor necrosis factor
UV Ultraviolet
VC Verrucous carcinoma

References

1. Bernstein SC, Lim KK, Brodland DG, Heidelberg KA. The many faces of squamous cell carcinoma. Dermatol Surg. 1996;22:243–54.
2. Gray DT, Suman VJ, Daniel Su WP, Clay RP, Harmsen WS, Roenigk RK. Trends in the population based incidence of squamous cell carcinoma of the skin first diagnosed between 1984 and 1992. Arch Dermatol. 1997;133:735–40.
3. Lohmann CM, Solomon AR. Clinicopathologic variants of cutaneous squamous cell carcinoma. Adv Anat Pathol. 2001;8:27–36.
4. Cassarino DS, Linden KG, Barr RJ. Cutaneous keratocyst arising independently of the nevoid basal cell carcinoma syndrome. Am J Dermatopathol. 2005;27:177–8.
5. Cassarino DS, De Rienzo DP, Barr RJ. Cutaneous squamous cell carcinoma: a comprehensive clinicopathologic classification—part two. J Cutan Pathol. 2006;33:261–79.
6. Cassarino DS, De Rienzo DP, Barr RJ. Cutaneous squamous cell carcinoma: a comprehensive clinicopathologic classification—part one. J Cutan Pathol. 2006;33:191–206.
7. Housman TS, Feldman SR, Williford PM, et al. Skin cancer is among the most costly of all cancers to treat for the Medicare population. J Am Acad Dermatol. 2003;48:425–9.
8. De Leeuw J, Van der Beek N, Neugebauer WD, Bjerring P, Neumann HA. Fluorescence detection and diagnosis of non-melanoma skin cancer at an early stage. Lasers Surg Med. 2009;41:96–103.
9. Weinstock MA, Bogaars HA, Ashley M, Litle V, Bilodeau E, Kimmel S. Nonmelanoma skin cancer mortality: a population-based study. Arch Dermatol. 1991;127:1194–7.
10. Weinstock MA. Death from skin cancer among the elderly: epidemiological patterns. Arch Dermatol. 1997;133:1207–9.
11. Gallagher RP, Hill GB, Bajdik CD, et al. Sunlight exposure, pigmentation factors, and risk of nonmelanocytic skin cancer. II. Squamous cell carcinoma. Arch Dermatol. 1995;131:164–9.
12. Gallagher RP, Ma B, McLean DI, et al. Trends in basal cell carcinoma, squamous cell carcinoma, and

melanoma of the skin from 1973 through 1987. J Am Acad Dermatol. 1990;23:413–21.

13. Glass AG, Hoover RN. The emerging epidemic of melanoma and squamous cell skin cancer. JAMA. 1989;262:2097–100.

14. Johnson TM, Rowe DE, Nelson BR, Swanson NA. Squamous cell carcinoma of the skin (excluding lip and oral mucosa). J Am Acad Dermatol. 1992;26:467–84.

15. Alam M, Ratner D. Cutaneous squamous cell carcinoma. N Engl J Med. 2001;344:975–83.

16. Rowe DE, Carroll RJ, Day Jr CL. Prognostic factors for local recurrence, metastasis, and survival rates in squamous cell carcinoma of the skin, ear, and lip: implications for treatment modality selection. J Am Acad Dermatol. 1992;26:976–90.

17. Preston DS, Stern RS. Nonmelanoma cancers of the skin. N Engl J Med. 1992;327:649–1662.

18. Ulrich C, Schmook T, Sachse MM, Sterry W, Stockfleth E. Comparative epidemiology and pathogenic factors for nonmelanoma skin cancer in organ transplant patients. Dermatol Surg. 2004;30:622–7.

19. Edge SE, Byrd DR, Compton CC, et al. Cutaneous squamous cell carcinoma and other cutaneous carcinomas. In: AJCC cancer staging manual, vol. 29. 7th ed. New York: Springer; 2010. p. 301–14.

20. De Villiers EM, Laverone D, McLaren K, Benton EC. Prevailing papillomavirus types in non-melanoma carcinomas of the skin in renal allograft recipients. Int J Cancer. 1997;73:356–61.

21. Cherpelis BS, Marcusen C, Lang PG. Prognostic factors for metastasis in squamous cell carcinoma of the skin. Dermatol Surg. 2002;28:268–73.

22. Barksdale SK, O'Connor N, Barnhill R. Prognostic factors for cutaneous squamous cell and basal cell carcinoma. Determinants of risk of recurrence, metastasis, and development of subsequent skin cancers. Surg Oncol Clin N Am. 1997;6:625–38.

23. Dubina M, Goldenberg G. Viral-associated nonmelanoma skin cancers: a review. Am J Dermatopathol. 2009;31:561–73.

24. Diepgen TL, Mahler V. The epidemiology of skin cancer. Br J Dermatol. 2002;146:1–6.

25. Jackson A. Prevention, early detection and team management of skin cancer in primary care: contribution to the health of the nation objectives. Br J Gen Pract. 1995;45:97–101.

26. Jensen P, Hansen S, Moller B, et al. Skin cancer in kidney and heart transplant recipients and different longterm immunosuppressive therapy regimens. J Am Acad Dermatol. 1999;40:177–86.

27. Penn I. Malignancy. Surg Clin North Am. 1994;74: 1247–57.

28. Moloney FJ, Comber H, O'Lorcain P, O'Kelly P, Conlon PJ, Murphy GM. A population-based study of skin cancer incidence and prevalence in renal transplant recipients. Br J Dermatol. 2006;154:498–504.

29. Harwood CA, Surentheran T, McGregor JM, et al. Human papilloma-virus infection and non-melanoma skin cancer in immunosuppressed and immunocompetent individuals. J Med Virol. 2000;61:289–97.

30. Miller D, Weinstock MA. Nonmelanoma skin cancer in the United States: incidence. J Am Acad Dermatol. 1994;30:774–8.

31. Setlow RB, Carrier WL. Pyrimidine dimers in ultraviolet irradiated DNA's. J Mol Biol. 1966;17:237–54.

32. Mitchell DL. The relative cytotoxicity of (6-4) photoproducts and cyclobutane dimers in mammalian cells. Photochem Photobiol. 1988;48:51–7.

33. Mitchell DL, Nairn RS. The biology of the 6-4 photoproduct. Photochem Photobiol. 1989;49:805–19.

34. Brash DE. UV mutagenic photoproducts in Escherichia coli and human cells: a molecular genetics perspective on human skin cancer. Photochem Photobiol. 1988;49:59–66.

35. Brash DE, Rudolph JA, Simon JA, et al. A role for sunlight in skin cancer: UV-induced p53 mutations in squamous cell carcinoma. Proc Natl Acad Sci USA. 1991;88:10124–8.

36. Tchou J, Kasai H, Shibutoni S, Chung M-H. Laval, Grollman AP, 8-Oxoguanine (8-hydroxyguanine) DNA glycosylase and its substrate specificity. Proc Natl Acad Sci USA. 1991;88:4690–4.

37. Boiteux S, Gajewski E, Laval J, Dizdaroglu M. Substrate specificity of the Escherichia coli Fpg protein (formamidopyrimidine–DNA glycosylase): excision of purine lesions in DNA produced by ionizing radiation or photosensitization. Biochemistry. 1992; 31:106–10.

38. Harris CC. Structure and function of the p53 tumor suppressor gene: clues for rational cancer therapeutic strategies. J Natl Cancer Inst. 1996;88:1442–55.

39. Kuerbitz SJ, Plunkett BS, Walsh WV, Kastan MB. Wildtype p53 is a cell cycle checkpoint determinant following irradiation. Proc Natl Acad Sci USA. 1992;89:7491–5.

40. Zahn Q, Carrier F, Fornace Jr AJ. Induction of cellular p53 activity by DNA-damaging agents and growth arrest. Mol Cell Biol. 1993;13:4242–50.

41. Yonish-Roauch E, Reznitzky D, Lotem J, Sachs L, Kimchi A, Oren M. Wild type p53 induces apoptosis of myeloid leukaemic cells that is inhibited by IL-6. Nature. 1991;352:345–7.

42. Nelson WG, Kastan MB. DNA strand breaks: the DNA template alterations that trigger p53-dependent DNA damage response. Mol Cell Biol. 1994;14:1815–23.

43. Bannin S, Moyal L, Shieh SY, et al. Enhanced phosphorylation of p53 by ATM in response to DNA damage. Science. 1998;281:1674–9.

44. Tibbetts SR, Brumbaugh KM, Williams JM, et al. A role for ATR in the DNA damage-induced phosphorylation of p53. Genes Dev. 1999;13:152–7.

45. Milne DM, Campbell LE, Campbell DG, et al. p53 is phosphorylated in vitro and in vivo by an ultraviolet radiation induced protein kinase characteristic of the c-Jun kinase, JNK1. J Biol Chem. 1995;270:5511–8.

46. She QB, Chen N, Dong Z. ERKs and p38 kinase phosphorylate p53 protein at serine 15 in response to UV radiation. J Biol Chem. 2000;275:20444–9.

47. Hwang BJ, Ford JM, Hanawalt PC, et al. Expression of the p48 xeroderma pigmentosum gene is p53-dependent

and is involved in global genomic repair. Proc Natl Acad Sci USA. 1999;96:424–8.

48. Amundson SA, Patterson A, Do KT, et al. A nucleotide excision repair master-switch: p53 regulated coordinate induction of global genomic repair genes. Cancer Biol Ther. 2002;1:145–9.

49. Carrier F, Georgel PT, Pourquier P, et al. Gadd45, a p53-responsive stress protein, modifies DNA accessibility on damaged chromatin. Mol Cell Biol. 1999;19:1673–85.

50. Aragane Y, Kulms D, Metze D, et al. Ultraviolet light induces apoptosis via direct activation of CD95 (Fas/APO-1) independently of its ligand CD95L. J Cell Biol. 1998;140:71–182.

51. Miyashita T, Reed JC. Tumor suppressor p53 is a direct transcriptional activator of the human bax gene. Cell. 1995;80:293–9.

52. Nakano K, Vousden KH. PUMA, a novel proapoptotic gene, is induced by p53, MOL. Cells. 2001;7:683–94.

53. Oda K, Arakawa H, Tanaka T, et al. p53AIP1, a potential mediator of p53-dependent apoptosis, and its regulationby Ser-46-phosphorylated p53. Cell. 2000;102:849–62.

54. Hill LL, Ouhtit A, Loughlin SM, et al. Fas ligand: a sensor for DNA damage critical in skin cancer etiology. Science. 1999;285:898–900.

55. Jost M, Kari C, Rodeck U. The EGF-receptor—an essential regulator of multiple epidermal functions. Eur J Dermatol. 2000;10:505–10.

56. Rosette C, Karin M. Ultraviolet light and osmotic stress: activation of the JNK cascade through multiple growth factor and cytokine receptors. Science. 1996;274:1194–7.

57. Nelson MA, Einspahr JG, Alberts DS, Balfour CA, Wymer JA, Welch KL, et al. Analysis of p53 gene in human precancerous actinic keratosis lesions and squamous cell cancers. Cancer Lett. 1994;85:23–9.

58. Campbell C, Quinn AG, Ro YS, Agus B, Rees JL. p53 mutations are common and early events that precede tumor invasion in squamous cell neoplasia of the skin. J Invest Dermatol. 1993;100:746–8.

59. Ziegler A, Jonason AS, Leffell DJ, et al. Sunburn and p53 in the onset of skin cancer. Nature. 1994;372:773–6.

60. Nakazawa H, English D, Randell PL, Nakazawa K, Martel N, Armstrong BK, et al. UV and skin cancer: specific p53 gene mutation in normal skin as a biologically relevant exposure measurement. Proc Natl Acad Sci USA. 1994;91:360–4.

61. Ren ZP, Hendrum A, Potten F, Nister M, Ahmadian A, Lundeberg J, et al. Human epidermal cancer and accompanying precursors have identical p53 mutations different from p53 mutations in adjacent areas of clonally expanded non-neoplastic keratinocytes. Oncogene. 1996;12:765–73.

62. Jonason AS, Kunala S, Price GJ, Restifo RJ, Spinelli HM, Persing JA, et al. Frequent clones of p53-mutated keratinocytes in normal human skin. Proc Natl Acad Sci USA. 1996;93:14025–9.

63. Ananthaswamy HN, Loughlin SM, Cox P, et al. Sunlight and skin cancer: inhibition of p53 mutations in UV-irradiated mouse skin by sunscreens. Nat Med. 1997;3:510–4.

64. Berg RJW, Van Kranen HJ, Rebel HG, et al. Early p53 alterations in mouse skin carcinogenesis by UVB radiation: Immunohistochemical detection of mutant p53 protein in clusters of preneoplastic epidermal cells. Proc Natl Acad Sci USA. 1996;93:274–8.

65. Ouhtit A, Gorny A, Muller HK, Hill LL, Owen-Schaub LB, Ananthaswamy HN. Loss of Fas-ligand expression in mouse keratinocytes during UV carcinogenesis. Am J Pathol. 2000;157:1975–81.

66. Zhang W, Remenyik E, Zelterman D, et al. Escaping the stem cell compartment: sustained UVB exposure allows p53- mutant keratinocytes to colonize adjacent epidermal proliferating units without incurring additional mutations. Proc Natl Acad Sci USA. 2001;98:13948–53.

67. Mudgil AV, Segal N, Andriani F, et al. Ultraviolet B irradiation induces expansion of intraepithelial tumor cells in a tissue model of early cancer progression. J Invest Dermatol. 2003;121:191–7.

68. Remenyik E, Wikonkal NM, Zhang W. Antigen-specific immunity does not mediate acute regression of UVB-induced p53-mutant clones. Oncogene. 2003;22:6369–76.

69. De Gruijl FR, Van der Leun JC. Development of skin tumors in hairless mice after discontinuation of ultraviolet irradiation. Cancer Res. 1991;51:979–84.

70. Candi E, Dinsdale D, Rufini A, Salomoni P, Knight RA, Mueller M, et al. TAp63 and DeltaNp63 in cancer and epidermal development. Cell Cycle. 2007;6:274–85.

71. Bachmann SA, Buechner M, Wernli S, Strebel P. Erb Ultraviolet light downregulates CD95 ligand and TRAIL receptor expression facilitating actinic keratosis and squamous cell carcinoma formation. J Invest Dermatol. 2001;117:59–66.

72. Raica M, Cimpean AM, Ribatti D. The role of podoplanin in tumor progression and metastasis. Anticancer Res. 2008;28:2997–3006.

73. Barbacid M. Ras genes. Ann Rev Biochem. 1987;56:779–95.

74. Bos JL. Ras oncogenes in human cancer: review. Cancer Res. 1989;49:4682–9.

75. Ananthaswamy HN, Pierceall WE. Molecular mechanisms of ultraviolet radiation carcinogenesis. Photochem Photobiol. 1990;52:1119–36.

76. Ananthaswamy HN, Price JE, Goldberg LH, Bales ES. Detection and identification of activated oncogenes in human skin cancers occurring on sun-exposed body sites. Cancer Res. 1988;48:3341–6.

77. Ananthaswamy HN, Price JE, Goldberg LH, Bales ES. Simultaneous transfer of tumorigenic and metastatic phenotypes by transfection with genomic DNA from a human cutaneous squamous cell carcinoma. J Cell Biochem. 1988;36:137–46.

78. Van der Lubbe JLM, Rosdorff HJM, Bos JL, Van der Eb AJ. Activation of N-ras induced by ultraviolet irradiation in vitro. Oncogene Res. 1988;3:9–20.

79. Pierceall WE, Goldberg LH, Tainsky MA, Mukhopadhyay T, Ananthaswamy HN. *Ras* gene mutation and amplification in human nonmelanoma skin cancers. Mol Carcinog. 1991;4:96–202.

80. Suarez HG, Nardeux PC, Andeol Y, Sarasin A. Multiple activated oncogenes in human tumor's. Oncogene Res. 1987;1:01–207.

81. Serrano M, Hannon GJ, Beach D. A new regulatory motif in cell-cycle control causing specific inhibition of cyclin D/CDK4. Nature. 1993;366:04–707.

82. Pomerantz J, Schreiber-Agus N, Liegeois NJ, Silverman A, Alland L, Chin L, et al. Cell. 1998;92:13–723.

83. Kubo Y, Urano Y, Fukuhara K, Matsumoto K, Arase S. Lack of mutation in the INK4a locus in basal cell carcinomas. Br J Dermatol. 1998;139:40–341.

84. Gibbons RJ. Histone modifying and chromatin remodelling enzymes in cancer and dysplastic syndromes. Hum Mol Genet. 2005;14:R85–92.

85. Bhalla KN. Epigenetic and chromatin modifiers as targeted therapy of hematologic malignancies. J Clin Oncol. 2005;23:3971–93.

86. Esteller M. The necessity of a human epigenome project. Carcinogenesis. 2006;276:1121–5.

87. Venza I, Visalli M, Tripodo B, et al. FOXE1 is a target for aberrant methylation in cutaneous squamous cell carcinoma. Br J Dermatol. 2010;162:1093–7.

88. Yu J, Ryan DG, Getsios S, Oliveira-Fernandes M, Fatima A, Lavker RM. MicroRNA-184 antagonizes microRNA- 205 to maintain SHIP2 levels in epithelia. Proc Natl Acad Sci USA. 2008;105:19300–5.

89. Dziunycz P, Iotzova-Weiss G, Eloranta JJ, et al. Squamous cell carcinoma of the skin shows a distinct microRNA profile modulated by UV radiation. J Invest Dermatol. 2010;130:2686–9.

90. Durham SE, Krishnan KJ, Betts J, Birch-Machin MA. Mitochondrial DNA damage in non-melanoma skin cancer. Br J Cancer. 2003;88:90–5.

91. Prior SL, Griffiths AP, Lewis PD. A study of mitochondrial DNA D-loop mutations and p53 status in nonmelanoma skin cancer. Br J Dermatol. 2009;161: 1067–71.

92. Harbottle A, Birch-Machin MA. Real-time PCR analysis of a 3895 bp mitochondrial DNA deletion in non-melanoma skin cancer and its use as a quantitative marker for sunlight exposure in human skin. Br J Cancer. 2006;94:1887–93.

93. Duensing S. Münger K Mechanisms of genomic instability in human cancer: insights from studies with human papillomavirus oncoproteins. Int J Cancer. 2004;109:157–62.

94. Meyer T, Arndt R, Nindl I, Ulrich C, Christophers E, Stockfleth E. Association of human papillomavirus infections with cutaneous tumors in immunosuppressed patients. Transpl Int. 2003;16:146–53.

95. Pfister H. Human papillomavirus and skin cancer. J Natl Cancer Inst Monogr. 2003;8:52–6.

96. Asgari MM, Kiviat NB, Critchlow CW, et al. Detection of human papillomavirus DNA in cutaneous squamous cell carcinoma among immunocompetent individuals. J Invest Dermatol. 2008;128:1409–17.

97. Forslund O, Ly H, Reid C, Higgins G. A broad spectrum of human papillomavirus types is present in the skin of Australian patients with non-melanoma skin cancers and solar keratosis. Br J Dermatol. 2003;149: 64–73.

98. Caldeira S, Zehbe I, Accardi R, Malanchi I, Dong W, Giarre M, et al. The E6 and E7 proteins of the cutaneous human papillomavirus type 38 display transforming properties. J Virol. 2003;77:2195–206.

99. Meyer T, Arndt R, Christophers E, Nindl I, Stockfleth E. Importance of human papillomaviruses for the development of skin cancer. Cancer Detect Prev. 2001;25:533–47.

100. Syrjänen S. The role of human papillomavirus infection in head and neck cancers, Ann Oncol. 2010;21: vii243–5.

101. Sober AJ, Burstein JM. Precursors to skin cancer. Cancer. 1994;75:645–50.

102. Rossi R, Mori M, Lotti T. Actinic keratosis. Int J Dermatol. 2007;46:895–904.

103. Goldberg LH, Joseph AK, Tschen JA. Proliferative actinic keratosis. Int J Dermatol. 1994;33:341–5.

104. Glogau RG. The risk of progression to invasive disease. J Am Acad Dermatol. 2000;42:S23–4.

105. Cockerell CJ, Wharton JR. New histopathological classification of actinic keratosis (incipient intraepidermal squamous cell carcinoma). J Drugs Dermatol. 2005;4:462–7.

106. Billano RA, Little WP. Hypertrophic actinic keratosis. J Am Acad Dermatol. 1982;7:484–9.

107. Lee MM, Wick MM. Bowen's disease. CA Cancer J Clin. 1990;40:237–42.

108. Saxena A, Kasper DA, Campanelli CD, Lee JB, Humphreys TR, Webster GF. Pigmented Bowen's disease clinically mimicking melanoma of the nail. Dermatol Surg. 2006;32:1522–5.

109. Cox NH, Eedy DJ, Morton CA. Guidelines for management of Bowen's disease: 2006 update. Br J Dermatol. 2007;156:11–21.

110. Kao GF. Carcinoma arising in Bowen's disease. Arch Dermatol. 1986;122:1124–6.

111. Anwar J, Wrone DA, Kimyai-Asadi A, Alam M. The development of actinic keratosis into invasive squamous cell carcinoma: evidence and evolving classification schemes. Clin Dermatol. 2004;22:189–96.

112. Kuo T. Clear cell carcinoma of the skin. A variant of the squamous cell carcinoma that simulates sebaceous carcinoma. Am J Surg Pathol. 1980;4: 73–583.

113. Martin HE, Stewart FW. Spindle-cell epidermoid carcinoma. Am J Cancer. 1935;24:273–98.

114. Silvis NG, Swanson PE, Manivel JC, Kaye VN, Wick MR. Spindle-cell and pleomorphic neoplasms of the skin. A clinicopathologic and immunohistochemical study of 30 cases, with emphasis on 'atypical fibroxanthomas'. Am J Dermatopathol. 1988;10:9–19.

115. Dotto JE, Glusac EJ. p63 is a useful marker for cutaneous spindle cell squamous cell carcinoma. J Cutan Pathol. 2006;33:413–7.

116. Ko CJ, McNiff JM, Glusac EJ. Squamous cell carcinomas with single cell infiltration: a potential diagnostic pitfall and the utility of MNF116 and p63. J Cutan Pathol. 2008;35(4):353–7.

117. Kirsner RS, Spencer J, Falanga V, Garland LE, Kerdel FA. Squamous cell carcinoma arising in osteomyelitis and chronic wounds: treatment with Mohs micrographic surgery vs amputation. Dermatol Surg. 1996;22:1015–8.

118. Sulica VI, Kao GF. Squamous-cell carcinoma of the scalp arising in lesions of discoid lupus erythematosus. Am J Dermatopathol. 1988;10:137–41.

119. Patel GK, Turner RJ, Marks R. Cutaneous lichen planus and squamous cell carcinoma. J Eur Acad Dermatol Venereol. 2003;17:98–100.

120. Weber F, Bauer JW, Sepp N, et al. Squamous cell carcinoma in junctional and dystrophic epidermolysis bullosa. Acta Derm Venereol. 2001;81:189–92.

121. Dupree MT, Boyer JD, Cobb MW. Marjolin's ulcer arising in a burn scar. Cutis. 2000;62:49–51.

122. Sabin SR, Goldstein G, Rosenthal HG, Haynes KK. Aggressive squamotous cell carcinoma originating as a Marjolin's ulcer. Dermatol Surg. 2004;30:229–30.

123. Schwartz RA. Verrucous carcinoma of the skin and mucosa. J Am Acad Dermatol. 1995;32:1–21.

124. Kao GF, Graham JH, Helwig EB. Carcinoma cuniculatum (verrucous carcinoma of the skin). A clinicopathologic study of 46 cases with ultrastructural observations. Cancer. 1982;49:2395–403.

125. Drachenberg CB, Blanchaert R, Ioffe OB, Ord RA, Papadimitriou JC. Comparative study of invasive squamous cell carcinoma and verrucous carcinoma of the oral cavity: expression of bcl-2, p53, and Her-2/neu, and indexes of cell turnover. Cancer Detect Prev. 1997;21:483–9.

126. Swanson SA, Cooper PH, Mills SE, Wick MR. Lymphoepithelioma-like carcinoma of the skin. Mod Pathol. 1988;1:359–65.

127. Okamura JM, Barr RJ. Cutaneous lymphoepithelial neoplasms. Adv Dermatol. 1997;12:277–95.

128. Arsenovic N. Lymphoepithelioma-like carcinoma of the skin: new case of an exceedingly rare primary skin tumor. Dermatol Online J. 2008;14:article 12.

129. Cranmer LD, Engelhardt C, Morgan SS. Treatment of unresectable and metastatic cutaneous squamous cell carcinoma. Oncologist. 2010;15:1320–8.

130. Sadek H, Azli N, Wendling JL, et al. Treatment of advanced squamous cell carcinoma of the skin with cisplatin, 5-fluorouracil, and bleomycin. Cancer. 1990;66:1692–6.

131. Miller AB, Hoogstraten B, Staquet M, et al. Reporting results of cancer treatment. Cancer. 1981; 47:207–14.

132. Fujisawa Y, Umebayashi Y, Ichikawa E, et al. Chemoradiation using low-dose cisplatin and 5-fluorouracil in locally advanced squamous cell carcinoma of the skin: A report of two cases. J Am Acad Dermatol. 2006;55(5 suppl):S81–5.

133. Guthrie Jr TH, McElveen LJ, Porubsky ES, et al. Cisplatin and doxorubicin. An effective chemotherapy combination in the treatment of advanced basal cell and squamous carcinoma of the skin. Cancer. 1985; 55:1629–32.

134. Guthrie Jr TH, Porubsky ES, Luxenberg MN, et al. Cisplatin-based chemo-therapy in advanced basal and squamous carcinomas of the skin: results in 28 patients including 13 patients receiving multimodality therapy. J Clin Oncol. 1990;8:342–6.

135. Wollina U, Hansel G, Koch A, et al. Oral capecitabine plus subcutaneous interferon alpha in advanced squamous cell carcinoma of the skin. J Cancer Res Clin Oncol. 2005;131:300–4.

136. Cartei G, Cartei F, Interlandi G, et al. Oral 5-fluorouracil in squamous cell carcinoma of the skin in the aged. Am J Clin Oncol. 2000;23:181–4.

137. Shin DM, Glisson BS, Khuri FR, et al. Phase II and biologic study of interferon alfa, retinoic acid, and cisplatin in advanced squamous skin cancer. J Clin Oncol. 2002;20:364–70.

138. Maubec E, Petrow P, Duvillard P, et al. Cetuximab as first-line monotherapy in patients with skin unresectable squamous cell carcinoma: final results of a phase II multicenter study [abstract]. J Clin Oncol. 2010;28:8510.

139. Laurent-Puig P, Cayre A, Manceau G, et al. Analysis of PTEN, BRAF, and EGFR status in determining benefit from cetuximab therapy in wild-type KRAS metastatic colon cancer. J Clin Oncol. 2009;27: 5924–30.

140. Bibeau F, Lopez-Crapez E, Di Fiore F, et al. Impact of Fc #RIIa-Fc#RIIIa polymorphisms and KRAS mutations on the clinical outcome of patients with metastatic colorectal cancer treated with cetuximab plus irinotecan. J Clin Oncol. 2009;27:1122–9.

141. Bauman JE, Eaton KD, Martins RG. Treatment of recurrent squamous cell carcinoma of the skin with cetuximab. Arch Dermatol. 2007;143:889–92.

142. Suen JK, Bressler L, Shord SS, et al. Cutaneous squamous cell carcinoma responding serially to single-agent cetuximab. Anticancer Drugs. 2007;18:827–9.

143. Glisson B, Kim S, Kies M, et al. Phase II study of gefitinib in patients with metastatic/recurrent squamous cell carcinoma of the skin. J Clin Oncol. 2006;24(18 suppl):5331.

144. Cohen EE, Rosen F, Stadler WM, et al. Phase II trial of ZD1839 in recurrent or metastatic squamous cell carcinoma of the head and neck. J Clin Oncol. 2003;21:1980–7.

145. Read W. Squamous carcinoma of the skin responding to erlotinib: three cases. J Clin Oncol. 2007; 25(18 suppl):16519.

146. Davies H, Bignell GR, Cox C, et al. Mutations of the BRAF gene in human cancer. Nature. 2002;417: 949–54.

147. Wan PT, Garnett MJ, Roe SM, et al. Mechanism of activation of the RAF-ERK signaling pathway by oncogenic mutations of B-RAF. Cell. 2004;116:855–67.

148. Flaherty KT, Puzanov I, Kim KB, et al. Inhibition of mutated, activated BRAF in metastatic melanoma. N Engl J Med. 2010;363:809–19.

149. Chapman PB, Hauschild A, Robert C, et al. Improved survival with vemurafenib in melanoma with BRAF V600E mutation. N Engl J Med. 2011;364:2507–16.

150. Ribas A, Kim K, Schuchter L, et al. BRIM-2: an open-label, multicenter Phase II study of RG7204 (PLX4032) in previously treated patients with BRAF V600E mutation-positive metastatic melanoma. J Clin Oncol. 2011;29 Suppl:8509 (abstract).

151. Kefford R, Arkenau H, Brown MP, et al. Phase I/II study of GSK2118436, a selective inhibitor of oncogenic mutant BRAF kinase, in patients with metastatic melanoma and other solid tumors. J Clin Oncol. 2010;28 Suppl:611s (abstract).

152. Arnault JP, Wechsler J, Escudier B, et al. Keratoacanthomas and squamous cell carcinomas in patients receiving sorafenib. J Clin Oncol. 2009;27:e59–61.

153. Dubauskas Z, Kunishige J, Prieto VG, et al. Cutaneous squamous cell carcinoma and inflammation of actinic keratoses associated with sorafenib. Clin Genitourin Cancer. 2009;7:20–3.

154. Wilhelm SM, Carter C, Tang L, et al. BAY 43-9006 exhibits broad spectrum oral antitumor activity and targets the RAF/MEK/ERK pathway and receptor tyrosine kinases involved in tumor progression and angiogenesis. Cancer Res. 2004;64:7099–109.

155. Whittaker S, Kirk R, Hayward R, et al. Gatekeeper mutations mediate resistance to BRAF-targeted therapies. Sci Transl Med. 2010;2:35ra41.

156. Poulikakos PI, Zhang C, Bollag G, Shokat KM, Rosen N. RAF inhibitors transactivate RAF dimers and ERK signal -ling in cells with wild-type BRAF. Nature. 2010;464:427–30.

157. Heidorn SJ, Milagre C, Whittaker S, et al. Kinase-dead BRAF and oncogenic RAS cooperate to drive tumor progression through CRAF. Cell. 2010;140:209–21.

158. Hatzivassiliou G, Song K, Yen I, et al. RAF inhibitors prime wild-type RAF to activate the MAPK pathway and enhance growth. Nature. 2010;464:431–5.

159. Halaban R, Zhang W, Bacchiocchi A, et al. PLX4032, a selective BRAF(V600E) kinase inhibitor, activates the ERK pathway and enhances cell migration and proliferation of BRAF melanoma cells. Pigment Cell Melanoma Res. 2010;23:190–200.

160. Nazarian R, Shi H, Wang Q, et al. Melanomas acquire resistance to B-RAF(V600E) inhibition by RTK or N-RAS upregulation. Nature. 2010;468:973–7.

161. Villanueva J, Vultur A, Lee JT, et al. Acquired resistance to BRAF inhibitors mediated by a RAF kinase switch in melanoma can be overcome by cotargeting MEK and IGF-1R/PI3K. Cancer Cell. 2010;18:683–95.

162. Tsai J, Lee JT, Wang W, et al. Discovery of a selective inhibitor of oncogenic B-Raf kinase with potent antimelanoma activity. Proc Natl Acad Sci USA. 2008;105:3041–6.

163. Bollag G, Hirth P, Tsai J, et al. Clinical efficacy of a RAF inhibitor needs broad target blockade in BRAF-mutant melanoma. Nature. 2010;467:596–9.

164. Caraglia M, Marra M, Pelaia G, Maselli R, Caputi M, Marsico SA, et al. Alpha-interferon and its effects on signal transduction pathways. J Cell Physiol. 2005;202:323–35.

165. Caraglia M, Vitale G, Marra M, Budillon A, Tagliaferri P, Abbruzzese A. Alpha-interferon and its effects on signaling pathways within the cells. Curr Protein Pept Sci. 2004;5:475–85.

166. Bromberg J. Signal transducers and activators of transcription as regulators of growth, apoptosis and breast development. Breast Cancer Res. 2000;2:86–90.

167. Yang CH, Murti A, Pfeffer SR, Kim JG, Donner DB, Pfeffer LM. Interferon alpha/beta promotes cell survival by activating nuclear factor kappa B through phosphatidylinositol 3-kinase and Akt. J Biol Chem. 2001;17:13756–61.

168. Tagliaferri P, Caraglia M, Budillon A, Marra M, Vitale G, Viscomi C, et al. New pharmacokinetic and pharmacodynamic tools for interferon-alpha (IFN-α) treatment of human cancer. Cancer Immunol Immunother. 2005;54:1–10.

169. You M, Yu DH, Feng GS. Shp-2 tyrosine phosphatase functions as a negative regulator of the interferon-stimulated Jak/STAT pathway. Mol Cell Biol. 1999;19:2416–24.

170. Song MM, Shuai K. The suppressor of cytokine signaling (SOCS) 1 and SOCS3 but not SOCS2 proteins inhibit interferon-mediated antiviral and antiproliferative activities. J Biol Chem. 1998;273:35056–62.

171. Caraglia M, Pinto A, Correale P, Zagonel V, Genua G, Leardi A, et al. 5-Aza-20-deoxycytidine induces growth inhibition and upregulation of epidermal growth factor receptor on human epithelial cancer cells. Ann Oncol. 1994;5:269–76.

172. Caraglia M, Tagliaferri P, Marra M, Giuberti G, Budillon A, Gennaro ED, et al. EGF activates an inducible survival response via the RAS→Erk-1/2 pathway to counteract interferon-a-mediated apoptosis in epidermoid cancer cells. Cell Death Differ. 2003;10:218–29.

173. Tagliaferri P, Caraglia M, Muraro R, Budillon A, Pinto A, Bianco AR. Pharmacological modulation of peptide growth factor receptor expression on tumour cells as a basis for cancer therapy. Anti-Cancer Drugs. 1994;5:379–93.

174. Caraglia M, Abbruzzese A, Leardi A, Pepe S, Budillon A, Baldassare G, et al. Interferon-alpha induces apoptosis in human KB cells through a stress-dependent mitogen activated protein kinase pathway that is antagonized by epidermal growth factor. Cell Death Differ. 1999;6:773–80.

175. Widmann C, Gibson S, Jarpe MB, Johnson GL. Mitogen-activated protein kinase, conservation of a three-kinase module from yeast to human. Physiol Rev. 1999;79:143–80.

176. Yan CYI, Greene LA. Prevention of PC12 cell death by N-acetylcysteine requires activation of the Ras pathway. J Neurosci. 1998;18:4042–9.

177. Aikawa R, Komuro I, Yamazaki T, Zou Y, Kudoh S, Tanaka M, et al. Oxidative stress activates extracellular signal-regulated kinases through Src and Ras in

cultured cardiac myocytes of neonatal rats. J Clin Invest. 1997;100:1813–21.

178. von Gise A, Lorenz P, Wellbrock C, Hemmings B, Berberich-Siebelt F, Rapp UR, et al. Apoptosis suppression by Raf-1 and MEK1 requires MEK- and phosphatidylinositol 3-kinase-dependent signals. J Mol Cell Biol. 2001;21:2324–36.

179. Zhou H, Li XM, Meinkoth J, Pittman RN. Akt regulates cell survival and apoptosis at a postmitochondrial level. J Cell Biol. 2000;151:483–94.

180. Lamberti A, Longo O, Marra M, Tagliaferri P, Bismuto E, Fiengo A, et al. C-Raf antagonizes apoptosis induced by IFN-a in human lung cancer cells by phosphorylation and increase of the intracellular content of elongation factor 1A. Cell Death Differ. 2007;14:952–62.

181. Naviglio S, Spina A, Marra M, Sorrentino A, Chiosi E, Romano M, et al. Adenylate cyclase/cAMP pathway downmodulation counteracts apoptosis induced by IFN-alpha in human epidermoid cancer cells. J Interferon Cytokine Res. 2007;27:129–36.

182. Boccellino M, Giuberti G, Quagliuolo L, Marra M, D'Alessandro AM, Fujita H, et al. Apoptosis induced by interferon-a and antagonized by EGF is regulated by caspase-3-mediated cleavage of gelsolin in human epidermoid cancer cells. J Cell Physiol. 2004;201:71–83.

183. Budillon A, Di Gennaro E, Caraglia M, Barbarulo D, Abbruzzese A, Tagliaferri P. 8-Cl-cAMP antagonizes mitogen-activated protein kinase activation and cell growth stimulation induced by epidermal growth factor. Br J Cancer. 1999;81:1134–41.

184. Lo Piccolo J, Granville CA, Gills JJ, Dennis PA. Targeting Akt in cancer therapy. Anti-Cancer Drugs. 2007;18:861–74.

185. Milano A, Iaffaioli RV, Caponigro F. The proteasome: a worthwhile target for the treatment of solid tumours? Eur J Cancer. 2007;43:1125–33.

186. Cilloni D, Martinelli G, Messa F, Baccarani M, Saglio G. Nuclear factor kB as a target for new drug development in myeloid malignancies. Haematologica. 2007; 92:1124–229.

187. Bruzzese F, Di Gennaro E, Avallone A, Pepe S, Arra C, Caraglia M, et al. Synergistic antitumor activity of epidermal growth factor receptor tyrosine kinase inhibitor gefitinib and IFN-α in head and neck cancer cells in vitro and in vivo. Clin Cancer Res. 2006;12:617–25.

188. Alvarado Y, Giles FJ. Ras as therapeutic target in hematological malignancies. Expert Opin Emerg Drugs. 2007;12:271–84.

189. Caraglia M, Marra M, Viscomi C, D'Alessandro AM, Budillon A, Meo G, et al. The farnesyltransferase inhibitor R115777 (ZARNESTRA) enhances the pro-apoptotic activity of interferon-a through the inhibition of multiple survival pathways. Int J Cancer. 2007;121:2317–30.

190. Wang D, Boerner SA, Winkler JD, LoRusso PM. Clinical experience of MEK inhibitors in cancer therapy. Biochim Biophys Acta. 2007;1773:1248–55.

191. Breuninger H, Black B, Rassner G. Microstaging of squamous cell carcinomas. Am J Clin Pathol. 1990; 94:624–7.

192. Immerman SC, Scanlon EF, Christ M, Knox KL. Recurrent squamous cell carcinoma of the skin. Cancer. 1983;51:1537–40.

193. Friedman NR, Day CL, Rowe DE. Prognostic factors for local recurrence, metastases, and survival rates in squamous cell carcinoma of the skin, ear, and lip. J Am Acad Dermatol. 1993;28:281–2.

194. Fagan JJ, Collins B, Barnes L, D'Amico F, Myers EN, Johnson JT. Perineural invasion in squamous cell carcinoma of the head and neck. Arch Otolaryngol Head Neck Surg. 1998;124:637–40.

195. Perez-Reyes N, Farhi DC. Squamous cell carcinoma of head and neck in patients with well-differentiated lymphocytic lymphoma. Cancer. 1987;59: 540–4.

196. Ulrich C, Kanitakis J, Stockfleth E, Euvrard S. Skin cancer in organ transplant recipients—where do we stand today? Am J Transplant. 2008;8:2192–8.

197. Ulrich C, Christophers E, Sterry W, Meyer T, Stockfleth E. Skin diseases in organ transplant patients. Hautarzt. 2002;53:524–33.

198. Safai B, Lynfield R, Lowenthal DA, Koziner B. Cancers—associated with HIV infection. Anticancer Res. 1987;7:1055–67.

Molecular Pathology of Melanocytic Skin Cancer

4

Giuseppe Palmieri, Peter Sarantopoulos, Raymond Barnhill, and Alistair Cochran

Key Points

- Melanoma as a result of accumulated alterations in genetic and molecular pathways among melanocytic cells, generating distinct subsets of melanomas with different biological and clinical behavior.
- Improvement of the classification and management of patients with melanoma, using conventional and innovative histopathological approaches.
- Development of therapeutic strategies specifically targeting molecular alterations involved in melanoma pathogenesis.

G. Palmieri, MD (✉)
Department of Cancer Genetics,
Institute of Biomolecular Chemistry,
National Research Council (CNR),
Traversa La Crucca, 3 – Baldinca Li Punti, Sassari, Italy
e-mail: gpalmieri@yahoo.com

P. Sarantopoulos • R. Barnhill
Department of Pathology and Laboratory Medicine,
David Geffen School of Medicine at UCLA,
and Jonsson Comprehensive Cancer Center,
Los Angeles, CA, USA

A. Cochran
Departments of Pathology,
Laboratory Medicine and Surgery,
David Geffen School of Medicine at UCLA,
and Jonsson Comprehensive Cancer Center,
Los Angeles, CA, USA

Molecular Complexity of Melanoma Pathogenesis

Cutaneous melanoma arises from melanocytes, neural crest-derived cells that are located in the basal layer of the epidermis and skin appendages in humans. Melanocytes, by synthesizing melanin pigments and exporting them to adjacent keratinocytes, play a key role in protecting the skin from the damaging effects of ultraviolet (UV) and other solar radiation [1]. Melanocytes can proliferate to form nevi (common moles), initially in the basal epidermis (junctional nevus) and later by limited local dermal infiltration (compound nevus) during embryonic life (congenital nevus) and in children and adults (acquired nevus), partly as a result of solar exposure in the latter two populations. Further progression of melanocytic tumors relates to factors that include intermittent exposure to UV radiation (though a direct relationship between risk of melanoma and UV exposure remains somehow unclear), a history of sunburn, and endogenous factors such as skin type and elevated numbers of nevi (especially the dysplastic or atypical moles) [2, 3].

Melanoma incidence is steadily rising worldwide [4]. In the USA, recent trends indicate that melanoma represents the single most common cancer among adults 25–29 years old. Lifetime risk of developing melanoma in Caucasians is estimated as 1 in 50 individuals [5, 6]. The incidence of melanoma varies according to the geographical origins of the population and the extent of quotidian exposure to the sun. Australia and the USA report a higher incidence of melanoma than the European countries (with the notable exception of Sweden) [7, 8]. There is a gradient of melanoma incidence from north to south in Europe, with highest frequencies in the northern counties. This suggests that initiation and development of melanoma is due to a combination of damaging effects of UV and predisposing genetic background [8].

Melanoma is characterized by a high tendency to metastasize and a striking resistance to therapies other than surgery. From a pathogenetic point of view, melanoma is a complex genetic disease. To date, several crucial cell-signaling pathways that correlate with the evolution of melanoma have been identified [9]. In an effort to simplify this web of functional interactions, classification may be based on the three main signal pathways (MAPK, CDKN2A, and PTEN/AKT), alterations in which can induce cell proliferation and/or overcome cell senescence controls, resulting in a growth advantage for the cells of the transforming melanocytic clone over surrounding cells. Signal transduction effectors (mainly, MITF and NF-kB), whose activity is specifically influenced by the activation of the upstream main pathways, may also participate in such a tumor classification.

Mitogen-Activated Protein Kinase (MAPK) Pathway

The *mitogen-activated protein kinase* (MAPK) signal transduction pathway regulates cell growth, survival, and invasion. MAPK signaling is initiated at the cell membrane, either by receptor tyrosine kinases (RTKs)-binding ligand or integrin adhesion to extracellular matrix, which transmits activation signals via RAS-GTPase on the cell membrane inner surface (Fig. 4.1). Active, GTP-bound RAS can bind effector proteins such as RAF serine-threonine kinase or phosphatidylinositol 3-kinase (PI3K) [10, 11].

The RAF kinase family consists of three members, ARAF, BRAF, and CRAF, all of which can activate MEK/ERK signaling [11]. In melanoma, the most commonly mutated component of this pathway is the *BRAF* gene, the prevalent *BRAF* mutation (in nearly 90 % of cases) being a substitution of valine with glutamic acid at position 600 (V600E) [12]. Mutated *BRAF* induces constitutive ERK signaling, stimulating proliferation and survival and providing essential tumor growth and maintenance functions [12]. BRAF is implicated in several aspects of melanoma induction and progression, although the presence of *BRAF* mutations in nevi [13, 14] strongly suggests that *BRAF* activation is necessary but not sufficient for the development of melanoma.

In a study aimed to better define the role of BRAF in melanomagenesis, a transgenic zebra fish expressing [V600E]BRAF showed dramatic development of patches of ectopic melanocytes (designated as fish-nevi) [15]. Remarkably, activated *BRAF* in p53-deficient zebra fish induced the formation of melanocytic lesions that rapidly developed into invasive melanomas that resembled human melanomas in terms of their histology and biological behaviors [15]. These data provide direct evidence that the p53 and BRAF pathways interact functionally during melanomagenesis.

The *BRAF* gene also cooperates with the cyclin-dependent kinase inhibitor p16[CDKN2A] (see below). Activating *BRAF* mutations have been reported to constitutively induce upregulation of *p16[CDKN2A]* and cell cycle arrest (this phenomenon appears to be a protective response to an inappropriate mitogenic signal). In particular, mutant BRAF protein induces cell senescence by increasing the expression levels of the p16[CDKN2A] protein, which, in turn, may limit hyperplastic growth caused by *BRAF* mutations [14]. Therefore, inactivation of *p16[CDKN2A]* gene may promote the melanocytic proliferation depending on oncogenic *BRAF*. In this sense, several factors seem to be able to induce the arrest of the cell cycle and cell senescence caused by *BRAF* activation [16, 17].

Finally, it has been showed that primary melanomas arising from chronically sun-damaged skin and from mucosal sites, which typically do not harbor *BRAF* and *NRAS* mutations, have increased copy number of the *CCND1/Cyclin D1* gene [18]. In contrast to primary melanomas, a subset (>15 %) of metastatic melanoma samples

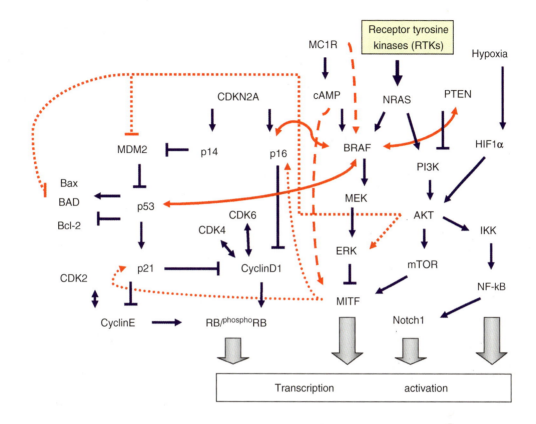

Fig. 4.1 Major pathways involved in melanoma. *Arrows*, activating signals; *interrupted lines*, inhibiting signals. *CDKN2A* cyclin-dependent kinase inhibitor of kinase 2A, *CDK*2/4/6 cyclin-dependent kinase 2/4/6, *MDM*2 murine double minute 2 (MDM2), *ERK* extracellular-related kinase, *MEK* mitogen-activated protein kinase/ extracellular related kinase, *MC1R* melanocortin-1 receptor, *cAMP* cyclic adenylate monophosphate, *MITF* microphthalmia-associated transcription factor, *BAD* BCL-2 antagonist of cell death, *IKK* inhibitor-of-kB-protein kinase, *PI3K* phosphatidylinositol 3-kinase, *PTEN* phosphatase and tensin homolog

with *BRAF* mutations also exhibit amplification of *CCND1/Cyclin D1*. These melanomas are resistant to BRAF inhibitors highlighting the need for combination therapy [19, 20].

CDKN2A

The cyclin-dependent kinase inhibitor 2 (*CDKN2A*; at chromosome 9p21) gene encodes two proteins, p16[CDKN2A] and p14[CDKN2A] (a product of an alternative splicing), that are known to function as tumor suppressors [21]. In particular, p16[CDKN2A] is part of the G1–S cell cycle checkpoint mechanism that involves the retinoblastoma-susceptibility tumor suppressor protein

(pRb). The p16[CDKN2A] inhibits CDK4, which, in turn, phosphorylates pRb and allows progression through the G1–S checkpoint (Fig. 4.1). On the other hand, p14[CDKN2A] interacts with the murine double minute 2 (MDM2) protein that targets p53 for degradation (Fig. 4.1) [22]. In particular, the p14[CDKN2A] protein exerts a tumor suppressor effect by inhibiting the oncogenic actions of the downstream MDM2 protein, whose direct interaction with p53 blocks any p53-mediated activity and targets the p53 protein for rapid degradation. Impairment of the p14[CDKN2A]-MDM2-p53 cascade, whose final effectors are the Bax/Bcl-2 proteins, has been implicated in defective apoptotic responses to genotoxic damage and, thus, to anticancer agents (in most cases, melanoma cells

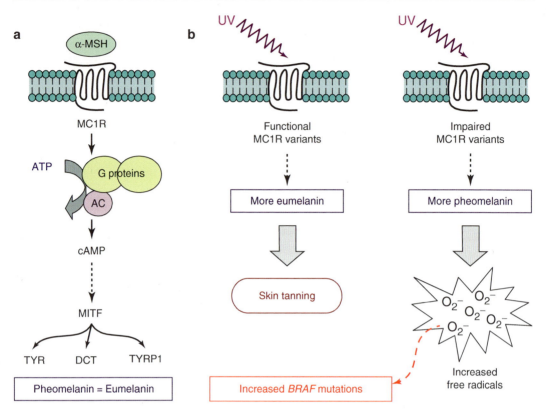

Fig. 4.2 Role of MC1R on pigmentation and melanoma pathogenesis. (**a**) Functional pathway downstream MC1R, leading to the activation of genes acting as major determinants of hair and skin pigmentation. (**b**) Effects of the increased production of eumelanin or pheomelanin. *αMSH* alpha melanocyte-stimulating hormone, *TYR* tyrosinase, *TYRP*1 tyrosinase-related protein 1, *DCT* DOPAchrome tautomerase

present concurrent high expression levels of Bax/Bcl-2 proteins, which may contribute to further increasing their aggressiveness and refractoriness to therapy) [23].

In normal conditions, expression levels of p53 within cells are low. In response to DNA damage, p53 accumulates and prevents cell division. Therefore, inactivation of the *TP53* gene results in an intracellular accumulation of genetic damage which promotes tumor formation [24]. In melanoma, such an inactivation is mostly due to functional gene silencing since the frequency of *TP53* mutations is low [25].

The *CDKN2A* mutations are more frequent in patients with a strong familial history of melanoma (three or more affected family members) relative to patients with no familial occurrence of melanoma [26]. A recent meta-analysis of studies conducted in independent populations indicated that multiple variants of the melanocortin-1 receptor (*MC1R*) gene increase the melanoma risk in *CDKN2A* mutation carriers [27].

The *MC1R* gene encodes a G-protein coupled receptor. In the skin, two types of melanin pigment, dark-protective eumelanin and red photo-reactive pheomelanin, are present [28]. MC1R plays an important role in determining the ratio of eumelanin and pheomelanin production (Fig. 4.2). After stimulation by UV, keratinocytes produce alpha melanocyte-stimulating hormone (MSH) that binds to the MC1R on melanocytes and shifts the balance of these two pigments in the direction of eumelanin [28]. In particular, stimulation of MC1R by MSH mediates activation of adenylate cyclase, subsequent elevation of cAMP levels, and activation of the microphthalmia transcription factor (MITF; see below) (Fig. 4.2a). Activated MITF binds to a conserved region found in the promoters of the *tyrosinase* (*TYR*), *tyrosinase-related protein 1* (*TYRP1*), and *DOPAchrome tautomerase* (*DCT*) genes, stimulating the transcriptional upregulation of these proteins and inducing maturation of the melanosomes [29]. This ultimately results in increased eumelanin production and darkening of the skin or hair.

New findings have shed light on the mechanisms by which MC1R contributes to melanoma risk. In vitro studies showed that acute UV irradiation of melanocytes with impaired MC1R results in an increased production of free radicals [30]. Melanomas that arise on body sites only intermittently exposed to sun, and which therefore lack marked signs of chronic solar damage, were found to have a high frequency of *BRAF* mutations [18]. One could speculate that induction of *BRAF* mutations may occur only when solar exposure is not sufficiently prolonged to induce the striking tissue changes that generate the hallmark signs of solar damage. Several *MC1R* variants, which are impairing relevant protein function, have been associated with *BRAF* mutation in melanoma arising in Caucasian populations from the USA and Europe [31–34]. On the basis of such indications, it is possible that increased production of free radicals following UV exposure in combination with impairment of *MC1R* may induce mutations in the *BRAF* gene (Fig. 4.2b).

Additional mechanisms promoting susceptibility to pathogenetic mutations of the *BRAF* gene may however exist since there is no demonstrable association between germ line *MC1R* status and the prevalence of somatic *BRAF* mutations in melanomas from Australian population, even after classifying the melanomas by their location relative to intermittent and chronic sun exposure [35].

PTEN-AKT

Phosphatase and tensin homolog deleted in chromosome ten (PTEN) has a key role in cellular signal transduction by decreasing intracellular phosphatidylinositol [3,4-bisphosphate (PIP2)

and 3,4,5-trisphosphate (PIP3)] that are produced by the activation of phoshoinosite 3-kinase (PI3K) [36]. Active RAS exerts the strongest stimulus for PI3K activation (Fig. 4.1), resulting in an increase of PIP3 intracellular levels and a consequent conformational change of AKT [37]. Activated AKT in turn phosphorylates its substrate, the serine/threonine kinase mTOR, leading to increased synthesis of target proteins that regulate cell division and apoptosis [37]. The mechanisms associated with the ability of AKT to suppress apoptosis include the phosphorylation and inactivation of many proapoptotic proteins, such as BAD (Bcl-2 antagonist of cell death) and MDM2, as well as the activation of NF-kB [38] (Fig. 4.1).

In primary melanomas, inactivation of *PTEN* gene is mainly due to hypermethylation-based epigenetic mechanisms, with a low incidence (less than 10 %) of somatic mutations [39]. *PTEN* inactivation has been mostly observed as a late event in melanoma, although a dose-dependent downregulation of PTEN expression has been implicated in early stages of tumorigenesis [36]. In addition, alterations of the BRAF-MAPK pathway are frequently associated with PTEN-AKT impairment [2, 40]. In summary, the combined effects of the loss of PTEN and activation of the PI3K/AKT pathway may result in aberrant cell growth, apoptosis escape, and abnormal cell spreading and migration.

Microphthalmia-Associated Transcription Factor (MITF)

The microphthalmia-associated transcription factor (MITF) is a basic helix–loop–helix leucine zipper transcription factor that is considered to be the master regulator of melanocyte biology, since it is involved in melanoblast survival and melanocyte lineage commitment. MITF is activated by the MAPK pathway as well as by the cAMP pathway (Fig. 4.1) and leads to transcription of genes involved in pigmentation (TYR, TYRP1, and DCT; see above) as well as cell cycle progression and survival. A genome-wide analysis of copy number alterations in cancer identified MITF as an amplified locus in melanoma; *MITF* amplification correlated with increased resistance to chemotherapy and decreased overall survival [41].

The connection between MITF and melanoma development is complex because it plays a double role of inducer/repressor of cellular proliferation. High levels of MITF expression lead to G1 cell cycle arrest and differentiation, through induction of the cell cycle inhibitors p16[CDKN2A] and p21 [42, 43] (Fig. 4.1). Very low or null MITF expression levels predispose to apoptosis, whereas intermediate MITF expression levels promote cell proliferation [41–43]. Therefore, it is thought that melanoma cells have developed strategies to maintain MITF levels in the range compatible with tumorigenesis. It has been shown that constitutive ERK activity, stimulated by [V600E]BRAF in melanoma cells, is associated with MITF ubiquitin-dependent degradation [44]. Nevertheless, continued expression of MITF is necessary for proliferation and survival of melanoma cells, because it also regulates CDK2 and Bcl-2 genes [45, 46]. It has been recently shown that oncogenic BRAF may control intracellular levels of the MITF protein through a fine balance of two opposite mechanisms: a direct reduction of MITF levels, by inducing protein degradation, and an indirect increase of MITF levels, by stimulating transcription factors which increase protein expression levels [47]. Oncogenic *BRAF* mutations are associated with *MITF* amplification in a low fraction (10–15 %) of melanomas [47] suggesting that other mechanisms are likely to be involved in ERK-dependent degradation of MITF.

Nuclear Factor-kB

Nuclear factor-kB (NF-kB) is important in inflammation and cell proliferation and survival [48]. A wide range of stimuli activates NF-kB which, upon activation, translocates to the nucleus to interact with kB sites located in regulatory regions of target genes [49].

Aberrant NF-kB regulation may cause alteration of the transcriptional activation of genes associated with cell proliferation, angiogenesis, tumor promotion, and suppression of apoptosis [50–52]. In melanoma, NF-kB is constitutively activated since expression of the inhibitor-of-kB (IkB) proteins, which form complexes sequestering NF-kB into the cytoplasm, seems to be significantly reduced in comparison to nevi [53]. In particular, activation of the AKT and/or MAPK pathways has been demonstrated to increase degradation of such complexes through activation of an IkB kinase (IKK) effector (Fig. 4.1), with subsequent release of NF-kB which may thus move to the nucleus and activate gene transcription [54–56].

From Molecular Mechanisms to Histopathological Markers

Increased knowledge of molecular mechanisms in melanoma has prompted interest in how this may be applied to improve clinical decision making on the basis of more accurate diagnosis, refined prediction of probable future clinical course (prognostication), and the likelihood of a meaningful response to specific treatment modalities. These assessments currently are based on consideration of patient's demographics, clinical presentation, and microscopic and immunohistochemical features of the individual melanoma. Clinical assessment relies on elicitation of a detailed clinical history and scrutiny of the skin tumor, possibly with the assistance of a dermoscope. If melanoma is suspected, the lesion is often examined in situ by ultrasound to assess depth of invasion [57]. Standard microscopic evaluation of tissue sections from a primary melanoma, stained by hematoxylin and eosin (HE), classifies the histology and cytology of any melanocytic proliferation present at the dermoepidermal interface, the presence and micrometer-measured extent of ulceration, and the measured thickness and depth of any dermal infiltration by tumor [58]. The tumor cells of junctional and dermal components are evaluated for pleomorphism, nuclear atypia, and the frequency and location of normal and abnormal mitoses. The associated stroma is assessed for the presence, density, and distribution of any peritumoral or intratumoral lymphocytic infiltrates. Evidence of vascular and/or lymphatic invasion sought and neurotropism and angiotropism recorded [59]. Prognosis is based on consideration of the presence and extent of ulceration, the micrometer-measured Breslow thickness, and the frequency of mitoses in the vertical growth phase [60].

Immunohistochemistry

Currently, immunohistochemistry (IHC) is routinely used to differentiate melanomas from benign melanocytic tumors that resemble melanoma in HE-stained tissue sections. We here provide a summary of current practice, but for a detailed account of this complex subject, see Ohsie et al. [61]:

- S-100, a 21 kDa acidic calcium-binding protein previously known to be expressed by glial cells, is a sensitive marker for cells of melanocytic lineage that is expressed in the nuclei and cytoplasm of the cells of 97–100 % of melanomas. S-100 is not a specific marker for melanocytic lesions; among others, fibroblasts in dermal scars may express S-100, a potentially major diagnostic pitfall in the evaluation of tissue for desmoplastic melanoma.
- HMB45, a marker of the premelanosomal glycoprotein gp100, is not as sensitive as S-100 but is more specific (69–93 %) with greater expression in primary (77–100 %) than in metastatic melanomas (58–83 %). Staining may be patchy or zonal with relatively strong HMB45 expression in the superficial component of primary melanomas and progressively weaker staining deeper. HMB45 may be less sensitive in amelanotic melanomas.
- MART-1 (melanoma antigen recognized by T-cells-1) and Melan-A are synonyms for a melanosomal differentiation-associated cytoplasmic protein that is recognized by T-cells. Two antibody clones are available: M2-7C10, generally referred to as MART-1, and A103, generally referred to as Melan-A. These antibodies show sensitivity (75–92 %) and specificity (95–100 %) for melanoma at a similar level to HMB45. Both antibodies stain metastatic melanomas less strongly than primary melanomas. MART-1 and Melan-A are associated with more diffuse and intense cytoplasmic staining than HMB45. They less often show weaker staining of melanoma cells located in the deeper dermis which facilitates interpretation.

- Tyrosinase is an enzyme hydroxylating tyrosine as the initial step in melanogenesis. In melanomas, positive staining to tyrosinase is seen as a strong diffuse finely granular pattern in the cytoplasm. The sensitivity of the antibody to tyrosinase for melanoma (84–94 %) exceeds that of HMB45, but sensitivity declines within metastatic lesions (79–93 %). Specificity for melanoma is also high (97–100 %), though tyrosinase is not entirely specific to cells of melanocytic lineage.
- MITF (see above) is located in the nucleus and a positive reaction is relatively easy to interpret. Sensitivity for melanoma is 81–100 %, with expression in S-100-negative melanomas. Initial reports claimed 100 % specificity for MITF, but recent reports indicate lesser specificity (88 %), especially in the case of spindle cell melanomas. Reactivity with some non-melanocytic tumors has been reported; this relative non-specificity somewhat offsets the interpretive advantages of nuclear staining.
- Cellular proliferation within melanocytic tumors, determined by enumeration of the frequency of mitoses per mm^2, may also be assessed using markers of the active phases of the cell cycle, such as Ki67 and PCNA. The general principle is that malignant melanomas have a higher frequency of Ki67-positive nuclei than benign nevi. Additionally, marker-positive nuclei in benign nevi are more frequently located in the superficial area of the lesion. Determination of the frequency of Ki67-positive melanoma cell nuclei can be challenging when there is an abundant population of lymphocytes, which have an inherently high proportion of Ki67-positive nuclei.

Representative examples about the use of the immunohistochemistry in differential diagnosis of melanocytic lesions are shown in Figs. 4.3, 4.4, and 4.5.

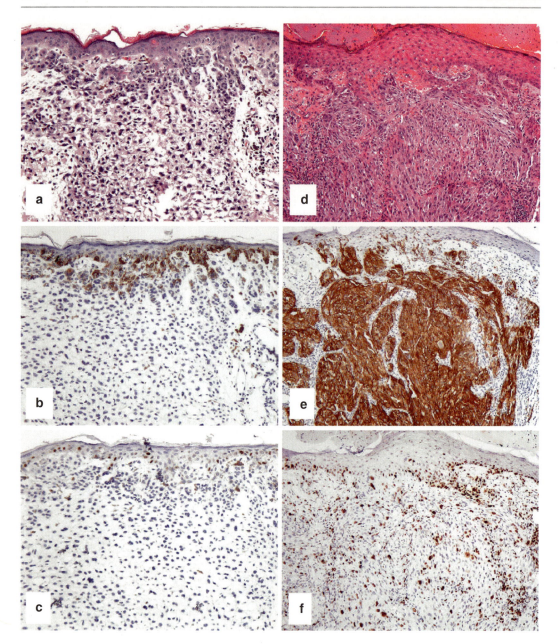

Fig. 4.3 IHC to help separate a compound nevus from a primary melanoma. (**a**) HE-stained compound nevus that arises at the epidermo-dermal junction and extends into the underlying dermis. (**b**) Only nevus cells at the junction stain with HMB-45. (**c**) A similar pattern with Ki67-positive nevus cells (admixed with keratinocytes at the junction but absent from the dermal component). (**d**) HE-stained primary melanoma arising from the overlying epidermis and extending into the dermis. In contrast to the nevus, (**e**) strong staining of epidermal and dermal melanoma cells with HMB-45 and (**f**) frequent junctional and dermal melanoma cells with Ki67-positive nuclei are observed

These standard clinical and histopathological IHC approaches are time tested, and using such approaches, experienced pathologists can readily and accurately identify more than 95 % of melanomas and separate them from melanocytic nevi. Problems arise in the interpretation of so-called borderline lesions (melanocytic tumors of unknown malignant potential—MELTUMP)

[62]. These are tumors in which the histology and/or cytology is typical neither of malignant melanoma nor melanocytic nevus. MELTUMPs include atypical Spitz lesions, atypical cellular blue nevi, deep penetrating nevi, and pigmented epithelioid melanocytomas. There is often very considerable diversity of opinion when such lesions are evaluated by multiple pathologists.

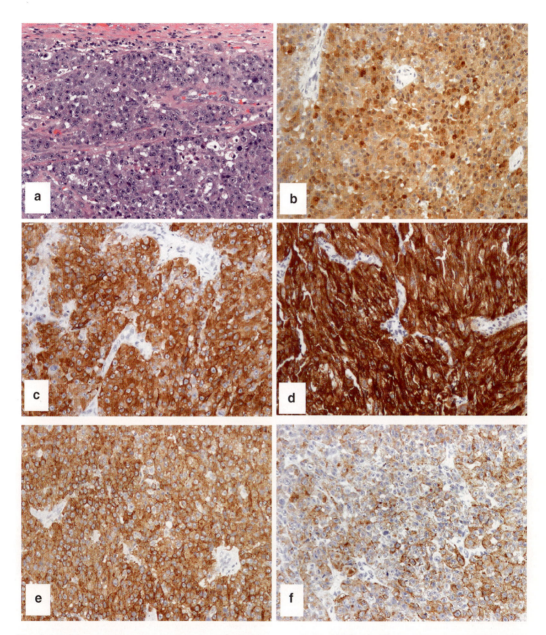

Fig. 4.4 IHC to confirm that a tumor is melanocytic. (**a**) HE-stained malignant epithelioid cellular neoplasm, cytologically and histologically suspicious for melanoma, without evidence of melanin synthesis. Differential immunohistochemical studies confirm that the tumor is melanocytic in histogenesis and likely malignant: (**b**) strong nuclear and cytoplasmic expression of S-100, (**c**) strong cytoplasmic expression of Mart-1, (**d**) very strong cytoplasmic expression of tyrosinase, (**e, f**) variable cytoplasmic expression of HMB-45, (**g**) strong nuclear expression of MITF, and (**h**) strong and frequent nuclear expression of Ki67. Note the differential expression of HMB-45 between a primary melanoma (e) and metastatic melanoma (f). This differential epitope expression is often (but not always) present

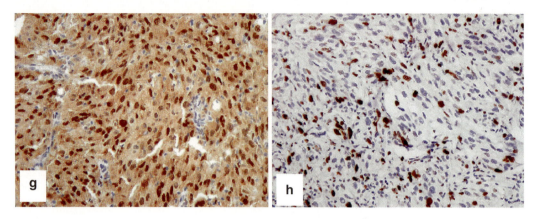

Fig. 4.4 (continued)

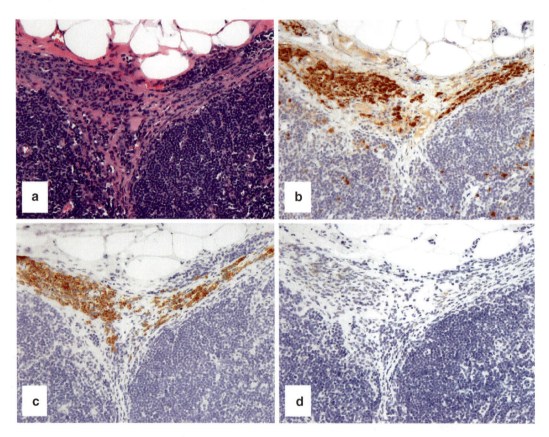

Fig. 4.5 IHC to identify capsular/trabecular nevus cells in a sentinel lymph node. (**a**) HE-stained section shows small blue-colored nevus cells in the nodal capsule (*pink*) and extending downwards in a connective tissue trabecu-lum. The nevus cells stain strongly with (**b**) S-100 and (**c**) MART-1, but weakly or not at all with (**d**) HMB-45. In contrast, melanoma cells stain strongly with S-100, Mart-1, and HMB-45

In these dilemmas, there is an urgent need for additional accurate diagnostic approaches that will supplement routine clinical and histological evaluation and increase diagnostic accuracy to a level where critical management decisions can be made with confidence.

Molecular techniques that can detect tumor type-specific abnormalities of genes (comparative

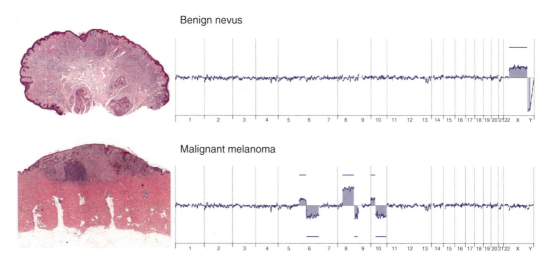

Fig. 4.6 Array comparative genomic hybridization. Histograms showing gains and losses in DNA copy number obtained from a benign melanocytic nevus and a malignant melanoma. The results plotted in these two histograms show no chromosomal aberrations for the melanocytic nevus, whereas there are chromosomal gains in 6p, 8q, and 10p and losses in 6q, 9p, and 10q for the melanoma. The x-axis represents the genomic position of chromosomes ordered from 1p (*left*) to 22 (*right*). The y-axis shows the relative gain or loss in DNA copy number for each neoplasm (Figure courtesy of Drs. Heinz Kutzner and Thomas Wiesner)

genome hybridization (CGH), gene microarrays), chromosomes (fluorescence in situ hybridization—FISH), and base pair constitution and sequence (gene sequencing) may become such helpful approaches.

Comparative Genomic Hybridization

The development of comparative genomic hybridization (CGH) technology provided for the first time a highly efficient means of assessing DNA copy number differences in neoplasms of interest on a genome-wide basis [63]. The initial methodology involved tumor DNA and reference DNA labeled with different fluorochromes and then simultaneously hybridized to chromosome metaphase spreads. The fluorescence ratio along the axis of each chromosome could then be measured indicating particular DNA gains or losses from the tumor sample at each chromosomal locus. The array CGH has since greatly increased the magnitude of resolution, allowing for significantly more precise definition of the area of chromosomal loss or gain (Fig. 4.6). With this technology, microarrays are constructed from

DNA derived from bacterial artificial clones, complementary DNAs, selected polymerase chain reaction products, and oligonucleotides.

In a study of melanomas and benign nevi by CGH, Bastian et al. reported that 96 % of melanomas had some type of chromosomal copy number change, whereas chromosomal copy number aberrations were rare in nevi [64]. The most common aberrations observed among melanomas were gains in 6p, 1q, 7p, 7q, 8q, 17q, 11q, and 20q and losses in 9p, 9q, 10q, 10p, and 6q. Among the analyzed nevi, only Spitz tumors (about 10 % of the total nevi examined) exhibited an identical isolated gain in chromosome 11p (none of 132 melanomas showed this gain in 11p) [64]. Subsequent investigations employing array CGH have shown that subsets of melanoma have distinct differences in the types and frequencies of chromosomal aberrations present [18, 64]. For example, acral and mucosal melanomas demonstrate a much higher frequency of focal amplifications and losses of DNA compared to the two melanoma subsets that arise in chronically sun-damaged (CSD) and intermittently sun-exposed skin (non-CSD), respectively. Further, CSD melanomas show frequent gains in 6p,

11q13, 17q, and 20q and losses in 6p, 8p, 9p, 13, and 21q, whereas non-CSD melanomas demonstrate gains in 6p, 7, 8q, 17q, and 20q and losses in 9p, 10, and 21q. The results of these studies not only provide insights into the molecular pathways of melanoma development but also a robust technique for analyzing histologically ambiguous melanocytic neoplasms. Ongoing work in a number of centers around the world is currently utilizing array CGH as a practical research technique to study difficult to classify melanocytic lesions using formalin-fixed paraffin-embedded (FFPE) material. The limitations of array CGH include the need to have at least 30–50 % pure tumor cells in the samplings from tumors of interest. Thus, small and/or superficial tumors or tumors with only small numbers of aberrant or malignant cells of interest may lie below the threshold for detection by CGH.

Fluorescence In Situ Hybridization

Based on the various CGH studies cited above, investigations have been undertaken to develop fluorescence in situ hybridization (FISH) probes in order to assess the most frequent chromosomal aberrations occurring in melanoma (see above). Recently a panel of four multicolor FISH probes targeting 6p25 (RREB1), 6 centromere, 6q23 (MYB), and 11q13 (CCND1) has been introduced for the analysis of melanocytic lesions from FFPE specimens [65]. In a study involving a training set of melanocytic nevi and melanomas and a subsequent validation set of melanocytic lesions, the four-probe panel showed a sensitivity of 87 % and specificity of 95 % for the recognition of melanoma.

The current FISH test has been applied to the separation of several challenging melanocytic tumors [64]. It has been used to separate primary melanomas from atypical nevi, particularly nevoid melanomas from nevi that are comprised of cytologically atypical nevocytes or that demonstrate a relatively high mitotic rate and/or the presence of atypical mitoses. Other studies have addressed separation of epithelioid cellular blue nevi from dermal metastases of melanoma; discrimination between cellular blue nevi, atypical cellular blue nevi, and malignant blue nevi; separation of desmoplastic melanomas from desmoplastic nevi; separation of pagetoid Spitz nevus from pagetoid (superficial spreading) melanoma; and distinction of Spitz tumors from melanoma and lymph nodal nevi from nodal metastases of melanoma. The application of FISH to these challenging melanocytic dilemmas has yielded somewhat diverse results and claims. Some authors report enthusiastically that FISH is a reliable adjuvant technique in the separation of nevi and melanomas, including Spitz nevi, while others have found less decisive outcomes.

In summary, practical experience with this panel of four FISH probes has shown its limitations and the need for further validation with the use of additional probes [66]. At present, the four-probe panel has an overall false-negative rate of about 25 % for melanoma and may be higher or lower for particular applications to challenging melanocytic neoplasms (see above). Thus, the use of FISH probes for melanocytic lesions remains a work in progress that requires more rigorous validation for each particular application. Nonetheless, if FISH testing is used with extreme prudence in particular diagnostic applications, it may provide useful ancillary information to supplement histological interpretation. Recent work has suggested that FISH positivity in melanomas greater than 2 mm in thickness may have predictive value for the development of metastases [67].

Gene Microarrays

This approach is based on the assessment of genes differentially expressed among tissues (mainly, normal or preneoplastic tissues versus malignant lesions). For such a purpose, tumor is carefully microdissected from adjacent normal tissue by laser capture microdissection and total mRNA isolated, amplified, and labeled. The labeled mRNA is then hybridized to a human gene chip array. Differential gene expression is accepted when there is a twofold or greater difference between the test and control samples and

$p < 5.00E\text{-}2$. This technique has been used to show significant gene expression differences between melanomas and nevi [68] or between primary melanomas and sentinel node metastases [69]. Studies in progress are applying this approach to assessment of nevoid and Spitzoid melanomas, atypical nevi, Spitz nevi, and atypical Spitzoid neoplasms.

Gene Sequencing

In this approach, the order of nucleotide bases in DNA molecules in the whole genome or exome is determined. In an initial study, scientists at the Sanger Institute sequenced a cell line derived from a metastatic melanoma and compared it to autologous normal tissue. Substitutions were identified that were related to ultraviolet damage [70]. The technique also identified insertions, deletions, and copy number variants. Comparable studies of biopsy material are in progress [71]. This approach seems likely to contribute to knowledge of melanoma causation and evolutionary pathogenesis. This approach is at present very expensive, but the techniques are in process of simplification and should in this way become less expensive and thus capable of more widespread application.

Actually, there is great interest in the detection of specific mutations that are associated with particular melanoma subtypes (that likely reflect differing paths of tumorigenesis) and that may indicate the likelihood of response to particular forms of therapy. These include *BRAF*, particularly the V600E mutation common in superficial spreading melanomas and indicative of tumors likely to respond to *BRAF* inhibitors such as vemurafenib; *c-KIT*, associated with lentiginous and uveal melanoma and with in vitro and clinical responses to treatment with imatinib mesylate; *NRAS* (despite the well-known role of RAS in tumor initiation and promotion, NRAS itself has not been successfully targeted); *GNAQ*, associated with blue nevi and uveal melanomas; and *BRCA1/2*, associated with uveal melanomas. This important area of study is in the process of rapid evolution. Key mutations are emerging, but the definitive slate of mutations to be screened in order to optimize therapy for the individual patient remains to be determined. It is likely that mutation testing will be incorporated in the standard laboratory workup of melanoma (and other tumors) in the near future.

Conclusions

Melanoma remains a prototype of solid cancers with an increasing incidence and extremely poor prognosis in advanced stages; an extremely complicate interaction of genetic and epigenetic alterations does contribute to limit the efficacy of current anticancer treatments. This scenario is further worsened by the fact that majority of melanomas do not seem to evolve from nevi and only a fraction of them is associated with dysplastic nevi [72], strongly suggesting that melanoma may mostly arise from normal-appearing skin without following a sequential accumulation of molecular events during tumorigenesis.

Recently, it has been suggested that melanomas may be derived from transformed melanocyte stem cells, melanocyte progenitors, or dedifferentiated mature melanocytes [73]. Although the origin of intradermic stem cells has yet to be determined, it has been postulated that the interaction with the tumor microenvironment (including surrounding and/or recruited fibroblasts and endothelial and inflammatory cells) may induce such cells to transform directly into the various cell variants (normal melanocytes, benign or intermediate proliferating melanocytic cells, malign or metastatic melanoma cells), without progressing through intermediates [73]. In the very near future, the biologic and molecular characterization of melanoma stem cells will also clarify whether the well-known drug resistance of melanoma resides in the existence of quiescent or drug-resistant cancer stem cells as well as whether the inhibition of self-renewing cancer stem cells prevents melanoma growth.

The only certainty is that targeting a single component in such complex signaling pathways is unlikely to yield a significant antitumor response in melanoma patients. For this reason, further evaluation of all known molecular targets along with the molecular classification of primary melanomas could become very helpful in predicting the subsets of patients who would be expected to be more or less likely to respond to specific therapeutic interventions. Now is the time to make our maximal efforts in translating all research knowledge into clinical practice.

Glossary

Molecular marker Key molecular alteration which may help diagnosis, staging, and/or prognosis of cancer patients.
Target therapy Treatment based on drugs specific for mutated/altered oncogenic protein playing a key role in molecular pathways involved in tumorigenesis.
Tumorigenesis Induction of malignant transformation due to a complex combination of genetic and molecular alterations.

References

1. Jhappan C, Noonan FP, Merlino G. Ultraviolet radiation and cutaneous malignant melanoma. Oncogene. 2003;22:3099–112.
2. Thompson JF, Scolyer RA, Kefford RF. Cutaneous melanoma. Lancet. 2005;365:687–701.
3. Cho E, Rosner BA, Feskanich D, Colditz GA. Risk factors and individual probabilities of melanoma for whites. J Clin Oncol. 2005;23:2669–75.
4. Curado MP, Edwards B, Shin HR, et al., editors. Cancer incidence in five continents, vol. IX, International Agency for Research on Cancer (IARC) Scientific Publications, No. 160. Lyon: IARC; 2007.
5. Rigel DS. Epidemiology of melanoma. Semin Cutan Med Surg. 2010;29:204–9.
6. Linos E, Swetter S, Cockburn MG, et al. Increasing burden of melanoma in the United States. J Invest Dermatol. 2009;129:1666–74.
7. Welch HG, Woloshin S, Schwartz LM. Skin biopsy rates and incidence of melanoma: population based ecological study. BMJ. 2005;331:481.
8. de Vries E, Coebergh JW. Melanoma incidence has risen in Europe. BMJ. 2005;331:698.
9. Palmieri G, Casula M, Sini MC, et al. Issues affecting molecular staging in the management of patients with melanoma. J Cell Mol Med. 2007;11:1052–68.
10. Giehl K. Oncogenic Ras in tumor progression and metastasis. Biol Chem. 2005;386:193–205.
11. Heidorn SJ, Milagre C, Whittaker S, et al. Kinase-dead BRAF and oncogenic RAS cooperate to drive tumor progression through CRAF. Cell. 2010;140:209–21.
12. Davies H, Bignell GR, Cox C, et al. Mutations of the BRAF gene in human cancer. Nature. 2002;417:949–54.
13. Pollock PM, Harper UL, Hansen KS, et al. High frequency of BRAF mutations in nevi. Nat Genet. 2003;33(1):19–20.
14. Michaloglou C, Vredeveld LC, Soengas MS, et al. BRAF^{E600}-associated senescence-like cell cycle arrest of human naevi. Nature. 2005;436:720–4.
15. Patton EE, Widlund HR, Kutok JL, et al. BRAF mutations are sufficient to promote nevi formation and cooperate with p53 in the genesis of melanoma. Curr Biol. 2005;15:249–54.
16. Wajapeyee N, Serra RW, Zhu X, et al. Oncogenic BRAF induces senescence and apoptosis through pathways mediated by the secreted protein IGFBP7. Cell. 2008;132:363–74.
17. Dhomen N, Reis-Filho JS, da Rocha Dias S, et al. Oncogenic Braf induces melanocyte senescence and melanoma in mice. Cancer Cell. 2009;15:294–303.
18. Curtin JA, Fridlyand J, Kageshita T, et al. Distinct sets of genetic alterations in melanoma. N Engl J Med. 2005;353:2135–47.
19. Smalley KS, Lioni M, Dalla Palma M, et al. Increased cyclin D1 expression can mediate BRAF inhibitor resistance in BRAF V600E-mutated melanomas. Mol Cancer Ther. 2008;7:2876–83.
20. Ascierto PA, De Maio E, Bertuzzi S, et al. Future perspectives in melanoma research. Meeting report from the "Melanoma Research: a bridge Naples-USA. Naples, December 6th–7th 2010". J Transl Med. 2011;9:32.
21. Pomerantz J, Schreiber-Agus N, Lie'geois NJ. The Ink4a tumor suppressor gene product, 19Arf, interacts with MDM2 and neutralizes DM2's inhibition of p53. Cell. 1998;92:713–23.
22. Zhang Y, Xiong Y, Yarbrough WG. ARF promotes MDM2 degradation and stabilizes p53: ARF-INK4a locus deletion impairs both the Rb and p53 tumor suppression pathways. Cell. 1998;92:725–34.
23. Palmieri G, Capone ME, Ascierto ML, et al. Main roads to melanoma. J Transl Med. 2009;7:86.
24. Levine AJ. p53, the cellular gatekeeper for growth and division. Cell. 1997;88:323–31.
25. Box NF, Terzian T. The role of p53 in pigmentation, tanning and melanoma. Pigment Cell Melanoma Res. 2008;21:525–33.
26. Meyle KD, Guldberg P. Genetic risk factors for melanoma. Hum Genet. 2009;126:499–510.
27. Fargnoli MC, Gandini S, Peris K, et al. MC1R variants increase melanoma risk in families with CDKN2A mutations: a meta-analysis. Eur J Cancer. 2010;46:1413–20.

28. Scott MC, Wakamatsu K, Ito S, et al. Human melano-cortin 1 receptor variants, receptor function and mel-anocyte response to UV radiation. J Cell Sci. 2002;115:2349–55.
29. Levy C, Khaled M, Fisher DE. MITF: master regula-tor of melanocyte development and melanoma onco-gene. Trends Mol Med. 2006;12:406–14.
30. Hauser JE, Kadekaro AL, Kavanagh RJ, et al. Melanin content and MC1R function independently affect UVR-induced DNA damage in cultured human mel-anocytes. Pigment Cell Res. 2006;19:303–14.
31. Landi MT, Bauer J, Pfeiffer RM, et al. MC1R ger-mline variants confer risk for BRAF-mutant mela-noma. Science. 2006;313:521–2.
32. Fargnoli MC, Pike K, Pfeiffer RM, et al. MC1R vari-ants increase risk of melanomas harboring BRAF mutations. J Invest Dermatol. 2008;128:2485–90.
33. Thomas NE, Kanetsky PA, Edmiston SN, et al. Relationship between germline MC1R variants and BRAF-mutant melanoma in a North Carolina popu-lation-based study. J Invest Dermatol. 2010;130: 1463–5.
34. Scherer D, Rachakonda PS, Angelini S, et al. Association between the germline MC1R variants and somatic BRAF/NRAS mutations in melanoma tumors. J Invest Dermatol. 2010;130:2844–8.
35. Hacker E, Hayward NK, Dumenil T, et al. The asso-ciation between MC1R genotype and BRAF mutation status in cutaneous melanoma: findings from an Australian population. J Invest Dermatol. 2010;130: 241–8.
36. Wu H, Goel V, Haluska FG. PTEN signaling path-ways in melanoma. Oncogene. 2003;22:3113–22.
37. Vivanco I, Sawyers CL. The phosphatidylinositol 3-kinase AKT pathway in human cancer. Nat Rev Cancer. 2002;2:489–501.
38. Plas DR, Thompson CB. Akt-dependent transforma-tion: there is more to growth than just surviving. Oncogene. 2005;24:7435–42.
39. Mirmohammadsadegh A, Marini A, Nambiar S, et al. Epigenetic silencing of the PTEN gene in melanoma. Cancer Res. 2006;66:6546–52.
40. Tsao H, Goel V, Wu H, et al. Genetic interaction between NRAS and BRAF mutations and PTEN/MMAC1 inactivation in melanoma. J Invest Dermatol. 2004;122:337–41.
41. Garraway LA, Widlund HR, Rubin MA, et al. Integrative genomic analyses identify MITF as a lin-eage survival oncogene amplified in malignant mela-noma. Nature. 2005;436:117–22.
42. Carreira S, Goodall J, Aksan I, et al. Mitf cooperates with Rb1 and activates p21Cip1 expression to regu-late cell cycle progression. Nature. 2005;433:764–9.
43. Loercher AE, Tank EM, Delston RB, Harbour JW. MITF links differentiation with cell cycle arrest in melanocytes by transcriptional activation of INK4A. J Cell Biol. 2005;168:35–40.
44. Wellbrock C, Marais R. Elevated expression of MITF counteracts B-RAF stimulated melanocyte and mela-noma cell proliferation. J Cell Biol. 2005;170:703–8.

45. McGill GG, Horstmann M, Widlund HR, et al. Bcl2 regulation by the melanocyte master regulator Mitf modulates lineage survival and melanoma cell viabil-ity. Cell. 2002;109:707–18.
46. Du J, Widlund HR, Horstmann MA, et al. Critical role of CDK2 for melanoma growth linked to its melanocyte-specific transcriptional regulation by MITF. Cancer Cell. 2004;6:565–76.
47. Wellbrock C, Rana S, Paterson H, et al. Oncogenic BRAF regulates melanoma proliferation through the lineage specific factor MITF. PLoS One. 2008;3: 2734.
48. Karin M, Cao Y, Greten FR, Li ZW. NF-kappaB in cancer: from innocent bystander to major culprit. Nat Rev Cancer. 2002;2:301–10.
49. Basseres DS, Baldwin AS. Nuclear factor-kappaB and inhibitor of kappaB kinase pathways in oncogenic initiation and progression. Oncogene. 2006;25: 6817–30.
50. Kim HJ, Hawke N, Baldwin AS. NF-kappaB and IKK as therapeutic targets in cancer. Cell Death Differ. 2006;13:738–47.
51. Jost PJ, Ruland J. Aberrant NF-kappaB signaling in lymphoma: mechanisms, consequences, and thera-peutic implications. Blood. 2007;109:2700–7.
52. Cilloni D, Martinelli G, Messa F, et al. Nuclear factor kB as a target for new drug development in myeloid malignancies. Haematologica. 2007;92:1224–9.
53. McNulty SE, del Rosario R, Cen D, et al. Comparative expression of NFkappaB proteins in melanocytes of normal skin vs. benign intradermal naevus and human metastatic melanoma biopsies. Pigment Cell Res. 2004;17(2):173–80.
54. Dhawan P, Singh AB, Ellis DL, Richmond A. Constitutive activation of Akt/protein kinase B in melanoma leads to up-regulation of nuclear factor-kappaB and tumor progression. Cancer Res. 2002;62:7335–42.
55. Rangaswami H, Bulbule A, Kundu GC. Nuclear fac-tor-inducing kinase plays a crucial role in osteopon-tin-induced MAPK/IkappaBalpha kinase-dependent nuclear factor kappaB-mediated promatrix metallo-proteinase-9 activation. J Biol Chem. 2004;279: 38921–35.
56. Uffort DG, Grimm EA, Ellerhorst JA. NF-kappaB mediates mitogen-activated protein kinase pathway-dependent iNOS expression in human melanoma. J Invest Dermatol. 2009;129:148–54.
57. Chami L, Lassau N, Chebil M, Robert C. Imaging of melanoma: usefulness of ultrasonography before and after contrast injection for diagnosis and early evalua-tion of treatment. Clin Cosmet Investig Dermatol. 2011;4:1–6.
58. Cochran AJ, Starz H, Ohsie SJ, et al. Pathologic reporting and special diagnostic techniques for mela-noma. Surg Oncol Clin N Am. 2006;15:231–51.
59. Barnhill RL, Lugassy C. Angiotropic malignant mela-noma and extravascular migratory metastasis: descrip-tion of 36 cases with emphasis on a new mechanism of tumour spread. Pathology. 2004;36:485–90.

60. Balch CM, Gershenwald JE, Atkins MB, et al., editors. AJCC cancer staging manual. 7th ed. American Joint Committee on Cancer. Springer: New York; 2010. p. 325–44.

61. Ohsie SJ, Sarantopoulos GP, Cochran AJ, Binder SW. Immunohistochemical characteristics of melanoma. J Cutan Pathol. 2008;35:433–44.

62. Elder DE, Xiaowei X. The approach to the patient with a difficult melanocytic lesion. Pathology. 2004;36:428.

63. Pinkel D, Albertson D. Array comparative genomic hybridization and its applications in cancer. Nat Genet Suppl. 2005;37:S11–7.

64. Bastian BC, Olshen AB, LeBoit PE, et al. Classifying melanocytic tumors based on DNA copy number changes. Am J Pathol. 2003;163:1765–70.

65. Gerami P, Jewell SS, Morrison LE, et al. Fluorescence in situ hybridization in melanoma. Arch Pathol Lab Med. 2011;135:830–7.

66. Gaiser T, Kutzner H, Palmedo G, et al. Classifying ambiguous melanocytic lesions with FISH and correlation with clinical long-term follow up. Mod Pathol. 2010;23:413–9.

67. North JP, Vetto JT, Murali R, et al. Assessment of copy number status of chromosomes 6 and 11 by FISH provides independent prognostic information in primary melanoma. Am J Surg Pathol. 2011;35:1146–50.

68. Koh SS, Opel ML, Wei J-P, et al. Molecular classification of melanomas and nevi using gene expression microarray signatures and formalin-fixed and paraffin-embedded tissue. Mod Pathol. 2009;22:538–46.

69. Koh SS, Wei J-P, Li X, et al. Differential gene expression profiling of primary cutaneous melanoma and sentinel lymph node metastases. Mod Pathol. 2012;25:828–37.

70. Pleasance ED, Cheetham RK, Stephens PJ, et al. A comprehensive catalogue of somatic mutations from a human cancer genome. Nature. 2010;463: 191–6.

71. Wei X, Walia V, Lin JC, et al. Exome sequencing identifies GRIN2A as frequently mutated in melanoma. Nat Genet. 2011;43:442–6.

72. Miller AJ, Mihm MC. Melanoma. N Engl J Med. 2006;355:51–65.

73. Zabierowski SE, Herlyn M. Melanoma stem cells: the dark seed of melanoma. J Clin Oncol. 2008;26:2890–4.

Basal Cell Carcinoma: Molecular and Pathological Features

5

Renato Franco, Anna Maria Anniciello,
Gerardo Botti, Michele Caraglia, and Amalia Luce

Key Points

- Basal cell carcinoma (BCC) is the most common non melanoma skin cancer worldwide.
- BCC occurrence depends upon a series of environmental factors, phenotype and genetic predisposition.
- UV rays are responsible of DNA damage, with subsequent mutations in certain genes within cells, such as the *p53* gene for BCC and SCC and the *patched (PTCH1)* gene for BCC.
- *p53* have been found in nearly 56 % of human BCC cases, while alterations of *PTCH1* have been found in 30 to 40 % of sporadic BCCs.
- Two hereditary disorders, Gorlin's syndrome (autosomal dominant) and xeroderma pigmentosum (autosomal recessive), are characterized by *PTCH1* gene mutations. *PTCH1* is a suppressor gene and its mutations leads to uncontrolled cell proliferation.

- BCC are commonly subdivided in undifferentiated (more frequent) and differentiated tumors.
- Surgical excision has a high cure rate for primary BCCs. Other curative techniques include curettage and electrocautery, cryosurgery, laser therapy, radiotherapy as well as topical immunomodulators, chemoterapy and electrochemotherapy. Up-to-date molecular targeting therapy is starting to be used.

Introduction

Basal cell carcinoma (BCC) is the most common skin cancer, being four- to five-times more frequent than squamous cell carcinoma and eight- to ten-times more frequent than melanoma [1]. BCC derives from basaloid epithelia located in the follicular bulges, in the anagen hair bulbs and the follicular matrix cells and in specific basaloid cells of the interfollicular epidermal areas. No precursor lesion has been identified [2–5].

BCC incidence is increasing worldwide: this trend has been exacerbated by further increase of both acute and prolonged exposure to the sunlight and the general population ageing. In addition a larger number of BCC diagnoses have been performed because of high individual sensibility to skin cancer prevention [6]. Despite low

R. Franco • A.M. Anniciello • G. Botti
Pathology Unit, National Institute
of Tumours Fondazione "G. Pascale",
Naples, Italy

M. Caraglia, MD, PhD(✉) • A. Luce
Department of Biochemistry and Biophysics,
Second University of Naples,
Via S.M. Costantinopoli, 16, Naples 80138, Italy
e-mail: michele.caraglia@unina2.it

mortality rates, BCC is associated with considerable morbidity and a significant burden for healthcare service [7].

BCCs are almost exclusively seen on hair-bearing skin. They occur rarely on the palms or on the soles, while its development on the mucous membrane is doubted [8]. BCC clinical presentation is generally a single lesion, although the presence of multiple lesions is not uncommon. Moreover, it is estimated that about 40 % of patients with one or more BCCs develop further BCCs within 10 years [9].

BCC seems to occur mainly in skin areas exposed to intense sun exposure and in sunburns before the age of 20, usually are diagnosed during adulthood, although they may be observed in children in specific clinical syndomes [10, 11]. In fact in the *unilateral basal cell nevus syndrome*, all lesions are present at birth [12]. Moreover, multiple BCCs could be observed in the rare *Gorlin-Goltz syndrome* which is a hereditary clinical condition characterised by a wide range of developmental abnormalities and predisposition to neoplasm [12, 13].

Epidemiology

The incidence and morbidity rates of BCC, squamous cell carcinoma and melanoma have been increasing in recent decades approximately of more than 4 % per year in all countries and social classes. It is estimated that approximately 50 % of fair-skinned individuals over 60 years old will develop some type of skin cancer [1, 14]. The higher incidence of such tumours is only partly justified by development of prevention campaigns of skin cancer, as well as greater attention of general practitioners to diagnosis and referral of patient. Men are more frequently affected than women, probably due to professional reasons [14].

BCC occurs more often in the elderly. In fact more than 50 % of the cases occur between 50 and 80 years of age. Moreover, an increasing incidence of BCC in individuals younger than 40 years has also been observed, accounting for more than 5 % of all diagnoses. There are

Table 5.1 BCC anatomic distribution in European patients

Author	Bernard [10]	Dessinotti [22]
Year/country	2008/France	2011/Greece
N	1,655	199
Head/neck	64.5 %	78 %
Trunk	25.1 %	15 %
Limbs	10.4 %	7 %

geographic variations in the incidence of BCC; in fact the incidence is higher in low latitudes, such as in some Australia regions (1,600/100,000 inhabitants/year) due to proximity to the Equator, than in Southern USA (300/100,000 inhabitants/year) and Europe (40–80/100,000 inhabitants/year) [1, 5, 15]. Two wide European series are reported in Table 5.1.

BCC is rarely described in black, Oriental and Hispanic people [16, 17]. In particular black people have a lower incidence of BCC in sun-exposed areas, but in unexposed skin regions, the incidence is similar to that observed in white people, being most of them of pigmented BCC subtype (>50 % of pigmented lesion as compared with 6 % in Caucasians) [7, 16, 18, 19].

Aetiology

The aetiology of BCC is still unclear, but its development seems to be related to combined contribution of endogenous and exogenous risk factors. Individual risk factors for BCC include gender, age, immunosuppression, genetic dysfunctions and pigmentary trait. Among exogenous risk factors, ultraviolet radiations (UVR) represent the primary established risk factor in BCC pathogenesis [20–23]. The relation between UV radiations and BCC development seems complex and remains highly controversial, with regard to the pattern of sun exposure and their occurrence in different period in life [18]. UVB radiation generates mutagenic photoproducts in DNA, such as cyclodipyrimidine dimers, and then mutations in specific genes related to critical cell functions, such as the p53 tumour suppressor gene. UVA rays have an indirect effect by generating cytotoxic and mutagenic free radicals, favouring the effect of UVB rays [20]. The mutagenic effects are directed also on critical genes, as p53 and PTCH1 [20, 22, 23]. Finally, UV rays have an indirect immunosuppressive action on the skin, harming the local antitumour monitoring activity of dendritic cell [12, 13]. Sun exposure, as predisposing factors, is particularly evident in patient with xeroderma pigmentosum, characterised by occurrence of multiple basal cell carcinoma and squamous cell carcinoma [12]. It has been also shown that occupational cumulative sun exposure is associated with BCC development in the older age group, whereas the prevalence of individuals with acute recreational sun exposure particularly in childhood and adolescence was significantly higher in the youngest age group of BCC [1, 24]. Prospective studies showed increased BCC risk with the number of sunburns after the age of 20 years old [10].

Additional factors favouring the development of both basal cell carcinoma and squamous cell carcinoma are large or numerous doses of roentgen rays, radiotherapy treatment, phototherapy (PUVA or UVB) and arsenic exposure [6, 16, 25–27] and, less commonly, burn scars and other scars. The role of dark hair dye colours, tobacco, alcohol, diets rich in fat and artificial tanning and photosensitising drugs in promoting BCC onset needs to be further clarified [26]. Thus, exposure to paraffin, coal, tar, pitch, industrial oils, agricultural chemicals, pesticides, ionising radiation and tattoos has been sporadically reported [24, 27–30]. The consumption of high daily doses of coffee (>6 cups) is associated with a reduction of up to 30 % in the prevalence of non-melanoma skin cancer in Caucasian women. Indeed, caffeine showed a photoprotective effect and reduced UVB-induced carcinogenesis by inducing apoptosis in the skin of mice. The same was observed in culture keratinocytes, in which caffeine increased the rate of apoptosis by inhibiting the ATR-Chk1 pathway [31–34].

The occurrence of consecutive BCCs is common, and the recurrence is more common in the first year. In 3 years the risk of a BCC patient to develop a further BCC ranges from 27 to 44 %, reaching 50 % in 5 years. Patients with more than ten BCCs have more than 90 % chance to develop a new lesion. Male patient older than 60 years, trunk localisation, superficial histological subtype and the presence of multiple actinic keratoses are predictive factors for the occurrence of new lesions [1, 5, 35, 36].

Pathogenesis

The Hedgehog Signalling Pathway in Gorlin-Goltz Syndrome: A Model of BCC Development

The Hedgehog signalling pathway is a well-conserved developmental pathway from insects to mammals [37]. Three homologues have been identified in humans, including the Sonic Hedgehog homologue (SHH), critical for the embryonic development and maintenance of the nervous system, axial skeleton, lungs, skin and hair. SHH is the ligand of a transmembrane receptor named PTCH1. The mechanism through which PTCH1 inhibits SHH signalling is complex [37]. PTCH1 represses the activity of the receptor Smoothened (SMO), which normally activates a family of transcription factors, termed glioma-associated transcription factors. Thus, the SMO protein, when unbound by PTCH, acts as a signal transducer, upregulating the expression of glioblastoma (GLI)1 and GLI2 signalling proteins, that eventuate in cell proliferation [38]. In addition Gli proteins control the expression of PTCH1, which provides a negative feedback of Hedgehog signalling, and GLI1 itself, which operates a positive feedback of Hedgehog ligand, thus regulating how much SHH is available to bind PTCH [39]. Upregulation of Gli proteins in BCC may play an important role in the initiation of BCC through the activation of the Bcl-2 gene [40, 41]. In addition GLI2 induces G1–S phase progression in contact-inhibited keratinocytes, apparently through the transcription factor E2F1 [42] (Fig. 5.1).

Almost invariably, BCCs in individuals with Gorlin-Goltz syndrome are caused by a mutation

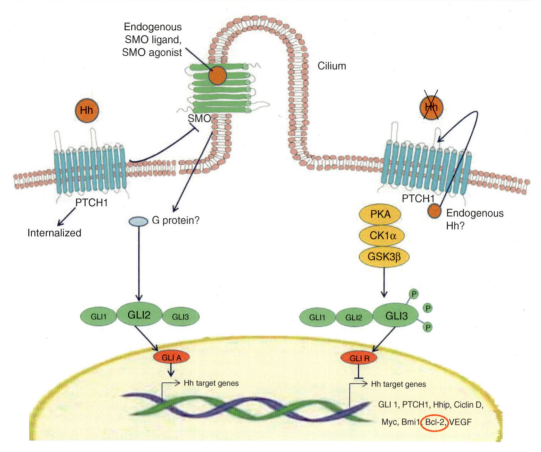

Fig. 5.1 Hedgehog pathway deregulation in BCC. Hedgehog signal transduction is induced by the patched 1 protein (PTCH) activated by the SHH ligand. Thus, binding of SHH to PTCH causes the loss of PTCH activity and the consequent activation of SMO, which transduces the SHH signal to the cytoplasm. Indeed, SHH signal is transmitted via GLI transcription factors, three separate zinc-finger proteins, GLI1 and GLI2 functioning as transcriptional activators and GLI3 as transcriptional repressor. SHH signalling cascade promotes generation of the activator GLIA, largely derived from GLI2, and the subsequent expression of a series of genes, especially Bcl-2. In the absence of a SHH ligand, PTCH blocks SMO activity, and full-length GLI proteins are processed to generate the repressor GLIR, largely contributed by GLI3 and the subsequent inhibition of SHH target gene transcription. Many drugs have been developed to control this pathway, which appears deregulated in many neoplasms, particularly for mutations occurring in PTCH and SMO proteins

of the PTCH1 gene [43]. In almost all BCCs, a constitutive SHH pathway activity is present, with 90 % exhibiting loss of PTCH1 and 10 % with activating mutations in SMO [44]. However, targeted expression of an activated *SMO* gene in mice model of BCC demonstrated that the neoplastic precursor was the resident progenitor cell of the interfollicular epidermis and upper infundibulum [5]. By contrast, in irradiated *PTCH1*+/− mice, BCC arose from stem cells of the follicular bulge [45]. The contrasting results are probably due to additional distinct functions of PTCH1 and SMO, influencing also tumourigenesis outside the SHH pathway. In fact PTCH1 can sequester cyclin B in the cytoplasm [46]. Furthermore, increasing SMO expression seems to be realised also by the loss of p53 functions [47]. Thus, the activation of the SHH pathway either through the loss of PTCH1 or through the expression of a mutated form of SMO is mechanistically distinct. Finally, although the SHH pathway can be activated in cells that do not

Fig. 5.2 Bcl-2 activation in Hedgehog pathway. Upregulation of Hedgehog pathway, through mutations of involved proteins, results in over-transcription of target genes, particularly Bcl-2, the most efficace antiapoptotic protein

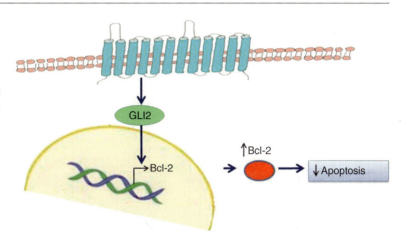

normally express SMO both through activated SMO overexpression and GLI2 overexpression, the loss of PTCH1 in cells that do not express SMO does not promote similar effects [45]. Finally, also deregulation of G1i2 expression could play a role in the tumour development. In fact increased GLI2 expression in skin stem cells promotes several tumours, depending on the cell of origin and GLI2 expression level [48].

Sporadic BCC

Deregulation of the SHH pathway is also frequently observed in the sporadic BCC. In fact mutations of SMOH or PTCH were reported in most sporadic BCCs, also induced by UVB [49, 50]. The overexpression of Bcl2, main target of SHH pathway, has been widely demonstrated in sporadic BCCs, particularly in indolent-growth subtypes (i.e. superficial and nodular BCCs) [51] (Fig. 5.2). Thus, Bcl-2-induced immortalisation of progenitor epithelia of the hair follicle and the inter-follicular epidermis through Bcl-2 predisposes to subsequent mutagenic 'hits' from UV light, particularly mutagenesis of p53, mainly observed in aggressive variants of BCC [52] (Fig. 5.3).

In fact p53 mutations have been documented in more than 40 % of aggressive BCCs; occurring in sun-exposed areas, 72 % of the mutations bear the signature of UV light induction [50]. Loss of basement membrane material around tumour cell nests signs the passage from indolent to aggressive BCC growth [52]. The activation of matrix metalloproteinases in this process of transformation guarantees the digestion of basal lamina around tumour nests, promoting the elaboration and/or release of cytokines, also inducing neoplastic cell proliferation [52].

Finally, BCC occurrence after solid organ transplant is significantly higher compared to the remaining population. In addition, in these patients a high frequency of aggressive histotypes and an increased tendency to recurrence and metastasis have been found [53–56]. The pathogenesis of post-transplant BCCs seems to be related to not known virus; in fact herpes virus-like DNA sequences have been demonstrated in some of these cases [53, 54].

Clinical Presentation

BCCs may have varying sizes from few millimetres to several centimetres. The most common site of occurrence is the head and neck district (Table 5.1). Clinically, five different presentations related to specific histopathological pattern have been described: (1) an opalescent or 'pearly' firm nodule, often with adjacent telangiectatic blood vessel, often observed in nodular basal cell carcinoma; (2) a scaly, erythematous, flat lesion with a distinct, sometimes 'pearl', border, observed in superficial basal cell carcinoma; (3) a flat lesion, sometimes depressed, white plaque with adjacent erythema in morphoeic basal cell carcinoma

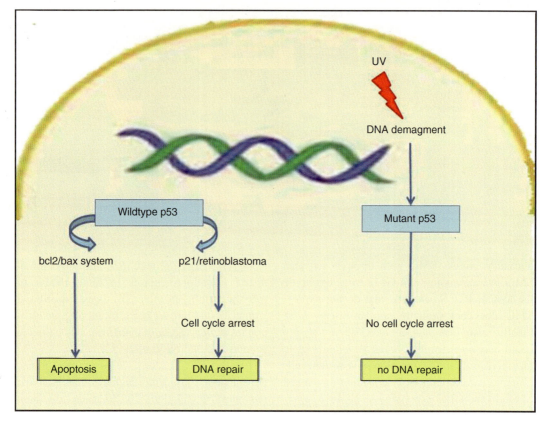

Fig. 5.3 UV light-induced mutant p53. Mutant p53 does not arrest cell cycle, consequently to sublethal genotoxic injury. In consequence, DNA repair does not occur and cells cumulate further genomic instabilities leading to an enhanced malignant potential

(this appearance is similar to lesion of morphoea); (4) depigmented subtype, morphologically similar to the nodular with sclerodermiform features and (5) a pink- or flesh-coloured nodule with a constricted inferior margin suggesting a seborrhoeic keratosis in fibroepithelioma, a rare form of BCC preferably located in the lumbosacral, pubic of genitocrural region [57–59].

The tumoural growth is generally slow, but rapid enlargement with ulceration and bleeding could occur. Local infiltration of perilesional extracutaneous tissues is rarely observed, dependent on tumoural anatomic sites, but metastasis is rarely recorded. Clinical differential diagnosis with other cutaneous tumours arises and only histological examination categorises the lesions correctly. For example, extensive pigmentation in BCC can be interpreted as a malignant melanoma.

Histopathology

Several histological subtypes of BCC are distinguished, and such a variety is related to the fact that basal cells can differentiate in both epidermis and adnexal structures.

BCC can be divided into two groups: undifferentiated and differentiated. The differentiated BCCs show a slight degree of differentiation toward the cutaneous appendage. However, a clear cut between the two groups cannot be made, because many undifferentiated basal cell carcinomas show focal differentiation in some areas and most differentiated basal cell carcinomas show areas lacking differentiation.

Some specific features are quite common to all BCC subtypes. Thus, six histological features are generally found in all BCCs: (1) *nests of basaloid cell*, resembling the epidermal basal row keratinocytes; (2) *peripheral palisading of the nests*, an expression of residual polarity of the tumoural basal cell; (3) *high mitotic rate*; (4) *individual necrotic keratinocytes*; (5) an unusual *cellular stroma composed of spindle cell* in a mucinous matrix with fine collagen fibrils and many mast cells; and (6) *cleft formation*, separating tumoural nests from their stroma, attributable to collagenase activity, mucin deposition and a reduction in the number of hemidesmosomes [60]. Some of these features can be attenuated in specific variants.

Additional common features are keratinisation and pigmentation. Pigmentation attributable to the proliferation of dendritic, heavily pigmented melanocytes along with the keratinocytes and the transfer of pigment also to neoplastic keratinocytes is mainly observed in superficial basal cell carcinoma [61].

The stroma is a determinant for BCC development, as it survives only when a broad representation of the stroma is present; for this reason the palms of the hands and soles of the feet will most likely not contain the elements necessary for the development of neoplasia. Stroma closed to tumoural nests contains many young fibroblasts, and areas of retraction of the stroma from the tumour island result in peritumoural lacunae.

BCC can be also found in clinical syndromes. The multiple basal cell carcinomas seen in the nevoid basal cell carcinoma syndrome (Gorlin-Goltz syndrome) present no distinctive features compared to ordinary basal cell carcinoma, even while they are still in the early nevoid stage and have not yet become invasive and destructive [62]. The BCCs encountered in the *Bazex syndrome* have a variable histological appearance. Some of them are indistinguishable from trichoepithelioma [52, 63]. Table 5.2 reports the frequency of the most common subtypes in two wide European series.

Undifferentiated BCCs

Among undifferentiated BCCs, two clinical groups can be considered, i.e. indolent-growth variants, as *superficial BCC* and *nodular BCC*, and aggressive variants, as *infiltrative BCC*,

Table 5.2 BCC histological subtypes in European patients

	Betti [7]	Scrivener [3]
Year/country	1995/Italy	2002/France
N	693	13,457
Solid/pigmented/adenoid	64.8 %	78.7 %
Infiltrative/sclerosing	16.6 %	15.1 %
Superficial	17.5 %	6.2 %
Mixed	NC	NC

NC unclassified

metatypical BCC and *morpheiform or sclerosing BCC* [52] (Figs. 5.4 and 5.5).

Superficial BCC is constituted by superficial basal keratinocyte nests, closed to epidermis or follicular epithelium, projecting through the papillary dermis. The peripheral cell layer of the tumour formation often shows palisading. The overlying epidermis usually shows atrophy. Fibroblast, often in a fairly large number, is arranged around the tumour cell proliferations [52].

Nodular BCC represents the most common subtypes of BCC and is characterised by discrete large or small nests of basaloid cells in either the papillary or reticular dermis. Adenoid features could be observed in nodular BCC [52, 57].

Infiltrative BCC is constituted by irregularly sized, angulated nests of tumour cells; a frequent mitotic activity and individual cell necrosis of the neoplastic cells. They can rapidly extend to subcutis and adjacent muscular and other structures [61].

Morpheiform or sclerosing BCC is characterised by columns of basaloid cells one to two cells thick, sparse in a densely collagenised stroma containing fibroblasts [58].

Two types of *metatypical BCC* are recognised: a mixed and an intermediary type. The mixed type is described as showing focal keratinisation, consisting of pearl with a colloidal or parakeratotic centre, and the intermediary type as showing two kinds of cells within a network of narrow strands, an outer row of dark-staining basal cell and an inner layer of larger cells, with intermediate features between basal cell and squamous cells [64, 65]. Metatypical BCCs are considered by some authors a transition from BCC to squamous cell carcinoma. Extensive squamous cell differentiations make the cancer more aggressive, with higher metastasis tendency

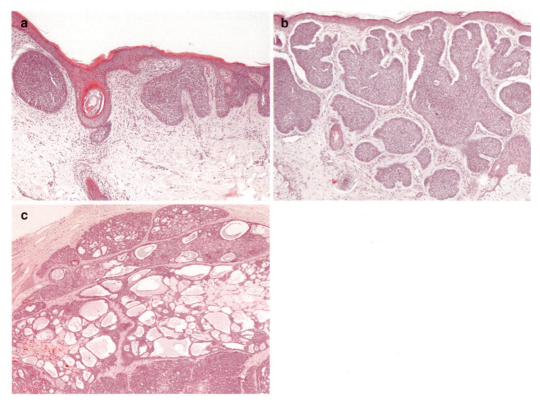

Fig. 5.4 Undifferentiated indolent BCC subtypes. (**a**) Superficial BBC is characterised by nests connected to epidermal surface (H&E 10×); (**b**) nodular BCC is characterised by nodular nests sparsed in the dermis (H&E 10×); (**c**) adenoid-cystic areas could be observed in nodular BCC (H&E 10×)

compared to classic variations of BCC [60, 64, 65]. Other authors considered this assumption erroneous, since different geneses of squamous cell carcinoma, a true anaplastic carcinoma of the epidermis, and BCC, a tumour composed of immature rather than anaplastic cells, make the occurrence of transitional forms quite unlikely. In this view it can be considered that so-called mixed types of metatypical BCC represent a keratotic basal cell carcinoma (see below) and that the intermediate types represent a basal cell carcinoma with differentiation into two types of cells (basal cell carcinoma with squamous differentiation) [60, 64].

Differentiated BCCs

Differentiated BCC subtypes are *keratotic BCC, infundibulocystic BCC, follicular BCC, pleomorphic BCC, BCC with sweat duct differentiation, BCC with sebaceous differentiation* and *fibroepithelioma of Pinkus* (Fig. 5.6). *Keratotic BCC* shows parakeratotic cells and horn cysts in addition to undifferentiated cells. The parakeratotic cells contain elongated nuclei in concentric whorls, or around the horn cysts. It is likely that they are cells with initial keratinisation somewhat similar to the nucleated cells in the keratogenic zone of normal hair shafts. The horn cysts, which are composed of fully keratinised cells, represent attempts of hair shaft formation [66].

In the *infundibulocystic BCC*, proliferating basaloid cells, typically in continuity with the overlying epidermis, proliferate as typical oblong nests surrounding keratin-filled structures. The tumour nests show a progressive squamoid differentiation lined by palisading cells and melanic pigmentation [67].

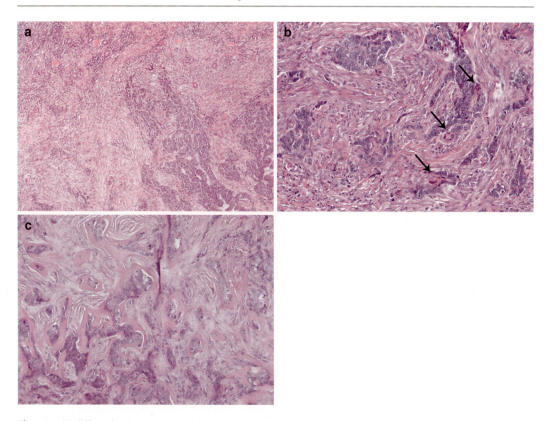

Fig. 5.5 Undifferentiated aggressive BCC subtypes. (**a**) Infiltrative BCC is characterised by angulated nests of tumour cells (H&E 20×); (**b**) focal squamous cell differentiation in metatypical BCC (*arrows*) (H&E 40×); (**c**) dense collagenised stroma in morpheiform BCC (H&E 10×)

On occasion, a BCC will show matrical differentiation, resulting in *follicular BCC* and resembling pilotricoma [68].

Some BCCs, particularly of nodular architecture, contain giant hyperchromatic nuclei, defining the subtype termed *pleomorphic BCC* or "basal cell epithelioma" with monster cells [69].

BCC with sweat duct differentiation shows in nodular BCC typical eccrine, and sometimes apocrine, differentiation with tubules lined by the cuboidal epithelium [70, 71]. Finally, the *BCC with sebaceous differentiation* is characterised by germinative cells representing more than 50 % of the transverse diameter of tumour lobules with sebocytes [72]. In fibroepithelioma of Pinkus, long thin branching, anastomosing strands of basal cell carcinoma are embedded in a fibrous stroma. Many of the strands show connections with the surface epidermis. Usually, the tumour is quite superficial and is well demarcated at its lower border. Fibroepithelioma combines features of the intracanalicular fibroadenoma of the breast, the reticulated types of seborrhoeic keratosis and superficial basal cell carcinoma [73]. Fibroepithelioma can change into an invasive and ulcerating basal cell carcinoma [74].

Histological uncommon variants are adamantinoid BCC, granular BCC and clear cell BCC. Adamantinoid BCC shows intercellular spaces were widened and cells were connected by stellate appendages [75]. The granular cell BCC shows in their cytoplasm numerous eosinophilic granules with tendency to coalesce [76, 77]. The clear cells contain vacuoles of different sizes filled with glycogen [78].

Some histological features represent relevant predictors of local recurrence, besides positive margins of resection. Morpheiform, infiltrating and metatypical features, poorly formed peripheral palisades, high degree of nuclear pleomorphism

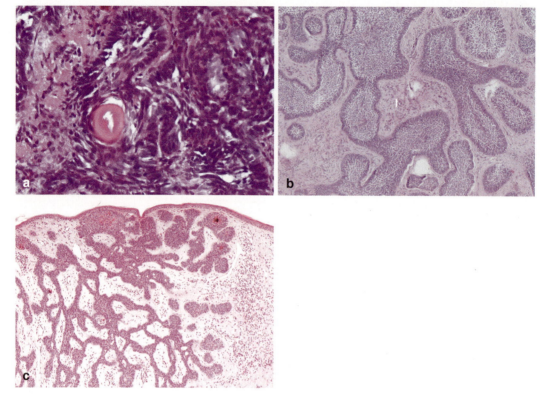

Fig. 5.6 Differentiated BCC subtypes. (**a**) Keratin formation in keratosis BCC (H&E 40×); (**b**) proliferating oblong nests in infundibulocystic BCC (H&E 20×); (**c**) long thin branching, anastomosing strands in Pinkus fibroepithelioma (H&E 10×)

and the perineural invasion represent high-risk features suggesting potential local recurrence [79].

Treatments

Surgical Management

The most commonly used treatments of BCCs are currently surgical-based.

The *surgical excision of BCCs with predetermined margins* guarantees a general control of more than 90 % of cases. In cases with positive margins, the re-excision not always contains residual tumours. In fact in a series of 74 patients, residual tumour has been observed in just 54 % of re-excised tissues [80]. In addition, the recurrence rates in studies with a 5-year follow-up of incomplete excision cases ranged from 21 to 41 % [81, 82]. Generally standard surgical excision with at least 3 mm of margins is considered a good treatment for all BCCs, arising with 5-year recurrence rates of anything up to 10 % [83].

Mohs micrographic surgery (MMS) provides an intraoperative control of margin status. Studies and reviews have found a 5-year cure rate of more than 90 % for primary tumours and for recurrent disease that are recorded for this type of treatment [84–87].

Curettage is widely used in the management of BCC. A preoperative biopsy is needed for the confirmation of clinical diagnosis of BCC. For standard curettage and electrocautery of lesions, recurrence rates have been reported to be between 7.7 and 19 % at 5 years [88, 89]. Cryosurgery involves the destruction of tissue using liquid nitrogen. Also in this case, it is advisable to biopsy first to confirm the diagnosis and determine the histological subtype. Recurrence rate in expert hands is generally very low [90].

Carbon dioxide laser ablation has also been used in the treatment of BCCs [83].

Nonsurgical Management

Radiotherapy can be used to treat primary, recurrent or incompletely excised BCCs, with a cure rate of more than 90 % for most skin lesions [91].

Imiquimod is an immune response modifier, binding to toll-like receptor. The effectiveness of imiquimod is induction of proinflammatory cytokines and subsequent cytotoxic T cell-mediated cell death. The use is suggested for superficial BCCs. Vehicle-controlled studies in the treatment of small BCC have reported reasonable results. A prospective study of 182 patients who received topical imiquimod applied 5×/week for 6 weeks gave clearance rates of 69 % at 5 years [92, 93]. Photodynamic therapy (PDT) causes the destruction of sensitised cells by an irradiating light source. Either 5-aminolevulinic acid (ALA) or methyl aminolevulinic (MAL) could be applied as prodrug to the skin. This is converted into protoporphyrin IX by the tumour cells. In the presence of intense red or blue light, a cytotoxic reaction occurs with reactive oxygen in the cell membranes of tumour cells containing protoporphyrin IX, and so the tumour cells die. This treatment in superficial BCCs has recorded a clearance of 87 % [94].

5-Fluorouracil is a fluorinated pyrimidine that blocks the methylation reaction of deoxyuridylic acid to thymidylic acid, destabilising DNA. It is sometimes used to treat small and superficial BCCs on low-risk sites [83]. Electrochemotherapy provides delivery into cells of non-permeant drugs with intracellular targets, as bleomycin and cisplatin. It is based on the local application of short and intense electric pulses that transiently permeabilise cell membrane. ECT has already been proven to be effective in diverse tumour histotypes, including basal cell carcinoma, with a good safety profile. ECT can be proposed as locoregional therapy for disseminated cutaneous lesions as alternative treatment strategy or as palliative care, in order to improve patients' quality of life [95].

Finally, molecular target therapies have been proposed. Since PDGFRα has been reported in BCCs to target molecules downstream the SHH signalling, the use of approved drugs inhibiting this receptor kinase, as sorafenib and imatinib, would be theoretically useful [96]. The combination of paclitaxel and carboplatin has been reported as effective for locally uncontrollable BCCs [97].

The interest for development of SHH inhibitors (SHHIs) has been generated by the evidence for SHH activation in many types of visceral cancers. Thus, uncontrollable BCCs represent potential targets for trials of SHHIs. The plant alkaloid cyclopamine is the first well-documented SHHI [98]. The topical application of cyclopamine promoted the regression of four sporadic BCCs [99]. Cyclopamine effectiveness is related to inhibition of SMO signalling, through direct binding to the protein [100–103]. In a phase 1 trial, GDC-0449, a selective inhibitor of SHH pathway, caused clinical response in eight out of nine patients with metastatic or locally advanced BCCs when administered orally [104]. The practical barriers to the development and use of HHIs in localised BCCs include the high cure rate with surgery, despite the unattractive aspects of such procedures described earlier.

Glossary

ALA-5	Aminolevulinic acid
BCC	Basal cell carcinoma
ECT	Electrochemotherapy
GLI	Glioblastoma
MAL	Methyl aminolevulinic
MMS	Mohs micrographic surgery
PDT	Photodynamic surgery
SHH	Sonic Hedgehog homologue
SMO	Smoothened
UV	Ultraviolet

References

1. Garner KL, Rodney WN. Basal and squamous cell carcinoma. Prim Care. 2000;27(2):447–58.
2. Roewert-Huber J, Lange Asschnfeldt B, Stockfleth E, et al. Epidemiology and aetiology of basal cell carcinoma. Br J Dermatol. 2007;157 Suppl 2:47–51.
3. Scrivener Y, Grosshans E, Cribier B. Variations of basal cell carcinomas according to gender, age, location and histopathological subtypes. Br J Dermatol. 2002;147:41–7.
4. Skelton LA. The effective treatment of basal cell carcinoma. Br J Nurs. 2009;18:346–50.
5. Youssef KK, Van Keymeullen A, Lapounge G, et al. Identification of the cell lineage at the origin of basal cell carcinoma. Nat Cell Biol. 2010;12:299–305.
6. Lear JT, Harvey I, de Berker D, Strange RC, Fryer AA. Basal cell carcinoma. J R Soc Med. 1998;91:585–8.
7. Betti R, Inselvini E, Carducci M, Crosti C. Age and site prevalence of histologic subtypes of basal cell carcinomas. Int J Dermatol. 1995;34(3):174–6.
8. Fusaro RM, Gol RW. Histochemically demonstrable carbohydrates of appendageal tumor of the skin. II. Benign apocrine gland tumor. J Invest Dermatol. 1962;38:37.
9. Armstrong BK, Kricker A. The epidemiology of UV induced skin cancer. J Photochem Photobiol B. 2001;63:8–18.
10. Bernard P, Dupuy A, Brun P, et al. Therapeutic modalities and economic assessment in the treatment of superficial basal cell carcinomas and multiple actinic keratoses by French dermatologists. Ann Dermatol Venereol. 2007;134(6–7):527–33.
11. Han J, Coldtz G, Hunter DJ. Risk factor for skin cancer: a nested casa control study within the Nurses Health study. Int J Epidemiol. 2006;35:1514–21.
12. Madan V, Hoban P, Stange RC, Fryer AA, Lear JT. Genetic and risk factor basal cell carcinoma. Br J Dermatol. 2006;154 Suppl 1:5–7.
13. Greinert R. Skin cancer: new marker for better prevention. Pathobiology. 2009;76:64–81.
14. Dipgen TL, Mattedi V. The epidemiology of skin cancer. Br J Dermatol. 2002;146 Suppl 61:1–6.
15. Bastiaens MT, Hoefnagel JJ, Bruin JA, et al. Differences in age, site, distribution and sex between nodular and superficial basal cell carcinoma indicate different types of tumors. J Invest Dermatol. 1998;110(6):880–4.
16. Vlajinac HD, Adanja BJ, Lazzar ZF, et al. Risk factors for basal cell carcinoma. Acta Oncol. 2000;39:611–6.
17. Gohara MA. Skin cancer in skins of color. J Drugs Dermatol. 2008;7:441–5.
18. Gloster Jr HM, Brodland DG. The epidemiology of skin cancer. Dermatol Surg. 1996;22:217–26.
19. Pennello G, Devesa S, Gail M. Association of surface ultraviolet B radiation levels with melanoma and non-melanoma skin cancer in United States blacks. Cancer Epidemiol Biomarkers Prev. 2000;9(3):291–7.
20. Dessinotti C, Antoniou C, Katsambas A, et al. Basal cell carcinoma: what's new under the sun. Photochem Photobiol. 2010;86:481–91.
21. Miller A, Tsao H. New insights into pigmentary pathways and skin cancer. Br J Dermatol. 2010;162:22–8.
22. Dessinotti C, Stratigos AJ, Rigopoupulos DAJ, et al. A review of genetic disorders of hypopigmentation: lessons learned from the biology of melanocytes. Exp Dermatol. 2009;18:741–9.
23. Hafner C, Landthaler M, Vogt T. Activation of the PI3K/AKT signalling pathway in non melanoma skin cancer is not mediated by oncogenic PIK3CA and AKT1 hotspot mutations. Exp Dermatol. 2010;19:e222–7.
24. Goldberg LH. Basal cell carcinoma. Lancet. 1996;347:663–7.
25. Hoban PR, Ramachandran S, Strange RC. Environment, phenotype and genetic: risk factors associated with BCC of the skin. Expert Rev Anticancer Ther. 2002;2:570–9.
26. Karagas MR, Nelson HH, Zencell MS, et al. Squamous and basal cell carcinoma of the skin in relation to radiation therapy and potential modification of risk by sun exposure. Epidemiology. 2007;18:776–84.
27. Cabrera HN, Gomez ML. Skin cancer induced by arsenic in the water. J Cutan Med Surg. 2003;7:106–11.
28. Ozyazgan I, Kontas O. Previous injuries or scars as risk factor for the development of basal cell carcinoma. Scand J Plast Reconstr Surg Hand Surg. 2004;38:11–5.
29. Spiewak R. Pesticides as cause of occupational skin disease in farmer. Ann Agric Environ Med. 2001;8:1–5.
30. Fredman DM, Sigurdson A, Dody MM, Mabuchi K, Linet MS. Risk of basal cell carcinoma in relation to alcohol intake and smoking. Cancer Epidemiol Biomarkers Prev. 2003;12:1540–3.
31. Sahl WJ, Glore S, Garrison P, Oakleaf K, Johnson SD. Basal cell carcinoma and lifestyle characteristics. Int J Dermatol. 1995;34:398–402.
32. Heffernan TP, Kawasumi M, Blasina A, Anderes K, Conney AH, Nghiem P. ATR-Chk1 pathway inhibition promotes apoptosis after UV treatment in primary human keratinocytes potential basis for the UV protective effects of caffeine. J Invest Dermatol. 2009;129:1805–15.
33. Lu YP, Lou YR, Xie JG, Peng QY, Zhou S, Lin Y, et al. Caffeine and caffeine sodium benzoate have a sunscreen effect, enhance UVB-induced apoptosis, and inhibit UVB-induced skin carcinogenesis in SKH-1 mice. Carcinogenesis. 2007;28:199–206.
34. Abel EL, Hendrix SO, McNeeley SG, Johnson KC, Rosenberg CA, Mossavar-Rahmani Y, et al. Daily coffee consumption and prevalence of nonmelanoma skin cancer in Caucasian women. Eur J Cancer Prev. 2007;16:446–52.
35. Martin RC, Edwards MJ, Cawte MJ, et al. Basosquamous carcinoma. Analysis of prognostic factors influencing recurrence. Cancer. 2000;88(6):1365–9. 136–42.

36. Richmond-Sinclair NM, Pandey N, Williams GM, Neale RE, van der Pols JC, Green AC. Clinical signs of photodamage are associated with basal cell carcinoma multiplicity and site: a 16 year longitudinal study. Int J Cancer. 2010;127:2622–9.

37. Hooper JE, Scott MP. Communicating with Hedgehogs. Nat Rev Mol Cell Biol. 2005;6:306–7.

38. Tang JY, So P-L, Epstein Jr EH. Novel Hedgehog pathway targets against basal cell carcinoma. Toxicol Appl Pharmacol. 2007;224:257–64.

39. Xie J, Murone M, Luoh SM, et al. Activating Smoothened mutations in sporadic basal-cell carcinoma. Nature. 1998;391:90–2.

40. Tojo M, Kiyosawa H, Iwatsuki K, et al. Expression of the GLI2 oncogene and its isoforms in human basal cell carcinoma. Br J Dermatol. 2003;148:892–7.

41. Hatta N, Hirano T, Kimura T, et al. Molecular diagnosis of basal cell carcinoma and other basaloid cell neoplasms of the skin by the quantification of GLI1 transcript levels. J Cutan Pathol. 2005;32:131–6.

42. Regl G, Kasper M, Schnidar H, et al. The zinc-finger transcription factor GLI2 antagonizes contact inhibition and differentiation of human epidermal cells. Oncogene. 2004;23:1263–74.

43. Johnson R, Rothman A, Xie J, et al. Human homolog of patched a candidate gene for the basal cell nevus syndrome. Science. 1996;272:1668–71.

44. Epstein EH. Basal cell carcinomas: attack of the hedgehog. Nat Rev Cancer. 2008;8:743–54.

45. Wang GY, Wang J, Mancianti ML, Epstein Jr EH. Basal cell carcinoma arise from hair follicle stem cells in PTCH1+/− mice. Cancer Cell. 2011;19:114–24.

46. Barnes EA, Kong M, Ollendorff V, Donoghue DJ. Patched1 interacts with cyclin B1 to regulate cell cycle progression. EMBO J. 2001;20:2214–23.

47. Wetmore C, Eberhart DE, Currann T. Loss of p53 but not ARF accelerates medulloblastoma in mice heterozygous for patched. Cancer Res. 2001;61:513–6.

48. Grachtchouk M, Pero J, Yang SH, et al. Basal cell carcinomas in mice arise from hair follicle stem cells and multiple epithelial progenitor populations. J Clin Invest. 2011;121:1768–81.

49. Reifenberger J, Wolter M, Weber RG, et al. Missense mutations in SMOH in sporadic basal cell carcinomas of the skin and primitive neuroectodermal tumors of the central nervous system. Cancer Res. 1998;58:1798–803.

50. Reifenberger J, Wolter M, Knobbe SB, et al. Somatic mutations in the PTCH, SMOH, SUFUH and TP53 genes in sporadic basal cell carcinomas. Br J Dermatol. 2005;152:43–51.

51. Crowson AN, Magro CM, Kadin M, et al. Differential expression of Bcl-2 oncogene in human basal cell carcinoma. Hum Pathol. 1996;27:355–9.

52. Crowson AN. Basal cell carcinoma: biology, morphology and clinical implications. Mod Pathol. 2006;19:S127–47.

53. Bavinck JNB, de Boer A, Vermeer BJ, et al. Sunlight, keratotic skin lesions and skin cancer in renal transplant recipients. Br J Dermatol. 1993;129:242–9. 91.

54. Rady RL, Yen A, Rollefson JL, et al. Herpes virus-like DNA sequences in non-Kaposi's sarcoma skin lesions of transplant patients. Lancet. 1995;345:1339–40.

55. Sitz KV, Keppen M, Johnson DF. Metastatic basal cell carcinoma in acquired immunodeficiency syndrome related complex. JAMA. 1987;257:340–3.

56. Oram Y, Orengo I, Griego RD, et al. Histologic patterns of basal cell carcinoma based upon patient immunostatus. Dermatol Surg. 1995;21:611–4.

57. Aoyagi S, Nouri K. Difference between pigmented and nonpigmented basal cell carcinoma treated with Mohs micrographic surgery. Dermatol Surg. 2006;32:1375–9.

58. Betti R, Gualandri L, Cerri A, et al. Clinical features and histologic pattern analysis of pigmented basal cell carcinoma in an Italian population. J Dermatol. 1998;25:691–4.

59. Mc Nuth NS. Ultrastructural comparison of the interface between epithelium and stroma in basal cell and control human skin. Lab Invest. 1976;35:132.

60. Farmer ER, Helwing EB. Metastatic basal cell carcinoma: a clinicopathologic study of seventeen cases. Cancer. 1980;46:748.

61. Howell JB. The basal cell nevus. Arch Dermatol. 1959;79:67.

62. Viksnis P, Berlin A. Follicular atrophoderma and basal cell carcinoma. Arch Dermatol. 1977;113:948.

63. Pilosila M, Kiistala R, Niemi KM, et al. The Bazex syndrome: follicular atrophoderma with multiple basal cell carcinoma, hypotricosis and hypohidrosis. Clin Exp Dermatol. 1981;89:598.

64. Mongomery H. Basal squamous cell epithelioma. Arch Dermatol Syph. 1928;18:50.

65. Borel DM. Cutaneous basosquamous carcinoma: review of the literature and report of 35 cases. Arch Pathol. 1973;95:293.

66. Foot NC. Adnexal carcinoma of the skin. Am J Pathol. 1947;23:1.

67. Kato N, Ueno H. Infundibulocystic basal cell carcinoma. Am J Dermatopathol. 1993;15:265–7.

68. Ali F, Brown A, Gottwald L, et al. Basal cell carcinoma with matrical differentiation in a transplant patient: a case report and review of the literature. J Cutan Pathol. 2005;32:445–8.

69. Elston DM, Bergfeld WF, Petroff N. Basal cell carcinoma with monster cells. J Cutan Pathol. 1993;20:70–3.

70. Hanke CW, Temofeew RK. Basal cell carcinoma with eccrine differentiation (eccrine epithelioma). J Dermatol Surg Oncol. 1986;12:820–4.

71. Misago N, Satoh T, Narisawa Y. Basal cell carcinoma with ductal and glandular differentiation: a clinicopathological and immunohistochemical study of 10 cases. Eur J Dermatol. 2004;14:383–7.

72. Misago N, Mihara I, Ansai S-I, et al. Sebaceoma and related neoplasms with sebaceous differentiation. Am J Dermatopathol. 2002;24:294–304.
73. Pinkus H. Premalignant fibroepithelial tumors of the skin. Arch Dermatol Syph. 1953;67:598.
74. Pinkus H. Epithelial and fibroepithelial tumors. Arch Dermatol. 1965;91:24–37.
75. Lerchin E, Rahbari H. Adamantinoid basal cell epithelioma. Arch Dermatol. 1975;111:1064.
76. Barr RJ, Graham JH. Granular basal cell carcinoma. Arch Dermatol. 1979;115:1064.
77. Mrak RE, Baker GF. Granular basal cell carcinoma. J Cutan Pathol. 1987;14:37.
78. Barnadas MA, Freeman RG. Clear cell basal epithelioma. J Cutan Pathol. 1988;15:1.
79. Dixon AY, Lee SH, Mc Gragor DH. Factor predictive of recurrence of basal cell carcinoma. Am J Dermatopathol. 1989;11:222.
80. Griffiths RW. Audit of histologically incompletely excised basal cell carcinomas: recommendations for management by re-excision. Br J Plast Surg. 1999;52:24–8.
81. Wilson AW, Howsam G, Santhanam V, et al. Surgical management of incompletely excised basal cell carcinomas of the head and neck. Br J Oral Maxillofac Surg. 2004;42:311–4.
82. De Silva SP, Dellon AL. Recurrence rate of positive margin basal cell carcinoma: results of a five-year prospective study. J Surg Oncol. 1985;28:72–4.
83. Smith V, Walton S. Treatment of facial Basal cell carcinoma: a review. J Skin Cancer. 2011;2011:380371.
84. Malhotra R, Wennberg AM, Larko O, Stenquist B. Five-year results of Mohs' micrographic surgery for aggressive facial basal cell carcinoma in Sweden. Acta Derm Venereol. 1999;79:370–2.
85. Huilgol SC, Huynh NT, Selva D. The Australian Mohs database, part II: periocular basal cell carcinoma outcome at 5-year follow-up. Ophthalmology. 2004;111:631–6.
86. Wennberg M, Lark'o O, Stenquist B. Five-year results of Mohs' micrographic surgery for aggressive facial basal cell carcinoma in Sweden. Acta Derm Venereol. 1999;79:370–2.
87. Leibovitch SC, Huilgol Selva D, Richards S, Paver R. Basal cell carcinoma treated with Mohs surgery in Australia II. Outcome at 5-year follow-up. J Am Acad Dermatol. 2005;53:452–7.
88. Rowe DE, Carroll RJ, Day CL. Prognostic factors for local recurrence, metastasis, and survival rates in squamous cell carcinoma of the skin, ear, and lip. Implications for treatment modality selection. J Am Acad Dermatol. 1992;26(6):976–90.
89. Kopf W, Bart RS, Schrager D. Curettage electrodesiccation treatment of basal cell carcinomas. Arch Dermatol. 1977;113:439–43.
90. Kuflik EG. Cryosurgery for skin cancer: 30-year experience and cure rates. Dermatol Surg. 2004;30:297–300.
91. Rowe DE, Carroll RJ, Day CL. Long-term recurrence rates in previously untreated (primary) basal cell carcinoma: implications for patient follow-up. Dermatol Surg Oncol. 1989;15:315–28.
92. Geisse J, Caro I, Lindholm J, Golitz L, Stampone P, Owens M. Imiquimod 5 % cream for the treatment of superficial basal cell carcinoma: results from two phase III, randomized, vehicle-controlled studies. J Am Acad Dermatol. 2004;50:722–33.
93. Gollnick H, Barona C, Fra RGJ, et al. Recurrence rate of superficial basal cell carcinoma following successful treatment with imiquimod 5 % cream: interim 2-year results from an ongoing 5-year follow-up study in Europe. Eur J Dermatol. 2005;15:374–81.
94. Morton CA, McKenna KE, Rhodes LE. Guidelines for topical photodynamic therapy: update. Br J Dermatol. 2008;159:1245–66.
95. Testori A, Tosti G, Martinoli C, et al. Electrochemotherapy for cutaneous and subcutaneous tumor lesions: a novel therapeutic approach. Dermatol Ther. 2010;23:651–61.
96. Xie J, Aszterbaum M, Zhang X, et al. A role of PDGFRα in basal cell carcinoma proliferation. Proc Natl Acad Sci U S A. 2001;98:9255–9.
97. Carneiro BA, Watkin WG, Mehta UK, Brockstein BE. Metastatic basal cell carcinoma: complete response to chemotherapy and associated pure red cell aplasia. Cancer Invest. 2006;24:396–400.
98. Binns W, Jame LF, Shupe JL, Everett G. A congenital cyclopian-type malformation in lambs induced by maternal ingestion of a range plant. Veratrum californicum. Am J Vet Res. 1963;24:1164–75.
99. Tabs S, Avci O. Induction of the differentiation and apoptosis of tumor cells in vivo with efficiency and selectivity. Eur J Dermatol. 2004;14:96–102.
100. Cooper MK, Porte JA, Young KE. Beachy Teratogen-mediated inhibition of target tissue response to Shh signaling. Science. 1998;280:1603–7.
101. Incardona JP, Gaffield W, Kapur RP, Roelink H. The teratogenic Veratrum alkaloid cyclopamine inhibits sonic hedgehog signal transduction. Development. 1998;125:3553–62.
102. Chen JK, Taipale J, Cooper MK, Beachy PA. Inhibition of Hedgehog signaling by direct binding of cyclopamine to Smoothened. Genes Dev. 2002;16:2743–8.
103. Chen JK, Taipale J, Cooper MK, et al. Effects of oncogenic mutations in Smoothened and Patched can be reversed by cyclopamine. Nature. 2000;406:1005–9.
104. Van Hoff DD, et al. Efficacy data of GDC-0449, a systemic Hedgehog (Hh) pathway antagonist, in a first-in-human, first-in-class, phase I study with locally advanced, multifocal or metastatic basal cell carcinoma patients. Proceedings of the 99th annual meeting of the American Association for Cancer Research. 2008; abstract LB-138.

Skin Adnexal Tumours: A Large Spectrum of Clinic-Pathological Lesions

Renato Franco, Maria Elena Errico, Federica Zito Marino, Anna Maria Anniciello, Gerardo Botti, Michele Caraglia, and Anna Grimaldi

Key Points

- Skin adnexal tumours are usually classified according to the skin appendage origin.
- More than 80 entities have been described. Most skin adnexal tumours are benign, and sometimes, many different terms are often used to describe the same tumour.
- They are usually encountered as single, sporadic tumours, but they may occasionally be multiple, hereditary and indicative of clinical syndromes, including visceral neoplasms.
- Clinical diagnosis is impossible. Thus, surgical excision is always required.
- Pathological routine examination is generally adequate for their correct classifications, but sometimes histochemical and immunohistochemical stains may occasionally serve as ancillary tools.

R. Franco • F. Zito Marino • A.M. Anniciello • G. Botti
Pathology Unit, National Institute of Tumours
Fondazione "G. Pascale", Naples, Italy

M.E. Errico
Pathology Unit, Paediatric Hospital
Santobono-Pausilipon, Naples, Italy

M. Caraglia, MD, PhD(✉) • A. Grimaldi
Department of Biochemistry and Biophysics,
Second University of Naples,
Via S.M. Costantinopoli, 16, Naples 80138, Italy
e-mail: michele.caraglia@unina2.it

Introduction

Cutaneous adnexal tumours (CATs) are one of the most challenging areas of dermatopathology. It includes a series of several benign and malignant neoplasms, more than 80 in a recent count, with morphological differentiation towards one of the three types of adnexal epithelial cells, resident in the normal skin, i.e. pilosebaceous unit, eccrine and apocrine glands. In addition more than one line of differentiation in CAT could be observed. The histogenesis of such mixed adnexal tumours is still uncertain, but the origin from pluripotent stem cells seems to be the most reliable [1]. They are usually encountered as single sporadic tumours, but they may be multiple, suggesting genetic syndromes, including also visceral cancers [2]. Thus, sometimes the diagnosis of CAT may contribute to early detection of cancer-prone syndrome [3]. Most CATs have a benign behaviour. For this reason, local complete surgical excision is considered curative. However, for each described benign CAT, a malignant counterpart has been encountered. Malignant CATs are very rare but very aggressive neoplasms, with a poor clinical outcome.

Practically the diagnostic approach to CAT requires surgical excision of skin lesion, and the pathologist's attention should be primarily directed to the identification of lesion origin, pilosebaceous, eccrine or apocrine glands; then to the characterisation of lesion, benign or malignant; and finally to histotypisation. The

A. Baldi et al. (eds.), *Skin Cancer*, Current Clinical Pathology,
DOI 10.1007/978-1-4614-7357-2_6, © Springer Science+Business Media New York 2014

spectrum of pilosebaceous lesions is wide. The classification of cutaneous sweat gland tumours is very difficult, mainly because the pathogenesis and exact origin of many lesions is still under investigation [4, 5]. In addition an ambiguous terminology is used to describe the same lesion in this category, rendering further more difficult the correct classification.

In this chapter, we will provide information about each category, deserving special issue to the most common entities.

General Consideration for Diagnosis of CATs

Surgical excision is generally required for the diagnosis of skin tumours. In the cases of potential CATs, clinical information useful to correctly classify the lesions includes patient's age, sex, location(s) of the lesion, the rate of tumour growth, whether the lesion is solitary or multiple, and, if present, any associated inherited or systemic diseases. Histological features at haematoxylin and eosin (H&E)-stained sections are considered generally adequate for correct classification of SAT. Thus, when tumour cells are characterised by coarsely vacuolated cytoplasm and starry nuclei, they are indicative of sebaceous differentiation, whilst follicular differentiation in adnexal tumours is generally characterised by the presence of basaloid bulbar follicular germinative cells proliferation, peripheral nuclear palisading and adjacent papillary mesenchymal cells, matrical shadow (ghost) cells and tumour is attached to the normal follicular structures. Apocrine tumours could be suspected when tumour cells show abundant eosinophilic cytoplasm, decapitation secretion and eccentric nuclei. In some instances, histochemical and immunohistochemical stains are needed in the definition of CATs. Thus, immunohistochemistry could aid to define the origin of tumour cells. Indeed monoclonal CEA and EMA are expressed by tumours with ductal differentiation. GCDFP-15 and androgen receptors are observed in apocrine lesions, whilst oestrogen and progesterone receptors are

Table 6.1 Immunohistochemical features of pilar tumours

Pilar tumours
Pilar adenoma immunoprofile is similar to basal-cell carcinoma (BCC) of skin: epithelial membrane antigen (EMA), carcinoembryonic antigen, S100, CD15 and CA72.4 are negative
Desmoplastic trichoepithelioma versus infiltrative BCC: EMA, CD15, chromogranin, CK20; these markers are largely negative in invasive BCC
IBCC stromal cells are stromelysin-3+

Table 6.2 Immunohistochemical features of sebaceous tumours

Sebaceous tumours
Absent expression of S-100, CA72.4, GCDFP-15, CEA compared with sweat gland tumours, which are positive for these markers
Sebaceous and sweat gland tumours CD15+ and BerEP4+
EMA characteristic 'bubbly' cytoplasmic decoration

Table 6.3 Immunohistochemical features of sweat gland tumours

Sweat gland tumours
Express CK, CEA, CA72.4, CD15 and p63
Epithelial membrane antigen more common in malignant neoplasms
Eccrine carcinomas S-100+, apocrine S-100–, GCDFP-15+
Paget's disease: CK7+, GCDFP-15+, BerEP4+, CA72.4+
Malignant melanoma: negative for Paget's disease markers, HMB-45+, melan-A+, S-100+
Bowen disease: AE1/AE3 and K903+, negative for Paget's disease and melanoma markers

expressed in different sweat gland lesions [6] (Tables 6.1, 6.2 and 6.3).

The diagnosis of malignancy often offers difficulties to the pathologist. Generally benign lesions are multilobulated and symmetric with smooth borders. Thus, tumour cells are almost monomorphous and no necrosis is observed. Malignant features include asymmetrical growth, infiltrative borders, irregular arrangement of the neoplastic cells, cytonuclear atypia and increased mitotic activity. Tumour necrosis and superficial ulcerations are commonly seen. The patients should be closely followed up for potential regional and distant metastasis.

Pilosebaceous Tumours

Histology of Pilosebaceous Apparatus

Skin appendages derives from ectoderm and are localised in the superficial and deep dermis and in the epidermal tissue. Classically they are divided into three distinct structures: (1) the pilosebaceous unit, (2) the eccrine sweat glands and (3) the apocrine glands. The distribution of these structures varies dependently from skin anatomic area. The pilosebaceous units are constituted by hair follicle and connected sebaceous glands. The hair follicle develops from the epidermis, as a deep invagination, and it forms the hair. The lower portion of hair follicle is located in the reticular dermis and subcutaneous fat and is constituted by connective papilla enclosed in the hair bulb. The cells lining the dermal papilla are involved in forming the hair shaft and internal root sheath. All sebaceous glands are associated to follicle, with the exception of the labia minor and glans penis. They are lobular glands, constituted by sebocytes, i.e. cells containing lipid vacuoles and lined by a single layer of dark, germinative cells. The product of sebocytes converges in short duct till hair follicle [6].

Pilosebaceous Tumours Classification

Among pilosebaceous proliferations, three categories have been considered: hamartomatous proliferation, benign tumours and malignant tumours. In each one of the categories, sebaceous and pilar derivations have to be recorded (Table 6.4).

Hamartomatous Proliferation

Hamartomatous proliferations recognise different clinic-pathological often unrelated lesions of (1) pilar origin (basaloid follicular hamartoma, basaloid epidermal proliferation and the group of *trichofolliculoma-like lesions*, including trichofolliculoma, sebaceous trichofolliculoma, folliculosebaceous cystic hamartoma, trichodiscoma/fibrofolliculoma and pilar sheath acanthoma) and of (2) sebaceous origin

(sebaceous hyperplasia and nevus sebaceous of Jadassohn) (Fig. 6.1).

The inherited or acquired *basaloid follicular hamartomas* histologically consist of anastomosing strands, branching cords of small basaloid cells admixed with squamous cells, deriving from hair follicles. It is often associated to other clinical conditions such as myasthenia gravis, basal-cell carcinoma (BCC) and systemic lupus erythematosus and alopecia [7–9]. The *basaloid epidermal proliferation* is morphologically similar to BCC, but it overlies dermatofibroma [10]. The group of trichofolliculoma-like lesions includes very similar hamartomatous proliferations. *Trichofolliculomas* develop at any age in the face and it consists of keratin-filled, unilocular or multilocular cysts open to the epidermis; from this main cavity, variable numbers of sebaceous glands bud out and branches develop [11]. In the *sebaceous trichofolliculoma*, the tumour is characterised by sebaceous gland opening to the cyst cavity [12]. Hamartomatous cysts are not open to the overlaying epidermis in the *folliculosebaceous cystic hamartoma* [13]. *Pilar sheath acanthoma* histologically consists of superficial broad invagination producing a crater-like cavity [6]. Finally, *trichodiscoma/fibrofolliculoma* is characterised by dilated follicular infundibulum, from which there is a proliferation of thin, trabeculated strands of basophilic epithelium within fibrous stroma [14]. *Sebaceous hyperplasia* is constituted by immature sebocytes organised in five or more lobules of a sebaceous gland opening into a single dilated follicular infundibulum. It is observed in middle-aged and elderly individuals, generally to the forehead and cheeks, as a small, yellow papule. Multiple sebaceous lesions (hyperplasia, adenoma, sebaceoma and carcinoma) can be associated to Muir–Torre syndrome [15]. The *nevus sebaceous of Jadassohn* (NSJ) is observed at birth as solitary yellowish, waxy hairless plaques and as nodular lesion in adults. It generally occurs in the head and neck region. Histologically it is characterised by mature elements of all lines of sebaceous differentiation and shows a wide range of morphological features. A variety of benign and

Table 6.4 Pilosebaceous tumours distribution

Hyperplastic and hamartomatous lesions		Benign neoplasms		Malignant neoplasms	
Hair and hair follicle	Sebaceous glands	Hair and hair follicle	Sebaceous glands	Hair and hair follicle	Sebaceous glands
Basaloid follicular hamartoma	Sebaceous hyperplasia	Trichofolliculoma	Sebaceous adenoma	Trichilemmal carcinoma	Sebaceous carcinoma
Basaloid epidermal proliferation	Nevus sebaceous of Jodassohn	Desmoplastic trichoepithelioma	Sebaceoma/sebaceous epithelioma	Trichoblastic carcinoma	Basal-cell carcinoma with sebaceous differentiation
Overlying dermal mesenchymal lesions		Trichoblastoma		Malignant proliferating trichilemmal cyst	
Trichofolliculoma		Trichoblastic fibroma		Pilomatrix carcinoma	
Sebaceous trichofolliculoma		Trichoadenoma			
Folliculosebaceous cystic hamartoma		Proliferating trichilemmal cyst/pilar tumour			
Trichodiscoma/fibrofolliculoma		Trichilemmoma			
Pilar sheath acanthoma		Desmoplastic trichilemmoma			
		Pilomatricoma/proliferative pilomatricoma			

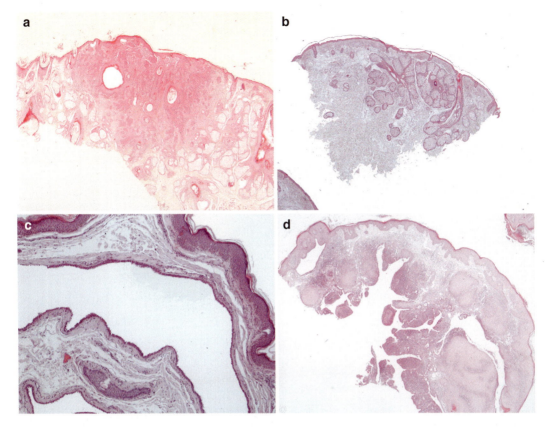

Fig. 6.1 Hamartomatous proliferation: (**a**) trichofolliculoma (H&E 2×), (**b**) sebaceous nevus (H&E 2×), (**c**) hidrocystoma (H&E 10×), (**d**) SCAT (H&E 2×)

malignant adnexal tumours have been described in association with NSJ. In a recent study of 596 cases of NSJ, malignancies were encountered in 1 % of cases, whereas benign skin tumours were identified in 13.6 % of cases of NSJ [16]. Allelic deletions of the human homologue of the Drosophila-patched gene are described in NSJ, justifying malignant tumours development within the lesions [17].

Benign and Malignant Pilosebaceous Tumours

Trichoepithelioma, Trichoadenoma and Desmoplastic Trichoepithelioma

Trichoepithelioma generally occurs in the head and neck region, as sporadic or as autosomal dominant disorder with multiple lesions (Fig. 6.2a). The gene related to Multiple Familial Trichoepithelioma (MFT) is probably CYLD located in the short arm of chromosome 9, in which several tumour-suppressor genes are located [18–20]. Histologically, trichoepithelioma is characterised by nests of uniform basaloid cells with peripheral palisading and formation of keratin cysts [21]. Rarely malignant trichoepithelioma have been reported [22]. Trichoadenoma is a rare benign follicular neoplasm characterised by proliferation of follicular germ with predominant keratin cysts and inconspicuous basaloid cells [6]. Desmoplastic trichoepithelioma (DTE) variant is characterised by compressed strands of basaloid germinative epithelium, with or without small horn cysts [23].

Trichoblastoma

Trichoblastoma develops in elderly individuals, commonly in the head and neck region [24]. Histologically it consists of nodules of cords and

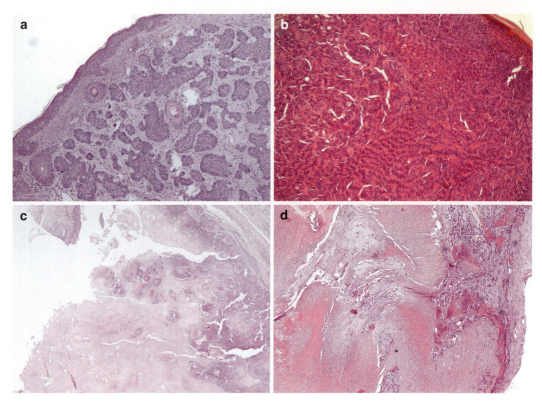

Fig. 6.2 Pilosebaceous benign tumors: (**a**) trichoepithelioma (H&E 10×), (**b**) trichoblastoma (H&E 20×), (**c**) pilar tumour (H&E 10×), (**d**) pilomatricoma (H&E 20×)

nests formed of solid basaloid germinative epithelial cells with peripheral palisading (Fig. 6.2b). Numerous melanocytes and melanin pigment are also frequently seen within the epithelial component [16]. Trichoblastic carcinoma is rarely described; it is a high-cellularity lesion with infiltration of underlying muscles [25].

Trichilemmoma

Trichilemmomas arise from the hair follicle outer root sheath, mainly of the bulb region. It develops in the face of adult individuals as solitary, small skin-coloured papule verrucous lesion. Multiple facial trichilemmomas are observed in Cowden syndrome (multiple hamartoma syndrome) [26] (Fig. 6.3a). Histologically, it consists of well-circumscribed and symmetric lesion connected to the epidermis, which show verruca vulgaris-like changes. Two forms are described: the prototypical early lesion with hyperplasia of the infundibular epithelium, with differentiation towards the outer root sheath, and the fully developed lesions

with lobules of uniform cells with clear cytoplasm and peripheral palisading pattern lobules. A desmoplastic trichilemmoma is also described [27]. Finally, very rare cases of trichilemmal carcinoma have been described [28] (Fig. 6.3b, c).

Proliferating Trichilemmal Cyst (Pilar Tumour)

Proliferating trichilemmal cyst (PTC) occurs on the scalps of elderly women, as nodulo-cystic lesion, usually ranging from 1 to 10 cm in diameter [29]. Histologically, PTC develops in the deep dermis and subcutaneous tissue, as well-defined, lobulated, solid and cystic mass of proliferating squamous epithelium, surrounded by thick hyalinised basement membrane (Fig. 6.2c). Malignant transformation is rarely described in PTC [30].

Pilomatricoma (Pilomatrixoma)

Pilomatricoma, or calcifying epithelioma of Malherbe, is a benign dermal and/or subcutaneous

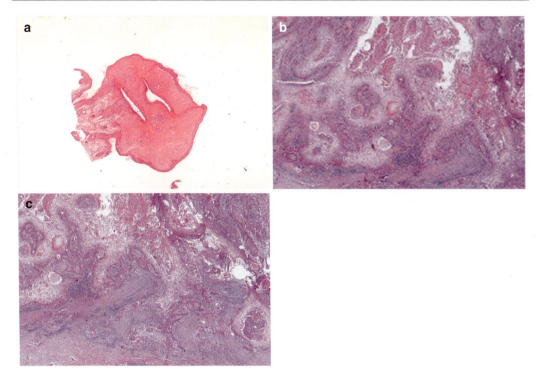

Fig. 6.3 Trichilemmal tumours: (**a**) trichilemmoma (H&E 2×), (**b**) trichilemmal carcinoma (H&E 20×), (**c**) trichilemmal carcinoma metastasis (H&E 20×)

tumour, most commonly observed in children and adolescents. Pilomatricoma is generally observed in the head and neck region and upper extremities. Multiple pilomatricomas are associated with different clinical syndromes, such as myotonic dystrophy Rubinstein–Taybi syndrome and Turner syndrome [31, 32]. Activation mutations of b-catenin are found in pilomatricoma [33]. Histologically pilomatricoma shows a well-circumscribed nodular lesion in the dermis and/or subcutis, surrounded by fibrous stroma, with early lesions characterised by basaloid cells lining a cystic cavity and contiguously transformed into nucleated shadow/ghost cells admixed with keratin and older lesions characterised by prominent shadow cell component, keratin debris and dystrophic calcification (Fig. 6.2d). Proliferating variant is characterised by prominent cellularity and scanty shadow cells. Pilomatrix carcinoma is a very rare tumour with high risk of local recurrence [34].

Sebaceous Neoplasms

Sebaceous adenoma occurs as dermal nodule. Histologically it shows lobules of predominate mature sebaceous cells and is peripherally located in germinal basaloid epithelial cells, with the absence of central draining duct. Sebaceoma is a histological variant of SA, with a prevalence of germinal basaloid epithelial cells and ductal differentiation. Also squamous metaplasia may rarely be seen.

Sebaceous carcinoma is frequently observed in the eyelid (ocular, palpebral sebaceous carcinoma), deriving from modified sebaceous gland, such as Meibomian glands or glands of Zeis, sometimes in the context of Muir–Torre syndrome. It is characterised by local recurrence and distant metastases. Histologically, asymmetry; poor circumscription; infiltrative growth pattern and preponderance of atypical, pleomorphic, basaloid cells arranged in solid sheets; and high mitotic activity characterise sebaceous carcinoma. Scattered sebocytes are often present. Tumour necrosis is related to poor prognosis [35]. Neoplastic cells are immunopositive for cytokeratin, low molecular CK, EMA, CA 15.3 and androgen receptor protein and immunonegative for CEA, S100 protein and GCDFP-15.70

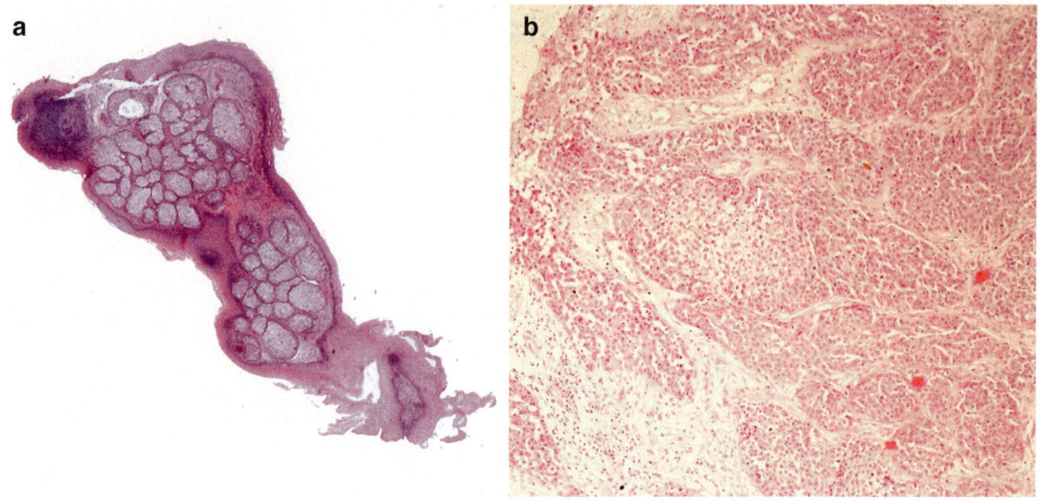

Fig. 6.4 Sebaceous neoplasm: (**a**) sebaceous adenoma (H&E 2×), (**b**) sebaceous carcinoma (H&E 20×)

[36]. Variants of sebaceous carcinoma are basaloid, spindle, squamoid cells and dedifferentiated (pleomorphic) (Fig. 6.4).

Sweat Gland Tumours

Histology of Sweat Glands (SG)

Eccrine SGs are widely distributed almost everywhere in the skin, with higher concentration in palms, soles and forehead; they develop from the fetal epidermis and are composed of three segments: intraepidermal duct (acrosyringium), intradermal duct and secretory portion. The ducts are lined with two layers of cells, whilst the secretory portion is composed of one layer of secretory cells, surrounded by myoepithelial cells.

Apocrine SGs are mainly localised in the axillary, groin and anogenital regions and, as modified glands, in the external ear canal (ceruminous gland), in the eyelid (Moll's glands) and in the breast (mammary glands). They develop as epithelial buds from the outer sheath of the hair germ (and therefore the apocrine duct usually leads to a follicular infundibulum), becoming functional only during puberty. The apocrine basal coils are located in the subcutaneous fat and are composed entirely of secretory cells; the ductal and secretory portions show the same composition of eccrine glands.

Apoeccrine SGs are mostly found in the axillary region, and within lesions of NSJ. Their presence explains the existence of some adnexal tumours having both eccrine and apocrine differentiation, including syringocystadenoma papilliferum (SCAP) and Fox–Fordyce disease. Some authors believe that these glands are synonymous to cutaneous mammary-like glands (MLG), which are now recognised as normal component of the skin in the anogenital region, including the perianal skin. MLG are characterised by features of eccrine, apocrine and specialised mammary glands.

General Consideration for Diagnosis of Cutaneous Sweat Gland Tumours

Cutaneous sweat gland tumours (CSGT) are uncommon, with a wide histological spectrum, complex classification and many different terms often used to describe the same tumour.

Historically CSGTs have been divided into apocrine and eccrine, but the histologic distinction is not always easy, and therefore, neoplasms with ductular differentiation often have debatable histogenesis; moreover, the description of apoeccrine glands and the existence of lesions with composite/mixed differentiation make the matter

Table 6.5 Sweat gland tumours origin classification

Origin/Differentiation	Hamartomas/benign neoplasms	Malignant neoplasms
Eccrine and apocrine	Hidrocystoma	
	Apocrine/eccrine nevus	
	Chondroid syringoma (mixed tumour)	
Eccrine	Poroma	Porocarcinoma
	Hidradenoma	Hidradenocarcinoma
	Spiradenoma	Spiradenocarcinoma
	Cylindroma	Malignant cylindroma
	Syringoma	Syringoid carcinoma
		Microcystic adnexal carcinoma*
		Aggressive Digital Papillary Adenocarcinoma*
		Adenoid cystic carcinoma
		Mucinous Carcinoma*
Apocrine	Syringocystadenoma papilliferum	Syringocystadenocarcinoma
	Hidradenoma papilliferum	Apocrine carcinoma
		Extramammary Paget's disease

*The histogenesis is not yet been elucidated

further complicated. Table 6.5 shows the classification of CSGT according to the current opinion about the predominant 'accepted' origin.

CSGT Classification

Benign/Hamartomatous Lesions

Hidrocystoma are cystic proliferation of SG, relatively rare, with predilection for the face and neck of middle-aged or older individuals. They have either apocrine or eccrine differentiation. The hidrocystomas represent retention cysts deriving from the gland duct [37]. Histologically hidrocystomas can be a uni- or multilocular lesion, usually lined by a double layer of epithelial cells. The inner layer consists of columnar cells with apical snouts or of flattened epithelium (Fig. 6.1c).

Syringocystadenoma papilliferum (*SCAP*) usually affects the young adults and occurs as a solitary or, less commonly, multiple lesions, most commonly in the face and scalp; they can occur in a pre-existing NSJ and rarely can be associated with other eccrine or apocrine tumours. Mutations in tumour-suppressor gene p16 may contribute to the pathogenesis of SCAP [38]. Histologically, SCAP is characterised by multiple epidermal invaginations and papillae with a fibrovascular core

and lined by two layers of epithelial cells (Fig. 6.1d). The luminal columnar cells exhibit decapitation secretion, as typical apocrine features.

Benign and Malignant Tumours

The differences among the benign CSGTs have only an academic value, since the precise categorisation of neoplasms rarely impacts on the clinical management. Indeed the surgical excision is generally curative.

SGs carcinomas are relatively less common than benign tumours, deriving mainly from eccrine SGs. They occur in adults, but they have also been reported in children. Malignant CSGTs arise mainly as de novo neoplasm, although malignant transformation of a pre-existent benign CSGTs has been described, usually as high-grade carcinoma [39]. Histologically, most malignant CSGTs preserve some features of their benign counterparts; clues for histologic distinction between benign and malignant tumours are irregularly permeating growth, nuclear atypia, perineural/vascular invasion by tumour cells, and foci of spontaneous tumour necrosis. Mitotic activity is not diagnostically helpful, being observed in benign tumours, too [40]. In addition to the malignant counterparts of the various types of CSGTs, several other distinctive CSG

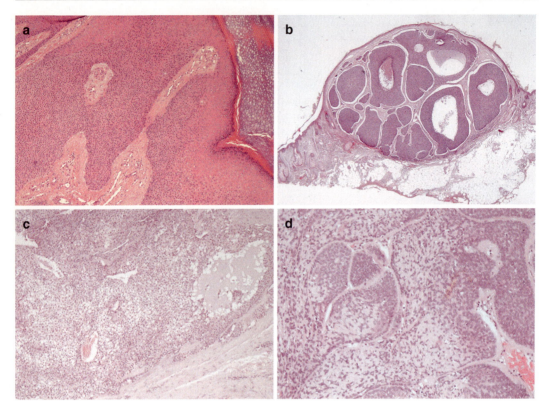

Fig. 6.5 Benign sweat gland tumours: (**a**) poroma (H&E 20×), (**b**) hidroadenoma (H&E 2×), (**c**) spiradenoma (H&E 20×), (**d**) cylindroma (H&E 20×)

carcinomas occur, i.e. microcystic adnexal carcinomas, aggressive digital papillary adenocarcinoma, adenoid cystic carcinoma and primary cutaneous mucinous carcinoma of the skin.

Herein we proposed the most common CSG tumours, accounting for each group both benign tumour and malignant counterpart.

Eccrine Tumours

Poroma/Porocarcinoma

Poromas (acrospiromas) are neoplasms with excretory eccrine duct differentiation; they usually arise in acral sites, particularly palms and soles. Histologically poroma consists of a proliferation of basaloid uniform tumour cells organised in ductal structures and occasional cysts, extending from the lower epidermis into the dermis (Fig. 6.5a).

Porocarcinoma is usually found in the lower extremities. It is characterised by asymmetrical, solid, growth pattern nodules of basaloid tumour cells, resembling those of poroma, but shows varying degrees of cytonuclear atypia, hyperchromatic

nuclei and prominent nucleoli. Porocarcinomas are aggressive tumours with potential local recurrence and metastasis. Indeed more than 14 mitoses per high power field, tumour depth of 7 mm and presence of lymphovascular invasion are associated with a more aggressive clinical course [24, 41]. Mutation of p53 gene with loss of its suppressor function has been widely reported [42].

Hidroadenoma/Hidradenocarcinoma

Hidradenoma is generally considered as an eccrine neoplasm. Clinically its presentation is a solitary, skin-coloured lesion and occurs more commonly in females. It has variable histomorphological patterns and consists of nests and nodules of small, monomorphous epithelial cells, with small ductular lumens, developing in the upper dermis. The lesion is characterised by pushy, but well-circumscribed, peripheral border (Fig. 6.5b). Recurrence of not fully excised hidradenoma is approximately observed in 12 % of all cases [40]. Most cases of hidradenocarcinoma arise de novo. Histologically tumour cells have similar features of hidradenoma, with cytonuclear atypia and foci of necrosis. Mitotic figures may be focally prominent. This carcinoma may metastasise [43].

Spiradenoma and Spirocarcinoma

Spiradenomas, derived from straight intradermal eccrine duct, usually present as a solitary, painful, nodular lesion in young adults, with a predilection of the trunk and upper extremities. They can be rarely observed in Brooke–Spiegler syndrome, a rare autosomal dominant inherited disorder, characterised by the development of multiple skin adnexal tumours [44]. Microscopically, spiradenomas are lobulated mass composed of multiple nests of small basophilic cells, admixed with squamoid cells and clear cells, with hyalinised basement membrane, and ductal differentiation (Fig. 6.5c).

Spiradenocarcinoma is a very rare malignant neoplasm, resulting from malignant transformation of spiradenoma, with loss of nodular growth pattern, infiltrative borders, cytonuclear pleomorphism and tumour necrosis. TP53 mutations have been identified in carcinomatous portion of these tumours [45].

Cylindroma and Malignant Counterpart

Cylindromas usually affect adult females, mainly involving the scalp and the face. They can be a solitary lesion or less commonly multiple nodules coalescing tumour (turban tumour), mainly observed in familial cylindromatosis and Brook–Spiegler syndrome. The pathogenesis of cylindroma is associated with mutation in the cylindromatosis tumour-suppressor gene (CYLD1), on chromosome 16q12–1319. Histologically, these tumours are characterised by numerous well-defined nodules of epithelial cells, lined by thick PAS positive basement membrane-like, hyalinised material, with a characteristic 'jigsaw puzzle' pattern (Fig. 6.5d).

Malignant cylindroma is a rare tumour arising from pre-existing benign cylindroma, characterised by infiltrative growth pattern with cytonuclear pleomorphism and loss of jigsaw appearance, hyaline sheath and peripheral palisading. The tumour has an aggressive behaviour [44].

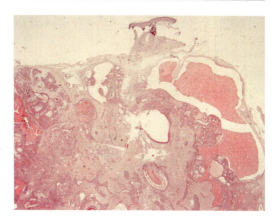

Fig. 6.6 Chondroid syringoma (H&E 20×)

Syringoma and Malignant Counterpart

Syringomas are small lesions, arising from the straight segment of the intradermal eccrine sweat duct, always multiple of the lower eyelid and upper cheeks. They are found more often in women and in adolescence or early adulthood and are constituted of tubules.

Chondroid syringoma is an uncommon tumour generally occurring in the head and neck region, most commonly the nose, cheek and upper lip. Histologically, it is a mixed tumour having both epithelial and mesenchymal stromal components. Thus, it is constituted of cords, ducts or tubules of bland epithelial cells, immersed in chondromyxoid stroma. Chondroid syringoma is classified into apocrine and eccrine types; in the apocrine type, lesions incorporating areas with pilar and sebaceous differentiation have been described suggesting that some tumours are best viewed as hamartomatous lesions of the pilosebaceous/apocrine unit [46] (Fig. 6.6). Rare malignant mixed tumours have been described, generally developing de novo [47, 48]. Histological diagnosis is foremost based on the biphasic nature of the neoplasm and an origin from MMT myoepithelial cells appears to be most plausible.

Microcystic Adnexal Carcinomas

Microcystic adnexal carcinomas are uncommon malignant neoplasms of mixed adnexal lineage with eccrine, apocrine and pilosebaceous features. It occurs as a solitary lesion in middle-aged adults, commonly in the face, with predilection to the upper and lower lip. Risk factors include previous radiation therapy and immunosuppression. There

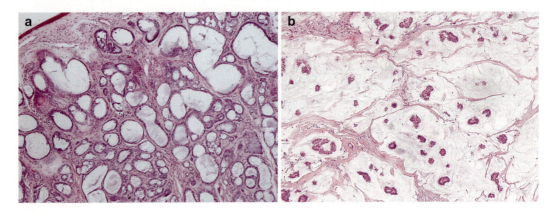

Fig. 6.7 (**a**) Microcystic carcinoma (H&E 20×), (**b**) mucinous carcinoma (H&E 20×)

is a single report of a 6q deletion [49]. Histologically microcystic adnexal carcinomas are characterised by cords and nests of bland basaloid or less commonly clear epithelial cells, infiltrating the dermis and subcutaneous tissue; keratin-filled microcysts and ductal structures are present. It exhibits prominent perineural and intraneural invasion and a locally aggressive behaviour, with occasional nodal and distant metastases [50] (Fig. 6.7a).

Aggressive Digital Papillary Adenocarcinoma

These are rare sweat gland neoplasms of eccrine origin. They occur in middle-aged adults, with male predilection and main acral location. Histologically the tumour is composed of multi-nodular, solid and cystic epithelial aggregates, consisting of cuboidal/low columnar cells. Multiple cystic spaces, containing eosinophilic material, with luminal papillary projections, are characteristically present. Cytologic atypia is usually not particularly evident; mitotic activity and necrosis are frequent findings. Digital papillary adenocarcinoma displays clinically aggressive behaviour. Therefore, all these tumours should be completely excised with or without amputation of the affected digit, as they may recur in 50 % of cases, with 14 % risk for metastasis [51].

Adenoid Cystic Carcinoma

Primary cutaneous adenoid cystic carcinoma (ACC) is a very rare malignant tumour of controversial histogenesis, although it has been regarded

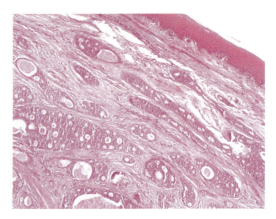

Fig. 6.8 Adenoid cystic carcinoma (H&E 20×)

as an eccrine tumour. The tumour affects older adults, with female predominance, and can occur in different anatomical sites, most commonly in the scalp, the chest and the abdomen [52]. Histologically, ACC is a poorly circumscribed dermal tumour, composed of islands, cords and strands of bland, basaloid cells. These tumours exhibit infiltrative pattern and are not connected to the epidermis (Fig. 6.8).

ACC has an indolent but progressive course, with 50 % of local recurrence rate; metastasis to regional lymph nodes and distant organs is exceedingly rare [53].

Mucinous Carcinoma

Primary cutaneous mucinous carcinoma is a rare low-grade malignancy tumour that affects older adults, especially men, and occurs most frequently in the head and neck and axillary regions, with a predilection to the eyelids. Histologically, the tumour is a well-demarcated, lobular dermal lesion, constituted of nests of bland epithelial cells, sometimes exhibiting a cribriform arrangement, embedded and 'floating' in multilocular pools of mucin (Fig. 6.7b). Cutaneous mucinous carcinoma is typically an indolent tumour with tendency for local recurrence; however, distant metastasis is rare [54, 55]. The histogenesis is not yet been completely elucidated.

Apocrine Tumours

Hidradenoma Papilliferum

Hidradenoma papilliferum is solitary, small and asymptomatic tumour that occurs almost exclusively in females, in vulvar and perianal region. In males, rare cases have been reported in nonanogenital locations, especially in the head and neck [56]. Hidradenoma papilliferum is a well-circumscribed solid or cystic dermal nodular lesion, formed of papillae or tubulopapillary structures, lined by epithelial cells with apical secretions, and outer myoepithelial cell component. The presence of histomorphological features similar to benign breast diseases are further evidence of its origin from MLG [56].

Apocrine Carcinoma

Apocrine carcinoma (AC) is a rare and highly aggressive cutaneous adenocarcinoma, more commonly seen in middle age; most tumours arise in the axilla, but other sites including eyelid (in Moll's glands), ear and scalp are described [57]. AC is thought to arise from apocrine glands, but an alternative, proposed origin could be the MLGs of the anogenital region [58]. These tumours have also been described in NSJ. Most ACs are slow-growing tumours, recording frequent relapse. Histologically, the tumour is composed of tubular and ductal structures with intraluminal papillary projections. It develops in the dermis with extension to the epidermis. Decapitation secretion is a diagnostic key, usually recognisable in differentiated tumours. Cytonuclear pleomorphism, increased mitotic activity and areas of tumour necrosis are also observed.

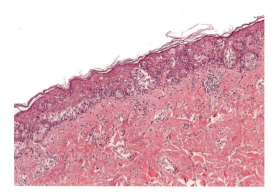

Fig. 6.9 Paget's disease (H&E 40×)

Extramammary Paget's Disease

Extramammary Paget's disease (EMPD) is commonly found in sites rich in apocrine glands, such as vulvar and perianal region of middle-aged females. It has also been described in the axillae, eyelids, external auditory canal, penis and scrotum. Microscopically it is characterised by intraepidermal proliferation of apocrine neoplastic cells, with dermal invasion observed in less than 20 % of cases (Fig. 6.9) [59].

Adnexal Tumours in Clinical Syndrome

As previously underlined, when adnexal tumours are multiple, they are expressions of complex genetic syndrome, often including visceral cancers. Thus, skin adnexal tumours diagnosis should warn the possibility of a clinical syndrome, often with lethal implications.

Trichilemmomas in Cowden's Syndrome

Cowden's syndrome (CS) is a multiple hamartoma syndrome [60]. Multiple mucocutaneous proliferative lesions are described in CS, including trichilemmoma, gingival, labial and lingual papillomatosis (85 % of cases), scrotal tongue (20 % of patients), acral keratoses in 73 % of patients and multiple skin tags (16 %) [61, 62]. Less frequently some soft tissue

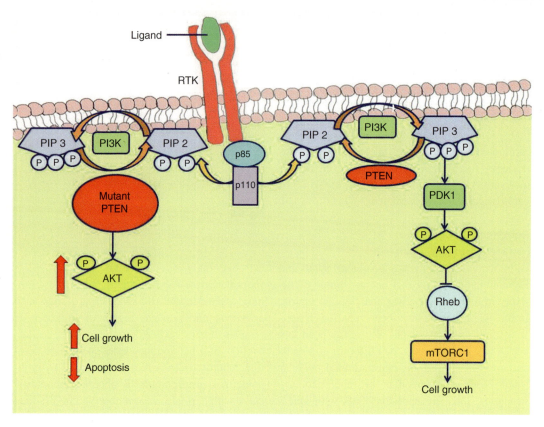

Fig. 6.10 PTEN deregulation in CS: phosphatidylinositol triphosphate (PIP-3) is normally dephosphorylated by PTEN to phosphatidylinositol (4,5)-diphosphate (PIP-2). Akt binding to PIP-3 allows its phosphorylation and activation. In the absence of PTEN, activated Akt phosphorylates via phosphoinositide-dependent kinase-1 (Pdk1). This results in cellular protection from several apoptotic stimuli. Activated Akt also downregulates p27 levels, stabilises cyclin D1 and mediates the activation of Rheb, playing critical roles in the activation of mTOR, thus leading to increased cellular proliferation. PTEN mutation in CS results in an activation of cell growth

tumours and other cutaneous tumours, including melanoma and carcinoma, are present [63]. The mucocutaneous lesions anticipate visceral lesions and occur at the mean age of 22 years. The incidence of extracutaneous lesions is different in male and female patients, being more frequent in the latter [64]. They include breast tumours, such as fibroadenomas and carcinomas, thyroid adenomas and follicular carcinomas, uterine leiomyomas, renal and endometrial carcinomas, hamartomatous polyps in gastrointestinal tract, central nervous gangliocytomas and medulloblastomas. Nonproliferative lesions are also present in CS, such as thyroid goitre, ovarian cysts, macrocephaly, kyphosis, arched palate, mental retardation, and epilepsy EEG abnormalities.

CS is an autosomal dominant disease with variable expressivity and penetrance [64]. CS is related to PTEN (Phosphatase and TENsin) tumour-suppressor gene mutation. This gene, localised on chr. 10q22–23, encodes a lipid phosphatase acting as tumour suppressor, mediating cell cycle arrest [65]. PTEN dysfunction leads to activation of the PI3K/mTORC1 intracellular signalling mutations (Fig. 6.10). It is detected in 80 % of patients with CS. PTEN germline mutations have also been found in two other syndromes with different clinical setting, the Bannayan–Riley–Ruvalcaba syndrome and Proteus-like syndrome (PLS) (20 %), manifesting with congenital malformations and constituting the syndromes under the term PTEN hamartoma/tumour syndrome [66]. The use of rapamycin (an mTOR inhibitor) in animal models

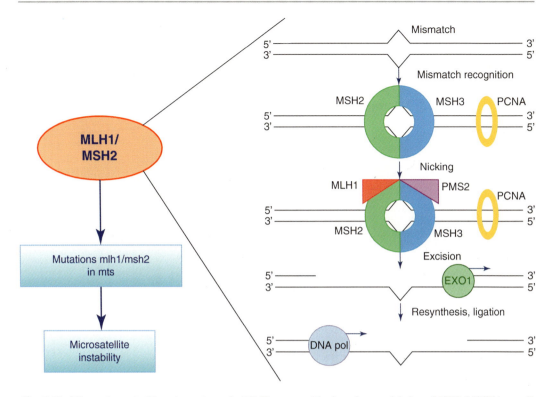

Fig. 6.11 Mismatch repair. The mismatch-repair (*MMR*) system is important for promoting the genetic stability of eukaryotes and prokaryotes. In eukaryotes, many homologues of bacterial MutS and MutL have been identified. MutS homologues (*MSHs*) form heterodimers with each other to carry out specific functions. The MutS, such as MSH2–MSH3 heterodimers, bind mismatches that are caused by insertions or deletions. MSH2–MSH6 heterodimers bind to single base-pair mismatches. Heterodimers of MutL homologues, such as MLH1–MLH3, are then recruited to this complex. Proliferating cell nuclear antigen (*PCNA*), which links the DNA polymerase to the DNA template during replication, interacts with this complex, which indicates that MMR might occur during DNA replication

favours the regression of advanced mucocutaneous lesions opening promising therapeutic perspectives in humans [67].

Sebaceous Tumours and Muir–Torre Syndrome

Muir–Torre syndrome (MTS) is characterised by the development of multiple sebaceous tumours and other visceral tumours [68].

All the spectrum of sebaceous tumours can be observed, from sebaceous adenoma till carcinoma. The incidence of sebaceous tumours in MTS patients is 14 %, and generally the onset of these cutaneous tumours appears prior to the internal malignancies [69]. Visceral cancers are multiple in 50 % of cases and the mean age of occurrence is 53 years [70]. They include colorectal cancer, urogenital cancers (ovaries, prostate, kidneys, ureters and bladder) and less frequently breast, upper gastrointestinal tract, lungs, larynx, parotid gland cancers and haematological malignancies.

MTS is transmitted as an autosomal dominant disease, with varying expressivity and penetrance. Most MTS patients carry truncating mismatch-repair genes MLH1, with subsequent microsatellite instability (Fig. 6.11) [71]. The clinical features and the genetic defects in MTS are very close to those found in Lynch syndrome/hereditary nonpolyposis colorectal cancer (HNPCC); thus, MTS is currently considered as an allelic subset of HNPCC [2, 72]. The diagnosis is based on demonstration of microsatellite instability and/or immunohistochemical screening for MLH1. Recently, it was reported that the mTOR inhibitor rapamycin/sirolimus can reduce the appearance of new sebaceous tumours of MTS [73].

Hair Follicle Cysts and Gardner Syndrome/Familial Adenomatous Polyposis

Gardner syndrome (GS) is characterised by unusual hair follicle cysts also in atypical sites, such as limbs, visceral carcinomas, mandible and skull osteomas and (sub)cutaneous tumours. It is considered a phenotypic variant of Familial Adenomatous Polyposis (FAP). The skin is generally affected by multiple epidermoid, trichilemmal, hybrid or pilomatrical cysts or pilomatricomas, on the face and the scalp, but, more rarely, other lesions can be present, such as post-traumatic desmoid tumours of the abdominal wall; nuchal fibroma; 'Gardner fibroma', as sheets of thick, haphazardly arranged collagen bundles with interspersed bland fibroblasts in the trunk; and lipomas, leiomyomas and neurofibromas [24, 37, 74].

As all FAP diseases, the diagnosis is based on the presence of more than 100 adenomatous colorectal polyps, or less than 100 polyps in addition to a first-degree relative with FAP. The disease is transmitted as an autosomal dominant disease with high penetrance, but about 25 % of patients have de novo mutations. The gene involved in GS is APC (Adenomatous Polyposis Coli), located on chr. 5q21-22 and encodes a protein inhibiting the Wnt signalling pathway by binding to beta-catenin and downregulating its activity. APC mutations produce protein truncation, with subsequent loss of activity, resulting in the cytoplasmic accumulation of beta-catenin that binds to several transcription factors of the TCF/LEF family, related to cell proliferation, differentiation, migration and apoptosis [75–77].

Visceral lesions include multiple adenomatous polyps of the colon and rectum (50–65 % of cases) that invariably undergo malignant transformation by 40 years of age; gastric and duodenal polyps (80 and 60 % of patients, respectively); desmoid tumours osteomas, affecting about 20 % of patients, occurring generally in the mandible and the skull; congenital hypertrophy of the retinal pigment epithelium (CHRPE), affecting 60–70 % of patients; dental lesions, present in 18 % of patients, such as odontomas, absent, surpernumerary or rudimentary teeth and multiple caries; thyroid carcinomas; and brain tumours (astrocytomas, glioblastomas, medulloblastomas), adrenal adenomas and pancreatic and hepatic carcinomas (hepatoblastomas).

Chemoprevention with the nonsteroidal antiinflammatory agent sulindac has demonstrated regression of colorectal adenomas, although its long-term efficacy is variable. Other selective COX-2 inhibitors (celecoxib, rofecoxib) have also been tried [78].

Trichodiscomas/Fibrofolliculomas/ Acrochordons and Birt–Hogg–Dube' Syndrome

The Birt–Hogg–Dube' syndrome (BHDS) is characterised by presence of more than ten cutaneous lesions, clinically suggestive of fibrofolliculomas, trichodiscomas or acrochorda, with at least one histological demonstration, transmitted as an autosomal dominant disease. Clinical manifestations are generally evident during the third life decade and include, besides cutaneous lesions, renal cell tumours, such as chromophobe ones and oncocytomas, spontaneous recurring pneumothorax, emphysema and pulmonary cysts and less commonly thyroid medullary carcinoma, follicular adenoma, multinodular goitre and colon polyps and adenocarcinomas [79–82]. The BHDS is determined by heterozygous (splice site, deletions, insertions, nonsense or missense) mutations of the gene BHD/FLCN, a tumour-suppressor gene located on chromosome 17p11.2, encoding folliculin (FLCN), expressed in multiple human tissues [83] (Fig. 6.12). FLCN interacts with FNIP1 and downregulates mTOR activity [84]. Thus, rapamycin has given interesting results in the treatment of mice model of BHDS tumours [85].

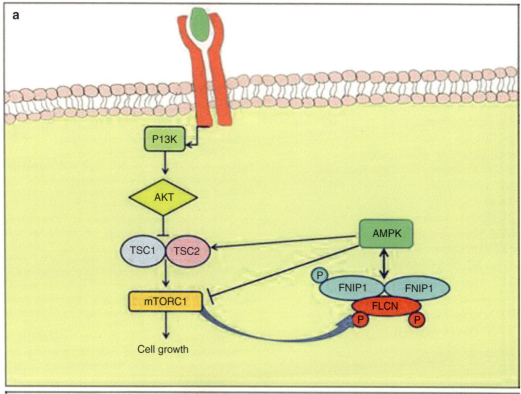

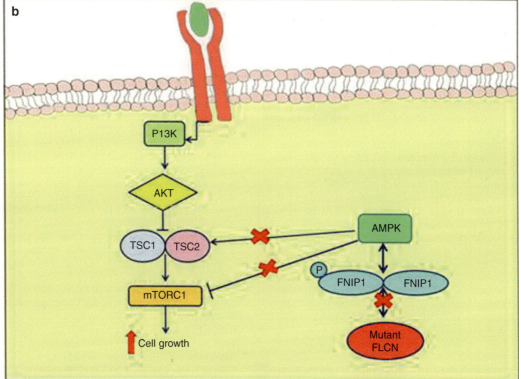

Fig. 6.12 FLCN pathway. (**a**) Normal FCLN protein complexes with FNIP1, FNIP2 and AMPK. This complex is phosphorylated by a rapamycin-sensitive kinase (mTORC1) and inhibits directly and indirectly mTOR-dependent proliferation. (**b**) When FLCN is altered, it fails to complex and allows activation of AKT, mTORC1

Glossary

APC Adenomatous polyposis coli
BCC Basal-cell carcinoma
BHDS Birt–Hogg–Dube' syndrome
CAT Cutaneous appendage tumors
CHRPE Congenital hypertrophy of the retinal pigment epithelium
CS Cowden syndrome
CSG Cutaneous sweat gland
CSGT Cutaneous sweat gland tumours
FAP Familial adenomatous polyposis
FLCN Folliculin
GS Gardner syndrome
H&E Haematoxylin and eosin
MFT Multiple familial tricoepithelioma
MLG Mammary-like glands
MTS Muir–Torre syndrome
NSJ Nevus sebaceous of Jadassohn
PTC Proliferating trichilemmal cyst
PTEN Phosphatase and TENsin

References

1. Rodriguez-Diaz E, Armio M. Mixed tumors with follicular differentiation: complex neoplasms of the primary epithelial germ. Int J Dermatol. 1994;34:782–5.
2. Winship I, Dudding T. Lessons from the skin-cutaneous features of familial cancer. Lancet Oncol. 2008;9:462–72.
3. Kanitakis J. Adnexal tumors of the skin as markers of cancer-prone syndrome. J Eur Acad Dermatol Venereol. 2010;24:379–87.
4. Klein W, Chan E, Seykora JT. Tumors of the epidermal appendages. In: Elder DE, editor. Lever's histopathology of the skin. 9th ed. Philadelphia: Lippincott Williams & Wilikins; 2005. p. 867–926.
5. Weedon D. Tumors of cutaneous appendages. In: Weedon D, editor. Skin pathology. 2nd ed. Edinburgh: Churchill Livingstone; 2002. p. 859–916.
6. Alsaad KO, Obaidat NA, Ghazarian D. Skin adnexal neoplasms—part 1: an approach to tumours of the pilosebaceous unit. J Clin Pathol. 2007;60:129–44.
7. Yoshida Y, Urabe K, Mashino T, et al. Basal cell carcinomas in association with basaloid follicular hamartoma. Dermatology. 2003;207:57–60.
8. Akasaka T, Kon S, Mihm Jr MC. Multiple basaloid cell hamartoma with alopecia and autoimmune disease (systemic lupus erythematosus). J Dermatol. 1996;23:821–4.
9. Morton S, Stevens A, Powell RJ. Basaloid follicular hamartoma, total body hair loss and SLE. Lupus. 1998;3:207–9.
10. Jih DM, Shapiro M, James WD, et al. Familial basaloid follicular hamartoma: lesional characterization and review of the literature. Am J Dermatopathol. 2003;25:130–7.
11. Stern JB, Stout DA. Trichofolliculoma showing perineural invasion. Trichofolliculocarcinoma? Arch Dermatol. 1979;115:1003–4.
12. Plewig G. Sebaceous trichofolliculoma. J Cutan Pathol. 1980;7:394–403.
13. Ramdial PK, Chrystal V, Madaree A. Folliculosebaceous cystic hamartoma. Pathology. 1998;30: 212–4.
14. Welsch MJ, Krunic A, Medenica MM. Birt-Hogg-Dube syndrome. Int J Dermatol. 2005;44:668–73.
15. Ponti G, Ponz de Leon M. Muir-Torre syndrome. Lancet Oncol. 2005;6:980–7.
16. Cribier B, Scrivener Y, Grosshans E. Tumors arising in nevus sebaceous: a study of 596 cases. J Am Acad Dermatol. 2000;42:263–8.
17. Xin H, Matt D, Qin JZ, et al. The sebaceous nevus: a nevus with deletions of the PTCH gene. Cancer Res. 1999;59:1834–6.
18. Harada H, Hashimoto K, Ko MS. The gene for multiple familial trichoepithelioma maps to chromosome 9p21. J Invest Dermatol. 1996;107:41–3.
19. Zhang XJ, Liang YH, He PP, et al. Identification of the cylindromatosis tumor suppressor gene responsible for multiple familial trichoepithelioma. J Invest Dermatol. 2004;122:658–64.
20. Zheng G, Hu L, Huang W, et al. CYLD mutation causes multiple familial trichoepithelioma in three Chinese families. Hum Mutat. 2004;23:400.
21. Kanitakis J, Bourchany D, Faure M, et al. Expression of the hair stem cell-specific keratin 15 in pilar tumours of skin. Eur J Dermatol. 1999;9:363–5.
22. Hunt SJ, Abell E. Malignant hair matrix tumor ("malignant trichoepithelioma") arising in the setting of multiple hereditary trichoepithelioma. Am J Dermatopathol. 1991;13:275–81.
23. Matsuki T, Hayashi N, Mizushima J, et al. Two cases of desmoplastic trichoepithelioma. J Dermatol. 2004; 31:824–7.
24. Jaqueti G, Requena L, Sanchez Yus E. Trichoblastoma is the most common neoplasm developed in nevus sebaceous of Jadassohn: a clinicopathologic study of a series of 155 cases. Am J Dermatopathol. 2000;22: 108–18.
25. Regauer S, Beham-Schmid C, Okuc M, et al. Trichoblastic carcinoma ("malignant trichoblastoma") with lymphatic and hematogenous metastases. Mod Pathol. 2000;13:673–8.
26. Brownstein MH, Mehregan AH, Bikowski JB, et al. The dermatopathology of Cowden's syndrome. Br J Dermatol. 1979;100:667–73.
27. Hunt SJ, Kilzer B, Santa Cruz DJ. Desmoplastic trichilemmoma: histologic variant resembling invasive carcinoma. J Cutan Pathol. 1990;17:45–52.
28. Chan KO, Kim IJ, Baladas HG, et al. Multiple tumour presentation of trichilemmal carcinoma. Dermatol Surg. 2003;29:886–9.

29. Casas JG, Woscoff A. Giant pilar tumor of the scalp. Arch Dermatol. 1980;116:1395.
30. Fernandez SH. Malignant proliferating trichilemmal tumour: a case report. Malays J Pathol. 1999;21:117–21.
31. Geh JL, Moss AL. Multiple pilomatrixomata and myotonic dystrophy: a familial association. Br J Plast Surg. 1999;52:143–5.
32. Noguchi H, Kayashima K, Nishiyama S, et al. Two cases of pilomatrixoma in Turner's syndrome. Dermatology. 1999;199:338–40.
33. Xia J, Urabe K, Moroi Y, et al. beta-Catenin mutation and its nuclear localization are confirmed to be frequent causes of Wnt signaling pathway activation in pilomatricomas. J Dermatol Sci. 2006;41:67–75.
34. Bremnes RM, Kvamme JM, Stalsberg H, et al. Pilomatrix carcinoma with multiple metastases: report of a case and review of the literature. Eur J Cancer. 1999;35:433–7.
35. Misago N, Mihara I, Ansai S, et al. Sebaceoma and related neoplasms with sebaceous differentiation: a clinicopathologic study of 30 cases. Am J Dermatopathol. 2002;24:294–304.
36. Bayer-Garner IB, Givens V, Smoller B. Immunohistochemical staining for androgen receptors: a sensitive marker of sebaceous differentiation. Am J Dermatopathol. 1999;21:426–31.
37. Sangueza OP. Hidrocistomas. Monogr Dermatol. 1993;6:146.
38. Boni R, Xin H, Hohl D, et al. Syringocystadenoma papilliferum: a study of potential tumor suppressor genes. Am J Dermatopathol. 2001;23:87–9.
39. Kazakow DV, Zelger B, Rütten A, et al. Morphologic diversity of malignant neoplasms arising in pre-existing spiradenoma, cylindroma, and spyradenocylindroma based on the study of 24 cases, sporadic or occuring in the setting of Brooke-Spiegler syndrome. Am J Surg Pathol. 2009;33:705–19.
40. Crowson AN, Magro CM, Mihm MC. Malignant adnexal neoplasms. Mod Pathol. 2006;19:S93–S126.
41. Urso C, Bondi R, Paglierani M, et al. Carcinomas of sweat glands: report of 60 cases. Arch Pathol Lab Med. 2001;125:498–505.
42. Akalin T, Sen S, Yuceturc A, et al. P53 protein expression in eccrine poroma and porocarcinoma. Am J Dermatopathol. 2001;23:402–6.
43. Waxtein L, Vega E, Cortes R, et al. Malignant nodular hidradenoma. Int J Dermatol. 1998;37:225–8.
44. Gerretsen AL, van der Putte SC, Deenstra W, et al. Cutaneous cylindroma with malignant transformation. Cancer. 1993;72:1618–23.
45. Granter SR, Seeger K, Calonje E, et al. Malignant eccrine spiradenoma (spiradenocarcinoma): a clinicopathologic study of 12 cases. Am J Dermatopathol. 2000;22:97–103.
46. Satter EK, Graham BS. Chondroid syringoma. Cutis. 2003;71:49–52.
47. Yamamoto O, Yasuda H. An immunohistochemical study of the apocrine type of cutaneous mixed tumors with special reference to their follicular and sebaceous differentiation. J Cutan Pathol. 1999;26:232–41.
48. Nather A, Sutherland IH. Malignant transformation of a benign cutaneous mixed tumour. J Hand Surg [Br]. 1986;11:139–43.
49. Wohlfahrt C, Ternesten A, Shalin P, et al. Cytogenetic and fluorescence in situ hybridization analysis of a microcystic adnexal carcinoma with del(6)(q23q25). Cancer Genet Cytogenet. 1997;98:106–10.
50. Ban M, Sugie S, Kamiya H, et al. Microcystic adnexal carcinoma with lymph node metastasis. Dermatology. 2003;207:395–7.
51. Duke WH, Sherrod TT, Lupton GP. Aggressive digital papillary adenocarcinoma (aggressive digital papillary adenoma and adenocarcinoma revisited). Am J Surg Pathol. 2000;24:775–84.
52. Chang SE, Ahn SJ, Choi JH, et al. Primary adenoid cystic carcinoma of skin with lung metastasis. J Am Acad Dermatol. 1999;40:640–2.
53. Van der Kwast TH, Vuzevski VD, Ramaekers F, et al. Primary cutaneous adenoid cystic carcinoma: case report, immunohistochemistry, and review of the literature. Br J Dermatol. 1988;118:567–77.
54. Requena L, Kiryu H, Ackerman AB. Neoplasms with apocrine differentiation. Philadelphia: Lippincott Williams & Wilkins; 1998.
55. Quereshi HS, Salama ME, Chitale D, et al. Primary cutaneous mucinous carcinoma: presence of myoepithelial cells as a clue to the cutaneous origin. Am J Dermatopathol. 2004;26:353–8.
56. Loane J, Kealy WF, Mulcahy G. Perianal hidradenoma papilliferum occurring in a male: a case report. Ir J Med Sci. 1998;16:726–7.
57. Miyamoto T, Hagari Y, Inoue S, et al. Axillary apocrine carcinoma with benign apocrine tumours: a case report involving a pathological and immunohistochemical study and review of the literature. J Clin Pathol. 2005;58(7):757–61.
58. Van der Putte SC, Van Gorp LH. Adenocarcinoma of the mammary-like glands of the vulva: a concept unifying sweat gland carcinoma of the vulva, carcinoma of supernumerary mammary glands and extramammary Paget's disease. J Cutan Pathol. 1994;21(2):157–63.
59. Obaidat NA, Alsaad KO, Ghazarian D. Skin adnexal neoplasms-part 2: an approach to tumours of cutaneous sweat glands. J Clin Pathol. 2007;60:145–59.
60. Fistarol S, Anliker M, Itin P. Cowden disease or multiple hamartoma syndrome – cutaneous clues to internal malignancy. Eur J Dermatol. 2002;12:412–21.
61. Salem O, Steck W. Cowden's Disease (multiple hamartoma syndrome). A case report and review of the English literature. J Am Acad Dermatol. 1983;8:686–96. 10.
62. Starinck T, van der Veen J, Arwert F, et al. The Cowden syndrome: a clinical and genetic study in 21 patients. Clin Genet. 1986;29:222–33.
63. Ruhoy S, Thomas D, Nuovo G. Multiple inverted follicular keratoses as a presenting sign of Cowden's syndrome: case report with human papillomavirus studies. J Am Acad Dermatol. 2004;51:411–5.
64. Pilarski R. Cowden's syndrome: a critical review of the clinical literature. J Genet Couns. 2009;18:13–27.

65. Waite K, Eng C. Protean PTEN: form and function. Am J Hum Genet. 2002;70:829–44.
66. Eng C. PTEN: one gene, many syndromes. Hum Mutat. 2003; 22:183–98.
67. Squarize C, Castilho R, Gutkind J. Chemoprevention and treatment of experimental Cowden's disease by mTOR inhibition with rapamycin. Cancer Res. 2008;68:7066–72.
68. Ponti G, Ponz de Leon M. Muir-Torre syndrome. Lancet Oncol. 2005;12:980–7.
69. Akhtar S, Oza K, Khan S, Wright J. Muir-Torre syndrome: case report of a patient with concurrent jejunal and ureteral cancer and a review of the literature. J Am Acad Dermatol. 1999;41:681–6.
70. Cohen P, Kohn S, Kurzrock R. Association of sebaceous gland and internal malignancy: the Muir-Torre syndrome. Am J Med. 1991;90:606–13.
71. Kruse R, Rutten A, Lamberti C, et al. Muir-Torre phenotype has a frequency of DNA mismatch-repair gene mutations similar to that in hereditary non-polyposis colorectal cancer families defined by the Amsterdam criteria. Am J Hum Genet. 1998;63:63–70.
72. South C, Hampel H, Comeras I, Westman J, Frankel W, de la Chapelle A. The frequency of Muir-Torre syndrome among Lynch syndrome families. J Natl Cancer Inst. 2008;100:277–81.
73. Levi Z, Hazazi R, Kedar-Barnes I, et al. Switching from tacrolimus to sirolimus halts the appearance of new sebaceous neoplasms in Muir-Torre syndrome. Am J Transplant. 2007;7:476–9.
74. Gaskin BJ, Fernando BS, Sullivan CA, et al. The significance of DNA mismatch repair genes in the diagnosis and management of periocular sebaceous cell carcinoma and Muir-Torre syndrome. Br J Ophthalmol. 2011;95:1686–90.
75. Groen E, Roos A, Muntinghe F, et al. Extra-intestinal manifestations of familial adenomatous polyposis. Ann Surg Oncol. 2008;15:2439–50.
76. Lipton L, Tomlinson I. The genetics of FAP and FAP-like syndromes. Fam Cancer. 2006;5:221–6.
77. Goss K, Groden J. Biology of the adenomatous polyposis tumor suppressor gene. J Clin Oncol. 2000; 18:1967–79.
78. Lynch PM. Chemoprevention with special reference to inherited colorectal cancer. Fam Cancer. 2008;7: 59–64.
79. Zbar B, Alvord W, Glenn G, et al. Risk of renal and colonic neoplasms and spontaneous pneumothorax in the Birt-Hogg-Dube syndrome. Cancer Epidemiol Biomarkers Prev. 2002;11:393–400.
80. Adley B, Smith N, Nayar R, Yang X. Birt-Hogg-Dube' syndrome. Clinicopathologic findings and genetic alterations. Arch Pathol Lab Med. 2006; 130:1865–70.
81. Leter E, Koopmans A, Gille JJ, et al. Birt-Hogg-Dube syndrome: clinical and genetic studies of 20 families. J Invest Dermatol. 2008;128:45–9.
82. Toro J, Wei M, Glenn G, et al. BHD mutations, clinical and molecular genetic investigations of Birt-Hogg-Dube' syndrome: a new series of 50 families and a review of published reports. J Med Genet. 2008;45: 321–31.
83. Warren M, Torres-Cabala C, Turner ML, et al. Expression of Birt-Hogg-Dube gene mRNA in normal and neoplastic human tissues. Mod Pathol. 2004;17:998–1011.
84. Hartman T, Nicolas E, Klein-Szanto A, et al. The role of the Birt-Hogg-Dube' protein in mTOR activation and renal tumorigenesis. Oncogene. 2009;28:1594–604.
85. Baba M, Furihata M, Hong S, et al. Kidney-targeted Birt-Hogg-Dube'gene inactivation in a mouse model: Erk1/2 and Akt-mTOR activation, cell hyperproliferation, and polycystic kidneys. J Natl Cancer Inst. 2008;100:140–54.

Claudio Clemente and Martin C. Mihm Jr.

The histological classification of melanocytic tumors is poorly correlated to the prognosis. The diagnostic criteria are not unequivocally accepted and often are poorly reproducible even among experts. The emphasis of the chapter is to present as clearly as possible the histological diagnostic features of each lesion along with the most important differential diagnostic considerations. A review of prognostication with emphasis on the latest recommendations of the American Joint Committee on Cancer, Melanoma subcommittee is presented.

Several areas of the pathology of the skin melanocytic tumors are, as yet, subject to doubts and disputes, and not all authors agree on the definition, the terminology, and the natural history of some histotypes. Also the diagnostic criteria are not unequivocally accepted and often are poorly

reproducible even among experts [1]. In recent years a great help to the clinical diagnosis of nevi and melanomas has come by dermatoscopy and image analysis, which is placed in an intermediate position between the clinical/macroscopic and the histopathological diagnoses. The diagnostic procedure for the definition of a melanocytic lesion begins from the clinical macroscopic and the dermoscopy images. It is important that the dermatologist/dermatoscopist sends to the pathologist, together with the biopsy, the clinical "in vivo" image in addition to the clinical diagnosis and the medical history, which are essential information for the final histopathological diagnosis. The pathologist samples the lesion according to the clinical and dermatoscopic informations received, and only with this procedure the pathologist may discuss with the dermatologist the different patterns of the lesion with a reciprocal exchange of important diagnostic informations [2].

The histological classification of melanocytic tumors is poorly correlated to the prognosis; however, it is important to identify every entity with a reproducible and well-identifiable name. More recently a new subset of melanocytic tumors, with unpredictable biologic behavior, was described. These tumors, difficult to insert into the specific histotypes, are reported as *melanocytic tumor of uncertain malignant potential, severely atypical melanocytic proliferations, borderline melanocytic tumor, nevomelanocytic tumor of undetermined risk, etc.* [3], but they might be included under the general term of *atypical melanocytic tumors*. A proposed

C. Clemente (✉)
Department of Pathology and Cytopathology,
San Pio X Hospital, Milan, Italy

Department of Pathology and Cytopathology,
IRCCS Policlinico San Donato, San Donato Group,
San Donato Milanese, Milan, Italy
e-mail: cclemente.ap@iol.it

M.C. Mihm Jr.
Pathology and Dermatology Department,
Harvard Medical School, Boston, MA, USA

Melanoma Program, Department of Dermatology,
Brigham and Women's Hospital, Boston, MA, USA

Melanoma Program,
Dana Farber and Brigham and Women's Cancer Center,
Boston, MA, USA

A. Baldi et al. (eds.), *Skin Cancer*, Current Clinical Pathology,
DOI 10.1007/978-1-4614-7357-2_7, © Springer Science+Business Media New York 2014

Table 7.1 Proposed morphological classification of melanocytic tumors

A. Melanocytic nevi

  1. Lentigo simplex

  2. Junctional, compound, and dermal nevus

  3. Congenital nevi

    (i) Proliferative nodules in congenital nevus

    (ii) Superficial atypical melanocytic proliferation

  4. Nevi, rare variants

    (i) Halo nevus

    (ii) Balloon cell nevus

    (iii) Recurrent melanocytic nevus

  5. Nevi of special sites

    (i) Genital nevi

    (ii) Acral nevus

B. Spindle and epithelioid cell nevi

  1. Pigmented spindle cell nevus (Reed nevus)

  2. Epithelioid and spindle cell nevus (Spitz nevus)

C. Dermal melanocytosis

  1. Blue nevus

  2. Cellular blue nevus

  3. Desmoplastic nevus

  4. Deep penetrating nevus

D. Dysplastic nevus

E. Atypical melanocytic tumors

  1. Atypical Spitz/Reed tumors

F. Atypical dermal melanocytosis

  1. Pigmented epithelioid melanocytoma

  2. Dermal melanocytic tumors of uncertain malignant potential (MELTUMP)

G. Melanoma

  1. Precancerous melanosis (in situ melanoma)

    (i) Lentigo maligna

  2. Superficial spreading melanoma

  3. Lentigo maligna melanoma

  4. Acral lentiginous melanoma

  5. Mucosal lentiginous melanoma

  6. Nodular melanoma

  7. Melanoma, rare variants

    (i) Melanoma in congenital nevus

    (ii) Desmoplastic melanoma

    (iii) Neurotropic melanoma

    (iv) Nevoid melanoma and minimal deviation melanoma

    (v) Malignant blue nevus

    (vi) Others

classification of the melanocytic tumors is reported in Table 7.1.

Melanocytic Nevi

Lentigo Simplex

Lentigo simplex is a small well-defined localized area of hyperpigmentation that is associated with proliferation of melanocytes along the dermoepidermal junction in contiguity (Fig. 7.1). This lesion characteristically is not associated with the nesting phenomenon of the nevus cells, and there are elongated retia, melanophages, and sparse dermal chronic inflammatory infiltrate. The main variants of lentigo simplex include *nevus spilus* which histologically may be indistinguishable from lentigo simplex or may show the features of lentigo simplex with occasional junctional nesting (*jentigo*). The principal differential diagnosis of lentigo simplex includes freckle, junctional nevus, or dysplastic nevus. The *freckle* is a nonproliferative lesion of melanocytes which is associated with hyperpigmentation of the basal skin layer. It usually is not associated with hyperplasia of the rete ridges. If junctional nests are present in a lentigo, it is impossible to exclude that the lesion represents an early *junctional nevus*. According to Hafner [4] the absence of BRAF, FGFR3, and PIK3CA mutations differentiates lentigo simplex from melanocytic nevus and solar lentigo. The *dysplastic nevus* characteristically is associated with a proliferation of nevocytes along the dermoepidermal junction but with cytologic atypia. The nests in lentigo simplex when present are small and lie at the tips of the rete ridges; the nests in dysplastic nevi vary in size, are associated with discohesion of nevocytes, and lie variously along the lateral side of the rete ridges and even between them in the superpapillary epidermis. Furthermore, there are stromal changes including increased vascularity and prominent inflammation associated with striking lamellations of collagen and often concentric eosinophilic fibrosis around

Fig. 7.1 Junctional nevus

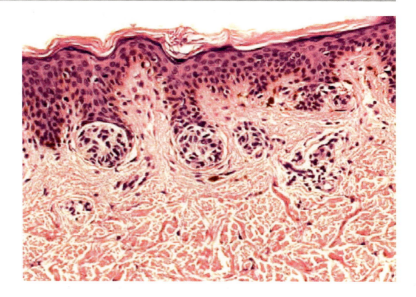

the rete ridges. *Senile lentigo* shows irregular rete hyperplasia with often irregular shapes at the base of the rete ridges. The most common shape is a "footlike" array with dense hyperpigmentation without melanocytic hyperplasia. *Lentigo maligna* is more strikingly different than lentigo simplex/senile but must be included because of the prominent single cell proliferation along the epidermis which may appear benign in early lesions. Lentigo maligna differs with a strikingly atrophic epidermis and sun-damaged dermis and often with a band-like or lichenoid inflammatory infiltrate admixed with melanophages. Furthermore in lentigo maligna the proliferation of melanocytes extends along the external root sheath of the hair follicles, even to the base of the hair follicle. *Mucosal lentigines* (labial, vulvar, penile) and acral lentigines may closely resemble lentigo simplex with increased number of intraepidermal basal pigmented melanocytes with dendritic morphology. Lentigines may be associated with systemic syndrome (LAMB, LEOPARD, Carney complex) [5].

Junctional, Compound, and Dermal Nevus

Junctional melanocytic nevi are focal pigmented lesions that by definition are flat to slight raised and exhibit intraepidermal nesting of nevomelanocytes usually localized to the tip of slightly hyperplastic rete ridges (Fig. 7.2). A nest of nevomelanocytes is considered to be five or more cells in a single cluster. Characteristically, the cells in the nests of junctional nevi are round to oval and lie contiguously together with scattered, usually coarse, melanin granules in their cytoplasm. The nucleus of the junctional nevus cells is larger than the normal nevomelanocyte and is round to oval, and usually a delicate nucleolus is evident. While the melanocytes in a nest are clumped together, because of separation artifact they usually are clearly separate from the adjacent keratinocytes with a space separating the nests from the keratinocytes. Often the nevus nests compress the adjacent keratinocytes that become elongated and fusiform with oval nuclei. No necrosis or apoptosis of the epidermal cells is present. At low-power magnification, one appreciates a well-circumscribed lesion that usually has hyperplasia of rete ridges with lentiginous proliferation of nevomelanocytes along the dermoepidermal junction but with nesting. The nevocytes have round to fusiform nuclei with tiny dot-like blue nucleoli. Their cytoplasm is clear and contains rather coarse melanin granules. Dendritic processes are not obvious although stubby small dendrites may be observed by high-power examination or with immunohistochemical stains

Fig. 7.2 Lentigo simplex

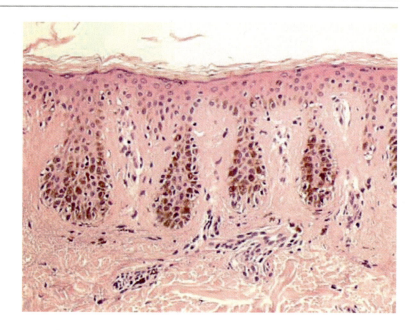

Fig. 7.3 Childhood junctional nevus

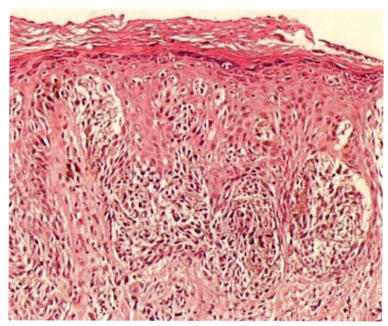

(HMB45). Occasionally the lesions, especially in acral sites, may not be associated with a lentiginous proliferation of melanocytes but with junctional nests. In such instances there may be trans-epidermal elimination of nests with their presence being noted even in the stratum corneum. The variants in junctional nevi include the *nevi of childhood* in which there may be prominence of single cells in the epidermis even to the level of the granular cell layer (pagetoid pattern), confined to the central part of the nevus (Fig. 7.3). Such intraepidermal proliferation, however, retains the benign characteristics of the cells in lentiginous array and in nests. *Congenital junctional* nevi are histologically indistinguishable from *acquired nevi* in small biopsies except that

Fig. 7.4 Melanoma, pagetoid spread

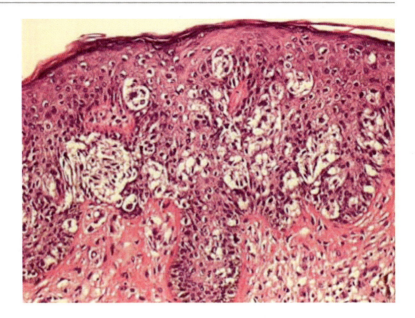

the predominance of deep dermal or periadnexal nests is more common in the congenital nevus than in the acquired nevus. *Acral junctional nevi* are often associated with a proliferation of single cells in the *stratum spinosum* characteristically overlying the junctional nests. The *lentiginous junctional dysplastic nevus* shows variation in morphology of the single cells and also in the size of the nests. Likewise, rather than showing a cohesive aggregate of nevus cells in the nests, the dysplastic nevocytes are characteristically discohesive in nests and show irregularities in nuclear size and shape in individual nests. *Superficial spreading melanoma* may show a prominent nesting pattern, but the cells are large and have prominent eosinophilic nucleoli and large cytoplasm filled with fine, dustlike, melanin granules; there is less retraction from keratinocytes of the nests; and it presents an "aggressive" proliferation with keratinocytes apoptosis (Fig. 7.4). Finally, the *pigmented junctional spindle cell nevus* is composed of a uniform population of spindle cells in well-defined and oriented nests, perpendicular or parallel to the skin surface. A *compound melanocytic nevus* refers to a lesion in which there is a proliferation of nevus cells in nests both in the epidermis and in the dermis. Low-power examination reveals a well-circumscribed symmetrical lesion. The intraepidermal component usually is

associated with well-developed nests present at the tips of the rete ridges with a regular and repetitive pattern. A lentiginous proliferation, similar to dysplastic nevus, is variably present in the compound nevus and in particular in the central area of congenital compound nevi (Fig. 7.5). Usually the intraepidermal component does not extend beyond the dermal component but if present, the extent beyond the dermal component is symmetrical on both sides of the lesion. The junctional nests are identical to those described under the junctional nevus. Intraepidermal junctional nevus cells have been described by the designation type A cells. These A cells are large round nevus cells with coarse melanin granules within them. In the dermal component of the lesion the picture is quite variable. In early lesions there are small nests of cells, many similar to type A cells, with large round nuclei present in the papillary dermis. These cells as they increase in number with lesion aging become smaller and round without pigment. They exhibit tiny nucleoli and are associated with fine fibroblast-like cells surrounding the nest. As the lesion ages, these cells are associated with a spindle-shaped cell that has been designated a type C cell at the base of the lesion. The type C cells are associated with increase in stroma with eosinophilic ground substance, an increased reticulum fibers present separating the type C cells

Fig. 7.5 Congenital compound nevus, lentiginous proliferation-like dysplastic nevus

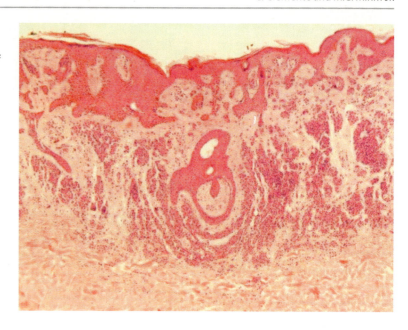

from one another. The type C cells can become arranged in highly complex patterns resembling neuroid structures or neurofibromas. Type A cells express S100 protein and HMB45. Type B cells may express either S100 or the Schwann cell-associated antigen but they are HMB45 negative. This variation in morphology and immunochemical findings is considered to be a maturation phenomenon of the nevus cells in their dermal component (Fig. 7.6). If the dermal component extends deeply into the dermis, in particular along adnexal structure, one must consider a *congenital nevus*. The differential diagnosis of the compound nevus includes *nevus spilus*. Some variants of nevus spilus have dermal nests and therefore represent variants of compound nevus. The *dysplastic nevus* usually is a type of compound nevus but with an irregular proliferation of atypical nevomelanocytes in the epidermis overlying the dermal component. There is no symmetry in this lesion so that the dermal component lies eccentrically in relationship to the epidermal component. Also in the compound nevus there is no atypia. *Nodular melanoma* can be differentiated from the compound nevus by the fact that there is, in addition to intraepidermal nesting, usually pagetoid aggressive spread of malignant melanocytes at the shoulder. Furthermore the characteristic maturation of type A to B to C cells is absent. In melanoma the deeper cells frequently exhibit finely granulated pigment in their cytoplasm, an atypical and rare finding in compound nevi. Also, the deeper component is not associated with a pushing border or expansive dermal nodule formation in nevi; this change is characteristic of melanoma. Mitotic activity in the dermal component is extremely rare in compound and dermal nevi, whereas it is common in melanomas [6]. Finally, compound nevi very rarely have a striking inflammatory response, whereas melanoma is commonly, especially below the intraepidermal component, associated with a lymphocytic host response. The term *dermal melanocytic nevus* refers to a lesion in which the nevus cells are completely confined to the dermal component with no intraepidermal involvement. The epidermis may be normal or flatted because of effacement of the rete ridges. There is no melanocytic proliferation or nesting in the typical dermal nevus. Occasionally, scattered single large nevomelanocytes are present overlying a dermal nevus but they are not considered significant unless there is a striking contiguous proliferation of them. The papillary dermis is unremarkable although occasionally there is some fibrosis of the papillary dermis. The nevic component of the dermal nevus exhibits nests of cells and sheets of cells that extend into the deep widened papillary dermis.

Fig. 7.6 Compound nevus: maturation

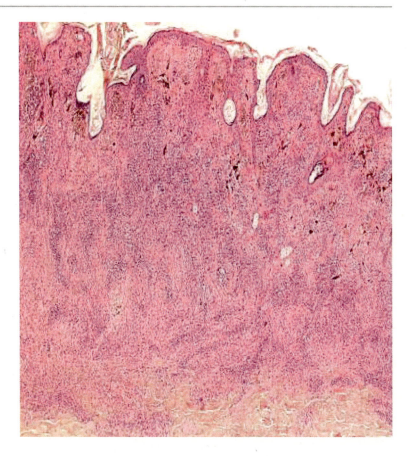

As the cells reach the papillary-reticular dermal junction, they frequently are noted to infiltrate as single cells into the superficial reticular dermis. The presence of nests of cells in the reticular dermis in an otherwise banal appearing dermal nevus is considered an abnormality of maturation (see section "Proliferative Nodules in Congenital Nevi", pag. 119). The characteristic lesion shows single cells that often have a fibroblast-like appearance. These cells are confined to the upper reticular dermis but presence in the deep reticular dermis suggests a congenital nevus. There is no evidence of preferential expansile growth in the form of expansile nodules in the deep component of a dermal nevus. The dermal nevus cells are usually type B and type C in nature. The superficial portions may be associated with nests of type B cells, while the deeper portions show the fibroblast-like changes associated with type C cells. Occasionally in the very superficial portions of the dermal component, type A cells as large round pigmented cells may be present within the upper papillary dermis. As the type C cells proliferate as S-shaped fibroblast-like cells with increasing ground substance, they resemble neurofibromas. Extensive organized stromal aggregates may resemble Wagner-Meissner corpuscles. Lesions containing prominent type C cell proliferation with extensive ground substance are dubbed "neuronevi" by Masson. In most such lesions one can still observe evidence of melanocytic proliferation, specifically nests of nevic cells. However, in some lesions there is no evidence of melanocytic activity. To differentiate such lesions from neurofibromas, one must observe the adventitial dermis of hair follicles and vessels. Neurofibromas infiltrate the adventitial dermis up the basement membrane of the external root sheath. Neuronevi on the whole respect the adventitial dermis. Mitoses do not occur in benign dermal nevi nor is the reevidence of expansile nodule formation deep in the nevus. "Aging" of dermal nevi has been associated with senescent changes which have been likened to the "ancient change" of schwannomas. Balloon cell changes also represent a possible senescent phenomenon due to degeneration of melanosomes. Sclerosis and infiltration by fat cells is related to involuting phase of the nevus. In such lesions there are hyperchromasia of nuclei, multinucleate giant cell formation, and large blue nucleoli; however, mitoses are absent. More than three mitoses in one section suggest to perform multiple levels to exclude a nevoid melanoma. In dermal nevus there is no evidence of necrosis and expansile clonal nodule formation and the nuclei do not contain the bright eosinophilic nucleoli of melanoma cells. One interesting change that occurs in dermal nevi is the presence of multiple large spaces lined by nevus cells. These spaces resemble vascular structures. The most important differential diagnostic consideration of the dermal nevus is melanoma. In melanoma there is no evidence of maturation of type B to type C cells. Rather, the lesion is composed of a uniform clonal population (single or multiple) of pleomorphic cells. In the depth of the lesion, often cells are larger rather than smaller in melanoma in contrast to the maturation of nevi. Mitoses are present throughout the lesion, in particular in the proliferative marginal areas, whereas in dermal nevi no mitotic activity is observed. A useful method in differentiating compound and dermal nevi from melanoma is to use the immunocytochemical stain with HMB45 and p16 antibodies. HMB45 usually does not stain the dermal deep component of ordinary acquired nevi. However, up to 30–40 % of the dermal component of dysplastic nevi can stain with HMB45 and all the dermal melanocytosis are positive. In such cases the histology of the lesion allows for the correct diagnosis. p16 is strong positive both in the nuclei and the cytoplasm of the nevi and negative in the vertical phase of the melanoma.

Congenital Nevi

Congenital nevi, by definition, are pigmented skin lesions present at birth. These lesions are divided in small (up to 1.5 cm in size), intermediate, and giant congenital nevi. Intermediate lesions are greater than 1.5 cm but can be removed by simple excision. Giant lesions, on the other hand, require often multiple staged excisions for removal. The histopathologic picture of a congenital nevus may be indistinguishable from an acquired nevus. According to Mark and Mihm [7], the following patterns are diagnostic of congenital origin: (*1*) *intramural or subendothelial nesting of nevus cells in small- to medium-size arteries, veins, and lymphatic vessels*; (*2*) *nevus cell nests in the papilla of the hair follicle*; (*3*) *nevus cells scattered in single cell array throughout the lower reticular dermis and subcutaneous fat*; (*4*) *nevus cells in arrector pili muscles*; and (*5*) *nevus cell in tight perivascular array mimicking an inflammatory infiltrate throughout the reticular dermis*. Thus, a congenital nevus may show areas of lentigo, areas of junctional nevus, areas of compound nevus, or areas of dermal nevus with limitation to the papillary-reticular dermal junction of the nevus cells. However, in many congenital nevi in striking contrast to acquired nevi, the nevocytes extend into the lower third of the dermis and may even involve the subcutaneous fat. The presence of this change is often also associated with involvement of skin appendages, vessels, and nerves. The dermal involvement in the lower reticular dermis and fat is predominantly composed of single cell array resembling the so-called Indian file. Involvement of the hair follicle includes nests in the lower two-third of the external root sheath, nests in sebaceous glands, or even nests of nevic cells in the papillae. Similarly, nests may occur in eccrine ducts or in eccrine glands. Subendothelial deposits of nevocytes may be observed in both the walls of arteries and veins. Finally, protrusion of nevus cells, delimitated by endothelial cells, into the lymphatics in the superficial and deep dermis may also be noted and distinguished by true lymphatic invasion by a melanoma (Fig. 7.7). Less specific is a pattern of nevic cells surrounding the appendages in the adventitial dermis and extending out into the collagen of the reticular dermis. At times the reticular dermal collagen may be strikingly abnormal in the congenital nevus.

Fig. 7.7 Congenital compound nevus: subendothelial deposits of nevus cells (pseudo-vascular invasion)

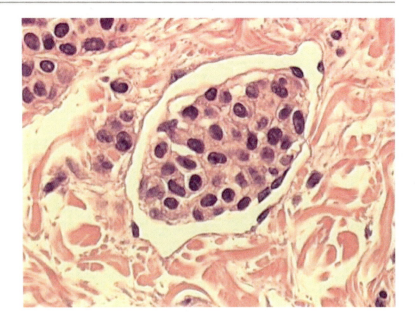

Thus, the collagen is infiltrated by the nevic cells, but the fibers of collagen are small in diameter, do not show striking interlacing as normal reticular dermal collagen fibers, and often lie parallel to the long axis of the epidermis. This type of reticular dermal change is more common in adult nevi in our experience than in the children's congenital nevi. High magnification reveals the cells to be of the type B cell in the superficial dermis but more of a type C cell appearance in the deeper dermis having a more fusiform aspect. Thus, the cells infiltrate singly amidst collagen fibers in the subcutaneous fat, have a rather fusiform appearance. However, at times throughout the entire dermis and into the subcutaneous fat, type B nevus cells may be noted. The giant congenital nevus [8], on the other hand, more commonly has extensive proliferation of nevus cells that are present throughout the entire dermis and into subcutaneous fat and may even be present in fascia and muscle beneath the cutaneous lesion. The histological alterations in these lesions, while composed of type B and type C cells or fusiform cells, are much more extensive and the changes involving appendages much more easily observed in the giant congenital nevus than in the small congenital nevi. Likewise in the large congenital nevi there are often quite prominent complex neuroid structures, areas of neurofibroma-like differentiation associated with chondroid and cartilage. Areas of cellular blue nevi and blue nevi may be observed in the giant congenital nevus as well as areas of spindle and epithelioid cell nevi. Frequently, when one is dealing with a congenital nevus that is extensive and deep, it is necessary to perform S100 stain to identify the depth margin of the lesion. If a congenital nevus is removed regardless of reason, the fascia and muscle below the skin must always be observed for the possibility of residual nevi nests.

Proliferative Nodules in Congenital Nevi

Congenital nevi can exhibit expansile nodular proliferations of nevus cells which are a cause for concern and present difficulties in the histopathologic diagnosis [9]. The more common nodule is composed of nevocytes that are type B in character; it is benign and shows no mitotic activity (Fig. 7.8). Any expansile aggregate of melanocytic origin must be carefully evaluated for features of malignancy which include severe nuclear atypia, the presence of necrosis of nevocytes with or without ulceration, the presence of an expansile destructive behavior of the nodule with deformity and obliteration of adjacent structures, and the presence of mitoses. Very importantly, there is usually a striking and abrupt border between the benign nevus cells and the atypical

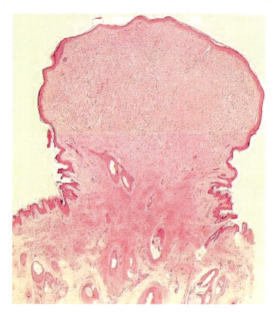

Fig. 7.8 Proliferative nodule in congenital nevus

melanocytic cells in the malignant lesions. Benign lesions show cells that tend to blend with the nevus cells in the adjacent congenital nevus. Thus, there appears to be a maturation from those cells in the midst of the lesion to the surrounding nevic cells. Malignant nodules are usually greater than 5.0 mm. in size. Lesions that show some mitotic activity (less than 7/mm^2), without necrosis, without ulceration, and without destructive deforming architectural features are considered as atypical and diagnosed the lesion as an *atypical nevomelanocytic proliferation* in a congenital nevus (see section "Atypical Melanocytic Tumors", pag. 139). The cellular components of these nodules may include populations of type B nevus cells or population of spindle and epithelioid cells. The histochemical stain for reticular fibers (silver impregnation method) can be useful in the differential diagnosis with melanoma; the positive fibers surround with a dense network every individual cell in the proliferative nodule; on the contrary, they are pushed to the periphery in the nodule of melanoma vertical growth. The congenital nevus of the scalp in the occipital region has been associated with intracranial nevocytic proliferations. Meningeal proliferations occur as well as proliferations of nevus cells

along penetrating arteries of the brain substance. Rarely, proliferations in the cisterna have led to internal hydrocephalus. The combination of an occipital congenital nevus and internal hydrocephalus is known as Touraine's syndrome. The principle differential diagnostic considerations include tumors of neural and fibroblastic origin. The common presence of neuro-differentiation resembling neurofibromas and schwannomas in giant congenital nevi may lead to an erroneous diagnosis if the entire clinical picture is not evident. We have found that in cases of peripheral nerve sheath tumors occurring in the setting of giant congenital nevi, one may find striking involvement of nerves by nevus cells in such cases. This change may help to identify the origin of the peripheral neural proliferation in a congenital nevus. However, taken along the peripheral nerve sheath, tumors can be indistinguishable from spontaneous neurofibromas or schwannomas and the clinical history may be necessary to identify the correct pathogenesis of the lesions. The dermatofibrosarcoma protuberans, especially the Bednar tumor or pigmented variant, can sometimes be confused with a fibroblastic variant of the congenital nevus. In congenital nevi, however, one does not find a storiform pattern. Also, the dermatofibrosarcoma protuberans is a large deforming nodule which displaces appendages. The fibroblastic variant of the congenital nevus is associated with a linear deposition of collagen fibers parallel to the long axis of the epidermis frequently, does not act as a deforming nodule, and hence leaves appendages unaltered.

Superficial Atypical Melanocytic Proliferation in Congenital Nevi

Another difficult histologic interpretation is the observation of striking epithelioid cells in the epidermis and superficial dermis of congenital nevi, especially in young patients that may simulate a superficial spreading melanoma. The nevus cells may show prominent nuclei with evident nucleoli and finely granular melanin in their cytoplasm. A careful evaluation of these proliferations reveals that the nuclei show very delicate and regular chromatin and that nuclear cytoplasmic ratios are small. Another important pattern is the

Fig. 7.9 Halo nevus

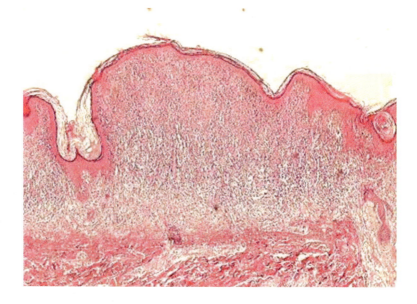

absence of pagetoid spread at the nevus shoulder. Also the dermal component shows a propensity to mature and blend with the underlying dermal nevus cells.

Nevi, Rare Variants

Halo Nevus

The *halo nevus* is defined as a pigmented lesion with usually benign clinical characteristics surrounded by a zone of depigmentation that is symmetrically disposed [10]. This rim of depigmentation gives rise to the name halo. Histologically there is a compound nevus usually associated to a very striking, band-like, infiltrative lymphocyte response that is present among the dermal component of the nevus (Fig. 7.9). In addition there is loss of melanin with tagging of lymphocytes along the dermoepidermal junction in the depigmented area. The halo nevus has also been known as *Sutton's nevus* or *leukoderma acquisitum centrifugum*. The halo is usually round or oval and the pigmented lesion is symmetrically disposed in the center of the lesion. The type of pigmented lesion that may give rise to a halo nevus includes ordinary acquired compound, junctional compound and dermal nevi, compound nevi of Spitz, dysplastic nevi,

and rarely congenital nevi. Halo blue nevi rarely occur. Characteristically the cells that infiltrate the nevus are T cell in type. Halo nevi are most commonly associated with compound nevus that is symmetrical, well circumscribed, and composed of intraepidermal nesting with type B cells and C cells in the dermis. At times one may see lymphocytes migrating into the junctional nests with lymphocyte nevus cell satellitosis. Lymphocyte nevus cell satellitosis is commonly observed in the dermal component. Altered nevus cells have an eosinophilic appearance to their cytoplasm and many binucleate with prominent nuclei forms are noted. On the whole most of the dermal nevus cells are larger than normal nevus cells. Mitotic figures are only rarely found in halo nevi and should alert suspicion of possibly an atypical proliferative lesion leading to examination of multiple sections. As far as pigmentation is concerned, the nevus cells may show residual melanin pigment. Occasionally scattered melanophages are noted around the inflamed dermal component as well as below the adjacent epidermis. Halo nevi must be distinguished from halo dysplastic nevi or from melanoma with vertical growth phase. In halo dysplastic nevi in addition to the brisk infiltrate, one observes a proliferation of atypical nevomelanocytes in the epidermis well away from the dermal component. These cells

Fig. 7.10 Balloon cell nevus

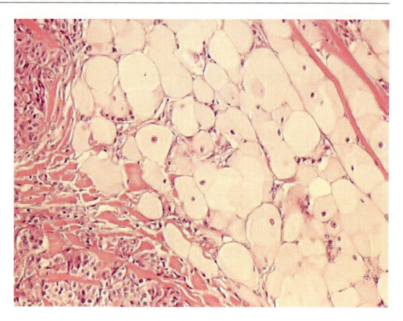

are present in lentiginous array and show irregular nesting. One must be aware, however, that most dysplastic nevi have some host response associated with them. The host response is usually not associated with lymphocyte nevus cell satellitosis of either the intraepidermal or the dermal component of the nevus or with the presence of lymphocytes along the dermoepidermal junction with lymphocyte nevus cell satellitosis. Melanoma can be differentiated histologically on the basis of the atypia of the cells, the presence of an expansile nodule growth in the dermal component and aggressive infiltration of the epidermis with pagetoid spread, and the presence of scattered mitoses with or without ulceration and necrosis. As far as the cytology of the individual cells is concerned, the halo nevus cells may be larger than normal nevus cells but show benign nuclear characteristics, whereas the melanoma cells show very pleomorphic nuclei with irregular chromatin patterns and with very prominent eosinophilic nucleoli. Likewise in the halo nevus, pagetoid spread is usually absent or minimal. Furthermore the intraepidermal component is a well-defined nested pattern as opposed to the melanoma which shows both irregular-sized nests and pagetoid spread. Nevus cells may be very difficult to discern in the midst of the inflammatory infiltrate. The S100 and particularly p16 stain

may be helpful in finding the nevus cells in a suspect lesion.

Balloon Cell Nevus

In *balloon cell nevus* more than 50 % of dermal nevomelanocytes manifest abundant clear, finely vacuolated cytoplasm and small hyperchromatic nuclei with a scalloped contour (Fig. 7.10) [11]. Multinucleation may be observed. The main differential diagnosis is that of balloon cell melanoma, based on the recognition of a malignant neoplastic cytology; in balloon cell melanoma, the majority of cells manifest pleomorphism, the nuclei appearing large with irregularly distributed chromatin, mitoses, and necrosis.

Recurrent Melanocytic Nevus

Usually the *recurrent nevus* is a compound nevus but in 32 % of cases it is a dermal nevus and a junctional nevus in 5 % of cases. Less than 10 % of recurrent nevi are dysplastic nevi. The recurrent nevus describes the appearance of pigmentation at the site of a previously removed benign (Fig. 7.11) lesion usually incompletely affected by shave biopsy [12]. The histological problem is frequently an intraepidermal melanocytic growth of atypical melanocytes in lentiginous array over the previous scar that suggests pagetoid melanoma [13]. Clinically, the recurrence occurs very

Fig. 7.11 Recurrent nevus and scar

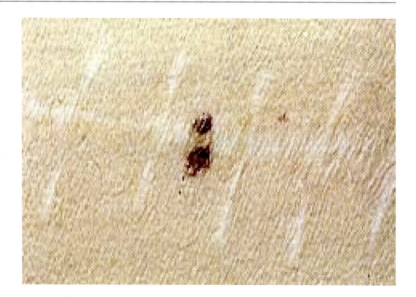

Fig. 7.12 Recurrent nevus

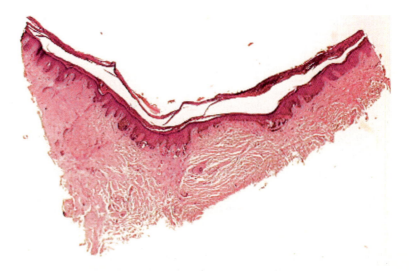

rapidly, usually in 1–2 months. This speed of recurrence is helpful in distinguishing a recurrent nevus from a recurrent melanoma which usually takes a much more protracted period of time even up to years for the recurrence to appear. The recurrent nevus presents a broad intraepidermal proliferation of melanocytes, sometimes greater than 6.0 mm in width with a combination of intraepidermal nests and single cells. The pagetoid spread of both nests and single cells is frequently observed. However, involvement in the stratum corneum does not commonly occur. Mitoses are characteristically absent in the intraepidermal component and in the superficial dermal component where single cells sometimes infiltrate the scar (Fig. 7.12). Nests predominate over single cells in this proliferation. The intraepidermal cells often have an epithelioid or round appearance with scattered melanin in their cytoplasm. This change resembles superficial spreading melanoma cells but the nuclear picture is that of a benign process with finely dispersed nuclear chromatin and small blue nucleoli. In the dermis beneath the proliferated lesion, there may be single round cells of a melanocytic nature but there are often numerous melanophages with scattered inflammation. Admixed with the depth of the scar or beneath it, one will find at the base of the scar nests of type B or type C nevus cells evidence of the residual dermal component of the lesion. Recurrent spindle and epithelioid cell nevi are one variant which may cause difficulty because of the propensity of the nevic cells to infiltrate the collagen of the scar. However, the spindle and epithelioid cell recurrences do not form expansile nodules but rather wedge-shaped proliferations with a mimicry of the inverted triangle of the benign spindle and epithelioid cell nevus. The recurrent dysplastic nevus is associated with epidermal atypia of a more marked degree. We have rarely seen epidermal hyperplasia with elongate rete in recurrent dysplastic nevi overlying the scar. The recurrent blue nevus shows characteristic dendritic cells that lie adjacent to the dermal fibrotic zone of the scar. Recurrent melanoma is the most significant differential diagnostic consideration in which one finds pagetoid spread of severely atypical epithelioid cells in the area adjacent to the scar in addition to the area overlying the scar. Likewise, if there be a dermal component, it is composed of an expansile nodule or vertical growth phase equivalent. One must always remember that recurrent nevi may be associated with single cell infiltration of the scar; this change should not be interpreted as melanoma. Review of prior material is essential when available.

Nevi of Special Site

The nevi of particular body sites (skin of genital, breast, acral, and belt area) and in physiologic states such as old or young age or pregnancy may show junctional or dermal proliferation that simulates dysplastic nevi and melanoma. This relatively frequent, recently recognized, and growing group of nevi has been termed, generically, *nevi of special sites*.

Nevi of Genital Skin

These nevi commonly affect the vulva of young women but occasionally occur on the male genitalia as well. Low-power examination reveals usually a well-circumscribed lesion with nevus cells in nests both intraepidermally and dermally. There is often easily visible a single cell basal

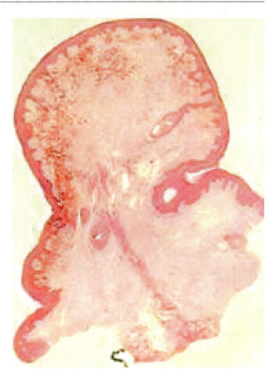

Fig. 7.13 Vulvar nevus: superficial dermal component

proliferation which may extend on both sides of the dermal component of the lesion when present; pagetoid spread, but of benign melanocytes, is found in approximately two-thirds of the patients. Keratinocytic hyperplasia is variable and does not show the regular rete ridge elongation of the dysplastic nevus [14]. Beneath the epidermis there is a coarse fibrosis without pattern that is distinctly different than the lamellar fibroplasia of the dysplastic nevus. The dermal component is usually confined to the upper half of the reticular dermis (Fig. 7.13) and consists of nests of nevus cells. High-power magnification usually shows a lentiginous and nested proliferation of nevomelanocytes but often spindle or epithelioid forms. These cells form oval discohesive theques that are present at both sides of the tips of the rete ridges and sometimes span the supra-papillary epidermis. Fusion of adjacent rete at their tips and even confluence of junctional nests in a plaque-like configuration may be noted. Extension along the basal layer of appendageal structures, especially the outer root sheath of the hair follicles, may be a striking feature. The high-power examination

Fig. 7.14 Acral nevus

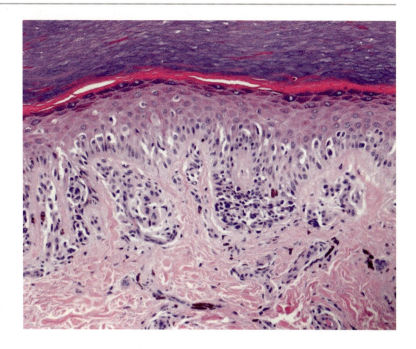

reveals that the spindle cells resemble some constituents of the compound nevus of Spitz, but these are smaller than the Spitz nevus cells and have less evident nuclear membrane and less prominent nucleoli. Chromatin however is evenly dispersed through the nucleus and there is a thin chromatin rim. Multinucleate giant cells in the intraepidermal component are a frequent finding. Often there are nests of pigmented epithelioid cells in the epidermis that are variably pigmented. These cells have small nuclei but often prominent nucleoli. As stated above, pagetoid spread may be observed but the pagetoid cells are not malignant in appearance and have a nuclear morphology similar to those in the intraepithelial and intradermal nests. The lesions tend to be symmetrical; if they have lateral extent, it appears symmetrically on both sides of the dermal component. Cells in the dermal component are disposed in nests which become smaller both in the size of the nests and in the size of the cells as they infiltrate into the papillary-reticular dermal junction and deeper into the reticular dermis. However, in some lesions one observes small nests of pigmented epithelioid cells entrapped in the collagen. The deeper cells mature into ordinary type B nevus cells. The lesion most commonly mistaken for the vulvar nevus is superficial spreading melanoma. One confidently can exclude superficial spreading melanoma by appreciating the characteristic spindle and epithelioid morphology of the intraepidermal component, the lack of cytologic features of malignancy including pleomorphism and prominent eosinophilic nucleoli, as well as an absence of mitotic activity. The second lesion to be considered is the *dysplastic nevus*. Dysplastic nevi may occur on vulvar skin as well as on male genital skin but they are very rare. The genital nevi are usually isolated lesions and are not associated with evidence of dysplastic nevi elsewhere.

Acral Nevus

The main morphological features distinguishing the *acral lentiginous nevi* from other acral non-lentiginous nevi are: elongation of rete ridges; continuous proliferation of melanocytes at the dermoepidermal junction; presence of single scattered melanocytes, or less commonly small clusters, within the upper epidermis; poor or absent lateral circumscription; melanocytes with abundant pale cytoplasm and round to oval, sometimes hyperchromatic, nuclei; and prominent nucleoli present at the dermoepidermal junction (Fig. 7.14). Some histological features of acral

Fig. 7.15 Pigmented
spindle cell nevus

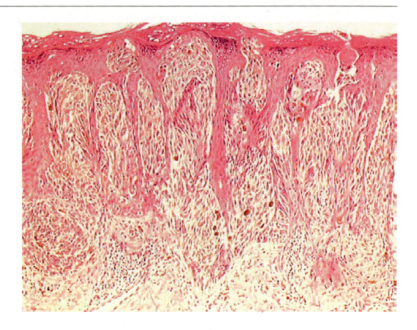

lentiginous nevi are similar to those of dysplastic nevi; however, anastomosing rete ridges, cytological atypia, and well-formed lamellar fibroplasia are usually absent. The histopathological criteria to distinguish these nevi from melanoma are the lack of pagetoid lateral spread, the absence of mitotic activity in the deep dermal component, and the evidence of dermal nevocytic differentiation. The identification of this benign acral nevus, which we have identified as the benign counterpart of acral lentiginous melanoma, is important in order to avoid misdiagnoses and consequent under- or over-treatment of doubtful pigmented lesions of acral skin [15].

Spindle and Epithelioid Cell Nevi

Pigmented Spindle Cell Nevus (Reed Nevus)

It is a benign tumor characterized by proliferation of spindle nevus cells intensely pigmented that are confined at the dermoepidermal surface or the top portion of the papillary dermis. Described by Reed in 1975 as pigmented spindle cell nevus, "non-Spitz" is also considered a variant of the epithelioid and spindle cell nevus. Its identification has clinical significance. The lesion

is usually a patch or plaque or a plaque with a small papule in contrast to the compound nevus of Spitz that is a papule or nodule. The spindle cell nevus is a symmetrical lesion, with sharp margins, characterized by a proliferation of spindle nevus cells, intensely pigmented, with typical superficial location limited to the dermoepidermal junction and sometimes extended to the superficial portion of the papillary dermis (Fig. 7.15). In the typical form the melanocytes are arranged in bundles or nests fairly regular in shape, size, and distribution and oriented in a vertical or horizontal pattern to occupy the junction and supra-basal portion of the epidermis and the superficial papillary dermis [16]. The extension to the dermis is often absent and, when present, is usually in bundles or small sharply demarcated nest and rarely to individual cells or in small groups irregularly shaped that may mimic melanoma in its spindle cell variant. In spindle cell nevus, however, the haphazard growth and pagetoid intraepidermal spread of melanocytes, especially at the lateral shoulder of the lesion, are absent. Pagetoid spread in the central nested area of the lesion is observed. The cell population often occurs uniformly in fusiform shape, with elongated nucleus and dispersed chromatin, small inconspicuous nucleoli, and little cytoplasm, with abundant melanin pigment, often in coarse granules. Epithelioid cells are rarely observed and even rarer is the presence of multinucleated giant cells. Mitosis may be present, even in large number, but at the junction the presence of a high mitotic index with evidence of atypical mitoses and depth should suggest the possibility of melanoma. The epidermal changes are characterized by elongation of the rete ridges and moderate hyperkeratosis. Frequently in the dermis, a lymphocytic infiltrate and numerous melanophages are present. Ulceration and foci of necrosis are usually absent. In addition to the previously described typical pattern, variants of the spindle cell nevus are reported: pigmented spindle cell nevus with prevalent epithelioid cells, atypical pigmented spindle cell nevus, plexiform pigmented spindle cell nevus, and combined spindle cell nevus. Plexiform pigmented spindle cell nevus is characterized by the extension of the melanocytic proliferation in the reticular dermis in the form of bundles of spindle cells intensively pigmented often in intimate association with adnexal structures, nerve or vascular, and interspersed by melanophages, isolated and in aggregates. This variant simulates the deep penetrating nevus, from which it differs, in particular, for the presence of an evident junctional proliferation of spindle cells in nests. The combined pigmented spindle cell nevus variant is characterized by the combination of a spindle cell nevus with another different nevus, more frequently dermal nevus or blue nevus. Although the spindle cell nevus shows cytoarchitectural aspects similar to epithelioid cell nevus (Spitz nevus) can be easily distinguished from this, especially for the presence of abundant melanin pigment and the presence of a junctional proliferation with little or minimal dermal extension. Differential diagnostic problems may arise with melanoma and dysplastic nevus, especially for the atypical variant of spindle cell nevus. The distinction from *dysplastic nevus* can be difficult when the spindle cell nevus presents cytoarchitectural focal atypia, in which case the marked tendency to arrange themselves in bundles of melanocytes and the general uniformity of the cell population are the main morphological aspects for a correct diagnosis of spindle cell nevus. The absence of a high

degree of architectural disorganization and severe cytological atypia; the intraepidermal spread of melanocytes confined mostly to the lower half of the epidermis, with rare isolated melanocytes in the superficial portions, but limited to the central portion of the tumor; and the presence of uniform cell population within the entire lesion represent the essential criteria for distinguishing spindle cell nevus from *melanoma*. The trans-epidermal migration of isolated cell or small nests is frequently present in pigmented spindle cell nevus and can simulate a pagetoid intraepidermal infiltration; however, the lack of malignant cytologic character, the absence of spread beyond the nests into the normal epidermis, and the absence of destruction of the epidermis are the most important characters in differential diagnosis with melanoma.

Epithelioid and Spindle Cell Nevus (Compound Nevus of Spitz Nevus)

This lesion is a benign tumor composed of spindle-shaped epithelioid melanocytes that occurs predominantly on the skin of the face or limbs in young individuals. It was described for the first time by Sophie Spitz [18] who designated the lesion as juvenile melanoma [17, 18] and, subsequently, as benign juvenile melanoma by Kopf and Andrade [19] or as pseudomelanoma. Today, these terms are to be avoided. In 1960, Kernen and Ackerman introduced the term epithelioid and spindle cell nevus [19], which is now universally accepted. This terminology, highly descriptive, on the one hand underlines the salient histopathological appearance, represented by a benign proliferation of fusiform and epithelioid melanocytes. The spindle and epithelioid cell nevus shows typically a symmetrical appearance often with a triangular pattern with the base in the upper dermis parallel to the long axis of the epidermis and the apex toward the depth (Fig. 7.16). The melanocytes are frequently large with spindle and/or epithelioid appearance (Fig. 7.17), arranged mainly in bundles or nests or alveolar structures. The cytoplasm is often abundant, dense, and large; is finely vacuolated and even wispy, eosinophilic, or amphophilic; and, in some cases diffusely pigmented with sparse and small melanin granules. The nucleus of melanocytes presents a dispersed chromatin and a well-demarcated nuclear membrane. The nucleolus is often centrally located, prominent, basophilic, or eosinophilic. There are sometimes multiple (two or three) nucleoli, sometimes with cytoplasmic invaginations (intranuclear pseudoinclusion). The spindle and epithelioid cell nevus can be junctional, compound, or dermal. The spindle and epithelioid cell compound variant is the most common. Each type of the cell population may consist primarily of fusiform melanocytes,

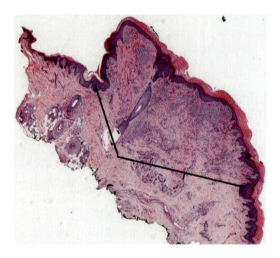

Fig. 7.16 Spitz nevus: reverse triangle

epithelioid cells, or both cell types. However, the pure epithelioid variant is most common in infancy. The presence of numerous epithelioid cells in an adult should prompt careful review and even levels if necessary to rule out a melanoma. It is not uncommon to find plurinucleate giant cells, also with four to five large nuclei. A useful rule of thumb is that the multiple nuclei are similar in a benign lesion. The malignant giant cell is associated with pleomorphic nuclei and nucleoli. The junctional component shows aggregate and nests of variable-size melanocytes unevenly distributed along the dermoepidermal junction (Fig. 7.18), often with major axis perpendicular to the skin surface. A halo, optically empty due to a fixation artifact phenomenon, separates the nests of the melanocytes from the epidermis. The junctional proliferation stops abruptly on the side margins and, if the nevus is compound, its lateral extension does not exceed the dermal component. The absence of lateral extension and dissemination supra-basal intra-epidermal-type "pagetoid" cells represents an important criterion for differentiating epithelioid and spindle cell nevus from melanoma, especially in adults. In the child, in fact, you can also see frequently involved even up to the stratum corneum of the epidermis with trans-epidermal elimination of individual melanocytes or nests. In the superficial dermal layer, typical mitoses can be observed but also very rare atypical

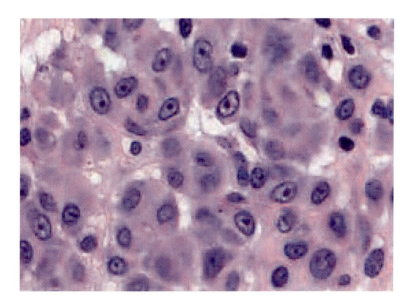

Fig. 7.17 Spitz nevus, epithelioid cells

Fig. 7.18 Spitz nevus, junctional and dermal proliferation

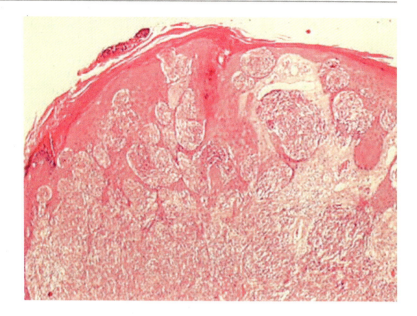

mitoses can sometimes be present even in the deep dermal portion; however, this character must be evaluated with caution because in the deep dermal portion, and along the proliferation margin, mitoses are more frequently present in melanoma. Marginal mitoses, namely, those within 250 μm of the peripheral border of the lesion, are of most concern and usually are associated with a metastatic potential of the lesion. In the dermal component, the melanocytes are arranged mainly in nests, bundles, or cords. The nests become smaller as they extend deeply and break up into single cells. These cells do not cause disruption of the dermal architecture so that the fibers appear to be falling apart. Rather, the cells appear as fibroblasts without destroying the architecture. Dr. Elston Helwig used to teach that the cells of the Spitz nevus look "at home in the dermis", much like the space between the collagen fibers of the reticular dermis separated without destroying a feature often available in single file. The size of the cells decreases in the reticular dermis, becoming more rounded with little cytoplasm (maturation). This kind of transformation is a morphological appearance characteristic and important for the diagnosis of epithelioid and spindle cell nevus. Two other histological features are important for the histological diagnosis: the uniformity of the cell population

morphology from side to side of the lesion and the presence of isolated single cells in a pseudo-infiltrative pattern at the base of the nevus, which reaches sometimes into the subcutaneous fat. The melanin pigment, when present, is in small quantities, most often in the superficial lesions, especially just below the epidermis. The spindle and epithelioid cell nevus is frequently accompanied by epidermal and stromal changes. Acanthosis, hyperkeratosis, pseudoepitheliomatous hyperplasia, and, less frequently, parakeratosis are frequently observed, especially in the epithelioid and spindle cell nevi of junctional or compound type, more rarely in the epithelioid and spindle cell dermal variant. The stromal alterations include frequently the presence of telangiectasia and edema of the papillary dermis, sometimes so marked as to create a clear zone of separation ("grenz zone") between the epidermis and the dermal component of nevus. Near the dermoepidermal junction, the "bodies of Kamino" can be found; these are rounded eosinophilic bodies present singly or in small clusters; they were interpreted as "apoptotic bodies," but they are now known to be portions of epithelial cell as well as nevus cell membranes admixed with cytosol. Lymphohistiocytic infiltrates are occasionally present and are scattered usually in the depth of the lesion. Dense infiltrates raise the question of a halo nevus or possibly an atypical lesion. Evidence of focal regression superficially with inflammation and fibrosis is usually a sign of a melanoma. *Halo Spitz nevi*, as any other halo nevus, have a prominent infiltrate that affects the entire lesion, not a focal portion. Numerous histopathological variants of the spindle and epithelioid cell nevus can be recognized. A *desmoplastic variant* [20] in which there is a striking pericellular fibrosis that encompasses the entire lesion. The brightly eosinophilic fibers highlight the often quite densely stained nevus cells. Clear epithelioid cell forms help to differentiate the lesion from a desmoplastic melanoma or sclerosing blue nevus. According to Hilliard [21], the staining pattern for p16 in desmoplastic melanomas and Spitz nevi in conjunction with the histopathologic features, S100 staining, Ki67proliferation index, and clinical scenario may aid in the difficult differential diagnosis between these two entities. There is also a *balloon cell variant* [22], a *lichenoid variant*, and as noted a *halo variant* [23]. Rarely a granulomatous response has been described. The *myxoid variant* [24], often with the presence of mast cells, is reported. The spindle and epithelioid cell nevus often poses problems of differential diagnosis with melanoma. In fact, some important characters for the histopathological diagnosis of malignancy, such as cellular atypia, intraepidermal spread, and the presence of mitosis, are not as conclusive if detected in epithelioid and spindle cell nevi. Knowledge of clinical features (age, location, mode of onset, duration, macroscopic and dermatoscopic appearance) is very important and sometimes essential for a correct interpretation of the lesion. One of the most important patterns is the cytology monomorphism present in Spitz nevus and absent in polyclonal proliferation of the melanoma. The junctional/superficial spindle and epithelioid cell nevus must be distinguished from dysplastic nevus and melanoma in situ. In favor of the dysplastic nevus are the proliferation of basal melanocytes with freckled "atypical" and polymorphic pattern and the presence of fused nests with major axis parallel to the skin surface, the elongation of the rete ridges, and the fibrosis of the superficial dermis.

The presence of a continuous proliferation of atypical melanocytes with a tendency to invade aggressively the more superficial layers of the epidermis, atypical mitoses, and marked dermal inflammatory infiltrate, referring to the diagnosis of melanoma in situ or invasive horizontal growth phase melanoma. The compound spindle and epithelioid cell nevus can pose problems of differential diagnosis with invasive superficial spreading melanoma. In particular the epithelioid and spindle cell nevi that have marked trans-epidermal migration in nests or single cells epidermal infiltration can simulate a "pagetoid" spread and those with numerous mitoses especially in the deepest portion of the lesion. The dermal epithelioid cell and dermal spindle nevus can be misinterpreted as nodular melanoma; in these cases the clonal proliferation without evidence of deep dermal maturation, the presence of atypical mitoses, and the cellular necrosis and apoptosis can be important characters to distinguish Spitz nevus from melanoma. The use of additional diagnostic methods such as immunohistochemical stains with monoclonal antibodies and/or polyclonal (anti-S100, NSE, HMB45), the determination of DNA content (ploidy) by means of flow cytometry or image analyzer, and the evaluation of cell proliferation (PCNA) still do not allow to differentiate with certainty nevus epithelioid and spindle cell melanoma. In our experience and in recent report [25], p16 expression in nodular spitzoid melanomas and Spitz nevi, in conjunction with clinical and histopathological evaluation, may be a useful tool in differentiating between these two entities. Melanoma cases are associated with loss of p16 immunoreactivity without any correlation with their Breslow thickness, whereas the Spitz nevi have a strong positive nuclear and cytoplasmic expression of p16 staining (Fig. 7.19). More recently, techniques of in situ hybridization of DNA in paraffin slides have demonstrated some chromosomal abnormalities suggestive of melanoma [26]. Furthermore, the technique of comparative genomic hybridization (CGH) has revealed that in Spitz one can find an increased copy of the short arm of chromosome 11 [27]. Less often changes in chromosome 6 have been

Fig. 7.19 Spitz nevus: nuclear and cytoplasm p16-positive stain

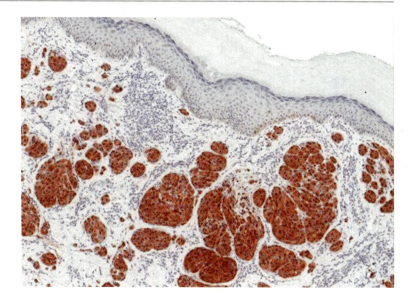

described [28]. These very limited changes are strikingly different than the myriad changes found in malignant melanoma.

Dermal Melanocytosis

The blue nevus and its variants (cellular, atypical, and combined) belong together with desmoplastic blue nevus, deep-penetrating nevus, Mongolian spot, and the Ota and Ito nevi, are a group of lesions defined as the "dermal melanocytoses" [29]. These lesions are characterized by the proliferation of pigmented dendritic or epithelioid melanocytes located in the papillary and reticular dermis and by a prevalent immunohistochemical positivity with HMB45 antibody stain.

The Common Blue Nevus

The blue nevus is a benign melanocytic tumor in which the depth of melanin pigment present in nevus cells in the deep dermis is responsible for the characteristic color of the lesion which takes its name (Fig. 7.20). The blue nevus occurs predominantly in young people, with equal frequency in both sexes. The sites most affected are the skin on the backs of hands and feet and buttocks. Lesions also may be found on the trunk

and on the scalp. Cases have been reported in extra-cutaneous site: oral cavity [30], uterus [31, 32], vagina [33], spermatic cord [34], and prostate (Fig. 7.21) [35, 36]; one case was described in a teratoma involving a mature cystic ovary [37] and in the bronchial tree [38]. Clinically, the lesions exhibit a blue, deep blue, blue-gray, or royal blue color. The blue nevus is characterized by three fundamental morphological aspects: (1) proliferation of dendritic melanocytes in the reticular dermis, (2) numerous melanophages, and (3) fibrogenetic stromal reaction. The dendritic melanocytes show typical elongate fusiform shape, with thin cytoplasmic extensions and prominent melanin pigment granules that sometimes obscure the nucleus. However, the pigment is always a brown finely granular one that differentiates the blue nevus cell from a melanophage in which the pigment is dense and coarse and often obscures the nucleus. In the blue nevus, the latter is oval to egg-shaped and displays finely dispersed chromatin, thin nuclear membrane, and inconspicuous nucleolus. Only rarely pleomorphism is present. The mode of cellular growth, individually or in small bundles, creeping between the collagen fibers of the dermis in a sometimes serpiginous pattern, without collagen fragmentation, is responsible for the apparent lack of cellularity of the lesion, which in low magnification can simulate the benign fibrous

Fig. 7.20 Blue nevus

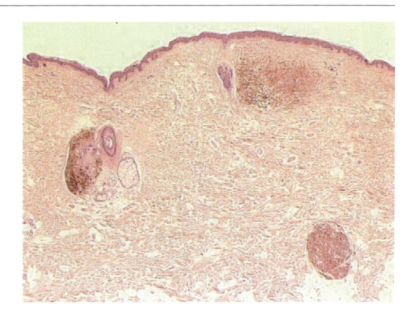

Fig. 7.21 Blue nevus
prostate, HMB45
immunostain

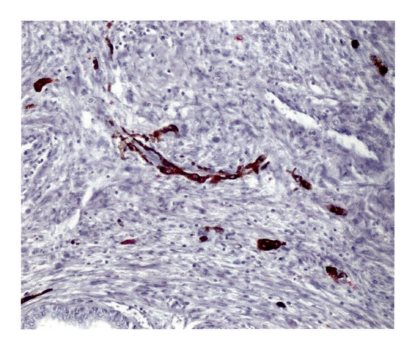

histiocytoma. Often one can observe a tendency of the nevus cells to arrange themselves around the skin appendages or along vessels or nerves. The fibrogenesis shows varying degrees, from mild to intense, until the formation of dense bundles that give the appearance of a desmoplastic or sometimes neuroid lesion. Commingled with the melanocytes melanophages with cytoplasm packed with large granules of melanin pigment are still present. In the typical form mitoses are usually not observed. The presence of a melanocytic proliferation-free zone immediately below the epidermis (grenz zone) is a characteristic feature. The epidermis may occasionally exhibit hyperplasia and hyperpigmentation of basal melanocytes very similar to the findings of a benign dermal fibrous histiocytoma. Frequently it is possible to observe multifocal areas of proliferation of the blue nevus. Among the variants of the blue nevus, one of the most common is the *combined blue nevus* where the lesion is presented in association with usually an acquired nevus. The ordinary nevus component may be a junctional, compound, or dermal nevus type. Less commonly, it may be a spindle and epithelioid cell Spitz nevus. Certainly one may find a combined congenital/blue nevus. The change may be present at birth. When it is acquired in the congenital setting, it appears as a change in the lesion. Because pigmented melanomas can occur in the deep portion of a congenital nevus and have a blue discoloration, we recommend always a biopsy of any acquired blue discolored area in one of these congenital lesions. The differential diagnosis of blue nevus is usually not a problem especially for the typical form. The differential diagnosis with other forms of dermal melanocytic proliferation must be considered. The nevus of Ota and Ito that, however, present a typical clinical pattern and location. The ectopic Mongolian spot is usually a congenital lesion that has similar coloration to the Mongolian spot in the lower posterior trunk. It is also a flat lesion with no consistency compared to blue nevi that are usually at least firm and slightly raised. The benign dermal fibrous histiocytoma, especially when there are marked hemosiderin deposits, and the tattoo should be also considered in differential diagnosis [39].

Cellular Blue Nevus

Cellular blue nevus is a characteristic melanocytic tumor frequently localized in sacral coccygeal and gluteal area with a marked cellularity involving not only the reticular layer but also the hypodermis often with a characteristic dumbbell-shaped pattern" (Fig. 7.22). The tumor frequently exhibits a multinodular growth, and three different patterns can be identified: (1) mixed biphasic, (2) alveolar, and (3) neuro-nevoid. The *mixed biphasic* is the most frequent and is composed of large nodules of spindle cells intermingled with nests of epithelioid cells resulting from cross section of spindle cell fascicles. These nodules are separated from one another by zones of

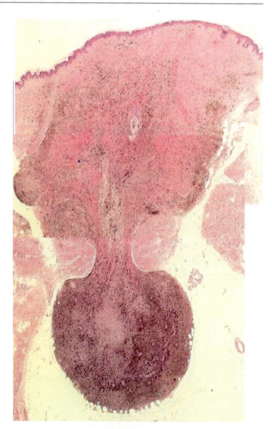

Fig. 7.22 Cellular blue nevus

fibrosis. These fibrous zones contain melanophages but also exhibit characteristic blue nevus cells. Rare mitoses can be observed in these nodules as can some pleomorphism. The *alveolar* type presents rounded nests, with sharp edges; polyhedral and spindle cells, often pigmented with vesicular nuclei; inconspicuous nucleoli; and typical clear cytoplasm. The nests are surrounded by pigmented dendritic melanocytes and melanophages commingled with little stromal collagen which can occasionally occur edematous. In the *neuro-nevoid* type, the cells present schwannian differentiation and tend to aggregate in bundles that simulate the appearance of peripheral nerves; collagen and macrophages can be abundant. At times the cellular blue nevi can be so strikingly proliferative with ulceration that they raise the question with a nodular melanoma. However, the presence of dendritic cells with melanophages in fibrous stroma between the nodular islands of cellular blue nevi helps to differentiate this tumor from nodular melanoma. Likewise, the islands of cells are filled with cells containing clear cytoplasm with coarse melanin granules scattered amidst the clear cytoplasm. Overall the nuclei are repetitively similar and mitotic figures may be observed but the mitoses are not atypical and are not frequent in number. In nodular melanoma which resembles cellular blue nevi, there is very high grade nuclear atypia associated with mitotic activity and necrosis.

Desmoplastic Nevus

Some nevi present or may become fibrous nodules for the presence of desmoplasia. The recognition of the desmoplastic nevus is important to distinguish from other benign skin lesions such as fibrous histiocytoma and dermal neurofibroma but also from desmoplastic melanoma [40]. The presence of desmoplasia in nevus may be related to regressive or reactive phenomena. The proliferation

is usually centered in the papillary dermis but can also be extended to the reticular dermis and junctional activity often is minimal or absent. The epidermis overlying the tumor may present pseudoepitheliomatous hyperplasia, irregular acanthosis, and hyperkeratosis. The nevus cells are arranged singly or in small clusters, nests, or cords, and spindle cells predominating type C cells and epithelioid types A and B are less frequent or rare but always readily apparent. Sometimes there are bizarre giant cells with or ganglion-like aspects. Not uncommon is the finding of intranuclear inclusions caused by invaginations of the cytoplasm to the nucleus. Mitoses are rare and atypical mitoses are absent. The melanin pigment is irregularly distributed granules of different sizes and quantitatively variable. Rare are the melanophages. The stroma consists of eosinophilic collagen bundles usually much thicker than those normally recognized in the papillary dermis. The stroma often surrounds and isolates individual cells. Characteristic is a convex lens patter with sharp margins (Fig. 7.23). In Table 7.2 the main characteristics between desmoplastic nevus and desmoplastic melanoma are compared.

Deep-Penetrating Nevus

The deep-penetrating nevus is a benign acquired melanocytic proliferation that often has a brown to blue/black coloration with histological features that resemble the combined nevus, a blue nevus and a spindle and epithelioid cell nevus [41].

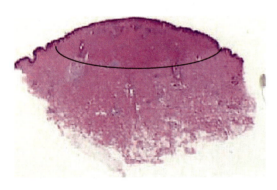

Fig. 7.23 Desmoplastic nevus, convex lens pattern

Table 7.2 Differential diagnosis between desmoplastic nevus and desmoplastic melanoma

	Desmoplastic nevus	Desmoplastic melanoma
Junctional activity	Poor or absent	Nests of melanocytes with acral or lentiginous pattern
Epidermis	Hyperkeratosis or irregular acanthosis	Atrophy and thinning
Margins	Well demarcated	Irregular (neurotropism)
Type of cells	Predominance of spindle cells rare epithelioid and giant cells	Epithelioid cells on the surface and spindle cells in depth
	Some bizarre ganglion-like cells	Rare polymorphism
Mitoses	Rare, superficial; no atypical mitoses	Present at all levels and atypical
Necrosis	Absent	Variable
Melanin pigmentation	Moderate	Usually scarce or absent

Fig. 7.24 Deep penetrating nevus

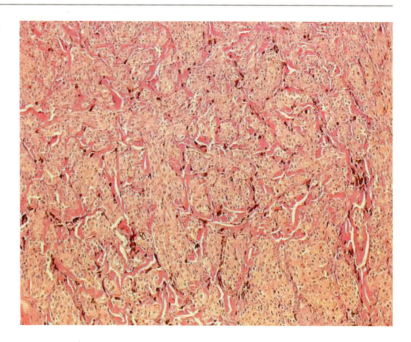

Necrosis, ulceration, and/or significant mitotic activity is usually absent. Low-power examination reveals a strikingly circumscribed but deeply penetrating lesion that is usually wedged shape. The base of the lesion lies along the long axis of the epidermis and the apex or apexes are present in the deep dermis and in the subcutaneous fat. The intraepidermal component consists of nests of nevus cells that are usually similar to the deep dermal proliferation. The dermal component of the lesion shows numerous fascicles and nests or cords of nevus cells surrounded by melanin-laden macrophages (Fig. 7.24). Most lesions have a focal scattered lymphoid infiltrate. The presence of a compound nevus with extensive deep infiltration with scattered melanophages and with an irregular border with theques of cells following neurovascular bundles is quite characteristic. There is some diminution in cell size from superficial to deep, but overall the cells remain about similar in size throughout, without evidence of maturation from the superficial to deep component of the nevus. The cells of the deep-penetrating nevus are S100 andHMB45 antigen positive; p16 may be variable with isolated positive nevus cell. They are negative for keratin and lysozyme except in the areas of the macrophages. The deep penetrating nevus poses a striking problem frequently in differential diagnosis from nodular melanoma [42]. Nodular melanoma usually presents large intraepidermal clonal nests of severely atypical cells. Melanomas are usually lesions with broad bases and with a narrower origin site, the converse of the deep penetrating nevus which has a broad base superficially and a tapered apex. Also melanomas tend to expand more laterally with expansile nodule formation in the dermis, whereas the deep penetrating nevus extends outward into the dermis along neurovascular bundles. Furthermore, melanoma shows much more pleomorphism and polyclonal nest. In the compound nevus of Spitz the fascicles become much smaller as they reach the mid to deep reticular dermis and there is often an insinuation of single cells in the lower reticular dermis.

Dysplastic Nevus

Dysplastic nevi are a type of acquired nevus usually greater than 6.0 mm in diameter, with irregular borders and irregular coloration, present in sun-exposed areas on the arms and trunk but importantly can also affect the scalp and covered areas of the body, namely, the female

Fig. 7.25 Dysplastic nevus

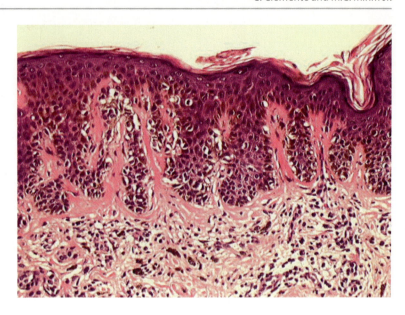

breasts and the bathing trunk areas. These lesions represent risk markers and potential melanoma precursors. They occur both sporadically or are inherited as an autosomal dominant. They rarely can be noted at birth. When sporadic, they can be single or only a few in number; when present in the familial setting, they can be numerous with some patients presenting with hundreds of lesions. The presence of a single dysplastic nevus is associated with a slight increase in incidence of melanoma. Multiple dysplastic nevi, especially in the familial setting have a substantial risk of increased incidence often as much as 125-fold compared to a person without the family involvement [43]. Genomic analysis of dysplastic nevi are associated with nonrandom mutations often involving chromosome 6. Dysplastic nevi exhibit an atypical proliferation of nevocytes with specific epidermal and dermal architectural features. In the heritable setting they are associated with the family history of atypical moles and/or melanoma and are referred to as the *dysplastic nevus syndrome*. The histopathological diagnosis of a dysplastic nevus requires an appreciation of both cytologic and architectural features [44]. The cytologic patterns have been described as lentiginous and epithelioid. The architectural features combine both epidermal and stromal changes and they are divided into major and minor criteria. The

presence of both major criteria and at least two of the minor criteria is requested for the diagnosis (Fig. 7.25). Dysplastic nevi may be junctional or compound. The important epidermal criterion is a hyperplasia and elongation of the rete ridges similar to the hyperplasia observed in lentigo simplex. The principal cytologic features are an atypical nevocytic proliferation with either a lentiginous pattern with small cells with irregular-shaped nuclei confined to the dermoepidermal junction or an epithelioid cell pattern with large round cells with fine melanin granules in their cytoplasm. These cells have also round nuclei with oval shape and small nucleolus. When the lesions are compound, they frequently show an irregular extent of the atypical proliferation beyond the dermal component. The stromal changes include patterns of collagen deposition around the rete ridges, increased vascularity, and inflammation. The histopathologic criteria have been formulated as follows:

Major criterion: A basilar proliferation of atypical nevocytes extending at least three rete ridges beyond any dermal nevocytic component. An organization of this proliferation in a lentiginous or epithelioid cell pattern

Minor criterion: The presence of lamellar fibroplasias or concentric eosinophilic fibrosis, neovascularization, inflammatory host response, and fusion of rete ridges

The major feature exhibits basilar proliferation of atypical nevocytes consists of a proliferation of nevocytes along the dermoepidermal junction in characteristically hyperplastic rete resembling lentigo simplex but with cytologic atypia. The atypia consists in pleomorphism of the melanocytic population with increase of the nuclear dimension, irregular chromatin pattern and presence of some cells with prominent nucleoli. In the junctional dysplastic nevus it is this change solely that is present and fulfills the requirement of the first major criterion. If there is a preexisting dermal component, then it is necessary to identify the extent at least three rete ridges beyond the dermal component. This change has also been referred to as the "shoulder" effect as described by Clark [45]. Similar pattern is present frequently in congenital and some acquired compound nevi but the intraepidermal proliferation beyond the dermal component in these nevi is absent. If present, the intraepidermal component is symmetrical on both sides of the lesion, whereas in the dysplastic nevus, it is asymmetrical. Occasionally pagetoid spread may be noted but consists of small nevocytes with hyperchromatic nuclei. The pagetoid spread is usually confined to the lower half of the epidermis. It is quite characteristic for an occasional single cell to be found in the papillary dermis beneath the atypical lentiginous proliferation. In epithelioid cell dysplasia the nevocytes have a characteristic appearance of ample cytoplasm surrounding usually round small nuclei. The cytoplasm contains fine melanin granules. The nuclei may have visible nucleoli which are small and blue or amphophilic, or the nuclei may be quite densely hyperchromatic. However, importantly the nuclear to cytoplasmic ratios are small. Often in epithelioid dysplasia the epidermis is slightly hyperplastic without the striking elongation of the rete ridges as seen in the lentiginous dysplasia. The epithelioid cells are present singly along the dermoepidermal junction, form nests of various sizes, and may be associated with pagetoid spread confined to the lower half of the epidermis without aggressive epidermis infiltration. Likewise, single cells may be noted in the papillary dermis with similar cytologic character to those in the epidermis. This change is especially important in scalp dysplastic nevi in children and adolescents where there is marked atypia of the intraepidermal nevomelanocytes with always scattered single cells in the dermis. Misinterpretation of this finding can lead to misdiagnosis and often quite radical unnecessary treatment. In both the lentiginous and epithelioid cell patterns, single cells or nests are present along the lateral side of the rete ridges with an irregular growth of nests toward the outside of the rete ridges; bridges between the elongated and filiform rete ridges are common. The minor criteria include the collagenous changes in the dysplastic nevus that may be divided into two types. The first is lamellar fibroplasias which describes a repetitive laying down of fine collagen fibers or lamellations of collagen at the tips of the rete ridges lying parallel to the long axis of the epidermis. These fibers are interspersed with what appear to be fibroblasts. However, these cells are S100 positive and probably represent transformed nevomelanocytes that have the capacity to lay down these fibers. The second type of collagenous change describes concentric eosinophilic fibrosis which is a dense application of bright eosinophilic tissue around the rete ridges with minimal cellularity. The second minor criterion for diagnosis of the dysplastic nevi is the frequent association with an increase in vascularity of capillary and venules in the papillary dermis. The third criterion is the presence of an inflammatory reaction consisting of a lymphocytic infiltrate scattered in the papillary dermis both in perivenular and intervenular arrays. The intensity of the reaction is related to the degree of atypia. More severe atypia is frequently associated to more striking inflammatory infiltrate. The importance of the infiltrate as a marker also of transformation of the dysplastic nevocytes has been described as occurring with the expression HLA-A,B,C (HLA) and beta-2 microglobulin (beta 2 m) [46]. The final aspect that serves as a minor criterion is the apparent fusion of the rete ridges at their tips by nests of nevic cells. While this change is most common in the lentiginous proliferation of nevomelanocytes, it can clearly also be observed in association with the epithelioid cell pattern. Frequently the bridging cells have a spindle configuration with the orientation of their nuclei parallel to the long axis of the epidermis. It is custom to grade melanocytic atypia in the dysplastic nevus as to slight, moderate, and severe. To define the nuclear atypia, we used to compare the dimension of the melanocytic cells to the keratinocytic nucleus of the stratum spinosum. Slight atypia refers to melanocytic nuclei that are approximately one and a quarter to one half the size of the spinous layer keratinocytic nucleus. Moderate atypia refers to nuclei that are one half to equal to the size of the spinous layer keratinocytic nucleus and severe atypia, the size of or up to 1 ½ to 2 times the size of the keratinocytic nucleus. In contrast the melanoma cells are very variable in their nuclear size. A characteristic of melanoma, pleomorphism, is demonstrated by sizes ranging from that of a slightly atypical nevocytic nucleus to several times the size of a spinous layer keratinocytic nucleus. Another approach to atypia is more descriptive. In this approach mild atypia shows a pleomorphism of small densely hyperchromatic cells confined to the dermoepidermal junction. The pleomorphism mainly has to do with irregularities and shape of the nuclei. Cytoplasmic retraction is marked. Moderate atypia refers to nuclei with more angular configurations even rectangular or triangular with a dense eosinophilic cytoplasm visible minimally around the nucleus. In severe atypia, the nuclei are larger, more hyperchromatic, but with nucleoli and with more ample cytoplasm. However, the cells do not show the type of open chromatin patterns of melanoma cells nor does the cytoplasm qualify for that of the finely granular pigment of melanoma cells. The epithelioid cells under this descriptive system of classification have small nuclei with very small nucleoli or markedly hyperchromatic small nuclei approximately ½ the size to 2/3 the size of squamous cell layer keratinocytic nuclei but are surrounded by ample cytoplasm and finely granular melanin within it. In both systems of classification of atypia, multinucleate giant cells may be observed. Mitosis is extremely rare. Another approach to grading is to use a two-grade system, namely, low grade and high grade. In this approach, high-grade atypia is equivalent to severe atypia. Low grade is identified as slight to moderate atypia using the above descriptions [47]. Finally, an antibody that reacts with adenylyl cyclase has been found to be useful

in grading. It stains the Golgi apparatus in benign nevi. In atypical lesions there is focal increase in Golgi staining but also variable staining of the nuclei and cytoplasm. In severe there are admixed nuclei that are diffusely and strongly positive [48]. With regard to therapy, the first rule is regardless of the degree of atypia, even if slight, any residual lesion should be re-excised. The reason for this strong recommendation is that there is an approximately 20 % error in the choice of the most atypical area by the clinician. In dysplastic nevi, there are cases in which the melanoma appears as the benign portion or as an area of regression. If a lesion has slight or moderate atypia even with positive margins and there is no residual, we recommend follow-up of the site with the question of re-excision left to the clinician. For any lesion that is severely atypical, we recommend a 5 mm margin. The atypia of the dysplastic nevus is in striking contrast to that of melanoma in situ. In dysplastic nevi the atypia is variable from cell to cell so that there is a discontiguous atypia present. Also the junctional proliferation is discontiguous in dysplastic nevus in contrast to horizontal growth of melanoma where the atypical cells are disposed side by side along the dermoepidermal junction replacing the basilar layer and are associated with aggressive pagetoid spread up to the level of the granular cell layer. It is this discontiguous uniform atypia that allows for the diagnosis of melanoma and differentiates this lesion from the dysplastic nevus in which there is no contiguous uniform atypia but random discontiguous atypia. One of the problems that is confronted in the dysplastic nevus is to separate severe atypia from melanoma in situ. We believe that this can best be effected by clearly appreciating the extent of atypia and the extent of pagetoid spread so that severely atypical dysplastic nevi with minimal pagetoid spread can clearly be classified as dysplastic nevi in our opinion. When the pagetoid spread extends beyond the upper half of the squamous cell layer, especially up the granular cell layer, then we believe that the diagnosis appropriately is focal melanoma in situ arising in association with the dysplastic nevus. A word of emphasis should be said concerning single cell infiltration of the papillary dermis. Dysplastic nevi characteristically may be associated as has been stated above with single cell infiltration of the papillary dermis more commonly in moderate to severe atypical proliferations and in the epithelioid cell proliferation. In such instances the cells are of the same character of the intraepidermal component and do not require a diagnosis of invasive melanoma. An appreciation of this type of infiltration in dysplastic nevi is extremely important to prevent over diagnosis of melanoma. Dysplastic nevi arising in association with a preexisting dermal component usually exhibit typical type B and type C nevus cell proliferation of the dermal component. However, in our experience, especially in persons with the dysplastic nevus syndrome, the dermal component may be quite hyperchromatic and fail to show type C nevus cell formation. These hyperchromatic nests of nevic cells frequently abut the papillary-reticular dermal junction and interestingly enough are often HMB45 positive. This type of atypia, so long as the nuclei show a rather banal chromatin pattern, there are no mitoses, and diminution in cell size with maturation is present, is not indicative of melanoma. At times these dermal nests may be associated with a linear fibrosis of eosinophilic collagen surrounding them and separating them from the overlying epidermis. This type of change should not be mistaken for melanoma with regression in which there are linear fine bands of collagen with increased vascularity that entrap and separate the nests of hyperchromatic cells. Nests of hyperchromatic melanoma cells entrapped in fibrous tissue usually are quite compact, have quite strikingly hyperchromatic nuclei, are highlighted by epithelioid cells with fine melanin in their cytoplasm, and show mitotic figures. If they are nested, the peripheral cells will be plump and hyperchromatic rather than those surrounding nevus nests that are thin and delicate fibroblast-like type C cells.

Atypical Melanocytic Tumors

Atypical Spitz/Reed Tumors

The problem of atypical Spitz nevomelanocytic/tumors is one of the most difficult that pathologists and dermatopathologists encounter. There are several very important issues. First, one must distinguish an atypical nevus from a malignant tumor. Secondly, if a tumor, an attempt must be made to predict if the lesion has a metastatic potential. Third, even if the lesion metastasizes, it may not spread systemically. Finally, can one identify conclusively a lesion that can kill the, especially in childhood and adolescence where most of the lesions occur. At times, one may be forced to write a descriptive diagnosis in a difficult case. There are several significant studies that discuss these difficulties. In a study in which nine cases selected for their diagnostic difficulty were circulated among "expert" pathologists, the reproducibility of the diagnosis of Spitz tumor was very poor [49]. In a subsequent study of 17 spitzoid lesions, there was no consensus as to diagnosis; some of these cases metastasize [50]. Of great significance, several lesions were diagnosed by most of the pathologists as Spitz nevus or Spitz tumor and proved fatal. Another study of mainly 72 cases of Spitz tumors and so-called "spitzoid" melanomas resulted in a 35–40 % overall disagreement rate among six reference pathologists [51]. Elder [52] reports the following criteria (Table 7.3) to distinguish Spitz tumor from nodular melanoma and pigmented spindle cell nevus from superficial spreading melanoma (Table 7.4).

Hybrid lesions, however, have characteristics that fall between those of classic Spitz tumor and vertical growth phase melanoma. These diagnostically challenging lesions have been termed *atypical Spitz tumors*, as has been proposed by Barnhill [50] and Spatz [53]. For such lesions, it has been proposed that points be assigned if certain features are present (designated by asterisks in Table 7.3). A patient over 10 years of age or a tumor diameter over 10 mm is assigned 1 point; fat involvement, ulceration, or a mitotic rate of 6–8 mitoses/mm^2 is assigned 2 points; and a mitotic rate of over 8 is assigned 5 points. On this scale, 0–2 points indicate low risk, 3–4 indicate intermediate risk, and 5–11 indicate high risk. Among the 30 children with Spitz tumor, 19 of whom had long disease-free follow-up, and 11 had a history of metastasis. The statement that "difficult" lesions are usually benign in terms of long-term follow-up [54], metastases and mortality do occur in some cases. In our opinion, equivocal lesions exhibiting the features listed

Table 7.3 Features for the differential diagnosis between Spitz nevus and nodular melanoma

	Spitz tumor	Nodular melanoma
Architecture		
*Diameter	Usually < 10 mm	Often > 10 mm
*Symmetry	Often present	Often absent
*Lateral borders	Sharply demarcated	Often poorly demarcated
*Irregular nesting	Uncommon	Common
*Ulceration	Absent	Sometimes present
*Deep extension (into fat)	Uncommon	In thick tumors
*Expansile nodule	Uncommon	Common (vertical growth phase)
*Cellularity	Variable, nested	Sheet-like, cohesive, polyclonal
Epidermal hyperplasia	Present	Absent, rarely present
Junctional proliferation	Discontinuous	Often continuous
Junctional nest orientation	Perpendicular to epidermis	Random
Pagetoid spread	Inconspicuous or absent	Often apparent
Pigment distribution	Little or no pigment	Patchy, asymmetric
Nesting pattern at base	Small, uniform	Larger, variable
Nuclear pleomorphism	Mild to moderate	May be severe
Maturation	Present	Absent
Regression	Usually absent	May be present
Cytology		
*Mitoses in lower third	Absent	Often present
*Maturation/zonation	Present	Generally absent
*Deep border	Infiltrating	Rounded, pushing, fascicular
Kamino bodies	Single and confluent	Inconspicuous or absent
Chromatin pattern	Delicate, evenly dispersed	Coarse, clumped
Necrosis	Absent	Often present

Modified from Elder [52]
The features marked with an * are reported by Barnhill [50] and Spatz [53] for the atypical Spitz tumor grading system

Table 7.4 Features for the differential diagnosis between pigmented spindle cell nevus from superficial spreading melanoma

	Pigmented spindle cell nevus	Superficial spreading melanoma
Architecture		
Diameter	Usually < 6 mm	Usually > 6 mm
Symmetry	Present	Usually absent
Lateral borders	Sharply demarcated	Pagetoid spread (shoulder)
Junctional nest shape	Ovoid, uniform	Variable in size and shape
Junctional nest orientation	Perpendicular to epidermis	Random
Pagetoid spread	Inconspicuous or absent	Present and conspicuous
Pigment distribution	Abundant, coarse	Less conspicuous, dusty
Cytology		
Cell size	Dermal cell < junctional cells	Dermal cell = junctional cells
Cell shape	Elongated spindle cells	Large epithelioid cells
Intraepidermal mitoses	Common	Common
Intradermal mitoses	Absent	Present only with vertical growth
Necrosis	Absent	Often present
Maturation	Present	Absent

Modified from Elder [52]

Table 7.5 Atypical Spitz tumor: features associated to death

Features associated with death:
Large bulky lesions usually deeply invasive
Ulceration
Necrosis
Severe pleomorphism
Numerous dermal and marginal mitoses
Intravascular invasion
Multiple positive lymph nodes in draining basin
Deeply invasive small cell melanomas of scalp [61]

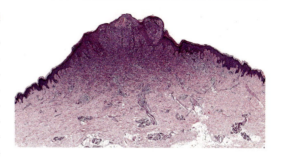

Fig. 7.26 Atypical Spitz tumor, asymmetry

in Table 7.3 as well as lesions that have any of the following characteristics (Table 7.5), if considered to fall short of an unequivocal diagnosis of melanoma, should be specially classified. The Penn group has chosen to call such lesions as a *MELTUMP* (*melanocytic tumors of unknown metastatic potential*) [3] followed by a differential diagnosis of melanoma with therapeutic discussion. In our approach we will diagnose such lesions as borderline tumors and then suggest based on our criteria whether the lesion should be excised and whether a sentinel lymph node biopsy should be considered. The possibility of more aggressive management of these lesions must be considered. Urso [55] found about 100 cases of metastasizing Spitz tumors. Although histologic data were not uniformly recorded, this review indicated that any number of the following histologic features could be found in a metastasizing lesion: (1) nodular growth in the dermis and/or large confluent, solid, cellular sheets with no collagen fibers interposed between cells; (2) extension of the neoplastic proliferation to the mid-deep dermis or to subcutaneous fat, especially if associated with absent or impaired maturation; (3) dermal mitoses, especially in the deeper part of the tumor; (4) asymmetry (Fig. 7.26); (5) heavy melanization in the deeper part of the tumor; (6) marked nucleolar and/or nuclear pleomorphism (Fig. 7.27); (7) necrosis; (8) epithelioid epidermal melanocytes below parakeratosis and/or epidermal ulceration; and (9) neoplastic cells in lymphatic vessels. Management of problematical spitzoid lesions should usually include a re-excision procedure and follow-up of the patient. A sentinel lymph node sampling

procedure may also be considered and in several reported studies was occasionally positive [55–59]. Interestingly, among 25 reported patients with atypical spitzoid lesions and positive sentinel nodes, not a single death occurred, although follow-up intervals have generally been short. In another series from the University of Michigan [60], in 69 patients with atypical Spitz tumors, 27 of whom had positive sentinel lymph nodes; there was no mortality in an average follow-up of 43.8 months. The only mortality occurred in a patient who refused a sentinel node biopsy. This study is supportive of the possibility of these lesions metastasizing as nevi. The other possibility is that the lesions are actually well-developed melanomas that will only demonstrate their potential later in life. John Kirkwood has stated: "We will only understand melanoma biology when we have 35 or more years of follow up." We agree with this wise statement. Nevertheless, it seems likely that atypical spitzoid lesions may be associated with excellent survival rates after positive sentinel node metastasis, especially in children. Many of these tumors, in our opinion, are best regarded as borderline lesions with a risk of metastasis estimated as determined above. During one of the annual meetings of the International Society of Dermatopathology in Graz, Austria (2008), a group of cases that were selected, because they were "bulky" tumors, were assembled by Cerroni and reviewed by a group of experts [3]. Most of the cases had some Spitz-like characteristics, but there were other cases that were included such as pigmented epithelioid melanocytomas, cellular blue nevi, and deep penetrating nevi. About one-third of these lesions had metastases, most

Fig. 7.27 Atypical Spitz tumor, cytologic pleomorphism

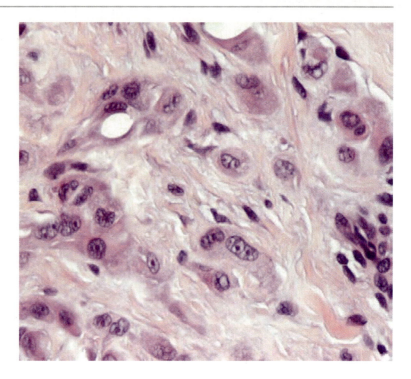

often to regional nodes, and in 20 % of the cases, the patients died, usually after a rather long disease-free interval. The use of the term *melanocytoma* was offered for these lesions. The definition of risk for aggressive behavior in these melanocytomas included the presence of mitoses, mitoses in the lower third of the lesion, and the presence of inflammation. It was suggested to tentatively classify these lesions into three risk groups: low risk, no inflammation, no mitoses; medium risk, presence of inflammation and/or mitoses not located at the base of the lesion; and high risk, presence of inflammation and/or mitoses near the base. Finally, in order to attempt to better understand fatal lesions, we studied 11 cases of children who died of melanoma originating in a tumor diagnosed before 13 years of age. We found the factors that were critical as listed in Table 7.5.

With regard to genomic studies, Bastian and his group reported that in 11 % of Spitz nevi there is an increase in the copy number of 11p, the site of the RAS gene, as determined by FISH [62]. In another study they found, in some Spitz nevi, a gain in 6p [27].

Atypical Dermal Melanocytosis

Pigmented Epithelioid Melanocytoma

Among the dermal melanocytoses, there are a group of tumors that are composed of epithelioid and dendritic melanocytes. These cells have very densely crowded cytoplasm filled with coarse melanin granules (Fig. 7.28) when compared to the delicate melanin granules of the blue nevus. These tumors were originally designated *animal-type melanoma* by Darier [63]; a series of six cases was reported by Crowson [64]. In this series one patient died; the others were still alive at last follow-up. This term was used because of the similarity of these lesions to the melanoma found in horses and other animals. Several years before this publication, Carney described his syndrome (myxomas [especially cardiac], spotty skin pigmentation, endocrine overactivity, and schwannomas) [65–67] that included the presence of what he termed "epithelioid blue nevi." In 1993 Carney, Zembowicz, and Mihm reviewed 41 cases of so-called animal-type melanoma and all the cases of Carney's epithelioid blue nevus.

Fig. 7.28 Pigmented epithelioid melanocytoma

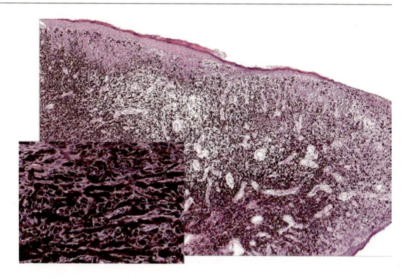

All concurred that there was no difference histologically between the two groups of cases. These authors then suggested a new nomenclature for these lesions, namely, the *Pigmented Epithelioid Melanocytoma (PEM)* [65]. Subsequently a genetic analysis found mutations of the protein kinase A regulatory subunit type, 1alpha (R1alpha), coded by the *PRKAR1A* gene, which is found in more than half of Carney complex patients, is also found in most PEMs but not in equine melanomas, nevi including deep penetrating and cellular blue nevi, or human melanomas [67]. The expression of R1alpha offers a useful test that could help to distinguish PEM from lesions that may mimic it histologically. Clinically these lesions present as blue-black nodules. They vary in size from a centimeter to several centimeters. They are usually asymptomatic. They affect both sexes equally and can be found anywhere on the body surface but are more common on the extremities. The lesions have a gradual growth course. They may occur at any time in life; a congenital example has been reported. They differ clinically from the Carney lesion by their occasional ulceration. In the follow-up about 40 % metastasize to regional lymph nodes without spread beyond the draining lymph node basin. It is noteworthy that no case of metastasis has been observed in Carney's syndrome. In all the reports of the PEM and animal-type melanoma, there has been only one death. The metastatic behavior

appears to be related to thickness. Lesions less than 2.0 mm in thickness virtually never spread. Even in these cases there is virtually no spread beyond the lymph node basin. The previously reported congenital nevus occurred in the scalp and involved the cranium and the dura. It was surgically excised. This little girl also had a tumor in the lung and the liver. These were not excised and she is alive and well when last checked at 11 years with no progression of tumor at any site. Morphologically the lesions resemble nodular melanoma but with very heavy pigmented melanocytes comprising the greatest portion of the lesion. The diagnostic cell is a large pigmented epithelioid melanocyte. The central mass of the lesion is composed of numerous melanocytes of both dendritic and epithelioid shapes. The dendritic processes are very thick and often have a thick spindled appearance. The cytoplasm is filled with numerous coarse melanin granules. Toward the periphery there are more prominent thick dendritic cells. The nuclei of the characteristic lesion are round to oval with a prominent rim of chromatin. There is a large blue nucleolus that stands amidst the dense melanin granularity. This feature clearly aids in differentiating the cells from the melanophages that have very vesicular nuclei with small gray nucleoli or the much larger red nucleoli of the melanoma cell. Usually the cells have bland morphology and mitoses are infrequent. Inflammatory infiltrates are usually quite limited. One very important feature that often causes confusion is the presence of dendritic melanocytes in the epidermis along the basal layer with prominent dendrites, a picture that is quite often present when the cells are in the papillary dermis. In some lesions there is also pagetoid spread. They have no relationship to aggressive behavior. When there is a doubt about the type of lesion, special stains such as Mart 1 or Melan-A compared to CD163 will allow identification of the melanocytes and exclude histiocytic cells. As far as atypia is concerned in the great majority of these lesions, the usual lesion is quite bland in spite of its cellularity. Mitoses are infrequent but can be observed. When there is significant atypia with frequent mitoses, then the differential diagnosis must include animal-type melanoma or a malignant blue nevus or melanoma arising in a neurocristic hamartoma. Although none of the patients died of the disease, clinical follow-up was short (mean, 32 months; range, up to 67 months) [68]. In subsequent follow-up of 5 years, there was no recurrence in the patients. What is problematic is that there were no histologic criteria separating PEMs with nodal involvement from those without nodal involvement, and the only feature more common in PEM in patients without the Carney complex than in epithelioid blue nevi of Carney complex was ulceration. These lesions should also be distinguished from unusually heavily pigmented examples of blue nevi. In our studies of these very difficult lesions, we have attempted to offer a novel approach to a lesion, the biologic potential of which is unknown until much longer follow-up is available. Its great resemblance to the melanoma of gray horses and Sinclair swine suggests that it may live symbiotically with the patient as in the case of man of the child with the congenital scalp PEM and the lung and liver nodules.

Dermal Melanocytic Tumors of Uncertain Malignant Potential

A variety of melanocytic tumors have been described that are usually bulky and exhibit nuclear atypia, mitotic activity, and other features suggestive of malignancy but do not fully qualify for an unequivocal diagnosis of malignancy. The Penn group has suggested that these lesions be designated as dermal melanocytic tumors of unknown malignant potential (MELTUMP) [3]. While this designation is very useful, it does not reflect any difference between tumors that notoriously do not metastasize, such as PEM, and tumors that more frequently metastasize such as the atypical Spitz tumor or the atypical plexiform deep penetrating nevus. Furthermore, in our consultative experience we find the term very liberally used for lesions with small vertical growth phase, even for lesions with radial growth phase and regression and sometimes for unusual radial growth phase lesions. The Penn group has also proposed the term SAMPUS for these lesions that designates a superficial atypical melanocytic proliferation of unknown biologic significance [69]. In our approach we will designate a lesion as borderline in nature and then give an estimation as to the risk of metastasis based on the various features including depth, presence of ulceration, mitoses per millimeter square, pleomorphism, and lymphatic invasion. We consider this to be more useful to the clinician and helpful in deciding whether further diagnostic therapy is necessary.

Melanoma

Since the original descriptions of subtypes of melanoma [70, 71], many advances have been made in the field of oncology since the advent of genetic studies. The classification has come under criticism as not being biologically base, but, interestingly enough, the most recent studies support the original classification. To wit, melanomas in sites of chronic sun exposure, such as lentigo maligna, do not exhibit the most common mutation in melanoma, the BRAF mutation, but rather do exhibit in many cases a c-kit mutation. Melanomas of the intermittently sun-exposed areas frequently express the BRAF mutation. Melanomas of non-sun-exposed skin, such as acral lentiginous or mucosal melanoma, also

Fig. 7.29 Melanoma in situ, pagetoid intraepidermal spread

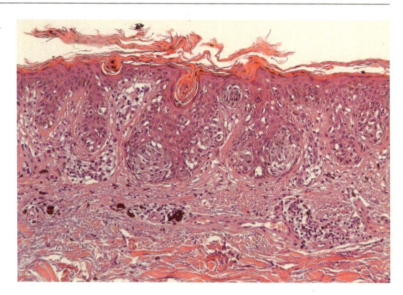

show, among other mutations, a c-kit mutation. As these aspects have also therapeutic importance, they imbue the basic classification with further significance [72].

Melanoma In Situ

Noninvasive melanoma or melanoma in situ refers to the in situ intraepidermal proliferation of malignant melanocytes usually 1.0–1.5 cm in size. The histopathologic changes of noninvasive superficial spreading-type melanoma are associated with two patterns. The first is one of epidermal hyperplasia without prominent rete ridges hyperplasia and a proliferation of pagetoid cells from the basilar region to the granular cell layer (intraepidermal aggressive pagetoid invasion) (Fig. 7.29). These so-called pagetoid cells have large ample cytoplasm filled with fine melanin granules. The nuclei are very variable in size but have marked irregular chromatin distribution and very prominent large eosinophilic nucleoli. Some of the nuclei are darkly hyperchromatic without visible chromatin patterns. The second pattern observed in superficial spreading melanoma is one that resembles the dysplastic nevus with elongation of the rete and with a confinement of the epithelioid cells to the dermoepidermal junction where they are disposed in a uniform contiguous array (Fig. 7.30). The cells usually replace the lower two or three layers of keratinocytes. Characteristically in dysplastic nevus the basilar proliferation is discontinuous. Some pagetoid spread is noted in this pattern but it usually is confined to the lower half of the epidermis and in the central area of the lesion. As far as *acral lentiginous melanoma in situ* is concerned, there is a uniform proliferation of cells with large nuclei and large cytoplasm. The large nuclei have prominent nucleoli that are either amphophilic or brightly eosinophilic. The cytoplasm is noted to extend by long dendrites even to the granular cell layer and filled with melanin granules emphasize the dendritic character of the cell. These cells are often contiguously arrayed along the dermoepidermal junction. Mitotic figures may be observed. Pagetoid spread is minimally present in the acral lentiginous melanoma in situ. A variant of acral lentiginous melanoma in situ is associated with a prominent proliferation of epithelioid cells without the prominent dendritic masses but with finely granular melanoma cells present throughout the epithelioid cells. This variant resembles superficial spreading melanoma in situ but is associated with marked epidermal hyperplasia, and the great majority of the cells are confined in the lower epidermis (Fig. 7.31). The greatest difficulty in interpretation of acral lentiginous melanoma in situ occurs when the cells are small without prominent cytoplasm and with small nuclei. Such lesions can best be

Fig. 7.30 Melanoma in situ, dysplastic nevus-like spread

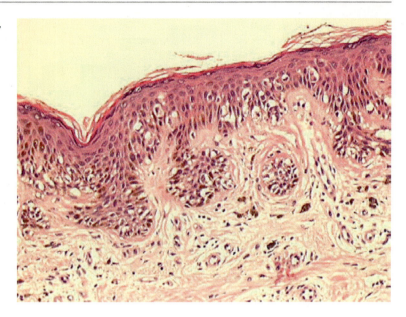

Fig. 7.31 Acral melanoma in situ

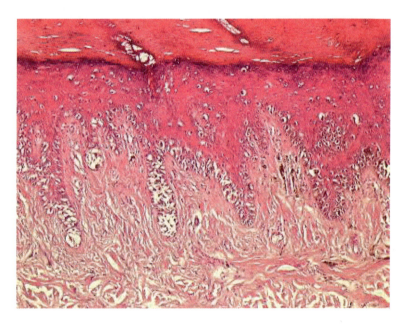

appreciated when one realizes that the cells uniformly replace the dermoepidermal junction and that the nuclei of the cells are similar one to another. Especially helpful in this type of proliferative process is the observation of mitoses. The epidermis is almost always markedly hyperplastic in acral lentiginous melanoma in situ and there may be an inflammatory infiltrate present in the dermis beneath. In instances where the melanocytic proliferation is difficult to detect and is associated with a markedly lymphoid infiltrate, one must be cautious not to mistake the lesion for an inflammatory process. The differential diagnosis of intraepidermal superficial spreading melanoma includes squamous cell carcinoma in situ with pagetoid appearing cells or Paget's disease. Squamous cell carcinoma in situ can be differentiated on the basis of

Fig. 7.32 Lentigo maligna

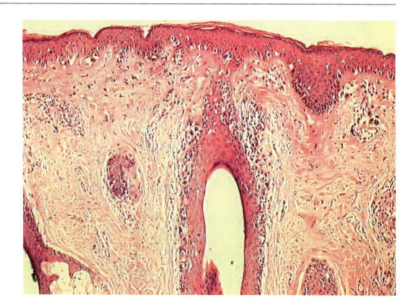

dyskeratosis of cells and the presence of intracellular bridges between the malignant anti-cytokeratin-positive cells. Likewise multinucleate giant cells often with dyskeratosis are common in squamous cell carcinoma in situ and are more uncommon in intraepidermal melanoma. Paget's disease is associated with cells that do not lie along the basilar region of the epidermis but rather above the basal cell layer. Careful histologic examination of lesions of Paget's disease reveals that there are small basal cells beneath the Paget cells. Likewise even if the cells of Paget's disease are pigmented, a rare finding, they have nuclei that have usually an open vesicular quality with prominent nucleoli. The cytoplasm of these cells is usually vacuolated. Striking pleomorphism of the cell is not noted. The use of mucicarmine or alcian blue stains will show mucin present in the Paget cells. Examination with immunoperoxidase stains for keratin and carcinoembryonic antigen will stain positively the Paget cells and negatively the melanoma cells.

Lentigo Maligna

We recognize an evolutionary concept of lentigo maligna (Fig. 7.32) melanoma that begins with a premalignant precursor, lentigo maligna, that goes on to an in situ phase and then invasive melanoma. Lentigo maligna describes a gradually spreading freckle-like lesion of the sun-exposed skin of the elderly which begins as a small flat tan macular pigmentation and may extend to several centimeters in size before invasive melanoma supervenes. This lesion, which has highly irregular coloration and irregular borders, is associated with a proliferation of irregular melanocytes confined to the epidermis in an atrophic epidermis. These cells are discontiguously arrayed and can extend down the hair follicle. This lesion has been variously defined by Jonathan Hutchinson lentigo melanosis or precancerous melanosis by Dubreuilh, but today it is commonly called Hutchinson's melanotic freckle or commonly termed *lentigo maligna*. Low-power examination reveals a proliferation of melanocytes along the dermoepidermal junction in a strikingly atrophic epidermis. In the early lesion there is a discontiguous proliferation of atypical cells randomly scattered above the markedly sun-damaged dermis. Frequently the cells may be noted to extend in scattered fashion down the superficial aspect down the hair follicle. These cells have pleomorphic nuclei. Some are round, others are rectangular, and others crescent shaped. As the lesion increases in size, there is continued proliferation but no confluence of cells, nesting, or pagetoid spread.

Fig. 7.33 Melanoma HGP

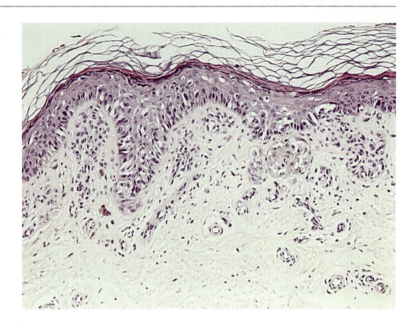

Superficial Spreading Melanoma

Superficial spreading melanoma represents the most common type of melanoma found in Caucasian persons. It is described histologically as showing large epithelioid cells in pagetoid array. In addition to the intraepidermal proliferative process with patterns of extensive pagetoid spread and the epithelioid cell proliferation in lesions with epidermal hyperplasia frequently resembling the dysplastic nevus, there supervenes infiltration of the papillary dermis by single cells or nests of cells. With this invasion a marked inflammatory response of lymphocytes is noted. Macrophages may also be scattered amidst the inflammatory infiltrate. The intradermal cells in the *horizontal* (*radial*) *growth phase* have the same histological characteristics as those in the epidermis, and the nests of cells are of similar size to those present in the epidermis (Fig. 7.33). The *vertical growth phase* can be detected by the appearance of cells in nests larger than the intraepidermal nests (Fig. 7.34). These clonal nests usually have a countable number of cells [25–50], which have a different cytologic appearance than those of the intraepidermal component. For example, if the intraepidermal component is characteristic with pagetoid cells with fine melanin pigment, the early vertical growth phase cells

may be small nevus-like melanoma cells or spindle cells or epithelioid cells without pigment. From this nest of cells which also show frequently quite prominent mitotic activity, the vertical growth phase continues to expand so that it either fills the papillary dermis (level III according to Clark classification) and widens it with subsequent invasion into the reticular dermis (level IV) or even into the subcutaneous fat (level V). Vertical growth phase melanoma cells are usually epithelioid or spindle in character but in most cases show a mixture of cells. In the invasive melanoma various prognostic parameters can be applied including thickness, tumor-infiltrating lymphocytes, mitotic rate, and presence or absence of regression to define the prognosis.

Differentiation from Melanoma with Regression and Recurrent Melanoma

Regressive fibrosis in melanoma is different from a scar, with a delicate pattern of thin collagen fibers in an edematous matrix containing scattered mononuclear cells with prominent ectatic venules oriented perpendicularly to the epidermis (Fig. 7.35). A scar is often hypovascular with laminated thick bundles of collagen in a parallel disposition to the epidermis. When vessels are present, they are small and may be closely aggregated. In regressed melanoma, there is usually

Fig. 7.34 Melanoma VGP

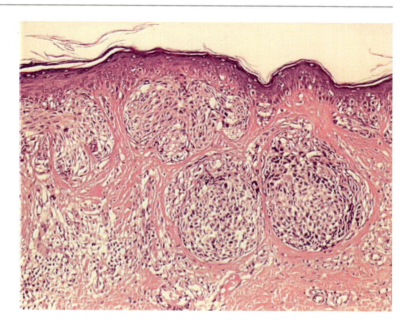

Fig. 7.35 Regressed
melanoma

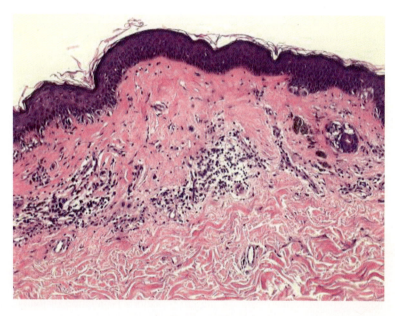

prominent inflammation that may be lichenoid
with conspicuous melanophages accumulation
(i.e., tumoral melanosis). In regressed melanoma,
there may be no discernible melanocytes. In
recurrent nevi, the epidermis shows melanocytic
hyperplasia and hypermelanosis. In regressed melanoma, a severely atypical intraepidermal or dermoepidermal melanocytic proliferation is found
outside the areas of regressive stromal fibrosis, in
contrast to recurrent nevi where the pattern and

cytology of melanocytic growth are typically banal
outside the scar. The residual dermal lesion in melanoma is usually severely atypical, while the residual dermal lesion in a recurrent nevus is not.

Lentigo Maligna Melanoma

Lentigo melanoma is characteristically a lesion of
sun-exposed areas of the elderly and classically

Fig. 7.36 Lentigo maligna
melanoma

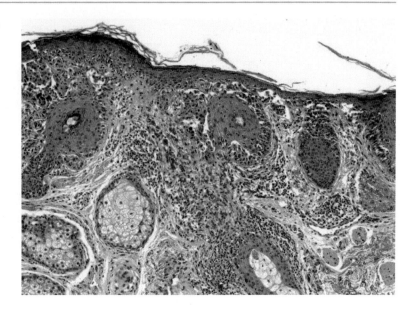

presents as a large freckle-like lesion on the face, surmounted by nodules. Histologically the nodules are often spindle cell in character. In a background of the severely atrophic epidermis with the lentiginous proliferation of atypical melanocytes, there supervenes single cell infiltration of the papillary dermis. We require the presence of an epithelioid cell usually with ruddy brown or dusky brown cytoplasm with large nucleus with prominent nucleolus to identify single cell infiltration. The presence of fibroblasts altered by chronic sun exposure with atypical forms, melanophages with dense pigment accumulation, and lymphocytes admixed with these melanophages often renders single cell infiltration difficult. Thus, the presence of an easily visible epithelioid cell allows for easy identification of single cell invasion. Nests of malignant cells invading the papillary dermis are usually fusiform in nature and are easily identified as distinct from the intraepidermal population. These single cells have more hyperchromatic nuclei, more prominent nucleoli, and usually a pigmented cytoplasm compared to the delicate cells that characterize the intraepidermal nests of lentigo maligna. The single cell infiltration and the infiltration of small nests of spindle cells are associated with a quite dense lymphocytic infiltrate with melanophages (Fig. 7.36). The vertical growth phase

with the equivalent of level III, IV, and V invasion in lentigo melanoma is commonly spindle cell in character. Although frequently there are admixed epithelioid cells with the spindle cell population and occasionally pure epithelioid populations may be also noted. There is one variant of vertical growth phase in lentigo maligna that is associated with numerous melanophages admixed with the spindle cells. The presence of this variant requires bleaching with potassium permanganate or other melanin bleach reagents in order to visualize the densely pigmented cells and to identify mitotic activity. Occasionally all the cells of the vertical growth phase of lentigo maligna melanoma are densely pigmented and must be bleached in order to separate them from aggregates of melanophages. The spindle cell population of lentigo maligna can be associated with a desmoplastic response. One of the problems with regard to lentigo maligna melanoma is the determination of margins, because of the variable activation of melanocytes in sun-exposed skin. We usually will declare a margin free if there is no significant contiguity of the atypical cells for at least 2 mm from the edge of the tumor. A recent study by Magro et al. has shown the usefulness of the s adenyl cyclase stain in helping to determine the margins [48]. This technique results in strong complete staining of the nuclei

Fig. 7.37 Acral lentiginous melanoma

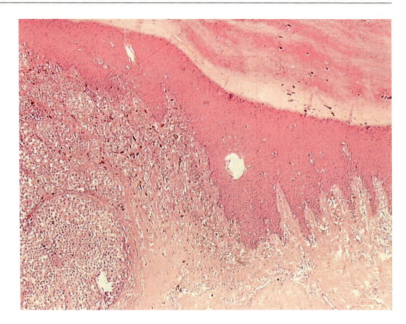

in malignant melanoma cells and is particularly helpful in detecting lentigo maligna melanoma in situ in the margin [73]

Acral Lentiginous Melanoma

Acral lentiginous melanoma presents as a flat, usually dark brown lesion with irregular areas of brown/black scattered over the surface and with an irregular border all surmounted by a nodule often with a hyperkeratotic surface. Histologically, the macular portion of the lesion shows a characteristic in situ proliferation of malignant melanoma cells contiguously arrayed along the dermoepidermal junction with long dendritic cytoplasmic extensions into the superficial epidermis (Fig. 7.37). The vertical growth phase can be composed of spindle cells, epithelioid cells, or a mixture of the two. Also, nevoid vertical growth phase can be occasionally seen as well as desmoplastic melanoma. A very important aspect of the vertical growth phase is that the cells can track along the eccrine adventitia into the reticular dermis and even into subcutaneous fat. Thus, this melanoma can rarely present as a flat lesion in which the entire tumor is spread along the eccrine apparatus into level V with poor prognosis.

Mucosal Melanoma Including Vulvar Melanoma

One of the most difficult types of melanoma involves the mucosa and has been termed *lentiginous mucosal melanoma*. This tumor usually demonstrates a striking pattern of atypical cells along the dermoepidermal junction in contiguous array. The nuclei of these cells are small and hyperchromatic and it is often difficult to visualize nucleoli in these hyperchromatic nuclei (Fig. 7.38). However, the aspect that allows for diagnosis is the presence of a contiguous proliferation of repetitively similar cells containing very dark nuclei with variable cytoplasm. Occasionally prominent dendritic processes filled with melanin can be noted and are very helpful in diagnosis. These dendritic processes extend up into the keratinizing layer of the mucosa. A brisk inflammatory infiltrate is often noted in the submucosa with scattered melanophages. Once again the presence of small cells without pigment associated with an inflammatory infiltrate may lead to the misdiagnosis of an inflammatory lesion. However, careful examination shows that the cells have uniformly dark nuclei, larger than lymphocytes and are associated with ample space around them to indicate cytoplasm of the malignant melanocyte. Mucosal lentiginous melanoma

Fig. 7.38 Lentiginous mucosal melanoma of rectum

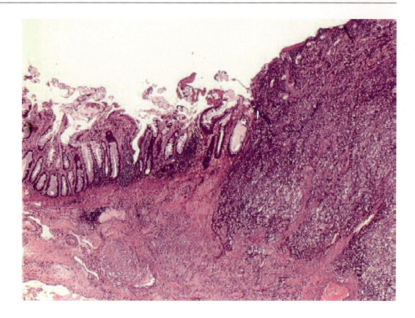

with radial growth phase presents as a large irregular pigmented macule of the mucosa surmounted often with a nodule or plaque as the vertical growth phase supervenes. In addition to the proliferation of uniformly atypical melanocytes contiguously placed along the dermoepidermal junction, sometimes with prominent dendritic forms it is present invasion of the submucosa by single cells in the radial growth phase. These single cells are often fusiform and are mistaken for fibroblasts, especially in the mouth and in the vagina. A brisk inflammatory infiltrate associated in both regions may be confused for inflammatory lesion especially if melanophages are admixed. Certainly, there is a pattern of mucosal melanoma that can resemble superficial spreading melanoma. It is much more easily diagnosed. Many mucosal and paramucosal melanomas can exhibit a mixed pattern. For example, in a series of 54 vulvar melanomas (personal observation), 15 % had a lentiginous pattern, 45 % had a pattern similar to superficial spreading melanoma, 20 % were mixed, 12 % were nodular, and the rest were unclassifiable. As the vertical growth phase appears, nests of cells are noted usually with often different histological appearance than the intraepidermal component. Thus the large epithelioid cells may be present or spindle cells at times a desmoplastic vertical growth phase is likewise

found. Neurotropism may be present with or without the desmoplastic response. These lesions almost never arise in association with a preexisting nevus.

Nodular Melanoma

Nodular melanoma is a rapidly growing raised pigmented lesion with no preexisting pigmented flat or radial growth phase. Low-power examination reveals a striking papulonodular excrescence that is frequently well defined, usually by a hyperplastic epidermis at each side but without any intraepidermal proliferation extending beyond the dermal component. There is no surrounding cell infiltration other than for an occasional cell adjacent to the nodule in the intraepidermal portion of the lesion. It is immediately appreciated that the tumor is composed of an expansile aggregate of melanocytes that variably infiltrate the reticular dermis and may even infiltrate the subcutaneous fat (vertical proliferation). Interestingly there is a certain symmetry to the nodular centrifugal proliferation because of its sharp demarcation. The dermal component of the lesion is associated with a highly pleomorphic population of cells that are usually epithelioid or more frequently mixed spindle and epithelioid but other cytotypes (balloon, nevoid, giant, etc.) may be present as clonal foci of proliferation. Well-differentiated pure spindle cell or nevoid populations are rare in nodular melanoma and should raise the possibility of minimal deviation or nevoid melanoma. The individual cells in nodular melanoma usually show striking pleomorphism and mitotic figures are often easily visible. This lesion may arise in association with a preexisting dysplastic nevus in which case there is an intraepidermal component of dysplasia. It may likewise arise in association with a preexisting dermal nevus in which remnants of the dermal nevus may be found scattered adjacent to the nodular proliferation. Many poorly differentiated skin tumors may simulate a nodular melanoma. The spindle cell squamous non-keratinizing carcinoma may be difficult to differentiate from a nodular melanoma but careful inspection of the epidermis will show the malignant cells to take origin there from and to have zonal processes extending between them. The presence of keratin by immunoperoxidase stains in the absence of S100 staining allows for conclusive diagnosis. Atypical fibroxanthoma can be difficult to distinguish from nodular melanoma but often shows more severe marked pleomorphism of the infiltrating cells with many bizarre atypical mitoses than in the usual nodular melanoma. However, one usually must rely on immunoperoxidase stains with the cells staining for macrophagic and lysosomal enzymes rather than for S100 and HMB45, the commonly positive stains in nodular melanoma. The reticulin stain may be helpful in that mesenchymal cells are all each surrounded by reticulum, whereas melanoma cells show nests surrounded by reticulum fibers. Leiomyosarcoma at times can pose a problem in differential diagnosis. If careful inspection of multiple levels fails to reveal pigment if one suspects melanoma, then appropriate immunoperoxidase stains with actin and desmin will allow for the correct diagnosis. The mixture between nevus and melanoma cell in particular in the deep part of a nodular melanoma may be important to identify to evaluate a correct thickness of the tumor; in these cases the immunohistochemical stain with p16 may be useful to differentiate nevus from melanoma cells and to define a correct thickness.

Melanoma, Rare Variants

Melanoma in Congenital Nevus

Melanoma in congenital nevi may occur anytime in life and in nevi of any size. However, most melanomas in giant nevi occur in early childhood in the first 5 years or in adulthood. Melanomas in small nevi or nevi of intermediate size occur almost exclusively in adult life. The most common melanoma presentation in the congenital nevus is a dermal nodule that is distinctly sharply demarcated from the surrounding nevi component. Low-power examination reveals this strikingly distinctive population of cells that almost invariably is more markedly hyperchromatic from the nevus cells and stands out in sharp contrast to them. p16 immunostain may be useful to distinguish the two different components (Fig. 7.39). Closer examination reveals that they are most commonly composed of spindle cells with admixed epithelioid cells with mitoses easily visible within them. Single cell necrosis is likewise present and there may be a host inflammatory response. The second commonest presentation is that of a pagetoid pattern of melanoma proliferation focally appearing in a congenital nevus. One must be very careful in the interpretation of this type of change and distinguish it from an epithelioid cell proliferation common especially in the first 2 years of life. The epithelioid cells that are benign have very delicate characteristics and are usually amelanotic. The epithelioid cells of melanoma have strikingly atypical nuclei with large eosinophilic nuclei and with finely granular melanin in their cytoplasm. As these cells infiltrate into the dermis, they do not blend or mature into the nevus cells of the congenital nevus but form an advancing sharply demarcated plaque or nodule contiguous with epidermal component and easily distinguishable from the dermal component. Pleomorphism of this nodule is easily noted as are numerous mitotic figures with variable host response. Individual

Fig. 7.39 Melanoma (left, negative p16 immunostain) and dermal nevus (periadnexal positive p16 immunostain)

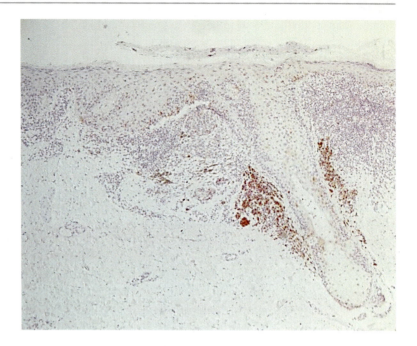

cell necrosis can also be observed. Any evidence of maturation of the cells into small nevus cells should dissuade one from diagnosing the lesion as malignant.

Desmoplastic Melanoma

Desmoplastic melanoma is a particular variant of melanoma characterized by a proliferation of predominantly spindle cells, collagen production, and spread of differentiation, or neurofibromatosis-type schwannian and brisk lymphoid cell dermal aggregates. Desmoplastic melanoma is considered as a separate entity because this cancer as well as raise some problems of diagnostic, clinical, histopathological, and therapeutic, shows a natural history that differs from that of a common melanoma. In desmoplastic melanoma we recognize two components: a junctional and intraepidermal lentiginous or pagetoid proliferation and a dermal component of spindle cells arranged in irregularly distributed bundles that extend from the papillary dermis to the reticular dermis, associated to a variable degree of proliferation of collagen, with irregular and ill-defined margins. The cells insinuate themselves between the collagen fibers as they are often not recognizable above the edge of the lesion. These characteristics are responsible for underdiagnosis of desmoplastic

melanoma and, above all, frequent errors in the evaluation of macroscopic and histologic margins of resection with inadequate surgical therapy that leads to frequent relapses. Collagen, which determines the characteristic appearance described as desmoplasia, is produced under the influence of TGF beta. The actual mechanism is unclear. Sometimes the production of collagen can be so marked as to simulate a fibromatosis. Other histological features described in desmoplastic melanoma include the presence of cells plurinucleate, or myxoid and storiform areas. The desmoplastic melanoma cells are in spindle-shaped arrangement in corrugated beams that simulate a neurofibroma or a schwannoma. The spindle cells are prevalent. Nuclear polymorphism is present and the nuclei are elongated and often S shaped. Sometimes it can be demonstrated fusiform and dendritic extensions of the cytoplasm of malignant melanocytes. Mitoses are rare and are often found only in areas of epithelioid cells present in the superficial papillary dermis. The neurotropism is a character that is considered important by many authors for the diagnosis but not always present. The neurotropism is a characteristic of desmoplastic melanoma, which seems associated with a high rate of recurrence but does not seem related in the same

Fig. 7.40 Desmoplastic melanoma, S100 immunostain of perineural invasion

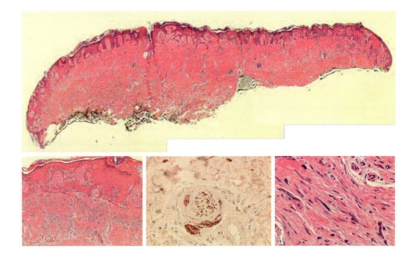

way the appearance of metastases. Frequently focal lymphocytes infiltrative aggregates are present (Fig. 7.40). Desmoplastic melanoma must be differentiated from a number of pigmented and unpigmented tumors characterized by proliferation of spindle cells in the dermis. If the pigment is present, must be taken into account the desmoplastic nevus and desmoplastic Spitz nevus, cellular blue nevus, malignant blue nevus, spindle cell melanoma, and metastatic malignant schwannoma; among non-pigmented as some sarcomas: the dermatofibrosarcoma protuberans, fibrosarcoma, leiomyosarcoma skin surface, the malignant schwannoma, and atypical fibroxanthoma; more rarely can be considered in the differential diagnosis of fibromatosis and hyperplastic scars with marked cellularity. Desmoplastic melanoma shows an intense and diffuse positivity for serum anti-S100 protein, but it is negative (except in rare superficial epithelioid cells) to HMB45, Leu 7, and NK1-beteb. p16 is very useful to differentiate desmoplastic nevus (p16 positive) from desmoplastic melanoma (p16 negative). The use of antibody anti-S100 protein is particularly important to highlight the perineural invasion and resection margin; otherwise, with the traditional histological examination alone, this could be underestimated. Also the skin of the re-resection for enlarging the margins must be examined by immunocytochemical S100 stain to exclude residual neoplastic foci and neural invasion.

Neurotropic Melanoma

Neurotropic melanoma is characterized by invasion and perineural extension. Unlike the desmoplastic melanoma, which may have perineural invasion, the neurotropic melanoma desmoplasia is poor or absent, while the tumor is characterized by a marked proliferation of spindle cells. The perineural invasion should be carefully sought, especially in peripheral portions of the tumor even at a distance from the margins, and must be differentiated from satellite and from lymphatic vascular neoplastic invasion. The perineural invasion may have very different quantitative aspects of a massive proliferation with expansive infiltration of the surrounding soft tissues or of individual cells; this pattern is often difficult to identify without the support of immunocytochemical staining with antiserum protein S100.

Nevoid Melanoma and Minimal Deviation Melanoma

Minimal deviation or nevoid melanoma describes a tumor proliferation of nevomelanocytes that resemble nevus cells but with mild atypia of the cells (Fig. 7.41). This lesion usually occurs in association with a preexisting nevus and is considered a histologic variant of melanoma which may have a more favorable prognosis than a fully evolved melanoma with the same measured depth. Lower-power magnification reveals an expansile nodule with or without reticular dermal

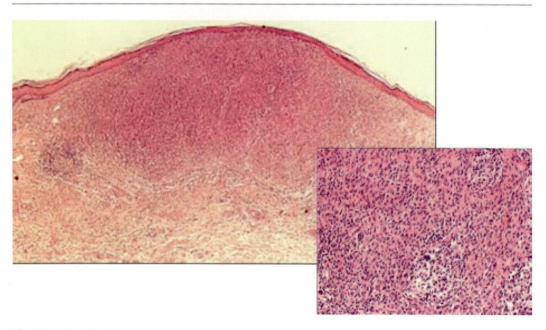

Fig. 7.41 Nevoid melanoma

involvement of usually quite pale cells unless there is a prominent pigment component. The pallor of the cells of the minimal deviation melanoma appreciated at low magnification is due to the banal nuclear characteristics without evidence of, or with low, hyperchromasia of the nuclei. The lesion is usually quite symmetrical usually oval in shape but with fascicles of cells extending into the reticular dermis. High-power evaluation of the cells resemble nevus, most commonly similar to the spindle and epithelioid cells of the Spitz nevus and often type B nevus cells. Some variants of minimal deviation melanoma consist of a proliferation of type A or type C cells. The most significant feature, at high-power examination, is the uniformity of the cells throughout the entire lesion, all resembling one type of nevus cell but with mild to moderate atypia. Thus, the cells are larger than normal nevus cells with more prominent nuclei and slightly increased in the nuclear to cytoplasmic ratio. If the cells are of the spindle and epithelioid cell type, they usually present nucleoli that are blue to amphophilic and are surrounded by a delicate chromatin rim. The cytoplasm of the spindle and epithelioid cells is a fine wispy cytoplasm, whereas the cytoplasm of the type B cells is more of a finely vacuolated and

hyalinized type. The cells from top to bottom and side to side are similar. Some diminution in cell size may be noted as the cells approach the reticular dermis, evidence of maturation (also called aberrant maturation). Mitotic figures are usually very rare. The presence of numerous mitoses excludes the diagnosis of minimal deviation melanoma. If reticular dermal involvement is present, fascicles of cells extend into the reticular dermis separating collagen and fibers but without destructive and deforming infiltration. Thus, the fascicles much more resemble the fascicles of the Spitz nevus in the reticular dermis than of fully evolved melanoma. There is no necrosis noted among the cells in the superficial or the deep component of the lesion and usually a host response is absent to minimally present with the exception of the rare presentation of a halo minimal deviation melanoma in which there is a brisk dense lymphocytic response with permeation throughout the lesion. Extension into the subcutaneous fat is unusual and speaks against the diagnosis of minimal deviation melanoma. While perineural infiltration may be observed, reactive fibrosis to the tumor is likewise absent. Occasionally in minimal deviation melanoma there is an intraepidermal component which consists of discrete nests of cells identical to those in the dermal nodule. If the intraepidermal component qualifies for radial growth phase melanoma of any type, superficial spreading, lentigo maligna, or other lentiginous types of melanoma, the diagnosis of minimal deviation melanoma is precluded. The variance of minimal deviation melanoma includes a halo minimal deviation melanoma in which there is brisk lymphocytic response throughout the entire tumor. This rare variant must be very carefully differentiated from melanoma with regression. Another variant is the desmoplastic minimal deviation melanoma which probably is a variant of type C cell proliferation with benign fibroblast-like cells forming an expansile nodule with fibrous response. The pigmented variant composed of pigmented spindle cells and associated with melanophages occurs; this lesion must be carefully distinguished from a spindle cell melanoma and can be done by appreciating that the melanoma cells usually have large nuclear to cytoplasmic ratios, are closely applied to one another, and have prominent nuclei and nucleoli with irregular heterochromatin. These spindle cells of the pigmented variant of minimal deviation melanoma have large amphophilic cytoplasm and large nuclei with small nucleoli and show very banal chromatin patterns. Of course the principal differential diagnosis with minimal deviation melanoma is fully evolved melanoma which can be distinguished on the basis of the pleomorphism of the cells, the high mitotic activity, the high nuclear atypia, the presence of single cell necrosis, and the presence of host lymphoid response. Minimal deviation melanoma of the spindle and epithelioid cell type can be differentiated from the compound Spitz nevus by the absence of maturation in minimal deviation melanoma, the presence of fascicles of cells rather than individual cells or small nests in the reticular dermis. Likewise the presence of an expansile nodule filling and widening the papillary dermis precludes the diagnosis of an ordinary compound nevus of Spitz. The deep penetrating nevus is differentiated from minimal deviation melanoma by the presence of a large epithelioid cells with finely granular melanin in their cytoplasm that fall on appendages and neurovascular bundles associated with a prominent melanophages aggregation. Careful examination of the deep penetrating nevus reveals that it does not form an expansile nodule but rather is composed of a network of cells among the neurovascular bundles. Minimal deviation melanoma is composed of an expansile nodule of spindle cells that resemble cells of the compound nevus of Spitz but that show slight atypia. Thus, the cells are somewhat larger than spindle cells but are uniformly so. The nuclei have elongate fusiform shapes but rather delicate nuclear chromatin. Fascicles of spindle cells infiltrate the reticular dermis but do not usually infiltrate subcutaneous fat. There is no mitotic activity is observed. If there is an intraepidermal component it is composed of cells identical to those in the dermis.

Malignant Blue Nevus

The malignant blue nevus is a very rare entity. In agreement with Maize and Ackerman (1987), the primary criterion for diagnosis of malignant blue nevus is the finding of a proliferation of fusiform melanocytes and intense pigmentation, with cytological characteristics of malignancy: marked cytologic atypia, nuclear polymorphism, and dense aggregates of malignant cells that expand and destroy the fibers of the reticular dermis extending to the hypodermis, without invasion of the epidermis. The typical "biphasic aspect" of the cellular blue nevus, due to the presence of nests of clear cells alternating with bands of pigmented spindle cell, fails in malignant blue nevus. Occasional is the finding of epithelioid cells and multinucleated giant. Foci of necrosis and atypical mitoses characterize the lesion, although the mitotic index is often low. The blue nevus must be distinguished from malignant cellular blue nevus. An asymmetric multinodular tumor bigger than 3 cm with frank cytological aspects of malignancy, atypical mitosis, and necrosis militates in favor of a malignant blue nevus. More complex is the distinction between malignant blue nevus and "atypical" cellular blue nevus because the differential diagnosis is placed on the degree of cytologic atypia, on these fairly subjective criteria, as well as on the presence of atypical mitoses. Precisely because of the lack of clear

Fig. 7.42 Rhabdoid melanoma

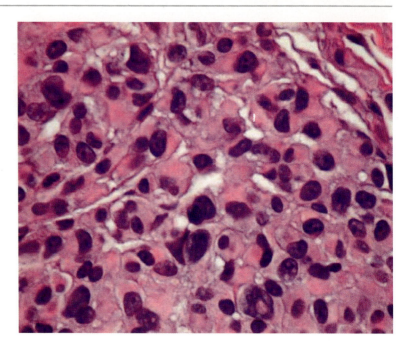

characteristics of malignancy, an atypical blue nevus can be regarded as "dermal melanocytic lesions of uncertain potential" and requires a radical surgical treatment and appropriate follow-up long term. Since there are no pathognomonic histopathological aspects of malignant blue nevus, the differential diagnosis of nodular melanoma or against metastatic requires copresence of residues or the onset of blue nevus at the site of a preexisting blue nevus. The use of immunocytochemical methods has not shown any interest, because the reactivity with S100 and HMB45 form has been demonstrated in both benign and malignant blue nevus [74]; p16 is negative. The presence of lymph node metastases with malignant cytologic features confirms the diagnosis.

Other Rare Melanomas
Small Cell Melanoma
Small cell melanoma is rare, but it is particularly important because it may easily be confused histologically with other small cell tumors, including lymphoma, Merkel cell carcinoma, undifferentiated carcinoma, Ewing's sarcoma, and peripheral neuro-ectodermal tumor. Cytologically small cell melanoma may also simulate benign nevus. Poorly differentiated small cell foci are frequently encountered in a melanoma that has arisen in a giant congenital nevus. The ulcerated small cell melanomas have frequently an aggressive course with an increased probability of positive sentinel lymph nodes (35 %). Small cell melanoma is also reported in the rectal/anorectal site.

Rhabdoid Melanoma
Rhabdoid features have been described primarily in metastatic melanoma, and rare cases of primary totally rhabdoid melanoma have been reported. Rhabdoid melanoma are characterized by large sheets of polygonal cells with abundant cytoplasm containing hyaline filamentous and eosinophilic inclusions (Fig. 7.42), an eccentric displaced vesicular nucleus, and large nucleoli. Ultrastructural analysis showed cytoplasmic whorls of intermediate filaments with entrapped rough endoplasmic reticulum, mitochondria, and lipid. The tumor cells are strongly immunoreactive with S100 protein, vimentin, and CD56 and are focally reactive with Mart-1 and, in some cases, keratins and desmin. Tumor cells were negative for Melan-A, tyrosinase, and HMB45. The differential diagnosis of the rhabdoid melanoma is wide and must be supported by a broad panel of immunohistochemical stains. In general non-melanocytic rhabdoid tumors are positive for vimentin, glial fibrillary acidic protein, desmin, actin, and AE1/AE3. Moreover,

Fig. 7.43 Myxoid melanoma

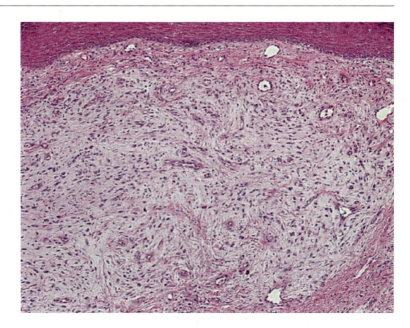

S100 protein expression has not been observed in renal rhabdoid tumors. Malignant peripheral nerve sheath tumor, especially the epithelioid variant, is positive for epithelial membrane antigen and synaptophysin and is only focally positive for S100 protein. Plasmacytoma or plasmablastic lymphoma and anaplastic large cell lymphoma would be positive for CD138 and CD30, respectively. Rhabdoid morphology has been described in carcinoma; however, the lack of expression of both high- and low-molecular-weight cytokeratins excludes an epithelial neoplasm as well as epithelioid mesothelioma. Rhabdomyosarcoma would express muscle markers, such as desmin and myoglobin, and it is quite easy to differentiate from rhabdoid melanoma.

Myxoid Melanoma (Fig. 7.43)

Myxoid melanoma is a rare variant with large malignant cells amidst a basophilic mucinous matrix. The myxoid stroma comprises mesenchymal acidic mucopolysaccharides, as opposed to neutral epithelial mucins and the epithelial mucin preparations (mucicarmine and PAS-diastase) are negative, whereas stains for acidic mucosubstances (i.e., Alcian blue at low pH) are positive. Myxoid melanomas are frequently amelanotic. Most often these tumors are metastatic deposits and a differential diagnosis with a primary lesion

may be difficult without the evidence of intraepidermal melanocyte proliferation. S100 decoration is frequently present but HMB45 and Melan-A positivity is less uniform, with both positive and negative results reported. The differential diagnosis of myxoid melanoma is broad, encompassing as it does other benign and malignant myxoid neoplasms that include soft tissue malignancies (myxoid liposarcoma, myxoid malignant fibrous histiocytoma, low-grade fibromyxoid sarcoma, low-grade myofibroblastic sarcoma, myxoid chondrosarcoma, myxoid peripheral nerve sheath tumors, myxoid rhabdomyosarcoma, malignant myoepithelioma, myxoid synovial sarcoma, myxoid follicular dendritic cell sarcoma, myxoid dermatofibrosarcoma protuberans, metastatic chordoma and its benign mimic parachordoma) as well as epithelial cancers (metastatic adenocarcinomas and malignant sweat duct tumors including malignant mixed skin tumor) and also sarcomatoid variant of anaplastic large cell Ki-1 lymphoma that can produce areas strikingly similar to myxoid melanoma.

Plasmacytoid Melanoma (Fig. 7.44)

The plasmacytoid cytological pattern is very rare in melanoma but sporadic cases are described; a case of primary melanoma of the oral cavity and a case of liver metastasis.

Fig. 7.44 Plasmacytoid
melanoma

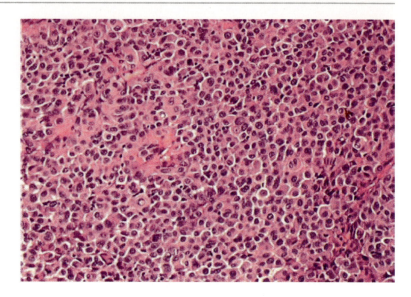

Follicular Melanoma

Follicular melanoma is a rare variant of melanoma with aggressive behavior. The melanoma
involves the hair follicle with pagetoid spread
into the follicular epithelium and invasion of papillary dermis. Only few cases are reported in
literature.

Metaplastic Change in Melanoma

Divergent differentiation or metaplastic change is
a rare phenomenon in melanoma and, when it
occurs, can be misinterpreted and lead to diagnostic uncertainty. These events in melanomas
are defined as the development of morphologically, immunohistochemically, and/or ultrastructurally recognizable non-melanocytic cell or
tissue components. Different types of divergent
differentiation are reported and include
fibroblastic/myofibroblastic, schwannian and
perineurial, smooth muscle, rhabdomyosarcoma-
tous, osteocartilaginous, ganglionic and gangli-
oneuroblastic, neuroendocrine, and probably
epithelial. A carefully chosen immunohistochemical panel and the input of electron microscopy
can help to clarify the nature of the cellular differentiation of these tumors and lead to a correct
final diagnosis. The clinical significance of such
aberrations is uncertain, nor are the underlying
mechanisms as yet well defined. Metaplastic foci
mimicking osteogenic sarcoma and cartilaginous
metaplasia have been described in one case of a

nasal mucosal primary and its metastasis and in
cases of subungual melanoma. Mesenchymal elements with rhabdomyoblastic, lipoblastic, and
neurogenous features have been also described in
those melanomas that arise in giant congenital
nevus.

Chondroid, Osteogenic Melanoma (Fig. 7.45)

This variant of metaplastic melanoma is quite
important as it most commonly, as a primary
tumor, affects the great toe or the thumb. There is
almost always a history of a trauma that is given
as the source of the swollen digit. Biopsy usually
will demonstrate an atypical chondroid or osteoid
with associated ossification and is usually misinterpreted as osteogenic sarcoma. Careful evaluation of the intervening stroma will usually raise
the suspicion of a spindle cell or epithelioid cell
tumor. Often there will be pigmentation. The
final clue is the observation of a radial growth
phase. Confirmation by S100 and Melan-A is
necessary to identify the malignant melanocytes
and differentiate them from S100 chondrocytes.

Signet Ring Melanoma (Fig. 7.46)

A signet ring primary melanoma is a very rare event,
being seen in some 0.5 % of melanomas. This variant must be considered with particular attention to
differentiate a metastatic non-melanocytic tumor,
particularly in pleural or peritoneal effusion, from a
signet ring melanoma. Cytologically the signet ring

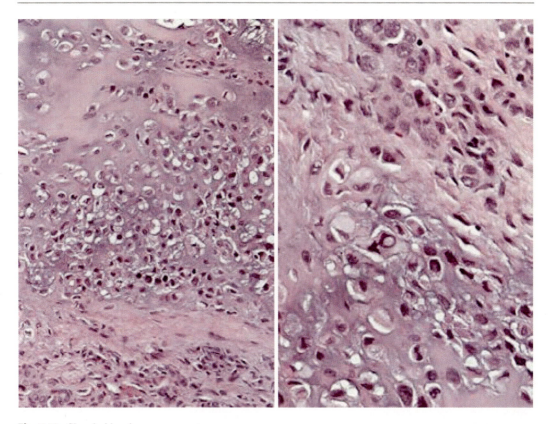

Fig. 7.45   Chondroid melanoma

Fig. 7.46   Signet ring
melanoma

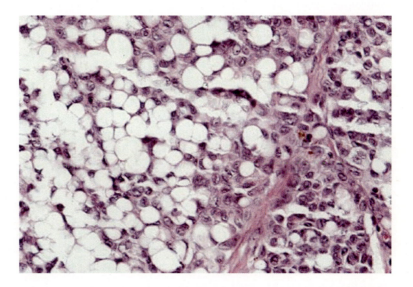

melanoma cell may present different morphology as small, large, or giant cells. An unusual histological variant with a combination of the signet ring cell melanoma with desmoplastic, pseudoglandular, and oncocytoid features is described. Ultrastructurally in the cytoplasm it is possible to demonstrate an accumulation of intermediate filaments, specifically vimentin. The signet ring cells are S100 protein and HMB45 positive; however, exceptions to this immunohistochemical profile are reported. Cases of S100-positive, HMB45-negative signet ring melanoma are described as are cases of HMB45-positive, S100-negative signet ring melanoma. In rare examples, intracytoplasmic neutral mucin may be observed. The histological differential diagnoses include all the tumors with prominent cytoplasmic vacuolation; tumors of vascular endothelium or adipose tissue, signet ring lymphoma, and epithelioid smooth muscle lesions as well as the more frequent signet ring adenocarcinoma are thus considered.

Spindle Cell Melanoma

Spindle cell melanoma is a rare variant that may present diagnostic difficulties particularly when staining with S100 is negative, weak, focal, or a combination of these and the other conventional melanocytic markers are negative. p75 NGF-R exhibits superior staining characteristics and greater sensitivity in identifying spindle cell melanoma than S100. p75 NGF-R may be a useful diagnostic and ancillary stain in addition to S100. Spindle cell melanoma has been described in urinary bladder, in primary melanoma associated to myxoid and cribriform pattern, in liver metastasis, and in melanoma on old burn scar. The c-kit expression, reported in literature, in the spindle cell melanoma could represent a major diagnostic pitfall.

Balloon Cell Melanoma

The balloon cell melanoma is a rare histological type of melanoma composed of nests and sheets of large polyhedrical and foamy cells with an abundant, clear, or finely vacuolated cytoplasm. Frequently its benign cytologic appearance presents a challenge for a correct histopathological diagnosis. In fact the tumor may simulate a balloon cell nevus but cytologic atypia, mitotic activity, and necrosis may be useful characters for the differential diagnosis. The presence of multinucleated giant balloon cells and deep maturation are features that suggest the diagnosis of balloon nevus. No intervening stroma is present between the malignant cells; the nuclei are irregular and large with prominent nucleoli. The cytoplasm is clear and in some case a PAS positivity and diastase sensitivity may be demonstrated due to the intracytoplasic accumulation

of glycogen. In most cases ultrastructural reports have demonstrated the presence of intracytoplasmic degenerating melanosomes or lipid similar to the balloon cell change of benign nevi. No case is described of balloon cell melanoma in situ. Immunohistochemical stains reveal reactivity with antibodies to S100 protein, Melan-A, HMB45, vimentin, and negative stain with p16. Numerous differential diagnoses must be considered including common acquired nevi, with which balloon cell melanoma may coexist, as well as other malignant non-melanocytic clear cell neoplasms as clear cell sarcoma of soft parts, atypical fibroxanthoma, granular cell carcinoma with clear cell change, metastatic renal cell carcinoma, clear cell basal cell carcinoma, malignant clear cell acrospiroma, sebaceous carcinoma, and clear cell squamous cell carcinoma.

Melanocarcinoma (Melanoma with Intermixed Epithelial Component or Divergent Differentiation)

A very rare variant with two distinct but intimately admixed components: melanocytic and epithelial described by Wen [75]. The immunohistochemical stains demonstrate the epithelial differentiation on the basis of cytokeratin (CAM5.2 and AE1/AE3) expression and melanocytic differentiation (HMB45, PNL2, MITF, and S100) of melanoma component. MITF is expressed in both components, raising the possibility of dual differentiation in a single tumor, rather than the alternative considerations of a collision tumor or a reactive pseudoepitheliomatous hyperplasia with eccrine duct lumen formation within a melanoma (Fig. 7.47). This unusual tumor with both melanocytic and epithelial components may represent a true melanocarcinoma, which becomes a plausible consideration, in view of melanoma plasticity and recent experimental evidence and speculation about the role of stem cells in melanoma.

Melanoma Prognostication

Great advances have been made in understanding the prognosis in melanoma. The first breakthrough was the classification of melanoma into subtypes and the definition of levels of invasion [70, 71].

Fig. 7.47 Melanocarcinoma: melanocytic and epidermoid differentiation

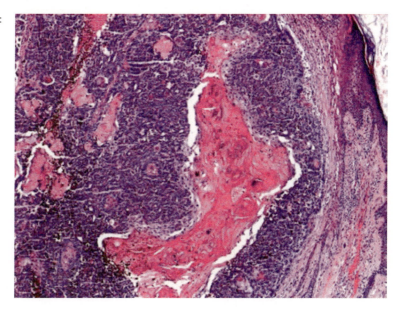

The measured thickness as introduced by Breslow is determined by measuring with a micrometer from the granular cell layer to the deepest tumor cell and expressing the result in millimeters [76]. This measurement and its relationship to prognosis are linear. It has been included in the 9th edition of the American Joint Committee on Cancer, Melanoma Committee Recommendations [77]. The other parameters that were included are ulceration and mitoses. The presence of mitoses would now replace the level of invasion. Hence, the designation "a" would indicate no ulceration or mitoses, and the designation "b" would indicate the presence of either mitoses or ulceration or both. Thus, the designation would be T1a or T1b, T2a, and following. Microscopic satellites also are to be included in the report. The number of mitoses is found by searching the field at 20× for the area of most mitoses. When that is found, it is considered the "hot spot" and it is counted in square millimeter. In most mitoses this area corresponds to 4 to 4 ½ 40× fields, counted consecutively in the manner to reflect as close to a square as possible. Then the amount is expressed in mitoses per mm squared. Less than one mitosis is not acceptable. The designation must be zero or the amount reached by counting in the above method. If there is only one mitosis, that area becomes the "hot spot" and is reported as 1 mitosis per mm. square. Microscopic satellites are reported as islands of tumor cells >0.05 mm in width that are separated by a significant distance from the vertical growth phase. The islands may be present below the vertical growth phase of around it. This finding is now reported as N2c. The other criteria that can be entered include tumor-infiltrating lymphocytes, regression, and vascular or neural invasion. Also, margins are reported and the presence of a preexisting lesion as appropriate. Another important feature relates to the sentinel lymph node positivity. It was determined immunohistochemical detection of nodal metastases is acceptable. With the much greater understanding of the morphology of melanoma cells by the community of pathologists, it was determined that one no longer must prove the presence of deposits by confirmation with hematoxylin and eosin-stained sections. Furthermore, the committee determined that, until more information is available, there should be no lower limit to the size of the deposit required to determine that a sentinel lymph node is positive. Even a single clearly malignant cell in the parenchyma should be so designated. Finally, it was decided that microscopic and macroscopic deposits in lymph nodes should only refer to the gross inspection of the tumor deposit. A macroscopic deposit is one that is clearly visible to the naked eye as observed in sectioning the lymph node. Other features that were considered but about which there was insufficient information to be cited in the mandatory report include the presence of tumor-infiltrating lymphocytes, regression, and neural and/or vascular invasion. For further details the reader is referred to a review of prognostic variable. For further details on these parameters, the reader is referred to the review by Piris and Mihm [78].

Conclusion

In this chapter we have attempted to review the various parameters of pigmented lesions in progression from the benign to the atypical to the malignant. There are many suggestions in the chapter about clues to diagnosis. We hope the reader will profit from this exercise and will also liberally use the references to further strengthen their understanding.

Glossary

Atypical melanocytic tumors a subset of melanocytic tumors, with unpredictable biologic behavior.

Dermal melanocytosis benign, flat, congenital birthmark with wavy borders and irregular shape

Dysplastic nevus a junctional or compound nevus with cellular and architectural dysplasia

Melanocytic nevi a pigmented lesion of the skin caused by a disorder involving melanocytes

Melanoma malignant tumor of melanocytes.

References

1. Hawryluk EB, Sober AJ, Piris A, Nazarian RM, Hoang MP, Tsao H, et al. Histologically challenging melanocytic tumors referred to a tertiary care pigmented lesion clinic. J Am Acad Dermatol. 2012;67(4): 727–35.
2. Crotty KA, Menzies SW. Dermoscopy and its role in diagnosing melanocytic lesions: a guide for pathologists. Pathology. 2004;36(5):470–7.
3. Cerroni L, Barnhill R, Elder D, Gottlieb G, Heenan P, Kutzner H, et al. Melanocytic tumors of uncertain malignant potential: results of a tutorial held at the XXIX Symposium of the International Society of Dermatopathology in Graz, October 2008. Am J Surg Pathol. 2010;34(3):314–26.
4. Hafner C, Stoehr R, van Oers JM, Zwarthoff EC, Hofstaedter F, Klein C, et al. The absence of BRAF, FGFR3, and PIK3CA mutations differentiates lentigo simplex from melanocytic nevus and solar lentigo. J Invest Dermatol. 2009;129(11):2730–5.
5. Rodríguez-Bujaldón A, Vazquez-Bayo C, Jimenez-Puya R, Galan-Gutierrez M, Moreno-Gimenez J, Rodriguez-Garcia A, et al. LEOPARD syndrome: what are café noir spots? Pediatr Dermatol. 2008;25(4):444–8.
6. O'Rourke EA, Balzer B, Barry CI, Frishberg DP. Nevic mitoses: a review of 1041 cases. Am J Dermatopathol. 2013;35(1):30–3.
7. Mark GJ, Mihm MC, Liteplo MG, Reed RJ, Clark WH. Congenital melanocytic nevi of the small and garment type. Hum Pathol. 1973;4:395–418.
8. Marchesi A, Leone F, Sala L, Gazzola R, Vaienti L. Giant congenital melanocytic naevi: review of literature. Pediatr Med Chir. 2012;34(2):73–6.
9. Phadke PA, Rakheja D, Le LP, Selim MA, Kapur P, Davis A, et al. Proliferative nodules arising within congenital melanocytic nevi: a histologic, immunohistochemical, and molecular analyses of 43 cases. Am J Surg Pathol. 2011;35(5):656–69.
10. Aouthmany M, Weinstein M, Zirwas MJ, Brodell RT. The natural history of halo nevi: a retrospective case series. J Am Acad Dermatol. 2012;67(4):582–6.
11. Schrader WA, Helwig EB. Balloon cell nevi. Cancer. 1967;20(9):1502–14.
12. Fox JC, Reed JA, Shea CR. The recurrent nevus phenomenon: a history of challenge, controversy, and discovery. Arch Pathol Lab Med. 2011;135(7):842–6.
13. Hoang MP, Prieto VG, Burchette JL, Shea CR. Recurrent melanocytic nevus: a histologic and immunohistochemical evaluation. J Cutan Pathol. 2001; 28(8):400–6.
14. Gleason BC, Hirsch MS, Nucci MR, Schmidt BA, Zembowicz A, Mihm Jr MC, et al. Atypical genital nevi. A clinicopathologic analysis of 56 cases. Am J Surg Pathol. 2008;32(1):51–7.
15. Clemente C, Zurrida S, Bartoli C, Bono A, Collini P, Rilke F. Acral-lentiginous naevus of plantar skin. Histopathology. 1995;27(6):549–55.
16. Díaz A, Valera A, Carrera C, Hakim S, Aguilera P, García A, et al. Pigmented spindle cell nevus: clues for differentiating it from spindle cell malignant melanoma. A comprehensive survey including clinicopathologic, immunohistochemical, and FISH studies. Am J Surg Pathol. 2011;35(11): 1733–42.
17. Paniago-Pereira C, Maize JC, Ackerman AB. Nevus of large spindle and/or epithelioid cells (Spitz's nevus). Arch Dermatol. 1978;114(12):1811–23.
18. Spitz S. Melanomas of childhood. Am J Pathol. 1948;24:591–609.
19. Kernen JA, Ackerman LV. Spindle cell nevi and epithelioid cell nevi (so-called juvenile melanomas) in children and adults: a clinicopathological study of 27 cases. Cancer. 1960;13:612–25.

20. Barr RJ, Morales RV, Graham JH. Desmoplastic nevus: a distinct histologic variant of mixed spindle cell and epithelioid cell nevus. Cancer. 1980;46(3): 557–64.

21. Hilliard NJ, Krahl D, Sellheyer K. p16 expression differentiates between desmoplastic Spitz nevus and desmoplastic melanoma. J Cutan Pathol. 2009;36(7):753–9.

22. Borsa S, Toonstra J, van der Putte SC, van Vloten WA. Balloon-cell variant of the Spitz nevus. Hautarzt. 1991;42(11):707–8.

23. Harvell JD, Meehan SA, LeBoit PE. Spitz's nevi with halo reaction: a histopathologic study of 17 cases. J Cutan Pathol. 1997;24(10):611–9.

24. Hoang MP. Myxoid Spitz nevus. J Cutan Pathol. 2003;30(9):566–8.

25. Al Dhaybi R, Agoumi M, Gagné I, McCuaig C, Powell J, Kokta V. p16 expression: a marker of differentiation between childhood malignant melanomas and Spitz nevi. J Am Acad Dermatol. 2011;65(2):357–63.

26. Martin V, Banfi S, Bordoni A, Leoni-Parvex S, Mazzucchelli L. Presence of cytogenetic abnormalities in Spitz naevi: a diagnostic challenge for fluorescence in-situ hybridization analysis. Histopathology. 2012;60(2):336–46.

27. Bastian BC, Wesselmann U, Pinkel D, Leboit PE. Molecular cytogenetic analysis of Spitz nevi shows clear differences to melanoma. J Invest Dermatol. 1999;113(6):1065–9.

28. Mihic-Probst D, Zhao J, Saremaslani P, Baer A, Komminoth P, Heitz PU. Spitzoid malignant melanoma with lymph-node metastasis. Is a copy-number loss on chromosome 6q a marker of malignancy? Virchows Arch. 2001;439(6):823–6.

29. Zembowicz A, Mihm MC. Dermal dendritic melanocytic proliferations: an update. Histopathology. 2004;45(5):433–51.

30. Lovas GL, Wysocki GP, Daley TD. The oral blue nevus: histogenetic implications of its ultrastructural features. Oral Surg Oral Med Oral Pathol. 1983;55(2): 145–50.

31. Patel DS, Bhagavan BS. Blue nevus of the uterine cervix. Hum Pathol. 1985;16(1):79–86.

32. Tobon H, Murphy AI. Benign blue nevus of the vagina. Cancer. 1977;40(6):3174–6.

33. Heim K, Müller-Holzner E, Pinzger G, Höpfl R. Multiple blue nevi of the vagina – a rare differential diagnosis to melanoma of the vagina. Gynakol Geburtshilfliche Rundsch. 1993;33 Suppl 1:289–90.

34. Rodriguez HA, Ackerman LV. Cellular blue nevus. Clinicopathologic study of forty-five cases. Cancer. 1968;21(3):393–405.

35. Nogueras Gimeno MA, Sanz Anquela JM, Espuela Orgaz R, Abad Menor F, Martínez Pérez E, Pérez Arbej JA, et al. Guinda Sevillano Blue nevus of the prostate C. Actas Urol Esp. 1993;17(2):130–1.

36. Jao W, Fretzin DF, Christ ML, Prinz LM. Blue nevus of the prostate gland. Arch Pathol. 1971;91(2):187–91.

37. Tsang P, Berman L, Kasznica J. Adnexal tumor and a pigmented nevoid lesion in a benign cystic ovarian teratoma. Arch Pathol Lab Med. 1993;117(8):846–7.

38. Ferrara G, Boscaino A, De Rosa G. Bronchial blue naevus. A previously unreported entity. Histopathology. 1995;26(6):581–3.

39. Harris GR, Shea CR, Horenstein MG, Reed JA, Burchette Jr JL, Prieto VG. Desmoplastic (sclerotic) nevus: an underrecognized entity that resembles dermatofibroma and desmoplastic melanoma. Am J Surg Pathol. 1999;23(7):786–94.

40. Sherrill AM, Crespo G, Prakash AV, Messina JL. Desmoplastic nevus: an entity distinct from Spitz nevus and blue nevus. Am J Dermatopathol. 2011;33(1):35–9.

41. Luzar B, Calonje E. Deep penetrating nevus: a review. Arch Pathol Lab Med. 2011;135(3):321–6.

42. Robson A, Morley-Quante M, Hempel H, McKee PH, Calonje E. Deep penetrating naevus: clinicopathological study of 31 cases with further delineation of histological features allowing distinction from other pigmented benign melanocytic lesions and melanoma. Histopathology. 2003;43(6):529–37.

43. Rhodes AR, Weinstock MA, Fitzpatrick TB, Mihm Jr MC, Sober AJ. Risk factors for cutaneous melanoma. A practical method of recognizing predisposed individuals. JAMA. 1987;258(21):3146–54.

44. Clemente C, Cochran AJ, Elder DE, Levene A, MacKie RM, Mihm MC, et al. Histopathologic diagnosis of dysplastic nevi: concordance among pathologists convened by the World Health Organization Melanoma Programme. Hum Pathol. 1991;22(4):313–9.

45. Clark Jr WH, Elder DE, Guerry 4th D, Epstein MN, Greene MH, Van Horn M. A study of tumor progression: the precursor lesions of superficial spreading and nodular melanoma. Hum Pathol. 1984;15(12):1147–65.

46. Ruiter DJ, Bhan AK, Harrist TJ, Sober AJ, Mihm Jr MC. Major histocompatibility antigens and mononuclear inflammatory infiltrate in benign nevomelanocytic proliferations and malignant melanoma. J Immunol. 1982;129(6):2808–15.

47. Monheit G, Cognetta AB, Ferris L, Rabinovitz H, Gross K, Martini M, et al. The performance of MelaFind: a prospective multicenter study. Arch Dermatol. 2011;147(2):188–94.

48. Magro CM, Crowson AN, Desman G, Zippin JH. Soluble adenylyl cyclase antibody profile as a diagnostic adjunct in the assessment of pigmented lesions. Arch Dermatol. 2012;148(3):335–44.

49. Schmoeckel C. How consistent are dermatopathologists in reading early malignant melanomas and lesions "precursor" to them? An international survey. Am J Dermatopathol. 1984;6(Suppl):13–24.

50. Barnhill RL, Argenyi ZB, From L, Glass LF, Maize JC, Mihm Jr MC, et al. Atypical Spitz nevi/tumors: lack of consensus for diagnosis, discrimination from melanoma, and prediction of outcome. Hum Pathol. 1999;30(5):513–20.

51. Cerroni L, Kerl H. Tutorial on melanocytic lesions. Am J Dermatopathol. 2001;23(3):237–41.

52. Elder DE, Murphy GF. Melanocytic tumors of the skin. Fourth series, Fascicle 12. Washington, D.C.: American Registry of Pathology in collaboration with the Armed Forces Institute of Pathology; 2010.

53. Spatz A, Calonje E, Handfield-Jones S, Barnhill RL. Spitz tumors in children: a grading system for risk stratification. Arch Dermatol. 1999;135:282–5.
54. McGovern VJ. Melanoma. Histologic diagnosis and prognosis. New York: Raven Press; 1983. p. 3–24.
55. Urso C. A new perspective for Spitz tumors? Am J Dermatopathol. 2005;27:364–6.
56. Lazzaro B, Elder DE, Rebers A, Power L, Herlyn M, Menrad A, et al. Immunophenotyping of compound and Spitz nevi and vertical growth-phase melanomas using a panel of monoclonal antibodies reactive in paraffin sections. J Invest Dermatol. 1993;100(3):313S–7.
57. Urso C, Borgognoni L, Saieva C, Ferrara G, Tinacci G, Begliomini B, et al. Sentinel lymph node biopsy in patients with "atypical Spitz tumors." A report on 12 cases. Hum Pathol. 2006;37(7):816–23.
58. Roaten JB, Partrick DA, Pearlman N, Gonzalez RJ, Gonzalez R, McCarter MD. Sentinel lymph node biopsy for melanoma and other melanocytic tumors in adolescents. J Pediatr Surg. 2005;40(1):232–5.
59. Lohmann CM, Coit DG, Brady MS, Berwick M, Busam KJ. Sentinel lymph node biopsy in patients with diagnostically controversial spitzoid melanocytic tumors. Am J Surg Pathol. 2002; 26(1):47–55.
60. Ludgate MW, Fullen DR, Lee J, Lowe L, Bradford C, Geiger J, et al. The atypical Spitz tumor of uncertain biologic potential: a series of 67 patients from a single institution. Cancer. 2009;115(3):631–41.
61. Barnhill RL, Flotte TJ, Fleischli M, Perez-Atayde A. Cutaneous melanoma and atypical Spitz tumors in childhood. Cancer. 1995;76(10):1833–45.
62. Bastian BC, LeBoit PE, Pinkel D. Mutations and copy number increase of HRAS in Spitz nevi with distinctive histopathological features. Am J Pathol. 2000; 157(3):967–72.
63. Darier J. Le melanome malin mesenchymateaux ou melano-sarcome. Bull Assoc Fr Cancer. 1925;14: 221–49.
64. Crowson AN, Magro CM, Mihm Jr MC. Malignant melanoma with prominent pigment synthesis: "animal type" melanoma – a clinical and histological study of six cases with a consideration of other melanocytic neoplasms with prominent pigment synthesis. Hum Pathol. 1999;30(5):543–50.
65. Zembowicz A, Carney JA, Mihm MC. Pigmented epithelioid melanocytoma: a low-grade melanocytic tumor with metastatic potential indistinguishable from animal-type melanoma and epithelioid blue nevus. Am J Surg Pathol. 2004;28(1):31–40.
66. Carney JA, Ferreiro JA. The epithelioid blue nevus. A multicentric familial tumor with important associations, including cardiac myxoma and psammomatous

melanotic schwannoma. Am J Surg Pathol. 1996;20(3): 259–72.
67. Zembowicz A, Knoepp SM, Bei T, Stergiopoulos S, Eng C, Mihm MC, et al. Loss of expression of protein kinase a regulatory subunit 1alpha in pigmented epithelioid melanocytoma but not in melanoma or other melanocytic lesions. Am J Surg Pathol. 2007;31(11): 1764–75.
68. Mandal RV, Murali R, Lundquist KF, Ragsdale BD, Heenan P, McCarthy SW, et al. Pigmented epithelioid melanocytoma: favorable outcome after 5-year follow-up. Am J Surg Pathol. 2009;33(12):1778–82.
69. Elder DE, Xu X. The approach to the patient with a difficult melanocytic lesion. Pathology. 2004;36(5): 428–34.
70. Clark Jr WH, From L, Bernardino EA, Mihm MC. The histogenesis and biologic behavior of primary human malignant melanomas of the skin. Cancer Res. 1969;29(3):705–27.
71. McGovern VJ. The classification of melanoma and its relationship with prognosis. Pathology. 1970;2(2): 85–98.
72. Broekaert SM, Roy R, Okamoto I, van den Oord J, Bauer J, Garbe C, et al. Genetic and morphologic features for melanoma classification. Pigment Cell Melanoma Res. 2010;23(6):763–70.
73. Magro CM, Yang SE, Zippin JH, Zembowicz A. Expression of soluble adenylyl cyclase in lentigo maligna. Arch Pathol Lab Med. 2012;136:1–7.
74. Rupec R, Eckert F, Ruzicka T. Malignant blue nevus. Hautarzt. 1993;44(3):164–6.
75. Wen YH, Giashuddin S, Shapiro RL, Velazquez E, Melamed J. Unusual occurrence of a melanoma with intermixed epithelial component: a true melanocarcinoma: case report and review of epithelial differentiation in melanoma by light microscopy and immunohistochemistry. Am J Dermatopathol. 2007; 29(4):395–9.
76. Breslow A. Thickness, cross-sectional areas and depth of invasion in the prognosis of cutaneous melanoma. Ann Surg. 1970;172(5):902–8.
77. Balch CM, Buzaid AC, Soong S-J, Atkins MB, Cascinelli N, Coit DG, Fleming ID, Gershenwald JE, Houghton A Jr, Kirkwood JM, McMasters KM, Mihm MF, Morton DL, Reintgen DS, Ross MI, Sober A, Thompson JA, Thompson JF. Final version of the American Joint Committee on Cancer staging system for cutaneous melanoma. J Clin Oncol. 2001;19(16):3635–48.
78. Piris A, Mihm Jr MC. Progress in melanoma histopathology and diagnosis. Hematol Oncol Clin North Am. 2009;23(3):467–80.
79. Kopf AW, Andrade R. Benign juvenile melanoma. Year Book of Dermatol. 1966;7–52.

Feliciano Baldi, Angeles Fortuño-Mar,
Alexander Bianchi, Alfredo D'Avino,
and Alfonso Baldi

Key Points

- DFSP is a low- to intermediate-grade soft tissue sarcoma originating from the dermal layer of the skin.
- DFSP comprises roughly .01 % of all malignant tumors and approximately 2–6 % of all soft tissue sarcomas.
- DFSP has a histologic appearance of a poorly circumscribed uniform population of bland spindle cells arranged in a monomorphous storiform or "herringbone" pattern, which extends into the subcutis, often with infiltration into and/or around the adipose tissue.

- The mainstay of treatment of DFSP is surgery.
- Merkel cells are normal constituent of the basal layer of the epidermis and the follicular epithelium and are thought to act as mechanoreceptors.
- The annual incidence of MCC ranges from 0.2 to 0.45 per 100,000, with a significant increase in the last years.
- MCC typical consists of small round blue cells. The tumor cells are monomorphous, the cytoplasm is usually scant, and the nuclei are relatively uniform.
- Early, radical surgery with margins of 2–5 cm is the recommended procedure for the treatment of primary MCC.

F. Baldi • A. Bianchi • A. D'Avino
Department of Biochemistry,
Section of Pathology,
Second University of Naples,
Naples, Italy

A. Fortuño-Mar, MD, PhD, MBA
Eldine Patologia Laboratory,
Valls, Tarragona, Spain
e-mail: af_mar@yahoo.es, afmar@comt.es

A. Baldi (✉)
Department of Environmental,
Biological and Pharmaceutical Sciences and
Technologies, Second University of Naples,
Via L. Armanni 5, Naples, Italy

Futura-onlus, Via Pordenone 2, 00182 Rome, Italy
e-mail: alfonsobaldi@tiscali.it

Dermatofibrosarcoma Protuberans

Dermatofibrosarcoma protuberans (DFSP) was first individuated as a clinical entity in 1924 by Darier and Ferrand. They described DFSP as a "progressive and recurring dermatofibroma" [1]. DFSP is a low- to intermediate-grade soft tissue sarcoma originating from the dermal layer of the skin. It is a nodular cutaneous tumor and is characterized by a storiform pattern. Historically it has been attributed to fibroblastic origin; however,

A. Baldi et al. (eds.), *Skin Cancer*, Current Clinical Pathology,
DOI 10.1007/978-1-4614-7357-2_8, © Springer Science+Business Media New York 2014

the histogenesis of this tumor is far from clear. It has been proposed, based on its consistent reactivity for CD34 and nerve growth factor receptor, that DFSP may be a particular form of nerve sheath tumor, but composed of cells other tan Schwann cell or perineural cells. Recent immunohistochemical evidence suggests that it may arise from the dendritic cell in the skin [2].

Epidemiology

DFSP comprises approximately 4 % of all soft tissue sarcomas [3, 4]. The estimated incidence is around 3 cases per one million persons per year [5], with a significant higher incidence among blacks [6]. DFSP usually presents during early or middle adult life between 20 and 50 years of age, although it has been described in both children and in the elderly [7]. The onset of the lesion is often in childhood, and there are an increasing number of reports about its appearing in the pediatric age group [8].

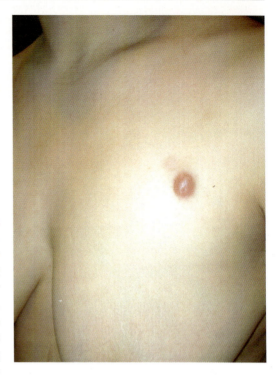

Fig. 8.1 Clinical presentation of a DFSP grown in the region of the trunk

Clinical Features

Although these tumors occur at almost any site, most lesions appear on the trunk, groin, or lower extremity, while a number of cases occur on the head and neck. DFSP is characterized by slow but persistent growth over a long period, with early tumors appearing as painless areas of cutaneous thickening with a plaque-like fashion (Fig. 8.1). Rarely, the lesion appears as an area of atrophy, and very rarely, multiple small subcutaneous nodules appear initially, rather than a plaque. Over time, they develop into a nodular mass and ultimately can develop into a large lesion, with occasionally ulceration of the skin. Typically DFSP is not adherent to underlying structures, with most tumors consisting of a solitary, protuberant, gray-white superficial mass involving the subcutis and skin, with an average size of less than 5 cm at time of diagnosis [9]. Occasionally, the area of the tumor displays a gelatinous appearance that corresponds at microscopic level to myxoid changes. DFSP often is confused with lipomas, epidermal cysts, scars,

keloid, dermatofibromas, nodular fasciitis, and insect bites [10] and this often causes a delayed diagnosis.

Diagnosis of Dermatofibrosarcoma Protuberans

Diagnosis is made using incisional biopsy [11]. An excisional biopsy is usually performed in all cases where it is possible to remove the entire lesion.

Magnetic resonance imaging (MRI) can be used to evaluate the local extent of the tumor.

Histopathology

DFSP has a characteristic histologic appearance of a poorly circumscribed uniform population of bland spindle cells arranged in a monomorphous storiform or "herringbone" pattern (Fig. 8.2a, b), which extends into the subcutis, often with infiltration into and/or around the adipose tissue. The epidermis over the lesion is usually normal

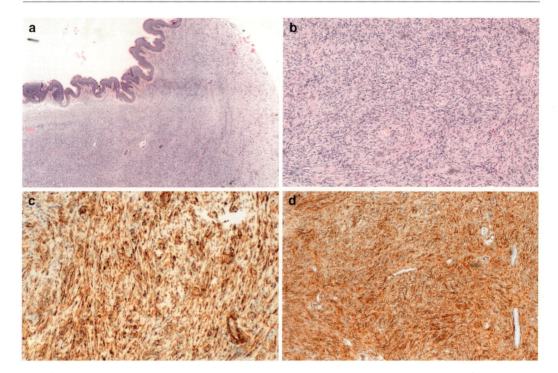

Fig. 8.2 (a) DFSP composed of slender fibroblasts arranged in a storiform pattern; (b) higher magnification, better showing a poorly circumscribed uniform popula- tion of bland spindle cells arranged in a monomorphous storiform pattern; (c) the neoplastic cells express CD34; (d) the neoplastic cells are positive for vimentin

or atrophic. Early lesions may demonstrate a "grenz zone," which is a tumor-free region separating the tumor from the epidermis. Cutaneous adnexa are often found entrapped within the tumors. Mitotic activity usually averages fewer than 5 mitotic figures per high-power field. Unusual variants of DFSP include the Bednar tumor that is characterized by melanin-containing cells [10] the myxoid DFSP that has deposits of interstitial mucin, and giant cell, and the atrophic type.

In contrast, the fibrosarcoma is characterized by long fascicles of spindle cells with more evident nuclear atypia and higher mitotic activity. Approximately 15 % of cases of DFSP contain a component of high-grade sarcoma. Immunohistochemical analysis can be utilized for the diagnosis. DFSPs are positive for vimentin, focally and inconstantly for actin, and strongly and consistently for CD34 (Fig. 8.2c, d). Staining for CD34, indeed, is commonly employed, and sensitivity has been reported as being between 84 and 100 % [11, 12]. Positivity for CD34 is lost within the areas of sarcomatous change.

Conversely, they are negative for S100 protein, HMB45, FXIIIa, and CD44.

Differential Diagnosis

Differential diagnosis with neurofibroma can be challenging since both DFSP and neurofibroma display CD34-positive cells, even if they are more abundant in DFSP; on the other hand, S100 protein is positive in neurofibromas and negative in DFSP. Concerning the differential diagnosis with dermatofibroma, the most important marker to be considered is CD34, since DFSP is consistently positive for CD34, while dermatofibroma lacks CD34-positive cells except for blood vessel endothelium.

Genetics

Most (90 %) of DFSP exhibit a chromosomal translocation between chromosomes 17 and 22. Consequence of this translocation is a fusion between the platelet-derived growth factor-B gene (PDGFB; chromosome 22) and the collagen 1 alpha 1 gene (COL1A1; chromosome 17), that leads to IPER-expression of the fusion oncogene and fully functional PDGFB [13, 14]. Detection of gene fusion by RT-PCR or FISH is helpful for confirming a diagnosis of DFSP.

Prognosis

DFSP is a locally aggressive tumor and despite sharing some histologic features with fibrohistiocytic tumors, it tends to grow in a more infiltrative fashion and has a greater capacity for local recurrence. Moreover, in rare instances, it gives distant metastases, but this is usually a late event.

Staging of Dermatofibrosarcoma Protuberans

DFSP is currently staged in accordance with the American Musculoskeletal Tumor Society Staging System which considers tumor grade and compartmentalization [15].

Treatment of Dermatofibrosarcoma Protuberans

The mainstay of treatment of DFSP is surgery [16]. In cases of very large or advanced DFSP, a multidisciplinary approach is recommended. Recent NCCN guidelines recommend margins of 2–4 cm using conventional surgical management. However, the use of Mohs surgery, allows complete excision with microscopic margins [17].

Merkel Cell Carcinoma

Merkel cells are normal constituent of the basal layer of the epidermis and the follicular epithelium and are thought to act as mechanoreceptors [18]. The Merkel cell carcinoma (MCC) was first described in 1972 as a sweat gland carcinoma by Toker [19]. Successively, the same investigator by means of electron microscopic studies identified dense-core neuroendocrine granules within the tumor cells, thus demonstrating their origin from Merkel cells [20]. The histogenesis of MCC, however, is still a debate, since certain differences exist between Merkel cells and MCC in terms of anatomical localization, of expression of neurofilaments, and of mitotic activity. Nevertheless, starting from the work of Johannessen in 1980, the term "Merkel cell carcinoma" was established [21].

Epidemiology

The annual incidence of MCC ranges from 0.2 to 0.45 per 100,000, with a significant increase in the last years [22]. MCC is principally a disease of the Caucasian race and both sexes are affected with a slight male predominance [23].

Clinical Features

MCC most commonly occurs as a solitary nodule in the elderly (Fig. 8.3), usually in sun-damaged skin, being the head and the neck region the most common site [24]. UV irradiation is recognized as one of the most important pathogenetic factors [25]. The clinical presentation of this tumor is rather nonspecific and especially small tumors can appear somewhat benign. Indeed, it is often mistaken for more common skin tumors of epithelial origin. MCC consists of nodular, firm, red-pink,

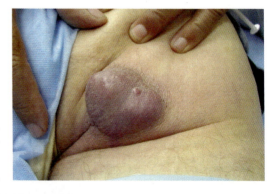

Fig. 8.3 Clinical presentation of a MCC grown in the perianal region (Dr Miguel López, Venezuela, personal observation)

non-ulcerated lesion, ranging from 1 to 4 cm in diameter. The natural history of MCC is variable, but typically tends to progress rapidly, with early and frequent metastasis to the regional lymph nodes. The overall survival rate is significant influenced by tumor size (≥2) [26]. Recurrences are frequent; however, there are some reports in the literature of spontaneous regression [27].

Diagnosis of Merkel Cell Carcinoma

The clinical presentation of this tumor is generally nonspecific; therefore, diagnosis of MCC is essentially based on peculiar histology representation on hematoxylin-eosin-stained slides together with the data from immunohistochemistry. Electron microscopy studies can confirm the presence of neuroendocrine granules in the tumor cells, as it is the case for normal Merkel cells.

Histopathology

MCC typically consists of small round blue cells. The tumor cells are monomorphous, the cytoplasm is usually scant, and the nuclei are relatively uniform with chromatin pattern finely granular (Fig. 8.4a). Histologically, MCC can be classified into three distinct subtypes: trabecular, intermediate, and small-cell type [28]. Trabecular is the least frequent type; tumor cells are organized in organoid clusters and trabeculae. In the intermediate subtype, the most common histologic subtype, there is a solid and diffuse growth pattern. The small-cell subtype is similar to small-cell tumors of other site, such as small-cell lung cancer. Microscopically, MCC is located in the dermis or sometimes in the subcutaneous tissue, with the epidermis usually uninvolved and with a thin grenz zone. Ultrastructurally, the tumor cells contain dense-core neurosecretory

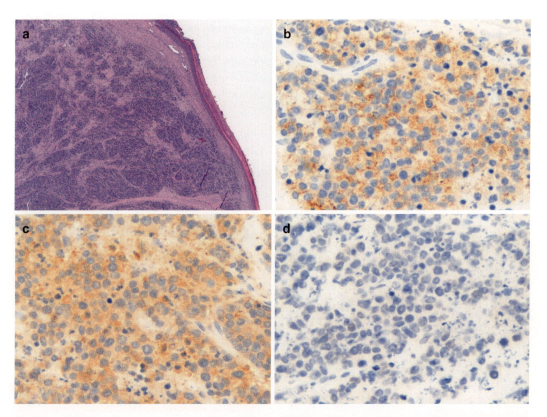

Fig. 8.4 (a) MCC composed of small round monomorphous blue cells centered in the dermis, with the overlying epidermis uninvolved; (b) the neoplastic cells express Cytokeratin 20; (c) the neoplastic cells are positive for synaptophysin; (d) the neoplastic cells do not express TTF-1

granules and tightly packed perinuclear intermediate filaments.

Immunohistochemistry can aid in the histological diagnosis of MCC, demonstrating the expression of both epithelial and neuroendocrine markers. Among the epithelial markers, the most important is cytokeratin-20, which is normally expressed only in the gastrointestinal epithelium, urothelium, and Merkel cells (Fig. 8.4b) [29]. Due to its neuroendocrine differentiation, MCC always stains positive for different neuroendocrine markers, such as neuron-specific enolase, chromogranin A, synaptophysin, and CD56 (Fig. 8.4c).

Differential Diagnosis

Pulmonary small-cell carcinoma and other malignant neuroendocrine tumors must be considered in the differential diagnosis with MCC. Cytokeratin-20 positivity in MCC serves to distinguish it from pulmonary small-cell carcinoma and also other malignant neoplasms, since it is not usually expressed in neuroendocrine carcinomas of other sites. On the other hand, thyroid transcription factor 1 (TTF1) is never expressed in MCC (Fig. 8.4d), while it is positive in tumors of the lung. Therefore, the combination of cytokeratin-20 and TTF1 staining is very useful for the differential diagnosis.

Genetics

Different types of chromosomal alterations have been shown in MCC [30]. The most common aberrations documented are trisomy of chromosomes 1, 6, and 11. Tumors displaying DNA alterations have a threefold risk of metastatic disease compared to tumors with no DNA alterations [31].

Prognosis

The prognosis is poor, with the 2-year survival rate ranging from 30 to 50 % [32]. Overall survival is strictly associated with the stage of the disease at the time of the diagnosis. Positive predictors of survival are female sex, localized disease, and younger age. Local recurrences are frequent (up to 44 % of patients), as well as distant dissemination (up to 40–50 % of patients), especially to the lungs, liver, and bone.

Staging of Merkel Cell Carcinoma

In most published series, MCC is not classified according to the TNM system. Actually, the most widely recognized staging system in the treatment of MCC is that proposed by Yiengpruksawan in 1991 [33].

Treatment of Merkel Cell Carcinoma

The recommended procedure for the treatment of primary MCC [34] is radical surgery with wide margins. Patients with regional node metastases or local recurrence must undergo excision of the primary lesion and lymph node dissection, associated with adjuvant radiation therapy [35].

Glossary

CD34 Glycoproteins found on immature hematopoietic cells and endothelial cells

Cytokeratin Any of a class of fibrous proteins that are intermediate filaments present usually in pairs chiefly in epithelial cells and that are sometimes used as markers to identify malignancies of epithelial origin

Nerve growth factor receptor Any of a family of plasma membrane integral proteins that bind nerve growth factors

Neuroendocrine tumor A tumor that forms from cells that release hormones in response to a signal from the nervous system

Soft tissue sarcoma A malignant tumor that begins in the muscle, fat, fibrous tissue, blood vessels, or other "soft" supporting tissues of the body

References

1. Darier J, Ferrand M. Dermatofibromes progressifs et recidivants ou fibrosarcomes de la peau. Ann Dermatol Syphiliga. 1924;5:545–62.
2. Haycox CL, Odland PB, Olbricht SM, Piepkorn M. Immunohistochemical characterization of dermatofibrosarcoma protuberans with practical applications for diagnosis and treatment. J Am Acad Dermatol. 1997;37:438–44.
3. Chang CK, Jacobs IA, Salti GI. Outcomes of surgery for dermatofibrosarcoma protuberans. Eur J Surg Oncol. 2004;30(3):341–5.
4. Kransdorf MJ. Malignant soft-tissue tumors in a large referral population: distribution of diagnoses by age, sex, and location. AJR Am J Roentgenol. 1995;164(1): 129–34.
5. Gloster HM. Dermatofibrosarcoma protuberans. J Am Acad Dermatol. 1996;35:355–74.
6. Criscione VD, Weinstock MA. Descriptive epidemiology of dermatofibrosarcoma protuberans in the United States, 1973 to 2002. J Am Acad Dermatol. 2007;56(6):968–73. Epub 2006 Dec 1.
7. Taylor HB, Helwig EB. Dermatofibrosarcoma protuberans: a study of 115 cases. Cancer. 1962;15: 717–25.
8. McKee PH, Fletcher CD. Dermatofibrosarcoma protuberans in infancy and childhood. J Cutan Pathol. 1991;18:241–6.
9. Bowne WB, Antonescu CR, Leung DH, Katz SC, Hawkins WG, Woodruff JM, et al. Dermatofibrosarcoma protuberans: a clinicopathologic analysis of patients treated and followed at a single institution. Cancer. 2000;88(12):2711–20.
10. Abeloff MD. Abeloff's clinical oncology. 4th ed. Philadelphia: Elsevier; 2008: Ch 74; Dupree WB, Langloss JW, Weiss SW. Pigmented dermatofibrosarcoma protuberans (Bednar tumor): a pathologic, ultrastructural and immunohistochemical study. Am J Surg Pathol. 1985;9:630–9.
11. Klijanienko J, Caillaud JM, Lagacé R. Fine-needle aspiration of primary and recurrent dermatofibrosarcoma protuberans. Diagn Cytopathol. 2004;30(4):261–5; Haycox CL, Odland PB, Olbricht SM, Piepkorn M. Immunohistochemical characterization of dermatofibrosarcoma protuberans with practical applications for diagnosis and treatment. J Am Acad Dermatol. 1997;37(3 Pt 1):438–44.
12. Abenoza P, Lillemoe T. CD34 and factor XIIIa in the differential diagnosis of dermatofibroma and dermatofibrosarcoma protuberans. Am J Dermatopathol. 1993;15(5):429–34.
13. Pedeutour F, Simon MP, Minoletti F, et al. Ring 22 chromosomes in dermatofibrosarcoma protuberans are low level amplifiers of chromosome 17 and 22l sequences. Cancer Res. 1995;55:2400–3.
14. Bridge JA, Neff JR, Sanberg AA. Cytogenetic analysis of dermatofibrosarcoma protuberans. Cancer Genet Cytogenet. 1990;49:199–202.
15. No authors listed. Soft tissue sarcoma. In: Greene PL, Page DL, Fleming ID, editors. AJCC cancer staging manual. 6th ed. New York: Verlag; 2002. pp. 193–200.
16. Arnaud EJ, Perrault M, Revol M, Servant JM, Banzet P. Surgical treatment of dermatofibrosarcoma protuberans. Plast Reconstr Surg. 1997;100(4):884–95.
17. Paradisi A, Abeni D, Rusciani A, Cigna E, Wolter M, Scuderi N, et al. Dermatofibrosarcoma protuberans: wide local excision vs. Mohs micrographic surgery. Cancer Treat Rev. 2008;34(8):728–36.
18. Briggaman RA, Wheeler CEJ. The epidermal-dermal junction. J Invest Dermatol. 1975;65:71–84.
19. Toker C. Trabecular carcinoma of the skin. Arch Dermatol. 1972;105:107–10.
20. Tang CK, Toker C. Trabecular carcinoma of the skin: an ultrastructural study. Cancer. 1978;42:2311–21.
21. Johannessen JV, Gould VE. Neuroendocrine skin carcinoma associated with calcitonin production: a Merkel cell carcinoma? Hum Pathol. 1980;11:586–8.
22. Hodgson NC. Merkel cell carcinoma: changing incidence trends. J Surg Oncol. 2005;89:1–4.
23. Boyle F, Pendlebury S, Bell D. Further insights into the natural history and management of primary cutaneous neuroendocrine (Merkel cell) carcinoma. Int J Radiat Oncol Biol Phys. 1995;31:315–23.
24. Tai PT, Yu E, Winquist E, Hammond A, Stitt L, Tonita J, et al. Chemotherapy in neuroendocrine/Merkel cell carcinoma of the skin: case series and review of 204 cases. J Clin Oncol. 2000;18:2493–9.
25. Koljonen V, Bohling T, Granhroth G, Tukiainen E. Merkel cell carcinoma: a clinicopathiological study of 34 patients. Eur J Surg Oncol. 2003;29:607–10.
26. Connelly TJ, Cribier B, Brown TJ, Yanguas I. Complete spontaneous regression of Merkel cell carcinoma: a review of the 10 reported cases. Dermatol Surg. 2000;26:853–6.
27. Haag ML, Glass LF, Fenske NA. Merkel cell carcinoma. Diagnosis and treatment. Dermatol Surg. 1995;21:669–83.
28. Miettinen M. Keratin 20: immunohistochemical marker for gastrointestinal, urothelial, and Merkel cell carcinomas. Mod Pathol. 1995;8:384–8.
29. Leong AS, Phillips GE, Pieterse AS, Milios J. Criteria for the diagnosis of primary endocrine carcinoma of the skin (Merkel cell carcinoma). A histological, immunohistochemical and ultrastructural study of 13 cases. Pathology. 1986;18:393–9.
30. Van Gele M, Leonard JH, Van Roy N, Van Limbergen H, Van Belle S, Cacquyt V, et al. Combined karyotyping, CGH and M-FISH analysis allows detailed characterization of unidentified chromosomal rearrangements in Merkel cell carcinoma. Int J Cancer. 2002;101:137–45.
31. Larramendy ML, Koljonen V, Bohling T, Tukiainen E, Knuutila S. Recurrent DNA copy number changes revealed by comparative genomic hybridization in primary Merkel cell carcinomas. Mod Pathol. 2004;17:561–7.

32. Linjawi A, Jamison WB, Meterissian S. Merkel cell carcinoma: important aspects of diagnosis and management. Am Surg. 2001;67:943–7.

33. Yiengpruksawan A, Coit DG, Thaler HT, Urmacher C, Knapper WK. Merkel cell carcinoma. Prognosis and management. Arch Surg. 1991;126:1514–9.

34. Brisset AE, Olsen KD, Kasperbauer JL, Lewis JE, Goellner JR, Spotts BE, et al. Strome se: Merkel cell carcinoma of the head and neck: a retrospective case series. Head Neck. 2002;24:982–8.

35. Kolsonen V. Merkel cell carcinoma. World J Surg Oncol 2006;4:7

Primary Cutaneous Lymphomas

9

Emanuela Bonoldi and Umberto Gianelli

Key Points

- The diagnosis of a PCL consists of a synoptic integration of clinical and biological data and must rely upon a comprehensive clinico-pathological correlation as a pivotal element in the diagnostic approach.
- Immunohistochemistry represents a highly valuable tool in order to determine the neoplastic nature of a cutaneous lymphoid infiltrate and to distinguish different lymphoma histotypes.
- The finding of B- or T-cell clonality, yet in the absence of morphological and immunohistochemical clues indicative of malignancy, should always be carefully considered and makes follow-up of the patient more intensive.
- Thanks to the joint effort of expert representatives of the EORTC cutaneous lymphoma study group and the WHO classification, a new classification WHO/EORTC was developed in 2005.

- Mycosis fungoides and primary cutaneous CD30-positive lymphoproliferative disorders represent the most common type of cutaneous T-cell lymphomas.
- Cutaneous B-cell lymphomas (CBCL) account for approximately 20–25 % of all primary cutaneous lymphomas. The most common histotypes is represented by cutaneous marginal zone B-cell lymphoma and cutaneous follicle centre lymphoma.

Main Problems in Evaluating Lymphoid Infiltrates of the Skin

The majority of lymphocytic infiltrates in the skin have noticeable common characteristics. Most infiltrates are of T-cell origin, represent reactive conditions and are not characterised by either significant cytologic or pattern atypia.

These infiltrates are immunologically driven and are the result of cytotoxic mechanisms or delayed-type hypersensitivity and antibody-related cellular immunity. Indeed, they appear more frequently in patients with underlying iatrogenic and/or endogenous immune dysregulation.

Examples of such benign conditions are comprised under the chapters of *spongiotic and*

E. Bonoldi (✉)
Pathology Unit, Hospital A. Manzoni,
Via dell'Eremo 9/12, Lecco 23900, Italy
e-mail: emanuela.bonoldi@policlinico.mi.it

U. Gianelli
Department of Pathophysiology and Transplantation,
University of Milan,
Milan, Italy

exematous dermatitis (allergic contact dermatitis and photoallergic reactions), *interface dermatitis* (erythema multiforme, acute graft vs. host disease, lichenoid dermatitis, with special regard to lichenoid drug eruptions and subacute cutaneous lupus erythematosus) or *diffuse and nodular lymphocytic dermal infiltrates* (polymorphous light eruption, non-scarring discoid/tumid lupus erythematosus, morphea, Jessner lymphocytic infiltrate of the skin).

Indeed, conditions of persistent lymphoid reactions may be characterised by either cytological atypia, thus mimicking lymphoma and potentially becoming biologically unstable, or by exhibiting clonal restriction and phenotypic aberrancy and therefore acquiring a limited tendency toward progression to overt lymphoma. Among these conditions are lymphoid reactions, which may resemble lymphoma. In reality, they are expressions of exuberant responses to immune dysregulation, both B- and T-lymphocyte proliferations, namely, the so-called lymphocytoma cutis, lymphomatoid drug eruptions, lymphomatoid lesions in collagen vascular diseases, primary cutaneous plasmocytosis and viral-associated lymphomatoid dermatitis.

Increased risk of malignant transformation in lymphoid proliferations following sustained activation of the immune system is strictly related to genetic instability of lymphocytes. Chronic infections, immunodeficiency status and autoimmune disorders favour mechanisms of clonal selection of transformed lymphocytes. The persistence of the trigger acts through different pathogenetic mechanisms, thus increasing proliferation and decreasing apoptosis. Selective advantages given to lymphoid clones may gain independence from antigen stimulation.

A model of infection-driven B-cell lymphoproliferation in the skin is represented by the activation of marginal zone lymphocytes by *Borrelia burgdorferi*, consequently giving rise to borrelial lymphocytoma and possibly to marginal zone lymphoma of the skin with pathogenetic mechanisms analogous to those described by other extranodal lymphomas, i.e. gastric MALT lymphoma associated to *Helicobacter pylori*, splenic marginal zone lymphoma associated with HCV infection and ocular adnexal MALT lymphoma associated with *Chlamydia psittaci infection*.

In regard to T-cell proliferations, an example of atypical lymphoid growth is displayed by lymphomatoid drug eruptions.

The molecular demonstration of clonality and of aberrant immunoprofile is not unusual in such conditions, and this data must be carefully taken into consideration when performing final diagnosis.

Recognition of antigen-mediated lymphoid proliferation is of the utmost importance to avoid the misdiagnosis of overt lymphoma and overtreatment. This is because withdrawal of the antigens responsible for the immune reaction and/or treatment of the immune dysregulation may lead to regression of the disease.

On the other hand, detection of oligoclonality or monoclonality, with or without loss of T antigen in the setting of morphological atypia, although not mandatorily leading to a diagnosis of malignancy, still represents an alarming condition. Such lesions should be identified as cutaneous lymphoid T-cell dyscrasia and in a small percentage of cases can progress to cutaneous T-cell lymphomas. This group of disorders encompasses a constellation of distinct entities (pityriasis lichenoides, pigmented purpuric dermatosis, syringolymphoid hyperplasia with alopecia, alopecia mucinosa, large plaque parapsoriasis and idiopathic erythroderma) and some inflammatory conditions which can present phenotypic abnormalities, mainly loss of CD7 and CD62L expression, most often observed in overt T-cell lymphomas.

On these basis, it is easy to understand that the differential diagnosis of a dense cutaneous lymphoid infiltrate characterised by morphological atypia, possibly accompanied by aberrant phenotype and clonal expansion or restriction, may still represent one of the most challenging problems in dermatopathology, despite advances in molecular pathology and immunohistochemistry. A final diagnosis consists of a synoptic integration of clinical and biological data and must rely upon a comprehensive clinicopathological correlation as a pivotal element in the diagnostic approach.

The main issues when facing a cutaneous lymphoid infiltrate are the following:

- To discriminate between reactive and neoplastic proliferation, with special regard to early neoplastic conditions.
- To identify reactive lesions more prone to developing malignancy.
- To identify the histotype of the neoplastic growth, which may be strictly correlated to specific clinical outcome.
- To distinguish primary diseases from concurrent and secondary skin involvement. In fact, the former have a favourable clinical behaviour and do not require aggressive treatment. Concurrent cutaneous B-cell lymphomas, involving other lymphoid and/or extranodal sites, present clinico-pathological and prognostic features much closer to primary ones.
- To discriminate between the different histological patterns of lymphomas linked to the age of the lesions and of the disorder itself (mycosis fungoides, for example, may show extremely heterogeneous clinical presentation and long history of smouldering lesions before there are overt manifestations of the disease).

Concerning the differential diagnosis between reactive and neoplastic lesions, the main cause of misinterpretation, making exclusion of malignant lymphoma possible to render only on morphological basis, encompasses the following items:

- Skin is by itself a natural homing for T-lymphocytes and exocytosis/epidermotropism of lymphocytes is a common finding.
- Morphological findings, especially in inflammatory disease, depend on the age of the lesion biopsied.
- Cytological atypia is not a hallmark of malignancy in skin lymphoid disorders. Presence of lymphocytes with "blastic" size and alarming nuclear features is a frequent finding in reactive disorders as well. These cells often express CD30 molecule as an activation marker without diagnostic implications.
- Cellular monomorphism, which is of paramount help in nodal lymphomas, is useless in the skin, where most of all indolent B-cell lymphomas display marked cellular pleomorphism.
- Predominance of a reactive population overwhelming the neoplastic growth is frequent in indolent B-cell lymphomas.
- In contrast to the nodal counterpart, the architectural pattern of growth can be of little help in both reactive and neoplastic entities.
- Immunomarkers like CD10 and BCL2 are very useful in the differential diagnosis between reactive germinal centres and follicular lymphomas in the lymph node, but results most often negative in the cutaneous counterpart, especially in early lesions.

Most Frequent Diagnostic Challenges in Everyday Practice

Benign Lymphoid Hyperplasia of the Skin and Cutaneous B-Cell Lymphoma

Cutaneous lymphoproliferative infiltrates with follicular growth pattern may be follicular lymphomas, marginal zone lymphomas or lymphoid hyperplasia of the skin (B-cell pseudolymphomas).

Besides clinical differences among these entities, there are morphological clues, together with immunophenotypical and molecular features, which can denote the distinctions.

According to Leinweber et al. [1], the main criteria suggestive of follicle centre lymphoma are:

- Absence of tingible body macrophages within follicles
- Reduced proliferation rate detected by immunohistochemistry
- Absence of the polarisation of the follicles evaluated with the aid of MIB-1
- Presence of small clusters of CD10- and/or Bcl6-positive cells outside the follicles
- Positivity for Bcl2 within follicular cells
- Monoclonality for JH chain of immunoglobulin, investigated by PCR

Cases presenting at least four of the mentioned criteria are considered to be malignant.

Additional features pointing to malignancy suggested by other authors [2] are as follows:

- Extensive expression of CD20 by cells showing loss of CD79a expression
- Equal kappa and light chain-restricted populations, potentially indicating an emerging lambda light chain-restricted population
- Absence of T-cell receptor-β (TCR-β) gene rearrangement due to the fact that T-cell clonality is not uncommonly detected in reactive disorders

The differential diagnosis is more difficult when dealing with cutaneous lymphoid hyperplasia and marginal zone lymphoma [3, 4] since these two disorders share similar clinical findings. Indeed, they both affect women more than men and present single or multiple slowly developing nodules involving the face, back and upper extremities. Morphologically, both entities may present reactive follicles; variable pattern of infiltration (diffuse, nodular, lichenoid and perivascular in different pattern combinations), either a bottom-heavy or top-heavy infiltrate; and the presence of a "grenz" zone.

More distinctive features for marginal zone lymphoma are:

- Aggregates or sheets of marginal zone cells
- Sheets or zones of plasma cells
- Lymphoepithelial lesions in the sweat and sebaceous glands
- Monotypic plasma cells
- Lysis or disintegration of CD23 or CD21 network of follicular dendritic cells
- B-cell/T-cell ratio ≥3:1
- Presence of IgH gene rearrangement

More distinctive features of cutaneous lymphoid hyperplasia are:

- Epidermal changes (focal spongiosis, with parakeratosis and exocytosis)
- Polytypic plasma cells with kappa/lambda <4/1
- Absence of IgH gene rearrangement

Primary Follicle Centre Lymphoma and Primary Marginal Zone Lymphoma of the Skin

The immunophenotypical profile is most important in differentiating these two entities. The typical differential features are the following:

- In primary follicle centre lymphoma the neoplastic cells are Bcl2−, Bcl6−, CD10+/− and CD23+/−
- Monotypic plasma cells are mostly located at the periphery of the infiltrate and are a major diagnostic criterion for marginal zone lymphoma [5]
- In marginal zone lymphoma the neoplastic cells are Bcl2+, BCL6−, CD10− and CD23−

Moreover clusters of CD123+ plasmocytoid dendritic cells are constantly observed in marginal zone lymphoma and not in other primary cutaneous lymphomas [6].

Marginal Zone Lymphomas with Marked Plasmacytic Differentiation and T-Cell-Rich Background Versus Peripheral T-Cell Lymphoma Versus Primary Cutaneous Plasmocytosis Versus Cutaneous Involvement by Castleman's Disease

More recently some authors have drawn attention to a variant of marginal zone lymphoma with marked plasmacytic differentiation and T-cell-rich background which had already been described by Magro et al. [7] and had been historically diagnosed as primary cutaneous immunocytoma or primary cutaneous plasmacytoma.

In the absence of a history of plasma cell myeloma, the diagnosis of cutaneous plasmacytoma should be made with great caution, and the presence of any lymphoid follicles, B cells or follicular dendritic cells in the infiltrate will lead to the exclusion of it.

Notwithstanding the notion that a T-cell component represents a phenomenon frequently reported in different primary cutaneous lymphoma, the occurrence in this variant of a marginal zone lymphoma of atypical-looking T-lymphoid cells that are small to medium in size, which may obscure the neoplastic B-cell proliferation, may lead to misdiagnosing peripheral T-cell lymphoma or mycosis fungoides.

Molecular study of IgH and TCR gamma gene rearrangement may be warranted to confirm the results.

Clinico-pathological studies have demonstrated that the T-cell-rich variants of marginal zone lymphoma have no prognostic implications.

Primary cutaneous plasmocytosis is a rare entity, sometimes occurring in concomitance with endocrinopathies and frequently accompanied by polyclonal hypergammaglobulinemia, which represents an analogy to mucosal-based plasmocytosis like Zoon's balanitis and plasma cell orofacialis. Polyclonality of plasma cells is mandatory for diagnosis.

Skin lesions associated with Castleman's disease are mainly in the context of POEMS syndrome. The histopathological findings consist of atrophic germinal centres with prominent hyalinised vessels associated with sheet-like proliferation of plasma cells, which may or may not show evidence of light chain restriction. Typically, the infiltrate is deeply located in the dermis possibly extending to subcutaneous tissue.

Early Lesions of Primary Cutaneous Follicle Centre Lymphoma Diffuse Type Versus Diffuse Large B-Cell Lymphoma

Primary cutaneous follicle centre lymphoma is usually described as a diffuse proliferation of large B predominantly cleaved lymphocytes, admixed with centroblasts, infiltrating the dermis and possibly the subcutis.

In the lymph node, a diffuse pattern of growth in the context of a follicle centre lymphoma is considered a marker of progression of the disease and connected to a diagnosis of diffuse large B-cell lymphoma with implications in treatment and prognosis.

On the other hand, in the skin, the biological and clinical behaviour of a primary follicle centre lymphoma is not affected by the pattern of growth.

Some authors [8, 9] have described the clinico-pathological features of early lesions of primary cutaneous follicle centre lymphoma diffuse type featured by patchy and diffuse lymphoid proliferation with a tendency to collect in perivascular and/or periadnexal districts thus mimicking reactive infiltrates. Giulia et al. [9] describe for the first time in detail the clinico-pathological

features of the early lesions of PCFCL diffuse variant, which actually represent the early manifestation of the so-called Crosti lymphoma of the back. They report a series of 24 patients with lesions located on back and shoulder (20 cases), arm (2 cases) and scalp (1 case). In most cases, the patients typically showed a larger infiltrated central lesion, surrounded by smaller papules or nodules sometimes far from the main affected area. All of them showed favourable outcome with radiotherapy following to surgical excision. Only one patient received chemotherapy. In three cases, the peripheral lesions underwent spontaneous regression, while in other cases recurrences happened. Biopsy specimens showed periadnexal and perivascular aggregates of small lymphocytes admixed with predominantly medium- to large-sized centrocytes and a minority of centroblasts. A follicular arrangement was never observed and CD21-positive dendritic reticular cells were fewer, and never clustered is commonly detectable in the follicular variant of this lymphoma. The authors suggest a different pathogenesis for this histotype and do not consider the diffuse variant as a progression of the follicular variant. Moreover, they stress the importance to distinguish it from diffuse large B-cell lymphoma leg type.

Diffuse Large B-Cell Lymphoma Versus Non-lymphoid Malignancies

Problems can arise in this differential diagnosis, in particular when appropriate tissue sampling is not provided or when the biopsy displays diffuse areas of necrosis or sclerotic band of collagen. Indeed, this group of disorders, including the leg type and the other types of NOS of diffuse large B-cell lymphomas, can be confused, at morphologic evaluation, with both T- and NK-cell lymphomas and with non-haematologic neoplasms. Merkel cell carcinoma and cutaneous metastatic carcinoma must be considered at times. The spindle cell variant of cutaneous diffuse large B-cell lymphomas (DLBCL) can be misinterpreted for spindle cell melanoma, spindle squamous cell carcinoma or spindle cell sarcomas. An extensive immunophenotyping of the neoplastic population helps to avoid misdiagnosis because expression of lymphoid markers has never been described in non-lymphoid tumours.

Other challenging situations can be observed in cases in which the neoplastic large B cells are few and sparse, but it is important to be aware that their presence does not by itself point to malignant lymphomas. Expression by these cells of BCL6 and CD10 is a helpful hint to malignancy.

Early Mycosis Fungoides Versus Inflammatory Lichenoid Reactions/T-Cell Dyscrasias

The histopathological diagnosis of early lesions of mycosis fungoides may be impossible in some cases since morphological features are similar to those described in many inflammatory skin diseases involving the interface and the papillary dermis (psoriasis, chronic contact dermatitis, drug-induced lesions). Immunohistochemical studies are not distinctive.

The best suggestion remains to stem the diagnosis from the comprehensive integration of clinical, histopathologic, immunophenotypic and molecular data. Limited to histopathologic evaluation, the diagnosis of mycosis fungoides can be suggested only when applying strictly the morphologic criteria published by the EORTC cutaneous lymphoma study group [10]. In those cases in which histopathology results do not match with clinical diagnosis, the pathologist should not hesitate to ask for further biopsies.

Available Diagnostic Tools: Advantages and Pitfalls

Immunohistochemistry

Modern immunohistochemical techniques allow the study of the phenotypic signature of different lymphoproliferative entities on routinely fixed paraffin-embedded tissue sections. Immunohistochemistry thus represents a highly valuable tool in order to determine the neoplastic nature of an infiltrate and to distinguish different lymphoma histotypes.

CD20, CD79a and PAX5 are conclusive in recognising mature B-cell lineage, just as BCL6 and CD10 mark germinal centre derivation and cytoplasmic Ig reactions may display monotypic or polytypic Ig expressions.

The immunohistochemical profiles of the most common histotypes, which can be obtained using commercially available antibodies and which are reported in the WHO classification of primary cutaneous lymphomas, are illustrated in the following section.

Recently, a group of monoclonal antibodies on different primary B-cell lymphomas has been demonstrated to help in better defining specific antigenic profiles for research and possibly diagnostic purposes, since they are exclusively or preferentially expressed by specific histotypes, with regard to primary FCL and primary MZL. No specific set of monoclonal antibodies was found to label primary cutaneous DLBCL [11].

The expression of IgM, together with FOXP1 and BCL2, can be used as additional tool in the everyday practice for the differentiation between PCFCL and PCLDLB leg type, with this last entity constantly positive for all these three monoclonal antibodies [12].

The demonstration of antigen loss by using an extensive panel for T-cell lineage (CD2, CD3, CD4, CD5, CD7, CD8) can be of utmost aid in supporting the neoplastic nature of a lymphoid proliferation. In particular loss of CD2, CD3 and/or CD5 is more specific than loss of CD7, but still of low sensibility.

The evaluation of CD4/CD8 ratio is relevant for the differential diagnosis between early-stage mycosis fungoides and inflammatory disorders, together with CD1a immunolabeling. This latter marker can demonstrate tiny aggregates of Langerhans cells in the epidermis mimicking Pautrier abscesses and representing a usual finding in immunomediated reactive lesions.

It has to be remembered that special care has to be taken in the comprehension of CD4 expression by the investigated population, because CD4 is also a marker of histiocytes.

Granzyme B, perforin, CD56 and TIA-1 are good markers of cytotoxic activity and find a useful application in the signature of different conditions encompassed in the CD30 lymphoproliferative diseases spectrum, extranodal natural killer/T-cell lymphomas and subcutaneous panniculitis-like T-cell lymphomas.

It is important to keep in mind that aberrant expression of B-cell lineage marker can be observed in T-cell lymphomas, for example, MUM-1; the post-germinal centre activation marker is expressed by "activated large cells" in both lymphomatoid papulosis and anaplastic large-cell lymphomas [13].

In conclusion, one must keep in mind that immunohistochemical characterisation of lymphoproliferative skin disorders is of extreme relevance to complete and support the diagnosis but must be analysed in the context of the clinical and morphological setting.

Molecular Pathology

The most efficient molecular methods to analyse B-cell clonality of formalin-fixed, paraffin-embedded samples seem nowadays represented by BIOMED-2 PCR-based protocol [14] which allows to overcome the two main problems affecting sensitivity and specificity in this field of pathology [15].

Firstly, the common occurrence of somatic hypermutation in primer binding sites in primary cutaneous lymphomas often makes the binding of primers ineffective, and secondly, only small amount of neoplastic cells may be present in such cases of lymphomas.

BIOMED-2 PCR can theoretically detect 1–5 clonal lymphocytes in a population of 100 lymphocytes in which the remaining are benign. This implies a considerable risk of false-positive results in otherwise benign disorders (pseudomonoclonality and oligoclonality). Suggestions to improve efficacy and efficiency of molecular analysis are to confirm the results by duplicate or triplicate tests on the same sample and/or to perform laser microdissection of the hotspots.

On the contrary, false-negative or polyclonal results can occur more frequently in overt B-cell lymphomas and less in T-cell lymphomas.

Finally, it has to be remembered that dual lineage rearrangement is not a rare event in lymphoid infiltrates of the skin. Such lineal infidelity can affect both B- and T-cell lymphomas and leads to the conclusion that IgH and TCR gene analysis is not equivalent to B- or T-lineage assessment and has to be interpreted cautiously for diagnostic purposes.

The finding of T-cell clonality, yet in the absence of morphological and/or immunohistochemical clues indicative of malignancy, should always be carefully considered and makes follow-up of the patient more intensive.

Classification of Cutaneous Lymphomas

Early classification of lymphomas did not discriminate between nodal and extranodal forms of non-Hodgkin lymphomas and was mainly based on morphological and immunophenotypical features of the tumour cells. Most forms of cutaneous lymphomas were considered as skin involvement of systemic diseases and were treated according to this concept.

The EORTC classification published in 1997 represented the first consensus classification for primary cutaneous lymphomas [16]. It adopted biological concepts borrowed from the REAL classification, emphasising the importance of integrating clinical, histological, immunophenotypical and genetic findings in the diagnostic approach and definition of different nosological entities.

Based on the data collected from large cutaneous lymphoma registries such as the Lymphoma Registry in Graz and the Dutch Cutaneous Lymphoma Working Group, three main categories were identified by indolent, intermediate and aggressive clinical behaviour.

The REAL classification was updated by the WHO classification of lymphoid neoplasms published in 2001. This scheme includes most cutaneous T-cell lymphomas of the previous

Table 9.1 WHO/EORTC classification of cutaneous lymphomas

Mature T-cell and NK-cell neoplasms	Mature B-Cell neoplasms
Mycosis fungoides	Cutaneous marginal zone B-cell lymphoma (MALT type)
Pagetoid reticulosis (localised disease)	Cutaneous follicle centre lymphoma
Follicular, syringotropic, granulomatous variants	Cutaneous diffuse large B-cell lymphoma
Granulomatous slack skin	Intravascular large B-cell lymphoma
Sezary syndrome	Lymphomatoid granulomatosis
CD30+ T-cell lymphoproliferative disorders of the skin	Chronic lymphocytic leukaemia
Lymphomatoid papulosis	Mantle cell lymphoma
Primary cutaneous anaplastic large-cell lymphoma	Burkitt lymphoma
Subcutaneous panniculitis-like T-cell lymphoma	
Primary cutaneous peripheral T-cell lymphoma (PTL), unspecified	Immature haematopoietic malignancies
(Subtypes of PTL, provisional)	
Primary cutaneous aggressive epidermotropic	Blastic NK-cell lymphoma
CD8-positive cytotoxic T-cell lymphoma	CD4+/CD56+ haematodermic neoplasm
Cutaneous gamma-/delta-positive T-cell lymphoma	Precursor lymphoblastic leukaemia/lymphoma
Primary cutaneous small/medium CD4+ T-cell lymphoma	T-lymphoblastic leukaemia
Extranodal NK/T-cell lymphoma, nasal type	T-lymphoblastic lymphoma
Hydroa vacciniformia-like lymphoma (variant)	B-lymphoblastic leukaemia
Adult T-cell leukaemia/lymphoma	B-lymphoblastic lymphoma
Angioimmunoblastic T-cell lymphoma	Myeloid and monocytic leukaemias
	Hodgkin lymphoma

classification, while cutaneous B-cell lymphomas differ significantly from those identified by both the REAL and WHO classifications.

Indeed, notwithstanding the improvement given by the EORTC approach, this classification did not gain wide approval among pathologists and oncologists because it had led considerable confusion on the therapeutic approach.

Thanks to the joint effort of expert representatives of the EORTC cutaneous lymphoma study group and the WHO classification, a new classification (WHO/EORTC) was developed in 2005 [17]. This proposal was widely accepted by clinicians and pathologists and included in the currently adopted WHO classification published in 2008, which represents the nowadays general classification of nodal and extranodal lymphoid tumours worldwide adopted [18–20].

This review illustrates the salient features of the most common entities in the context of the recent WHO/EORTC classification of primary cutaneous lymphomas (Table 9.1).

Mature T-Cell and NK-Cell Neoplasms

Mycosis Fungoides and Subtypes

Clinical features: Mycosis fungoides (MF) represents the most common type of cutaneous T-cell lymphomas. It has been classified according to the type of skin lesions (patches, plaques and tumours), the presence or absence of large-cell transformation and/or extracutaneous involvement. It pursues an indolent clinical course with slow progression, and sometimes, subsequent biopsies are needed for a proper diagnosis, especially in the early manifestations of the disease. The male to female ratio is 2:1 with adults/elderly mostly affected. Skin lesions vary from large erythematous patches preferentially involving non-sun-exposed areas to reddish brown infiltrated plaques with wrinkled surface, to nodules solitary or generalised, sometimes ulcerated. A combination of patches, plaques and tumours is common in the well-developed

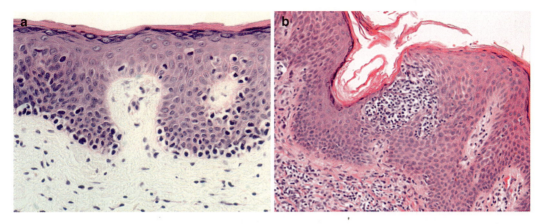

Fig. 9.1 Mycosis fungoides, patch stage. (**a**) Atypical lymphocytes arranged along the interface line. (**b**) Intraepidermal collection of atypical cells forming Pautrier microabscess

disease. Large-cell transformation occurs in more than 50 % of tumour stage MF. The most frequent sites of extracutaneous involvement in the later stages of the disease are lymph nodes, lung, spleen and liver. Several clinical variants of MF have been described. Some of them represent distinct clinico-pathological entities, while others are peculiar kind of skin involvement described by case reports. MF is rare in childhood (0.5–5 % of all cases) and presents mainly with early-stage lesions sometimes with concurrent or prior history of pityriasis lichenoides chronica. Sezary syndrome (SS) is actually considered an aggressive form of peripheral T-cell lymphoma involving elderly adults which may be or not preceded by idiopathic erythroderma and presents with generalised lymphadenopathy and pruritic erythroderma. The disorder is characterised by the presence of the so-called Sezary cell in the peripheral blood, the lymph nodes and the skin.

Histopathology: The histological features of MF are prototypical and correlate with the different clinical lesions. *Patch stage*: The diagnostic architectural hallmarks consist in the so-called string of pearls (at least four T-lymphocytes contiguously aligned within the basal layer), associated with Pautrier microabscesses (collection of at least four atypical T cells within the epidermis and papillary dermal fibrosis, with coarse horizontally disposed wiry bundles of collagen). MF cells (Lutzner cells)

are lymphocytes of medium-large size (approximately the diameter of a basal keratinocyte nucleoli), with irregular convoluted nuclei (cerebriform nuclei) (Fig. 9.1a and b). These epidermotropic T cells are larger than those present in the papillary dermis and show a discrete halo. Often in Pautrier microabscesses they are intermingled with dendritic Langerhans cells. Absence or little spongiosis is mandatory. A clinico-pathological algorithm has been published [10] reporting different parameters to make diagnosis most reproducible. *Plaques stages*: The neoplastic cells represent the main contributor to dermal infiltrate unlikely patch stage. Epidermotropism is prominent sometimes associated with syringotropism and Pautrier microabscesses most frequent (Fig. 9.2). The tumour cells are highly atypical and form a dense band-like infiltrate within the papillary dermis and perivascular aggregates in the middle dermis. *Tumour stage*: A pan-dermal dense neoplastic infiltrate is typical of this stage with extension to the subcutaneous fat and possible sparing of the epidermis. *Large-cell transformation*: It is defined by the presence of more than 25 % large neoplastic cells forming clusters.

Immunophenotype: MF cell typically expresses CD2, CD3, CD4 and CD5. The diagnosis of MF is most challenging for the pathologist in the early stages because most dermal lymphocytes are reactive. Plenty of studies have tried to determine reproducible cut-offs of the CD8-/CD3-positive

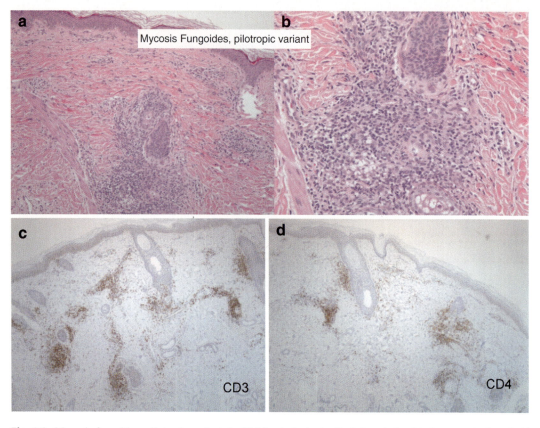

Fig. 9.2 Mycosis fungoides, pilotropic variant. (**a, b**) Morphologic detail of the relationship between the lymphoid infiltrate ad the pilo-sebaceous unit. (**c, d**) The lymphoid cells express the CD3 and CD4 antigen

cells in order to help discriminating early MF from reactive dermatoses. Assessing of CD4 cells has been avoided because of cross-reaction with histiocyte population. Different studies show that CD8/CD3 is significantly lower in MF when compared with controls, and other reports suggest that CD4/CD8 more than 2 is specific for MF. Actually semiquantification of lymphocyte subsets is unlikely to be routinely used. On the contrary, of more importance is the detection of T-cell-associated antigen loss, with special regards to CD7 and at less extent CD5 downregulation. The suggested immunohistochemical baseline includes a pan-B-cell marker (CD79a). With disease progression CD30 expression may be detectable in the large-cell component. Neoplastic cells of erythrodermic MF and SS share the same immune signature, but CD7 antigen loss is less frequent in the latter entity. Moreover, large cells in SS are often MUM1 positive.

Genetics: T-cell receptor genes are clonally rearranged in most of the cases of MF in plaques or tumour stage, while only about 50 % of the patch stages do not show any TCR gene rearrangement. Complex karyotypes are present in tumour stages of the disorders with many structural and numerical alterations described.

Primary Cutaneous CD30-Positive Lymphoproliferative Disorders

CD30 T-cell lymphoproliferative disorders comprise a spectrum of conditions ranging from lymphomatoid papulosis (Lyp) to anaplastic large-cell lymphoma (ALCL) and including borderline cases [21]. This group accounts for 30 % approximately of cutaneous T-cell lymphomas and has to be distinguished by cases of transformed mycosis fungoides expressing CD30 antigen (a member of the tumour necrosis factor receptor family).

Extensive CD30 expression by the neoplastic population is mandatory for diagnosis of these entities which share a common pathogenetic pathway strictly involving the role of CD30/CD30L in activation of TRF2 (TNF receptor-associated factor) up to NF-kB signal transduction leading either to proliferation of apoptosis.

Owing to this mechanism, these lymphoproliferative disorders run a more favourable course and are amenable of regression. Most probably, past diagnosis of "regressing atypical histiocytosis" and "cutaneous Hodgkin disease" would be nowadays renamed as PC CD30 LPD.

It is of the utmost relevance to keep in mind that CD30-positive lymphocytes isolated or in clusters can be observed in a variety of inflammatory skin conditions, such as viral infections, arthropod bite reactions, lymphomatoid drug reaction and lupus pernio [22].

Lymphomatoid Papulosis (Lyp)

Clinical features: Red papules and nodules smaller than 1.5–2 cm or pink papulo-nodules, single or in clusters, predominantly affecting the trunk and limbs mostly of adults but even of children. The lesion may ulcerate in the centre and result in a scar. A waxing and waning course of the eruption is typical with tendency to spontaneous involution in 3–4 months and subsequent recurrences. The incidence of concurrent lymphoma or progression to lymphoma ranges between 4 and 20 % confirming the benign clinical course of this disorder. Yet, other malignant skin lymphomas, in particular mycosis fungoides, anaplastic large-cell lymphoma and Hodgkin lymphoma, may precede or follow Lyp.

Histopathology: Three main histologic subtypes have been described, with features merging one in the other and varying in relation to the age of the biopsied lesion.

Type A Lyp presents as a bottom-heavy striking polymorphous infiltrate with a distinct perivascular, perineural and eccrinotropic pattern, composed of small reactive lymphocytes, histiocytes and rare Sternberg-like atypical cells. An epidermal reaction with neutrophilic exocytosis and even necrosis and ulceration sustained by heavy vasculitis is frequent. Sometimes a granulomatous component with eosinophilia is evident so mimicking arthropod bite reaction. In *type B* Lyp, which is the less frequent variant, the infiltrate is still mixed, but large atypical cells begin to dominate and show a lichenoid distribution, resembling the plaque stage of mycosis fungoides. *Type C* Lyp lesions are featured by monotonous infiltrates of the large atypical cells and few small lymphocytes intermingled.

Immunophenotype: The large atypical cells of types A and C are CD30 positive and usually CD4+, so sharing the same signature of ALCL. In contrast, the large cells of Lyp B do not express CD30. Markers pointing to natural killer differentiation are generally negative, while cytotoxic antigen can be variably expressed.

A rare CD8+ form of Lyp has been described, histologically characterised by a granulomatous eccrinotropic infiltrate.

Genetics: t(2;5) translocation responsible of the protein ALK (anaplastic lymphoma kinase) has been occasionally reported. On the contrary T-cell gene rearrangement has been described in up to 60–70 % cases of Lyp.

Cutaneous Anaplastic Large-Cell Lymphoma

Clinical features: Usually single, but sometimes multiple, persistent large often ulcerative nodule, which does not undergo spontaneous regression. A cut-off of 2 cm in diameter has been proposed by some investigators to distinguish from Lyp. The median age of presentation is 60 years. A type C Lyp/borderline CD30-positive lymphoproliferative disease has been described, usually associated with a history of Lyp either concurrent or prior.

Secondary skin involvement of primary nodal ALCL, occurrence of ALCL in the setting of other lymphomas (mycosis fungoides and Hodgkin lymphoma) and ALCL in the context of

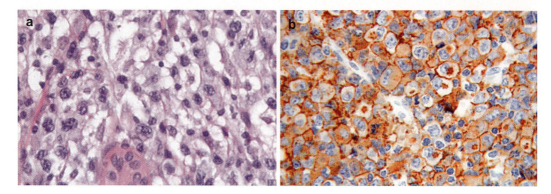

Fig. 9.3 Cutaneous anaplastic large-cell lymphoma. (**a**) Large pleomorphic cells, growing in a diffuse sheet-like pattern. (**b**) The neoplastic cells strongly express the CD30 antigen

post-transplant T-cell lymphoproliferative disorders represent other categories of this disease.

Histopathology: The common pattern shows a cohesive sheet-like growth, extending to the subcutis, of large cells, even multinucleated, with eccentric horseshoe-shaped nucleus and prominent eosinophilic Golgi region (Fig. 9.3). A small-cell variant exists with scattered atypical hallmark cells intermingled with dominant small-intermediate-sized atypical lymphocytes. Angiocentricity and angiodestruction by the neoplastic cells are frequent findings. Epidermotropism is reported. The epitheliomorphic feature of the cells can represent a challenging problem of differential diagnosis on morphological grounds with undifferentiated carcinoma. Other histological subtypes are the sarcomatoid, giant, neutrophilic-rich and histiocyte-rich variants. Mixed patterns are frequent. Histological variant does not influence prognosis with the exception of small-cell subtype, which runs a worse clinical course.

Immunophenotype: Immunohistochemical analysis shows a T-helper cell phenotype (CD3+, CD4+) of most cases, with a consistently positive CD30 staining and loss of pan-T-cell antigens. A null phenotype is not infrequent. EMA and ALK-1 are constantly negative in true primary ALCL of the skin. Clusterin a ubiquitous highly glycosylated protein, commonly positive in nodal ALCL, is variably detectable in the primary cutaneous disorder and cannot be used to distinguish the two entities. Nevertheless its cytoplasmic dot-like expression is typical of

ALCL only and can be useful in the differential diagnosis with other T-cell malignancies. In the small-cell variant, the small lymphoid cells are typically negative.

Genetics: The majority of cases display clonal T-cell rearrangement. The (2;5)(p23;q35) translocation and its variants are rarely present in primary cutaneous ALCL, contrarily to the nodal counterpart.

Blastic NK-Cell Lymphomas

T-NK cutaneous lymphomas are a heterogeneous group of rare disorders, featured by overlapping immunophenotypical signature and morphology between T-cell lineage and NK cells.

The two main entities are extranodal NK/T cell of nasal type and blastic plasmocytoid dendritic cell neoplasm.

This last entity is a rare and intriguing disease affecting middle-aged patients, with aggressive biological behaviour and poor outcome due to massive bone marrow involvement and leukemic progression. The neoplastic growth shows the following immunophenotypic profile: CD43+, CD101+, CD123+ and TCL1+. Variable expression of CD68, TdT, BDCA-2, TIA1 and CD34 has been reported. The normal counterpart is the plasmocytoid dendritic cell precursor, possibly strictly related to a common myeloid/NK precursor cell.

Fig. 9.4 Cutaneous marginal zone B-cell lymphoma. (**a**) Polymorphic lymphoid proliferation with bland cytologic atypia. (**b**) Peripheral plasma cellular components

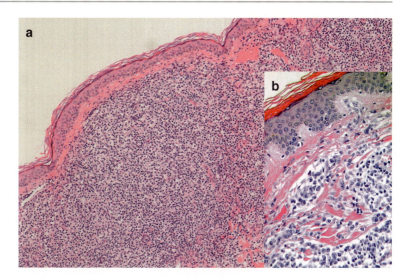

Mature B-Cell Neoplasms

Cutaneous B-cell lymphomas (CBCL) account for approximately 20–25 % of all primary cutaneous lymphomas and probably occur far more frequently than is generally believed. They share an overall favourable prognosis and their proper identification is important to avoid overtreatment. The most relevant prognostic factors are histological type and size of the lesions.

Cutaneous Marginal Zone B-Cell Lymphoma (MALT Type)

Clinical features: Cutaneous marginal zone B-cell lymphoma (CMZL) affects patients in the fifth to sixth decades, with a male predominance, and may present with single or multiple red to violaceous papules, plaques and nodules involving the upper extremities or the trunk. Skin recurrences are frequent. In endemic areas *Borrelia burgdorferi* appears to be causal agent in some cases.

Histopathology: The pattern of growth may be perivascular, nodular or diffuse, involving the dermis and extending to the subcutis without epidermal infiltration (Fig. 9.4). Tumour cells surround and colonise reactive germinal centre and are composed of variable number of marginal zone B cells, with centrocyte-like or monocytoid morphology, mixed with plasma cells characteristically arranged at the periphery of the lymphoid nodules and subepidermally, together with scattered transformed B cell (sometimes more than 20 %). Plasma cell differentiation may be prominent. Intranuclear Dutcher bodies are commonly found. The presence of very immature plasma cells points to a possible secondary cutaneous involvement. Aggregates of CD123 dendritic plasmocytoid cells can be observed. Lymphoepithelial lesions are occasionally evident in eccrine ducts or secretory coils.

Immunophenotype: The marginal zone cells display a CD20+, bcl-2+, CD43+/–, CD10–, bcl-6–, CD5–, ciclina D1- and CD23 – phenotype. CD10 and bcl-6 are particularly useful in the differential diagnosis with primary follicle centre cell lymphoma. Light chain restriction of the lymphoplasmacytoid and plasma cells is detected in at least 80 % of the cases.

Genetics: IgH genes are clonally rearranged in more than 80 % of cases. t(14;18)(q32;q31) involving IgH and MALT1 genes is reported in about 30 % of cases. FAS gene mutation is present in a minority of cases. Recent studies [23] support the existence of a subset of CMZL characterised by monocytic plasma cells with class switch heavy chain expression and prominent mast cell component.

Fig. 9.5 Cutaneous follicle centre lymphoma: monomorphic neoplastic nodule, lacking a mantle zone and "tingible bodies" macrophages

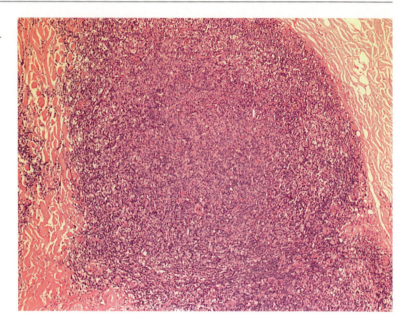

Cutaneous Follicle Centre Lymphoma

Clinical features: Cutaneous follicle centre lymphoma (CFCL) manifests mainly in middle-aged adults, with no gender predominance, and represents the most common subtype of PCL. The presentation consists of firm erythematous plaques, nodules or tumours distributed on the trunk and/or head and neck districts. The previous term "Crosti lymphoma" or "reticulohistiocytoma of the dorsum" refers to a distinctive clinical presentation of this entity.

Histopathology: The infiltrate is composed of mature B cells of germinal centre derivation (centrocytes and centroblasts in variable proportion), arranged in superficial perivascular and deeper nodular or diffuse pattern of growth. The neoplastic follicles lack mantle zone, polarisation of the germinal centre and tangible bodies macrophages (Figs. 9.5 and 9.6). The proportion of large cells and the presence of a diffuse pattern of growth do not influence the prognosis (Figs. 9.7 and 9.8). A morphological spindle cell variant has been described which may be confused with a mesenchymal neoplasm (Fig. 9.9).

Immunophenotype: Neoplastic cells show positivity for B-cell markers (CD19, CD20, CD22) and bcl-6 protein, with CD10 variably expressed. On the contrary, bcl-6 expression is always maintained even in diffuse growth. In contrast to nodal follicular lymphomas, Bcl-2 is rarely demonstrated or faintly positive in the neoplastic follicles. A strong expression of CD10 and bcl-2 should address to a possible secondary nodal follicular lymphoma. The proliferation rate measured with the ki-67 index is typically low in the neoplastic proliferation. The presence of a network of CD21- and CD23-positive follicular dendritic cells helps in the differential diagnosis with CMZL. The presence of bcl-6 +/CD10+ centrocytes in the interfollicular region may help to define the neoplastic nature of the follicular infiltrate.

Genetics: Clonal IgH gene rearrangement is demonstrable in 90 % of the cases. On the contrary, t(14;18)(IgH;Bcl-2) is rarely shown by PCR but can be documented in up to 40 % by FISH analysis in those cases characterised by follicular pattern.

Primary Cutaneous Diffuse Large B-Cell Lymphoma

The WHO/EORTC classification scheme distinguishes primary cutaneous diffuse large B-cell lymphoma (PCDLBCL) leg type and other NOS type. The differential diagnosis of PCDLBCL is

Fig. 9.6 Cutaneous follicle centre lymphoma: nodular lymphoid proliferation with sparing "grenz zone" and deep extension

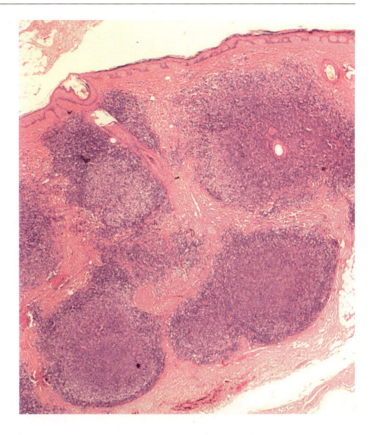

broad and difficult to define histologically, because it encompasses histo-morphological spectrum of lymphoproliferative diseases and other malignant neoplasms mimicking lymphomas. The recognition of different histotypes of PCDLBCL has been an important advancement in the management of the patients because of variations in the biological behaviour of different entities. Indeed prognosis of PBDLBCL variably depends on specific factors both clinical (anatomic site and extent of the disease) and immunological (immunophenotype). Patients who present with solitary or few lesions have a much better prognosis than those with multiple lesions.

Primary Cutaneous Diffuse Large B-Cell Lymphoma: Leg Type

Clinical features: PCDLBCL leg type is the most common form of PCDLBCL and accounts for 5–10 % of all cutaneous B-cell lymphomas. It

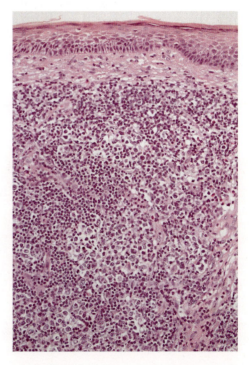

Fig. 9.7 Cutaneous follicle centre lymphoma: centroblasts predominate in the neoplastic nodule

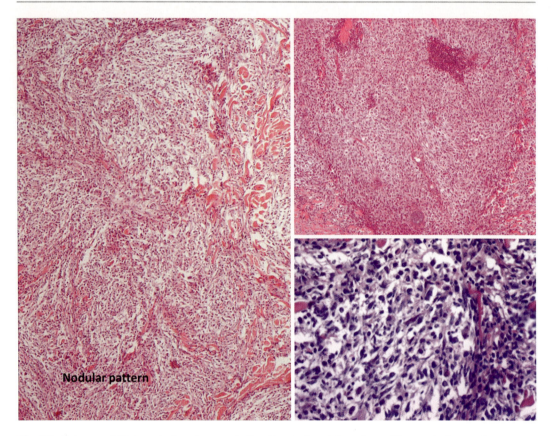

Fig. 9.8 Cutaneous follicle centre lymphoma, spindle cell variant: nodular pattern of the neoplastic growth

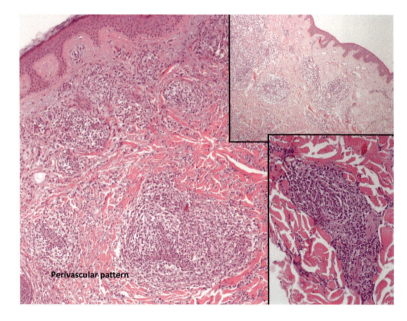

Fig. 9.9 Cutaneous follicle centre lymphoma, spindle cell variant: perivascular pattern of the neoplastic growth

Fig. 9.10 Primary cutaneous diffuse large B-cell lymphoma – other type (NOS): the large-cell component is composed predominantly of centroblasts

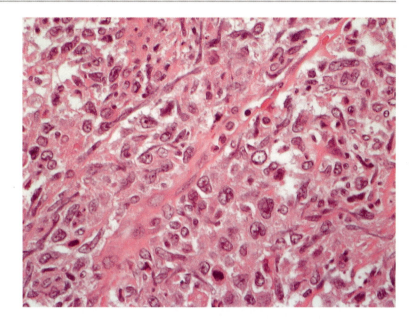

frequently develops on the legs of elderly patients presenting with red nodules or plaques sometimes ulcerated, solitary or multiple. It exhibits an unfavourable prognosis, with frequent relapses and systemic dissemination. A minority of cases are recognised on non-leg sites.

Histopathology: The infiltrate is composed predominantly of centroblast- and immunoblast-like tumour cells, with round non-cleaved nuclei and prominent nucleoli, with brisk mitotic activity and numerous apoptotic cells (Fig. 9.10). Epidermotropism is unusual and proliferation involves mainly the dermis with a diffuse pattern.

Immunophenotype: The neoplastic B cells express pan-B-cell markers (CD20, CD79a) and are nearly always strongly positive for bcl-2, IRF4/MUM1 and FOXP1. Bcl-6 stains positively in most cases, while CD10 is usually negative.

Genetics: Clonality studies show clonal rearrangement of IgH genes. FISH analysis frequently shows translocations involving C-MYC, BCL-6 and IgH genes. T(14;18) is not found in this lymphoma, and the marked BCL-2 positivity by immunohistochemistry may be explained by amplification of the BCL-2 gene.

Primary Cutaneous Diffuse Large B-Cell Lymphoma: Other Type (NOS)

This category is very heterogeneous comprising morphological variants, which in most cases represent cutaneous involvement by systemic diseases, with special regard to intravascular large B-cell lymphoma, T-cell-rich large B-cell lymphoma and plasmablastic diffuse large B-cell lymphoma [24].

Intravascular Large B-Cell Lymphoma

Clinical features: Intravascular large B-cell lymphoma (ILBCL) is an aggressive and usually disseminated disease typically affecting elderly patients. Patients with involvement limited to the skin (so-called cutaneous variant) show a better outcome than those who present multiorgan involvement. Cutaneous presentation is polymorphous, including painful telangectatic lesions, panniculitis, erythematous streaks, plaques and tender nodules.

Histopathology: The large neoplastic lymphoid cells are trapped in vascular lumina within the dermis and the subcutis, making deep biopsies mandatory for diagnostic purposes. Mitotic index is constantly high.

Immunophenotype: Tumour cells beyond positivity for pan-B-cell markers may co-express CD10 and CD5. Overexpression of bcl-2 is not accompanied by BCL2 gene rearrangement.

Genetics: Immunoglobulin genes are clonally rearranged.

Glossary

Epidermotropism Tendency to infiltrate the epidermis

Extranodal A localisation of lymphoproliferative neoplasms different from a lymph node

Grenz zone An area savings the epidermis

Mono(poly)clonality Belonging to a single (or multiple) cell clone(s)

References

1. Leinweber B, Colli C, Chott A, Kerl H, Cerroni L. Differential diagnosis of cutaneous infiltrates of B lymphocytes with follicular growth pattern. Am J Dermatopathol. 2004;26:4–13.
2. Magro CM, Crowson AN. Primary cutaneous follicle center cell lymphoma. In: Magro CM, Crowson AN, Mihm MC, editors. The cutaneous lymphoid proliferations. New York: Wiley; 2007.
3. Baldassano MF, Bailey EM, Ferry JA, Harris NL, Duncan LM. Cutaneous lymphoid hyperplasia and cutaneous marginal zone lymphoma: comparison of morphologic and immunophenotypic features. Am J Surg Pathol. 1999;23:88–96.
4. Arai E, Shimizu M, Hirose T. A review of 55 cases of cutaneous lymphoid hyperplasia: reassessment of the histopathologic findings leading to reclassification of 4 lesions as cutaneous marginal zone lymphoma and 19 as pseudolymphomatous folliculitis. Hum Pathol. 2005;36:505–11.
5. Kempf W, Sander CA. Classification of cutaneous lymphomas – an update. Histopathology. 2010;56:57–70.
6. Kutzner H, Kerl H, Pfaltz MC, Kempf W. CD123-positive plasmacytoid dendritic cells in primary cutaneous marginal zone B-cell lymphoma: diagnostic and pathogenetic implications. Am J Surg Pathol. 2009;33(9):1307–13.
7. Magro CM, Porcu P, Ahmad N, Klinger D, Crowson AN, Nuovo G. Cutaneous immunocytoma: a clinical, histologic, and phenotypic study of 11 cases. Appl Immunohistochem Mol Morphol. 2004;12:216–24.
8. Santucci M, Pimpinelli N. Primary cutaneous B-cell lymphomas. Current concepts. I. Haematologica. 2004;89:1360–71.
9. Gulia A, Saggini A, Wiesner T, Fink-Puches R, Argenyi Z, Ferrara G, et al. Clinicopathologic features of early lesions of primary cutaneous follicle center lymphoma, diffuse type: implications for early diagnosis and treatment. J Am Acad Dermatol. 2011;65:991–1000.
10. Santucci M, Biggeri A, Feller AC, Massi D, Burg G. Efficacy of histologic criteria for diagnosing early mycosis fungoides: an EORTC cutaneous lymphoma study group investigation. European Organization for Research and Treatment of Cancer. Am J Surg Pathol. 2000;24(1):40–50.
11. Fanoni D, Tavecchio S, Recalcati S, Balice Y, Venegoni L, Fiorani R, et al. New monoclonal antibodies against B-cell antigens: possible new strategies for diagnosis of primary cutaneous B-cell lymphomas. Immunol Lett. 2011;134:157–60.
12. Demirkesen C, Tüzüner N, Esen T, Lebe B, Ozkal S. The expression of IgM is helpful in the differentiation of primary cutaneous diffuse large B cell lymphoma and follicle center lymphoma. Leuk Res. 2011;35:1269–72.
13. Robson A. Immunocytochemistry and the diagnosis of cutaneous lymphoma. Histopathology. 2010;56:71–90.
14. van Dongen JJ, Langerak AW, Brüggemann M, Evans PA, Hummel M, Lavender FL, et al. Design and standardization of PCR primers and protocols for detection of clonal immunoglobulin and T-cell receptor gene recombinations in suspect lymphoproliferations: report of the BIOMED-2 Concerted Action BMH4-CT98-3936. Leukemia. 2003;17:2257–317.
15. Melotti CZ, Amary MF, Sotto MN, Diss T, Sanches JA. Polymerase chain reaction-based clonality analysis of cutaneous B-cell lymphoproliferative processes. Clinics (Sao Paulo). 2010;65:53–60.
16. Willemze R, Kerl H, Sterry W, Berti E, Cerroni L, Chimenti S, et al. EORTC classification for primary cutaneous lymphomas: a proposal from the Cutaneous Lymphoma Study Group of the European Organization for Research and Treatment of Cancer. Blood. 1997;90(1):354–71.
17. Willemze R, Jaffe ES, Burg G, Cerroni L, Berti E, Swerdlow SH, et al. WHO-EORTC classification for cutaneous lymphomas. Blood. 2005;105(10):3768–85.
18. Kim YH, Willemze R, Pimpinelli N, Whittaker S, Olsen EA, Ranki A, et al. TNM classification system for primary cutaneous lymphomas other than mycosis fungoides and Sezary syndrome: a proposal of the International Society for Cutaneous Lymphomas (ISCL) and the Cutaneous Lymphoma Task Force of the European Organization of Research and

Treatment of Cancer (EORTC). Blood. 2007;110: 479–84.

19. Senff NJ, Noordijk EM, Kim YH, Bagot M, Berti E, Cerroni L, et al. European Organization for Research and Treatment of Cancer and International Society for Cutaneous Lymphoma consensus recommendations for the management of cutaneous B-cell lymphomas. Blood. 2008;112:1600–9.

20. Pileri Jr A, Patrizi A, Agostinelli C, Neri I, Sabattini E, Bacci F, et al. Primary cutaneous lymphomas: a reprisal. Semin Diagn Pathol. 2011;28:214–33.

21. Duvic M. CD30+ neoplasms of the skin. Curr Hematol Malig Rep. 2011;6:245–50.

22. Werner B, Massone C, Kerl H, Cerroni L. Large CD30-positive cells in benign, atypical lymphoid infiltrates of the skin. J Cutan Pathol. 2008;35:1100–7.

23. Edinger JT et al. Cutaneous marginal zone lymphomas have distinctive features and include 2 subsets. Am J Surg Pathol. 2010;34(12):1830–41.

24. Plaza JA, Kacerovska D, Stockman DL, Buonaccorsi JN, Baillargeon P, Suster S, et al. The histomorphologic spectrum of primary cutaneous diffuse large B-cell lymphoma: a study of 79 cases. Am J Dermatopathol. 2011;33:649–55.

Comparative Oncology of Skin Cancer

10

Ira Gordon

Key Points

- Naturally occurring skin cancers of companion animals can serve as useful models of our understanding of these diseases in people.
- The most common skin tumors in dogs include mast cell tumor, lipoma, sebaceous gland tumor, histiocytoma, squamous cell carcinoma, melanoma, fibrosarcoma, and basal cell tumor.
- The most common skin tumors in cats include basal cell tumor, mast cell tumor, fibrosarcoma, squamous cell carcinoma, and sebaceous gland tumor.

Cancer is the leading cause of death in people from 45 to 65 years of age and the leading cause of death for geriatric pets [1, 2]. The annual incidence of skin cancer in dogs and cats is estimated to be 90.4 and 34.7 per 100,000 pets at risk [3]. This annual incidence is high compared to humans with an annual incidence of only 5.2 per 100,000 people at risk [1, 4–6]. Studying this animal population with skin cancer provides an

I. Gordon, DVM
Department of Radiation Oncology Branch,
National Cancer Institute,
10 Center Drive MSC 1002, Bethesda,
MD 20817, USA
e-mail: gordoni2@mail.nih.gov

opportunity to improve our knowledge about the biology, epidemiology, pathogenesis, and treatment of skin cancer across species, contributing to advances in human and animal health through a comparative oncology approach.

The Study of Skin Cancer and Advantages of the Comparative Oncology Approach

The complex biology and therapeutic challenges associated with skin cancer necessitates continued research. Considerable knowledge about skin cancer comes from clinical experience and clinical studies of human patients. As with all cancer research, in vitro and in vivo studies also contribute to our knowledge and guide decisions that will hopefully lead to new options and breakthroughs in the treatment of skin cancer. Progress can be slow, and approaches that seem promising based on in vitro and in vivo studies frequently do not end up translating into significant improvements when attempted in the clinic. These approaches are still a valuable and necessary component of skin cancer research. Newer mouse models of cancer and advanced in vitro research techniques will continue to improve our understanding of skin cancer. Developments in the fields of surgical oncology, radiation oncology, and drug development toward treatments that more effectively target skin cancer while sparing normal tissues improve our ability to effectively manage patients with this disease.

A. Baldi et al. (eds.), *Skin Cancer*, Current Clinical Pathology,
DOI 10.1007/978-1-4614-7357-2_10, © Springer Science+Business Media New York 2014

The naturally occurring cancers seen in companion animals represent an additional cancer model that can contribute to our understanding of these diseases. A comparative oncology approach to the study of skin cancer integrates knowledge and studies of these naturally occurring cancers in pets with other basic and clinical research. Studying the similarities and the differences between neoplastic conditions of animals and humans can provide additional knowledge and insight into the biology of cancer. Furthermore, assessing novel approaches to the diagnosis and treatment of skin cancer in animals may provide important evidence into the application of these approaches for humans. Most comparative oncology studies in companion animals focus on dogs because of the large number of pet dogs that develop cancer as well as their similar size and living environment compared to humans. In some instances, studying skin cancer of cats, horses, and other animals can also contribute information through a comparative approach. The remainder of this chapter focuses on discussing the features of skin cancer in companion animals and humans that are notably similar and those that are different.

There are many characteristics of companion animals that make them valuable as models of skin cancer. Compared to laboratory animals such as mice, dogs represent a more natural outbred population and are more genetically and physiologically similar to people [7]. Pet animals live in the same environmental conditions as people with similar exposures to environmental carcinogens. The tumors they develop occur naturally rather than by transplantation or artificial induction by mutations or controlled exposures to carcinogens. These tumors are often driven by similar genetic aberrations to those seen in human tumors. Importantly, skin tumors in companion animals develop within the framework of a syngeneic surrounding stroma and a functioning immune system. Companion animals are frequently managed with the same interventions as people including surgery, chemotherapy, and radiation therapy. Despite these treatments, just as with skin cancer in humans, tumors in companion animals show progression, resistance to therapy, and metastasis. Overcoming these features of cancer remains critical to future advances in skin cancer therapy, and they are very difficult to study in other preclinical cancer models.

As the field of cancer therapy moves toward more molecularly targeted treatments, a comparative oncology approach must consider which tumors driven by the same or similar genetic aberrations. For many cancer-associated genes, the sequences of dogs and humans are closer to each other than mice and humans [7]. Companion animal cancers are more comparable to human tumors in terms of tumor size and cell kinetics than rodent tumors. Due to their larger size, serial biopsies, imaging, and collection of reasonable volumes of samples such as blood, urine, and cerebrospinal fluid are more feasible than in rodents.

For these reasons, there is a great deal of additional knowledge and insight about human cancer that can be gained by studying skin cancer in companion animals. Clinical trials involving companion animals are now commonplace and can prioritize biologic questions that address questions that apply to comparative oncology.

Common Types of Skin Cancer in Animals

The incidence of specific types of skin cancer varies between animal species. In dogs, the most common cutaneous neoplasms are mast cell tumor, lipoma, sebaceous gland tumor, histiocytoma, squamous cell carcinoma, melanoma, fibrosarcoma, and basal cell tumor. In cats, the most common cutaneous neoplasms are basal cell tumor, mast cell tumor, fibrosarcoma, squamous cell carcinoma, and sebaceous gland tumor [3].

Epithelial Tumors

Basal cell tumors represent a heterogeneous group of cutaneous epithelial tumors without squamous and adnexal differentiation. The term basal cell tumor classically can be used to describe any neoplasm originating from basal cells (whether benign or malignant) [8]. Newer reclassification schemes have suggested the use of the term basal cell tumor to refer to only benign proliferations of basal cells. These tumors are common in cats and less common in dogs [9]. In cats, they typically occur on the skin of the head and neck and present as well-circumscribed intradermal and subcutaneous masses. The overlying epidermis often shows alopecia or ulceration. Centrally, these tumors often have cystic degeneration. In cats and dogs, these tumors do not metastasize and complete surgical excision is curative. Their malignant counterpart, basal cell carcinoma, is more locally invasive and may rarely metastasize.

Papillomas are benign proliferations of the epidermis. There are many different papillomaviruses that have been identified in each species of animal. Papillomas may regress spontaneously in some species due to a cell-mediated immune response. In dogs, a formalin-inactivated vaccine has been shown to protect against canine oral papillomavirus (COPV) infection [10]. Because the capsid structure of all papillomaviruses is morphologically identical and there is a high degree of similarity at the structural and biological level between COPV and malignancy-associated human papillomaviruses, the canine disease was useful for evaluating prophylactic and therapeutic interventions for control of human papillomavirus infection and malignant sequelae [10]. A skin tumor seen in horses called the equine sarcoid is the result of a nonproductive infection with bovine papillomavirus. This tumor is not related to human sarcoidosis and does not appear to have an analogous condition in humans.

Modified sebaceous glands are present in many parts of the body and can become neoplastic. Specific examples of these seen in animals include sebaceous hyperplasia/adenoma/epithelioma, meibomian gland adenoma, and perianal adenoma. Sebaceous hyperplasia typically appears as less than 1 cm cauliflower-like raised lesions that can become ulcerated. Surgery for these lesions is curative. Sebaceous adenocarcinomas are rare in animals and are typically larger, inflamed, and ulcerated.

Squamous cell carcinoma (SCC) is associated with several factors in animals including prolonged exposure to ultraviolet light, lack of epidermal pigment at the tumor site, and sparse haircoat at affected sites [11]. SCC is common in dogs, cats, horses, cattle, and other animals. The most common sites for SCC in cats are the pinna, eyelids, and planum nasale (Fig. 10.1). In dogs, the most common sites are the head, abdomen, and limbs. Cutaneous SCC in animals is usually a slow growing and invasive tumor that is slow or late to metastasize. Many treatments have been described for animals with cutaneous SCC including surgery, radiation therapy (external

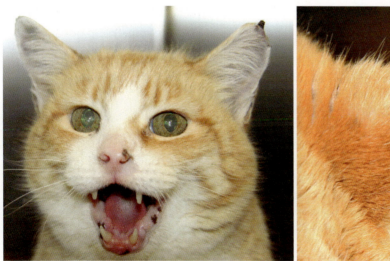
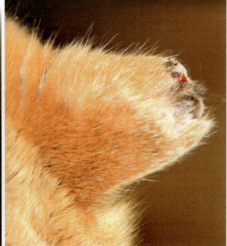

Fig. 10.1 A cat with squamous cell carcinoma. Ulcerated, crusting lesions on the planum nasale and pinna in regions of nonpigmented fur and skin (Image provided by Michael Kent, DVM)

beam, strontium-90 plesiotherapy), retinoids, immunotherapy (imiquimod), intralesional chemotherapy (cisplatin, carboplatin, 5-fluorouracil), photodynamic therapy, and topical chemotherapy (5-fluorouracil).

Multicentric squamous cell carcinoma in situ (Bowen's-like disease) is seen in cats and has been described in the dog [12, 13]. In contrast to invasive squamous cell carcinoma in cats, exposure is not related to ultraviolet light exposure and lesions frequently occur in haired, pigmented skin.

Melanocytic Tumors

Melanocytic tumors are common in dogs and horses. Gray horses are extremely prone to development of melanocytic tumors. In dogs, location of the tumor is of critical importance to the malignant potential of these tumors. Generally, tumors arising from the haired skin are benign, whereas those arising from mucocutaneous junctions are malignant. Benign cutaneous melanomas typically show little nuclear or cellular pleomorphism and have fewer than three mitotic figures per ten high-power fields (HPF). The majority of cases of malignant melanoma in dogs occur at mucocutaneous junctions or in the oral cavity.

Round Cell Tumors

Cutaneous lymphoma is seen in dogs and cats. The clinical appearance of cutaneous lymphoma shows marked variability and may manifest as patches, plaques, or tumors. Similar to cutaneous lymphoma in humans, cases in dogs and cats are typically classified as epitheliotropic and nonepitheliotropic. In epitheliotropic lymphomas, T-cells have an affinity for epidermis and adnexal epithelium. Nonepitheliotropic lymphomas are B- or T-cell origin and have clusters or sheets of neoplastic lymphocytes. Cutaneous lymphoma tends to be progressive and multicentric and will progress to involve regional lymph nodes and viscera (Fig. 10.2).

Other cutaneous round cell tumors are seen with varying frequency in animals including several tumors seen commonly in animals that are not seen frequently in humans. Although

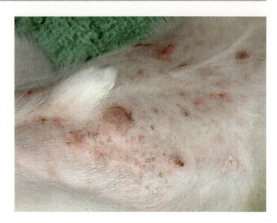

Fig. 10.2 Multifocal skin lesions over the abdomen of a dog with cutaneous lymphoma (Image provided by Michael Kent, DVM)

multiple myeloma in animals can have cutaneous involvement, cutaneous plasma cell tumors are usually de novo proliferations that are not associated with primary bone marrow disease. Most cutaneous plasmacytomas in dogs are benign and cured by surgical excision. Cutaneous mast cell tumors are among the most common cutaneous neoplasms seen in dogs and cats and can be focal or multicentric. There are species variations in the biologic behaviors of mast cell tumors, but tumors of mast cells are very rare in humans. Cutaneous histiocytomas are unique to dogs and are benign spontaneously regressing tumors. Its malignant counterpart, the histiocytic sarcoma, is seen in dogs but rarely described in humans.

Comparative Clinical and Pathologic Aspects of Specific Animal Skin Cancers

Melanoma

Melanoma is a common and malignant disease seen in human and veterinary medicine. Histopathology is the most common means of diagnosis although the disease has a highly variable appearance histologically that can complicate diagnosis. Aspects of the histologic appearance of a lesion are often used to predict the biologic behavior of the tumor. Melanocytic tumors in humans and animals have important clinical and pathologic similarities and differences.

Clinical Aspects of Melanoma

Clinically, melanoma is reported to account for 3 % of all neoplasms and 7 % of all malignant tumors in dogs [14]. The common sites for melanoma in dogs are quite different from humans where the vast majority are cutaneous. The most frequently affected sites in dogs are the oral cavity (56 %), lip (23 %), skin (11 %), and digit (8 %) [12, 15]. Oral melanoma is the most common oral tumor in dogs and the vast majority are malignant (Fig. 10.3). Dogs with oral melanoma may present when a mass is observed but more commonly present for signs of dysphagia, halitosis, ptyalism, or bleeding [15, 16]. The most common metastatic sites for oral melanoma to spread to are the regional lymph nodes, lung, and viscera although melanoma metastases have been documented at nearly any site [17–20]. In dogs and humans, there is an increased frequency of oral melanoma in males compared to females [17, 21–24].

Only approximately 5 % of cutaneous melanomas in dogs are malignant in notable contrast to humans [11, 12, 15]. Certain breeds of dog have an increased incidence of melanoma, usually dogs

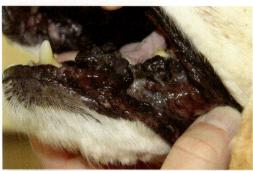

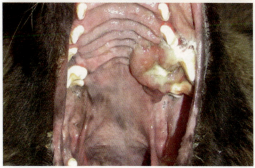

Fig. 10.3 Pigmented oral melanoma (*top*) and amelanotic oral melanoma in dogs (Image provided by Michael Kent, DVM)

with darkly pigmented skin. Predisposed breeds include the Miniature Schnauzer, Scottish Terrier, and Standard Schnauzer [25, 26]. This is an interesting contrast to humans where cutaneous melanoma appears to be less common in individuals from races with darkly pigmented skin [27–29].

Cutaneous melanoma is common in horses. Over 90 % are benign at initial presentation, but the majority of these are believed to have the potential to undergo malignant transformation over time [15, 30–37]. Gray and white horses are markedly predisposed and develop melanoma with increasing prevalence as they age, often developing multifocal cutaneous sites of involvement [32, 38].

Melanoma is uncommon in cats, but they do develop oral, cutaneous, and ocular forms [39–44]. Over 50 % of melanomas in cats are malignant. Melanoma is also seen in many other domestic species of animal including cattle, sheep, goats, alpaca, and swine [45–48]. The Sinclair miniature breed of pig has a genetic predisposition to develop melanoma and has been used as a model for human spontaneous cutaneous melanoma [49–51].

In animals, the location of a melanoma lesion is an important prognostic indicator. Melanoma involving the oral cavity, mucocutaneous junctions, and the subungual region is considered malignant regardless of histologic features. In humans, melanomas involving the oral cavity or mucocutaneous junctions are also malignant.

Gross Pathology and Histopathology of Melanoma

Regardless of species, melanoma varies widely in gross appearance. Masses may be any color including gray, brown, black, or red [13, 15, 52]. Cutaneous melanoma can appear as a smooth dome, a nodule, a plaque, or a lobulated mass [53]. Cutaneous melanomas in horses are usually flat and firm although multiple lesions may coalesce creating a cobblestone appearance [32]. The skin over a lesion may be alopecic or ulcerated. Masses can be compressive but more commonly are infiltrative and unencapsulated. They may be poorly defined without forming a discrete mass and they may efface normal structures.

Histologically, cutaneous melanomas in animals are not differentiated the same way as human melanoma. The term "nevus" which is used to describe pigmented melanocytic lesions of the epidermis and dermis in humans is not used in veterinary pathology [15, 26]. Consequently, veterinary pathologists do not typically differentiate dysplastic nevi, from melanoma in situ, from early invasive melanoma. Most of the melanomas in animals are invasive masses in contrast to the thin, superficial, spreading type of melanoma that is seen most commonly in humans [15]. Human and canine melanoma can both be described by whether the neoplastic cells are spindle cells, epithelioid cells, round cells, or a mixture of these morphologies. Oral melanoma in dogs and humans is malignant and has a poor prognosis regardless of histologic type and morphology.

Poorly differentiated and amelanotic melanomas present a diagnostic challenge for the pathologist. A number of immunohistochemical methods have been developed to improve the diagnosis of melanoma although currently available markers are either not specific for melanoma or are only variably expressed by melanoma. Therefore, the diagnosis often depends on the expertise of the pathologist in combination with immunohistochemical findings. Nearly all melanomas are vimentin positive and cytokeratin negative in humans, dogs, and cats, but this is not specific for melanoma as many sarcomas have a similar pattern [44, 54–56]. S100 is a calcium-binding protein found in the cytoplasm and nucleus. Most melanomas are S100 positive, but this is also not specific for melanoma [44, 56, 57]. Similarly, neuron-specific enolase is used to help identify melanocytic tumors but is not specific [16, 58]. Melan-A is the most specific IHC marker for melanoma and is usually strongly positive in melanocyte cytoplasm [16]. One study of 122 canine oral melanomas showed that 92 % were Melan-A positive including a number of amelanotic tumors [16].

Squamous Cell Carcinoma

Clinical Aspects of Squamous Cell Carcinmoma

Squamous cell carcinoma is the most common malignant tumor of the skin in cats and second most common in dogs following mast cell tumors [59]. Due to its association with sun damage, incidence correlates to geography and climate.

Squamous cell carcinomas may present either as plaques, erosive lesions, or nodular masses of varying size [59]. Initial plaques will often progress to large erosive or nodular lesions (Fig. 10.4). Multiple lesions are common. The planum nasale is a common tumor site for cats with squamous cell carcinoma but is much less common in dogs. White-faced cats and short-coated dogs with light coat color have the highest incidence of squamous cell carcinoma [60, 61].

Gross Pathology and Histopathology of Squamous Cell Carcinoma

Most squamous cell carcinomas in dogs and cats are well differentiated, arising from superficial

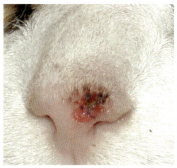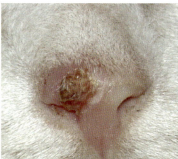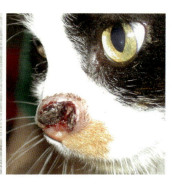

Fig. 10.4 From *left to right*, the planum nasale of three cats with progressively more invasive squamous cell carcinoma (Image provided by Michael Kent, DVM)

hair follicles without involvement of the epidermis [13]. The adjacent epidermis often has some degree of keratinocyte hyperplasia or dysplasia associated with solar damage. Poorly differentiated squamous cell carcinoma lesions tend to have high mitotic activity. For anaplastic lesions, immunohistochemistry to detect high molecular weight cytokeratins may be helpful in differentiating this tumor [59].

Lesions of multicentric squamous cell carcinoma in situ have irregular epidermal hyperplasia with marked hyperkeratosis and parakeratosis. They frequently have hyperpigmentation of the stratum corneum. There is often marked disruption of normal epithelial stratification. The differentiation between multicentric squamous cell carcinoma in situ and actinic keratosis is usually made clinically based on the location of lesions.

Basal Cell Carcinoma

Clinical Aspects of Basal Cell Carcinoma

Basal cell carcinomas are common in cats and uncommon in dogs. Basal cell carcinomas in cats sometimes coexist with actinic keratosis and/or squamous cell carcinoma but most occur in regions of the skin that are not exposed to ultraviolet radiation. It is common for the overlying epidermis to be alopecic, ulcerated, or blue/black in color due to pigment within the tumor [13]. The metastatic rate of basal cell carcinomas in dogs and cats is very low.

Gross Pathology and Histopathology of Basal Cell Carcinoma

Basal cell carcinomas can be divided into three histologic types: solid basal cell carcinoma, keratinizing basal cell carcinoma (also called basosquamous carcinoma or basal cell carcinoma with follicular differentiation), and clear cell basal cell carcinoma [59].

Solid basal cell carcinomas are circumscribed, irregular masses of epithelial aggregates. Necrosis is often present in the centers of epithelial islands. The epithelial cells of basal cell carcinomas may produce mucin. Melanization of the epithelial cells is common in solid basal cell carcinomas [59].

Keratinizing basal cell carcinoma is an irregular dermal mass that is commonly ulcerated. These tumors usually do not have melanization or ulceration as described for solid basal cell carcinomas. The centers of the epithelial islands in these tumors exhibit squamous differentiation and keratinization [59].

Clear cell basal cell carcinoma is a rare variant of basal cell carcinoma seen occasionally in cats. These tumors have similar architecture to solid basal cell carcinomas, but the epithelial cells are large and polygonal with clear or finely granular cytoplasm. This appearance occurs due to the presence of numerous phagolysosomes within the cells [59].

Actinic Skin Cancers in Animals and Humans

A causal relationship between exposure to ultraviolet radiation and the development of cutaneous squamous cell carcinoma, basal cell carcinoma, and malignant melanoma is well established in humans [62]. The skin of companion animals is partially protected by their coat, but chronic solar damage can still occur in regions with little or no pigment (Fig. 10.5). Susceptible regions include the skin of the planum nasale, the abdomen, and areas of the ears, face, and limbs.

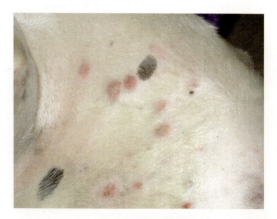

Fig. 10.5 Multifocal cutaneous squamous cell carcinoma lesions along the light skinned, thin coated trunk of a dog (Image provided by Michael Kent, DVM)

An association between sun exposure and oculofacial squamous cell carcinoma in white-faced cattle, horses, and cats has been observed [59]. There is also evidence for a similar association of sun exposure and squamous cell carcinoma in certain breeds of dogs. Dogs also have an association with solar exposure and cutaneous hemangiosarcoma. The increased frequency of this particular actinic tumor may be due to the thin epidermis of dogs allowing more dermal damage from ultraviolet radiation. In contrast to humans, basal cell carcinomas do not appear to have an increased incidence in dogs or cats in sun-exposed locations. There is also no evidence for an association between solar dermatosis and cutaneous melanoma in dogs and cats [59].

Comparative Molecular Pathology of Skin Cancer

In the modern era of oncology, it has become increasingly important to understand the molecular biology underlying the pathogenesis of each tumor. As it relates to comparative oncology, this suggests that it is not sufficient to assume that just because tumors in animals and humans have similar histopathologic features, they necessarily share the same molecular drivers of oncogenesis. However, many of the genes and pathways that are aberrantly expressed or regulated in human cancers have also been found in animals. The list of known mutations and gene expression changes seen in companion animal cancers continues to grow. The following section describes some of the biologic factors that have been shown to be associated with skin tumors in dogs and cats and the possible comparative relevance.

Mutations and altered expression of the p53 tumor suppressor gene are among the most common changes seen in cancer in animals and humans. Specific skin cancers that have been reported to altered p53 expression in dogs include papilloma, squamous cell carcinoma, and melanoma [63–68]. In canine melanoma, alterations in p53 appear to occur later in the progression of melanoma and can include gene deletion, gene silencing, disruption of p53 DNA-binding domains, or altered stability or subcellular localization of the protein. Altered p53 expression has also been shown in cats and horses with squamous cell carcinoma and horses with melanoma [67, 69].

Vascular endothelial growth factor (VEGF) is an important growth factor and regulator of angiogenesis that plays a role in a wide variety of human tumors. VEGF is expressed in canine squamous cell carcinoma but not in basal cell tumors [70]. An autocrine pathway for VEGF signaling in canine squamous cell carcinoma has been proposed [71]. In canine melanoma, one study showed that 95 % of melanoma tissues expressed VEGF and that serum and plasma levels of VEGF were higher in dogs with melanoma than a control population. Furthermore, high circulating VEGF levels correlated to shorter survival time in definitively treated dogs [72].

Bcl-2 is a key regulator of programmed cell death that has an anti-apoptotic function. Bax is a proapoptotic protein of the same family. This gene family has been shown to play a role in the growth of the circumscribed, superficial cutaneous basal cell tumors in cats, in part, due to high expression of bcl-2 and low expression of bax in basal cell tumors [73]. These tumors are slowly proliferating based on low Ki-67 labeling index but are insensitive to apoptotic stimuli due to their levels of bax and bcl-2; less than 1 % of tumor cells are found to be undergoing apoptosis by TUNEL assay [73].

β-catenin is an intercellular junction protein involved in the Wnt signaling pathway present in the epidermis of normal skin with a cytoplasmic and membrane distribution. Deregulation of the Wnt/β-catenin signaling pathway is associated with abnormal cellular proliferation and differentiation. Membrane β-catenin expression has been shown to be reduced or absent in many cases of canine squamous cell carcinoma [74]. A similar distribution is seen in human squamous cell carcinoma. A similar loss of membrane β-catenin expression has been demonstrated in canine melanoma [75].

Cyclooxygenase (Cox) is an enzyme involved in arachidonic acid metabolism leading to the formation of prostaglandins. One isoform (Cox-1) is constitutively expressed in most tissues and appears to play a homeostatic role. A second isoform (Cox-2) is an induced enzyme expressed in inflammatory and other pathologic conditions including many cancers. Overexpression of Cox-2 leads to production of high levels of prostaglandins, specifically prostaglandin E_2 (PGE$_2$). PGE$_2$ increases angiogenesis, tumor cell proliferation, and resistance to apoptosis. Moderate to high expression of Cox-2 has been demonstrated in canine, feline, and equine squamous cell carcinoma and canine melanoma [76–79]. Cox-2 expression has also been shown to be induced in basal and suprabasal keratinocytes of dogs and cats with actinic keratosis [80].

Survivin is a protein belonging to the inhibitor of apoptosis (IAP) family and also plays a role in cell-division pathways. In normal human and canine epidermis, survivin expression is low or absent and confined to basal keratinocytes. In canine and human squamous cell carcinoma, nuclear survivin expression is present and a subset of cases show cytoplasmic survivin expression as well. Survivin is also expressed in advanced melanomas in humans and is a potential therapeutic target. A study in dogs evaluating siRNA knockdown of canine melanoma cells inhibited cell growth and increased apoptotic cell death [81].

A mutation in the Birt-Hogg-Dubé (BHD) tumor suppressor gene is associated with hereditary multifocal renal cystadenocarcinoma and nodular dermatofibrosis in German Shepherd dogs [82]. This condition is characterized by multifocal cutaneous nodules consisting of dense collagen fibers with concurrent uterine leiomyomas and multifocal tumors in the kidneys. Birt-Hogg-Dubé syndrome in humans is a rare disorder that is frequently associated with mutation to the same gene and is characterized by multiple benign skin tumors and lung tumors. Transforming growth factor-beta-1 has also been shown to be overexpressed in the cutaneous lesions of dogs with nodular dermatofibrosis [83].

Activation of telomerase is a mechanism that allows many types of neoplastic cells to avoid senescence. Telomerase levels are undetectable or low in canine somatic tissues but are elevated in 95 % of canine tumors including cutaneous tumors [84, 85].

SART-1 is a squamous cell carcinoma antigen that is recognized by cytotoxic T lymphocytes and is a potential target for immunotherapy. mRNA of the canine orthologue of SART-1 has been identified in canine squamous cell carcinoma and has a very similar sequence to human SART-1. It is not currently known whether canine SART-1 induces a T-cell response [86].

Metallothionein is an important transcription factor regulator that has increased expression in human melanoma. Metallothionein [87–89] expression has also been demonstrated in a subset of canine and feline cutaneous melanomas [90]. Cyclin-dependent kinase inhibitor 2A (also known as ink-4a) is a tumor suppressor protein. Mutations of the gene encoding ink-4a (P16^{Ink4A}) are among the most frequent genetic abnormalities seen in human tumors, including over 50 % of malignant melanomas [91]. Loss or dramatic reduction of this protein has been demonstrated in canine melanoma [65]. The WAF1 p21 tumor suppressor gene is important for melanocyte growth and differentiation and has been seen to be mutated or poorly expressed in human melanoma. Similarly, loss, dramatically reduced expression, and altered subcellular localization of this protein have been shown in canine melanoma [65]. PTEN is a tumor suppressor gene that is mutated or silenced in many human cancers including malignant melanoma. Loss or dramatic reduction of PTEN has been demonstrated in canine melanoma [65]. N-ras is a protooncogene that when mutated is a potent inducer of tumorigenesis due to activation of growth-related signal transduction pathways. N-ras mutations have been detected in many human tumors including melanoma. N-ras mutations have also been found in canine malignant melanoma [92].

The Future of the Comparative Oncology of Skin Cancer

Comparative oncology continues to be a growing field of study [3, 93]. As more is learned about the clinical, pathologic, and molecular aspects of skin cancer in animals and people, there are more opportunities for us to gain valuable insight through a comparative approach. Further work in this field will hopefully lead to continued improvements to the care and treatment of humans and animals with skin cancer.

Glossary

Basal cell tumors (adenoma and carcinoma) Tumors originating from skin basal cells, characterized by local invasiveness and almost lack of metastatic potential

Companion animals house pets (dogs and cats)

Cox-2 cyclooxygenase type 2 Is a enzyme that is frequently overexpressed in pet tumors; it increases angiogenesis, tumor cell proliferation and resistance to apoptosis. It is frequently targeted in veterinary oncology using cox-inhibitors

Melanoma A melanocitic tumor localized in the skin or muco-cutaneous regions. The cutaneous localization is associated with aggressive behavior in 10% of the horses while it is benign in pets. The mucocutaneous location is associated with local invasiveness and distant metastases in pets

p53 A tumor suppressor genes frequently mutated in tumors of companion animals

Sarcoid An equine neoplasm caused by non productive papillomavirus infection

Squamous cell carcinoma a rapidly growing, usually sun-induced tumor of skin and nasal planum, more common among pets with depigmented areas of the body

VEGF Vascular endothelial growth factor is a growth factor and promoter of angiogenesis that is frequently overexpressed in canine cancer (squamous cell carcinoma and melanoma) and is sometimes associated with patient outcome

References

1. Vail DM, MacEwen EG. Spontaneously occurring tumors of companion animals as models for human cancer. Cancer Invest. 2000;18:781–92.
2. Office of Statistics and Programming NCfIPaC, Centers for Disease Control and Prevention. Leading Causes of Death by Age Group, United States – 2007.
3. Withrow SJ, Vail DM, Page R. Withrow and MacEwen's Small Animal Clinical Oncology, 5th ed. St. Louis: Saunders, 2012.
4. Teclaw R, Mendlein J, Garbe P, et al. Characteristics of pet populations and households in the Purdue Comparative Oncology Program catchment area, 1988. J Am Vet Med Assoc. 1992;201:1725–9.
5. Dorn CR. Epidemiology of canine and feline tumors. Compend Contin Educ Pract Vet. 1976;12:307–12.
6. Priester WA, McKay FW. The occurrence of tumors in domestic animals. Natl Cancer Inst Monogr. 1980;(54):1–210.
7. Paoloni M, Khanna C. Translation of new cancer treatments from pet dogs to humans. Nat Rev Cancer. 2008;8:147–56.
8. Goldschmidt MH. Basal- and squamous-cell neoplasms of dogs and cats. Am J Dermatopathol. 1984;6:199–206.
9. Diters RW, Walsh KM. Feline basal cell tumors: a review of 124 cases. Vet Pathol. 1984;21:51–6.
10. Bell JA, Sundberg JP, Ghim SJ, et al. A formalin-inactivated vaccine protects against mucosal papillomavirus infection: a canine model. Pathobiology. 1994;62:194–8.
11. Meuten MJ. Tumors in domestic animals. 4th ed. Ames: Iowa State Press; 2002. p. 45–118.
12. Goldschmidt MH, Shofer FS. Skin tumors of the dog and cat. Oxford: Butterworth Heinemann; 1998.
13. Gross TL, Ihrke PE, Walder EJ. Veterinary dermatopathology: a macroscopic and microscopic evaluation of canine and feline skin disease. St. Louis: Mosby; 1992. p. 336–40.
14. Cotchin E. Melanotic tumours of dogs. J Comp Pathol. 1955;65:115–29.
15. Smith SH, Goldschmidt MH, McManus PM. A comparative review of melanocytic neoplasms. Vet Pathol. 2002;39:651–78.
16. Ramos-Vara JA, Beissenherz ME, Miller MA, et al. Retrospective study of 338 canine oral melanomas with clinical, histologic, and immunohistochemical review of 129 cases. Vet Pathol. 2000;37:597–608.
17. Todoroff RJ, Brodey RS. Oral and pharyngeal neoplasia in the dog: a retrospective survey of 361 cases. J Am Vet Med Assoc. 1979;175:567–71.
18. Theon AP, Rodriguez C, Madewell BR. Analysis of prognostic factors and patterns of failure in dogs with malignant oral tumors treated with megavoltage irradiation. J Am Vet Med Assoc. 1997;210:778–84.
19. Williams LE, Packer RA. Association between lymph node size and metastasis in dogs with oral malignant melanoma: 100 cases (1987–2001). J Am Vet Med Assoc. 2003;222:1234–6.
20. Proulx DR, Ruslander DM, Dodge RK, et al. A retrospective analysis of 140 dogs with oral melanoma treated with external beam radiation. Vet Radiol Ultrasound. 2003;44:352–9.
21. Jemal A, Devesa SS, Hartge P, et al. Recent trends in cutaneous melanoma incidence among whites in the United States. J Natl Cancer Inst. 2001;93:678–83.
22. Aronsohn MG, Carpenter JL. Distal extremity melanocytic nevi and malignant melanomas in dogs. J Am Anim Hosp Assoc. 1990;26:605–12.
23. Barker BF, Carpenter WM, Daniels TE, et al. Oral mucosal melanomas: the WESTOP Banff workshop proceedings. Western Society of Teachers of Oral Pathology. Oral Surg Oral Med Oral Pathol Oral Radiol Endod. 1997;83:672–9.

24. Rogers 3rd RS, Gibson LE. Mucosal, genital, and unusual clinical variants of melanoma. Mayo Clin Proc. 1997;72:362–6.

25. Conroy JD. Melanocytic tumors of domestic animals with special reference to dogs. Arch Dermatol. 1967;96:372–80.

26. Goldschmidt MH. Benign and malignant melanocytic neoplasms of domestic animals. Am J Dermatopathol. 1985;7(Suppl):203–12.

27. McGovern VJ. Epidemiological aspects of melanoma: a review. Pathology. 1977;9:233–41.

28. Goubran GF, Adekeye EO, Edwards MB. Melanoma of the face and mouth in Nigeria. A review and comment on three cases. Int J Oral Surg. 1978;7: 453–62.

29. Sigg C, Pelloni F. Frequency of acquired melanonevocytic nevi and their relationship to skin complexion in 939 schoolchildren. Dermatologica. 1989;179: 123–8.

30. Kunze DJ, Monticello TM, Jakob TP, et al. Malignant melanoma of the coronary band in a horse. J Am Vet Med Assoc. 1986;188:297–8.

31. Gorham S, Robl M. Melanoma in the gray horse: the darker side of equine aging. Vet Med. 1986;81: 446–8.

32. Johnson PJ. Dermatologic tumors (excluding sarcoids). Vet Clin North Am Equine Pract. 1998;14:625–58, viii.

33. Kirker-Head CA, Loeffler D, Held JP. Pelvic limb lameness due to malignant melanoma in a horse. J Am Vet Med Assoc. 1985;186:1215–7.

34. Rodriguez F, Forga J, Herraez P, et al. Metastatic melanoma causing spinal cord compression in a horse. Vet Rec. 1998;142:248–9.

35. Schott HC, Major MD, Grant BD, et al. Melanoma as a cause of spinal cord compression in two horses. J Am Vet Med Assoc. 1990;196:1820–2.

36. Sundberg JP, Burnstein T, Page EH, et al. Neoplasms of Equidae. J Am Vet Med Assoc. 1977;170:150–2.

37. Valentine BA. Equine melanocytic tumors: a retrospective study of 53 horses (1988 to 1991). J Vet Intern Med. 1995;9:291–7.

38. Levene A. Equine melanotic disease. Tumori. 1971; 57:133–68.

39. Munday JS, French AF, Martin SJ. Cutaneous malignant melanoma in an 11-month-old Russian blue cat. N Z Vet J. 2011;59:143–6.

40. Schobert CS, Labelle P, Dubielzig RR. Feline conjunctival melanoma: histopathological characteristics and clinical outcomes. Vet Ophthalmol. 2010;13:43–6.

41. Ramos-Vara JA, Miller MA, Johnson GC, et al. Melan A and S100 protein immunohistochemistry in feline melanomas: 48 cases. Vet Pathol. 2002;39:127–32.

42. Patnaik AK, Mooney S. Feline melanoma: a comparative study of ocular, oral, and dermal neoplasms. Vet Pathol. 1988;25:105–12.

43. Roels S, Tilmant K, Ducatelle R. p53 expression and apoptosis in melanomas of dogs and cats. Res Vet Sci. 2001;70:19–25.

44. van der Linde-Sipman JS, de Wit MM, van Garderen E, et al. Cutaneous malignant melanomas in 57 cats: identification of (amelanotic) signet-ring and balloon cell types and verification of their origin by immunohistochemistry, electron microscopy, and in situ hybridization. Vet Pathol. 1997;34:31–8.

45. Hamor RE, Severin GA, Roberts SM. Intraocular melanoma in an alpaca. Vet Ophthalmol. 1999;2: 193–6.

46. Oxenhandler RW, Adelstein EH, Haigh JP, et al. Malignant melanoma in the Sinclair miniature swine: an autopsy study of 60 cases. Am J Pathol. 1979; 96:707–20.

47. Richerson JT, Burns RP, Misfeldt ML. Association of uveal melanocyte destruction in melanoma-bearing swine with large granular lymphocyte cells. Invest Ophthalmol Vis Sci. 1989;30:2455–60.

48. Parsons PG, Takahashi H, Candy J, et al. Histopathology of melanocytic lesions in goats and establishment of a melanoma cell line: a potential model for human melanoma. Pigment Cell Res. 1990;3:297–305.

49. Millikan LE, Boylon JL, Hook RR, et al. Melanoma in Sinclair swine: a new animal model. J Invest Dermatol. 1974;62:20–30.

50. Hook Jr RR, Aultman MD, Adelstein EH, et al. Influence of selective breeding on the incidence of melanomas in Sinclair miniature swine. Int J Cancer. 1979;24:668–72.

51. Hook Jr RR, Berkelhammer J, Oxenhandler RW. Melanoma: Sinclair swine melanoma. Am J Pathol. 1982;108:130–3.

52. Meleo KA. Tumors of the skin and associated structures. Vet Clin North Am Small Anim Pract. 1997;27:73–94.

53. Mulligan RM. Melanoblastic tumors in the dog. Am J Vet Res. 1961;22:345–51.

54. Perniciaro C. Dermatopathologic variants of malignant melanoma. Mayo Clin Proc. 1997;72:273–9.

55. Rabanal RH, Fondevila DM, Montane V, et al. Immunocytochemical diagnosis of skin tumours of the dog with special reference to undifferentiated types. Res Vet Sci. 1989;47:129–33.

56. Sandusky GE, Carlton WW, Wightman KA. Diagnostic immunohistochemistry of canine round cell tumors. Vet Pathol. 1987;24:495–9.

57. Sandusky Jr GE, Carlton WW, Wightman KA. Immunohistochemical staining for S100 protein in the diagnosis of canine amelanotic melanoma. Vet Pathol. 1985;22:577–81.

58. Koenig A, Wojcieszyn J, Weeks BR, et al. Expression of S100a, vimentin, NSE, and melan A/MART-1 in seven canine melanoma cells lines and twenty-nine retrospective cases of canine melanoma. Vet Pathol. 2001;38:427–35.

59. Walder EJ. Comparative aspects of nonmelanoma skin cancer. Clin Dermatol. 1995;13:569–78.

60. Dorn CR, Taylor DO, Schneider R. Sunlight exposure and risk of developing cutaneous and oral squamous cell carcinomas in white cats. J Natl Cancer Inst. 1971;46:1073–8.

61. White SD. Diseases of the nasal planum. Vet Clin North Am Small Anim Pract. 1994;24:887–95.

62. Gallagher RP, Lee TK, Bajdik CD, et al. Ultraviolet radiation. Chronic Dis Can. 2010;29 Suppl 1:51–68.

63. Albaric O, Bret L, Amardeihl M, et al. Immuno-histochemical expression of p53 in animal tumors: a methodological study using four anti-human p53 antibodies. Histol Histopathol. 2001;16:113–21.

64. Gamblin RM, Sagartz JE, Couto CG. Overexpression of p53 tumor suppressor protein in spontaneously arising neoplasms of dogs. Am J Vet Res. 1997;58:857–63.

65. Koenig A, Bianco SR, Fosmire S, et al. Expression and significance of p53, rb, p21/waf-1, p16/ink-4a, and PTEN tumor suppressors in canine melanoma. Vet Pathol. 2002;39:458–72.

66. Mayr B, Schellander K, Schleger W, et al. Sequence of an exon of the canine p53 gene–mutation in a papilloma. Br Vet J. 1994;150:81–4.

67. Roels S, Tilmant K, Van Daele A, et al. Proliferation, DNA ploidy, p53 overexpression and nuclear DNA fragmentation in six equine melanocytic tumours. J Vet Med A Physiol Pathol Clin Med. 2000; 47:439–48.

68. Teifke JP, Lohr CV, Shirasawa H. Detection of canine oral papillomavirus-DNA in canine oral squamous cell carcinomas and p53 overexpressing skin papillomas of the dog using the polymerase chain reaction and non-radioactive in situ hybridization. Vet Microbiol. 1998;60:119–30.

69. Teifke JP, Lohr CV. Immunohistochemical detection of P53 overexpression in paraffin wax-embedded squamous cell carcinomas of cattle, horses, cats and dogs. J Comp Pathol. 1996;114:205–10.

70. Maiolino P, De Vico G, Restucci B. Expression of vascular endothelial growth factor in basal cell tumours and in squamous cell carcinomas of canine skin. J Comp Pathol. 2000;123:141–5.

71. Al-Dissi AN, Haines DM, Singh B, et al. Immunohistochemical expression of vascular endothelial growth factor and vascular endothelial growth factor receptor associated with tumor cell proliferation in canine cutaneous squamous cell carcinomas and trichoepitheliomas. Vet Pathol. 2007;44:823–30.

72. Taylor KH, Smith AN, Higginbotham M, et al. Expression of vascular endothelial growth factor in canine oral malignant melanoma. Vet Comp Oncol. 2007;5:208–18.

73. Madewell BR, Gandour-Edwards R, Edwards BF, et al. Bax/bcl-2: cellular modulator of apoptosis in feline skin and basal cell tumours. J Comp Pathol. 2001;124:115–21.

74. Bongiovanni L, Malatesta D, Brachelente C, et al. Beta-Catenin in canine skin: immunohistochemical pattern of expression in normal skin and cutaneous epithelial tumours. J Comp Pathol. 2011;145:138–47.

75. Han JI, Kim DY, Na KJ. Dysregulation of the Wnt/beta-catenin signaling pathway in canine cutaneous melanotic tumor. Vet Pathol. 2010;47:285–91.

76. Mohammed SI, Khan KN, Sellers RS, et al. Expression of cyclooxygenase-1 and 2 in naturally-occurring canine cancer. Prostaglandins Leukot Essent Fatty Acids. 2004;70:479–83.

77. Pestili de Almeida EM, Piche C, Sirois J, et al. Expression of cyclo-oxygenase-2 in naturally occurring squamous cell carcinomas in dogs. J Histochem Cytochem. 2001;49:867–75.

78. Pronovost N, Suter MM, Mueller E, et al. Expression and regulation of cyclooxygenase-2 in normal and neoplastic canine keratinocytes. Vet Comp Oncol. 2004;2:222–33.

79. Thamm DH, Ehrhart 3rd EJ, Charles JB, et al. Cyclooxygenase-2 expression in equine tumors. Vet Pathol. 2008;45:825–8.

80. Nardi ABD, Raposo TMM, Huppes RR, et al. Cox-2 inhibitors for cancer treatment in dogs. Pak Vet J. 2011;31:275–9.

81. Moriyama M, Kano R, Maruyama H, et al. Small interfering RNA (siRNA) against the survivin gene increases apoptosis in a canine melanoma cell line. J Vet Med Sci. 2010;72:1643–6.

82. Lingaas F, Comstock KE, Kirkness EF, et al. A mutation in the canine BHD gene is associated with hereditary multifocal renal cystadenocarcinoma and nodular dermatofibrosis in the German Shepherd dog. Hum Mol Genet. 2003;12:3043–53.

83. Vercelli A, Bellone G, Abate O, et al. Expression of transforming growth factor-beta isoforms in the skin, kidney, pancreas and bladder in a German shepherd dog affected by renal cystadenocarcinoma and nodular dermatofibrosis. J Vet Med A Physiol Pathol Clin Med. 2003;50:506–10.

84. Yazawa M, Okuda M, Kanaya N, et al. Molecular cloning of the canine telomerase reverse transcriptase gene and its expression in neoplastic and non-neoplastic cells. Am J Vet Res. 2003;64:1395–400.

85. Yazawa M, Okuda M, Setoguchi A, et al. Measurement of telomerase activity in dog tumors. J Vet Med Sci. 1999;61:1125–9.

86. Takaishi Y, Yoshida Y, Nakagaki K, et al. Expression of SART-1 mRNA in canine squamous cell carcinomas. J Vet Med Sci. 2008;70:1333–5.

87. Weinlich G. Metallothionein-overexpression as a prognostic marker in melanoma. G Ital Dermatol Venereol. 2009;144:27–38.

88. Weinlich G, Bitterlich W, Mayr V, et al. Metallothionein-overexpression as a prognostic factor for progression and survival in melanoma. A prospective study on 520 patients. Br J Dermatol. 2003;149:535–41.

89. Weinlich G, Eisendle K, Hassler E, et al. Metallothionein – overexpression as a highly significant prognostic factor in melanoma: a prospective study on 1270 patients. Br J Cancer. 2006;94:835–41.

90. Dincer Z, Jasani B, Haywood S, et al. Metallothionein expression in canine and feline mammary and melanotic tumours. J Comp Pathol. 2001;125:130–6.

91. Sharpless E, Chin L. The INK4a/ARF locus and melanoma. Oncogene. 2003;22:3092–8.

92. Mayr B, Schaffner G, Reifinger M, et al. N-ras mutations in canine malignant melanomas. Vet J. 2003;165:169–71.

93. MacEwen EG. Highlights and horizons in veterinary oncology. Compend Contin Educ Pract Vet. 1999;21:902–4.

Clinical-Pathological Integration in the Diagnosis of Skin Cancer

Alon Scope and Ashfaq A. Marghoob

Key Points

- Separation of dermatopathology from clinical dermatology creates a gap with potential pitfalls in diagnosis.
- The clinician should communicate to the pathologist pertinent clinical (e.g. size of lesion) and procedural information (e.g. if biopsy is incisional).
- The clinician should always reconcile the histopathological diagnosis with his clinical diagnosis.

Clinical dermatology and dermatopathology are currently separate subspecialties within the realm of dermatological diagnosis. This was not always the case. At the end of the nineteenth century, Paul Gershwisn Unna noted the following: "The dermatologist is fortunate in being able to study the clinical picture with his histologically-trained eye and the microscopic picture with his dermatologically-trained eye" [1, 2]. After all, clinical der-

matology is a form of gross pathological diagnosis that complements the microscopy-based pathological diagnosis. However, in 1974, dermatopathology was established as a board-certified specialty that can be practiced by certified dermatologists and pathologists. The separation of dermatopathology from clinical dermatology had the advantage of offering more profound specialization in microscopic skin pathology. However, the separation of gross from microscopic diagnosis of skin pathology creates a gap with potential pitfalls in diagnosis; to this end, good communication between clinician and pathologists can narrow this gap and allow for diagnostic integration.

The following are steps taken in the diagnosis of skin cancer, from the bedside to the pathology laboratory and back: (1) *Clinical examination* – the clinician identifies a suspicious lesion based on data from history, clinical, and dermoscopic examination and decides to perform a biopsy. With these data in mind, the clinician fills a biopsy requisition slip. (2) *Biopsy* – the clinician selects the appropriate biopsy technique and performs the biopsy. (3) *Pathology laboratory processing* – the biopsied specimen undergoes processing at the pathology laboratory resulting in a glass slide-mounted specimen. (4) *Microscopic analysis* – the pathologist analyzes the slide and renders a diagnosis which is communicated to the clinician. (5) *Clinical decision* – the clinician reconciles the final pathological diagnosis with the pre-biopsy clinical diagnosis, makes a decision about the need for further treatment, and communicates the results to the patient.

A. Scope, MD (✉)
Department of Dermatology,
Sheba Medical Center,
4 Hacarmel Street, Apt 35,
Ramat Gan, Ganey Tikva 55900, Israel
e-mail: scopea1@gmail.com

A.A. Marghoob
Hauppauge Dermatology Section,
Memorial Sloan-Kettering Skin Cancer
Center Hauppauge,
Long Island, NY, USA

A. Baldi et al. (eds.), *Skin Cancer*, Current Clinical Pathology,
DOI 10.1007/978-1-4614-7357-2_11, © Springer Science+Business Media New York 2014

For each step, let us examine possible pitfalls in diagnosis that can be potentially evaded by improving clinical-pathological communication.

Clinical Examination

We will not belabor on how to identify lesions suspicious for skin cancer, as the topic will be discussed widely in this book. During clinical examination, the physician obtains data that could be pertinent to the pathologist for achieving an accurate final histopathological diagnosis. For example, the clinician that has thoroughly examined the patient knows whether the biopsied lesion is solitary or a mere sample of widespread rash, what is the history of the patient and lesion (e.g., patient with history of melanoma, lesion is a rapidly changing nodule), and what is the size and clinical appearance of the lesion. In addition, clinical and dermoscopic examination offer a unique en face overview of the entire lesion, revealing the distribution of structures and colors within the lesion, an overview that will not be available to the pathologist at the microscope which receives very limited vertical samples of the lesion [3]. Thus, all pertinent data available to the clinician should be communicated to the pathologist via the biopsy requisition slip (Table 11.1). As we will discuss, the availability of these data can influence the final diagnosis rendered by the pathologist.

Biopsy

The clinician selects the biopsy technique [4]. According to the American Academy of Dermatology guidelines for the diagnosis of melanoma, "Whenever possible, excise the lesion for diagnostic purposes using narrow margins" [5]. Excision is defined as complete removal of a skin lesion for the purpose of performing histopathological examination; the most common technique used is elliptical excision. Excision offers advantages for pathological diagnosis. The whole lesion is submitted to the pathology laboratory for analysis so the chance of sampling error is reduced; melanoma staging is more accurate since the

Table 11.1 Pertinent information for the biopsy requisition slip

Category	Details
Identifying information/ demographics	Date of procedure
	Name of patient
	Unique patient identifying number (e.g., national ID number, medical record number)
Lesion details	Anatomic location of lesion
	Size of lesion
	Dermatological description of lesion type (e.g., macule, papule, plaque)
	Whether lesion is solitary or representative sample of multiple lesions
Biopsy technique	Excisional or incisional biopsy
	If excisional – technique used if other than elliptical excision (e.g., saucerization with intent for complete removal of lesion)
	If incisional – technique used (e.g., shave biopsy, punch biopsy), extent of the biopsy relative to the size of lesion (e.g., small 3 mm shave sample from a large 3 cm plaque)
Diagnosis	Most probable clinical diagnosis
	Differential diagnoses, if applicable
Requests for nonroutine processing	Request for special stains
Addition helpful details	Patient history (e.g., history of melanoma)
	Lesion history (e.g., rapid change, presence of ulceration, recurrence at previous biopsy site)
	Annotation of suspicious foci within lesion (using drawing or photograph of lesion)

lesion is not truncated at the base; primary removal of the lesion is achieved, so recurrence of skin cancer is less likely even in the case of melanoma erroneously diagnosed as a nevus; finally, correct orientation of the lesion for processing at the pathology laboratory is straightforward.

When performing an incisional biopsy such as shave or punch biopsy, a sample from a skin lesion is obtained for histopathologic examination, without an explicit intent of completely removing the lesion. With regard to indication for incisional biopsy, the

American Academy of Dermatology notes: "An incisional biopsy technique is appropriate when the suspicion for melanoma is low, when the lesion is large, or when it is impractical to perform an excision" [5]. The aim in these cases is to establish the diagnosis and plan, if necessary, more definitive therapy. The appeal of incisional biopsy for clinicians is that it is technically simpler and faster than excision, usually leaves smaller scars, and, in the case of shave biopsy, does not require a sterile technique and does not require stitch removal.

However, incisional biopsy can limit the extent of pathological diagnosis. First, with a shave technique, the lesion can be transected at the base, making it difficult for a pathologist to differentiate a solar keratosis from a superficial squamous cell carcinoma or causing an underestimation of the Breslow thickness in melanoma. In fact, Ng et al. reported that shave and punch biopsies underestimate the final Breslow depth of melanoma by approximately 8 and 20 %, respectively [6]. Second, a diagnostic error is more likely to occur with incisional biopsy due to the limited sampling of the lesion [7, 8]. Finally, in case of diagnostic error associated with an incisional biopsy of skin cancer, there is a greater chance of adverse event due to progression of the residual cancer [7].

Pathology Laboratory Processing

Briefly, the formalin-fixated biopsy specimen is processed at the pathology laboratory as follows: the biopsied specimen is often further sectioned into smaller pieces (e.g., "bread-loafing" of excisional specimen); each piece is put into a cassette and embedded in paraffin, resulting in paraffin blocks; each paraffin block is trimmed until the edge is straight, and then thinly sectioned samples of tissue are mounted on a glass slide; the slide specimens are stained with hematoxylin and eosin. It has been estimated that the glass-mounted specimens available for the pathologist's analysis represent a mere 2 % of the lesion [3].

As previously noted, the separation between clinical examination of the lesion and the processing at pathology laboratory can entail some limitations. First, the sampling technique at the laboratory grossing bench is often not related to clinical or dermoscopic features of the lesion. Second, tissue is discarded during processing at the pathology laboratory. The concern is that the laboratory sampling of the tissue will be somewhat random and fail to provide the pathologist with the areas that were most concerning to the clinician. To this end, different techniques have been suggested to alert the grossing pathologist to clinically suspicious foci, including annotations of the specimen with dye, stitch, or superficial scoring, adding an annotated photograph of the lesion with the requisition slip and using ex vivo dermoscopy at the grossing bench [9, 10].

Microscopic Analysis

The pathologist analyzes the slide specimen and renders a diagnosis which is communicated to the clinician. It is imperative for clinicians to understand that pathology is another form of morphological diagnosis with accuracy less than 100 %. Like any type of diagnosis, it is subjective and error-prone. The more information the pathologist receives about the patient and lesion, the better the sampling of lesion at the bedside and pathology laboratory; the more the pathologist is trained and experienced with dermatopathology, the greater the chance of accurate diagnosis.

There are several pitfalls in pathological diagnosis of skin cancer that can be mended by better clinical-pathological communication [11]. Some examples follow.

First, histopathological diagnosis of melanoma in situ on sun-damaged skin, also termed lentigo maligna, can be challenging. The early signs of melanoma – proliferation of solitary melanocytes along the basal layer of the epidermis, small nest formation, and slight extension down to infundibula, in association with solar elastosis in the dermis – can be quite subtle. In particular, if the pathologist receives a 3 mm section of tissue with such subtle changes and is not made aware that this section is a small incisional sample of a 2-cm pigmented patch on the face of an elderly individual, the pathologist may be inclined to diagnose the lesion as a junctional nevus. Pathologists may assume that the biopsy specimen represents the size of most or the entire clinical lesion; the apparent small size of biopsy specimen may tilt diagnosis toward benign. In addition, the area sampled may not be the "worst" or most diagnostic area on histopathology. For example, Somach el al. showed that 40 % of excisions of lentigo maligna demonstrated more pronounced histopathologic features of melanoma than previous incisions of the same lesions [8]. The knowledge that the lesion is a large pigmented patch on sun-damaged face of an elderly individual, clinically unlikely to be a junctional nevus, will likely raise the pathologist's suspicion that the lesion may represent a melanoma in situ. In case of doubt, the pathologist may request the clinician for further, larger sampling of the lesion.

Second, nodular melanomas may masquerade histopathologically as Spitz nevi or congenital nevi. In particular, the risk of misdiagnosis of nodular melanoma increases if an incisional biopsy is performed. Principle attributes for the histopathologic evaluation of melanocytic neoplasms include the lesion's symmetry, lateral circumscription, and maturation of cells with progressive descent into the dermis [12]; these attributes can only be fully assessed when the lesion is completely excised. Alerting the pathologist that the lesion is a rapidly growing nodule in adult, if such information is available to the clinician, can increase the pathologist's index of suspicion for a nodular melanoma.

Clinical Decision

The clinician should always reconcile the histopathological diagnosis with his clinical diagnosis. If the clinical impression and pathological diagnosis are commensurate, the diagnosis is more likely to be accurate. The clinician should give further consideration to histopathological diagnoses that are discordant with the clinical diagnosis.

Referring back to the example of 2-cm pigmented patch on the face of an elderly adult, the clinical differential diagnosis is likely between melanoma, solar lentigo, lichen planus like keratosis, and pigmented solar keratosis. Nevus is less likely. If the clinician receives a diagnosis of "junctional dysplastic nevus" that does not fit well with the clinical differential diagnosis, this clinical-pathological discordance should be further investigated. The pathologist that issued the diagnosis should be alerted by the clinician of the possible clinical-pathological discordance (Figs. 11.1 and 11.2). The converse is also true, and discordance noted by the pathologist should be communicated to the clinician. Stevens and Cockerell suggest the following: "If a given lesion demonstrates features of melanoma clinically, and the pathologic diagnosis does not confirm the clinical impression, the possibility that the sample may not have been representative should be considered and a second or sometimes even third sample should be taken. Furthermore, the pathologic diagnosis should be assessed critically and, if necessary, additional sections should be cut or a second, more expert opinion should be sought" [13]. Careful follow-up of the patient is also important. During the patient's post-biopsy visit, the clinician should examine the surgical scar for residual or recurrent lesion (Fig. 11.1). Focal recurrence of pigmentation at the edge of the scar could uncover an incompletely removed melanoma that was misdiagnosed as nevus (Fig. 11.2). Finally, if the clinical index of suspicion for malignancy is high, conservative re-excision could be considered, particularly in cases of incisional biopsy or excisional biopsy in which the lesion reaches the surgical margins.

In conclusion, the "gold standard" of diagnosis is integration of clinical and histopathological diagnoses via good communication between clinician and pathologist. The clinician should share with the pathologist pertinent clinical details, whether the biopsy is an incisional or excisional sample, and whether there are focal areas of concern within the lesion. Finally, clinical-pathological diagnostic discordance should be noted by the clinician and communicated to the pathologist and vice versa.

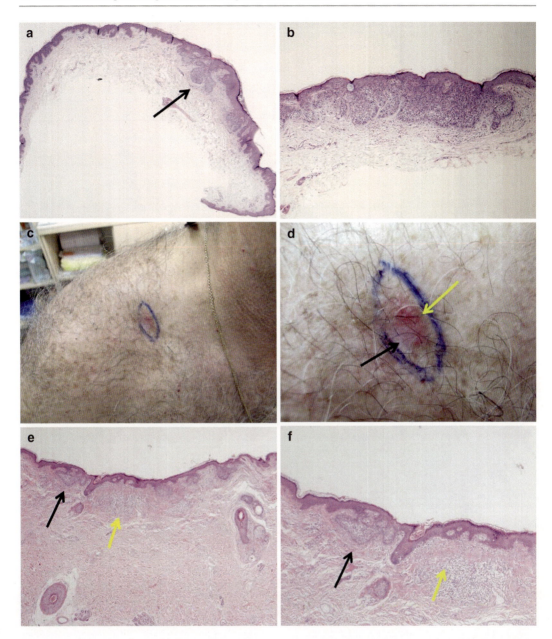

Fig. 11.1 (**a**) Shave biopsy specimen showing a basaloid aggregate at the superficial dermis, emanating from the undersurface of the epidermis (*black arrow*); the edges of the biopsy specimen appear uninvolved by the neoplasm (hematoxylin and eosin, 4×). (**b**) The neoplasms comprise of aggregations of basaloid cells with peripheral palisading of nuclei and clefting from the surrounding dermis which shows fibroplasia. The diagnosis rendered was superficial basal cell carcinoma; margins are free (hematoxylin and eosin, 10×). (**c**) Clinical image at follow-up of the patient shortly after biopsy results were received. The biopsy site at the right shoulder is highlighted with ink. (**d**) Close-up clinical image of the lesion reveals that the shave biopsy scar (*black arrow*) is a small part of a larger lesion, seen as a reddish plaque (*yellow arrow*). Hence, the biopsy was incisional, and based on clinical integration, the margins cannot be free. The lesion was subsequently excised. (**e**, **f**) Histopathology specimen from the excisional biopsy showing residual aggregates of basal cell carcinoma (*black arrow*) adjacent to the scar of the previous biopsy (*yellow arrow*)

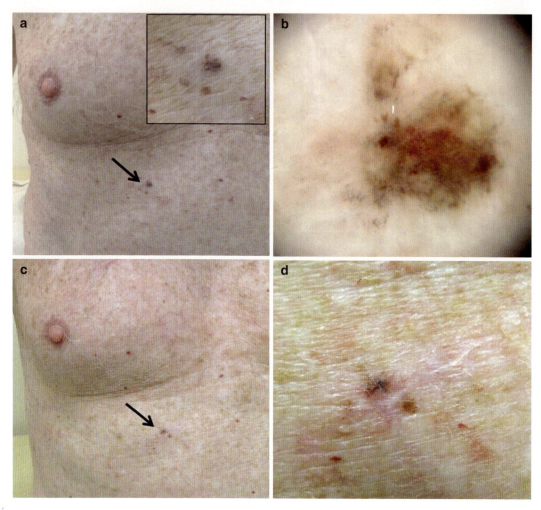

Fig. 11.2 (**a**) A 73-year-old man with previous history of melanoma was found on skin examination to have an irregular 5 mm pigmented macule on the right upper abdomen (*arrow*); inset shows a close-up clinical image. (**b**) Dermoscopically, the lesion was homogenous-globular in pattern, showing irregular distribution of colors, including brown and gray, and of dermoscopic structures, including pigmented blotch, globules, and granularity. Based on clinical and dermoscopic findings, the lesion was suspicious for melanoma. The lesion was excised and the histopathological diagnosis was junctional dysplastic nevus, margins involved. (**c**) At follow-up, 6 months after the biopsy, recurrent pigmentation is seen (*arrow*). (**d**) On clinical close-up, irregular pigmentation is seen at the edge of the scar. The clinical and dermoscopic findings at baseline, taken together with the recurrence of pigmentation at the edge of the scar, make the lesion highly suspicious for melanoma. A pathological revision of the original excision was requested. (**e**) Upon revision, the diagnosis was changed to melanoma in situ. Histopathological examination shows a proliferation of solitary melanocytes along the basal layer of the epidermis, with focal confluence, as well as junctional nests, with underlying dermis showing solar elastosis (hematoxylin and eosin, 10×)

e

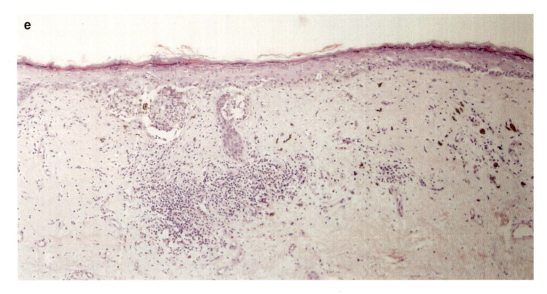

Fig. 11.2 (continued)

Glossary

Elliptical excision Is a technique in which the full thickness of the skin is removed in an elliptical shape

Excisional biopsy Is defined as complete removal of a skin lesion for the purpose of performing histopathological examination

Incisional biopsy Is the one where a sample from a skin lesion is obtained for histopathologic examination, without an explicit intent of completely removing the lesion, like in shave or punch biopsy

Saucerization biopsy Refers to a deep shaving biopsy

References

1. Unna PG. Histopathology of the skin (Ger). In: Orth J, editor. Hand-book of special pathological anatomy. Berlin: A. Hirschwald; 1894. p. 729–30.
2. Hollander AW. Development of dermatopathology and Paul Gerson Unna. J Am Acad Dermatol. 1986;15(4):727–34.
3. Dyson SW, Bass J, Pomeranz J, Jaworsky C, Sigel J, Somach S. Impact of thorough block sampling in the histologic evaluation of melanomas. Arch Dermatol. 2005;141(6):734–6.
4. Marghoob AA, Terushkin V, Dusza SW, Busam K, Scope A. Dermatologists, general practitioners, and the best method to biopsy suspect melanocytic neoplasms. Arch Dermatol. 2010;146(3):325–8.
5. Sober AJ, Chuang TY, Duvic M, Guidelines/Outcomes Committee, et al. Guidelines of care for primary cutaneous melanoma. J Am Acad Dermatol. 2001;45(4):579–86.
6. Ng PC, Barzilai DA, Ismail SA, Averitte Jr RL, Gilliam AC. Evaluating invasive cutaneous melanoma: is the initial biopsy representative of the final depth? J Am Acad Dermatol. 2003;48(3):420–4.
7. Ng JC, Swain S, Dowling JP, Wolfe R, Simpson P, Kelly JW. The impact of partial biopsy on histopathologic diagnosis of cutaneous melanoma: experience of an Australian tertiary referral service. Arch Dermatol. 2010;146(3):234–9.
8. Somach SC, Taira JW, Pitha JV, Everett MA. Pigmented lesions in actinically damaged skin. Histopathologic comparison of biopsy and excisional specimens. Arch Dermatol. 1996;132(11):1297–302.
9. Braun RP, Kaya G, Masouye I, Krischer J, Saurat JH. Histopathologic correlation in dermoscopy: a micropunch technique. Arch Dermatol. 2003;139(3):349–51.
10. Scope A, Busam KJ, Malvehy J, Puig S, McClain SA, Braun RP, et al. Ex vivo dermoscopy of melanocytic tumors: time for dermatopathologists to learn dermoscopy. Arch Dermatol. 2007;143(12):1548–52.
11. Marghoob AA, Changchien L, DeFazio J, Dessio WC, Malvehy J, Zalaudek I, et al. The most common challenges in melanoma diagnosis and how to avoid them. Australas J Dermatol. 2009;50(1):1–13.
12. Macy-Roberts E, Ackerman AB. A critique of techniques for biopsy of clinically suspected malignant melanomas. Am J Dermatopathol. 1982;4(5):391–8.
13. Stevens G, Cockerell CJ. Avoiding sampling error in the biopsy of pigmented lesions. Arch Dermatol. 1996;132(11):1380–2.

Cytology

Angeles Fortuño-Mar

Key Points

- The cytologic smear, is a simple, reliable and inexpensive method for the diagnosis of skin tumours.
- It is a non-scarring pretreatment diagnostic test that leaves no scars. It has no contraindications.
- Scrape cytology is used in superficial lesions; FNA (fine needle aspiration) cytology is used in nodular lesions.
- Useful in the early diagnosis of actinic keratosis, basal and squamous cell carcinomas, malignant melanoma and Merkel's, Paget's, sebaceous, DFSP (dermatofibrosarcoma protuberans) and metastatic disease.

Introduction

The cytologic smear, is a simple, reliable and inexpensive method which has been used for many years in the diagnosis of bullous and vesicular dermatoses. The utility of the examination of exfoliative cells for the diagnosis of cancer was first appreciated by G. Papanicolaou. The cytologic smear can be useful as a diagnostic aid for skin tumours based on the fact that neoplastic cells tend to exfoliate easier because of their diminished cell cohesion. Cytodiagnosis of skin tumours can be performed by different techniques, including fine needle aspiration (FNA) and scrape cytology [1].

A relative latecomer to the field, cytodiagnosis in dermatology has not achieved as much popularity as the cytological assessment of lesions. This may be due to the reluctance of cytologists to attempt skin scrapes – which they are inexperienced at interpreting – or to the preference of the dermatologist for the more traditional small biopsies, which they feel are more reliably diagnosed on histology and for which, with skin, there is such ease of access [2].

A. Fortuño-Mar, MD, PhD, MBA
Eldine Patologia Laboratory,
Valls, Tarragona, Spain
e-mail: af_mar@yahoo.es, afmar@comt.es

Technical Considerations

Two methods are in common use for cytological assessment of a skin lesion: examination of a skin scrape and FNA. For superficial lesions involving the epidermis, a skin scrape is the method of choice. FNA is used for the diagnosis of palpable nodular lesions.

Technical Procedures

Direct Skin Scrape

The skin scrape was first used in the late 1940s in the differential diagnosis of bullous lesions by Tzanck [3]. It consists of a scraping of an ulcer base in search for multinucleated giant cells.

Any surface crust topping the lesion should be lifted with the blade or curette. It is then directed towards the periphery of the lesion for sampling, as the centre is likely to be inflamed and necrotic. Cutting action may be necessary for dislodging tissue from the lesion, but this should be done as gently as possible.

With non-crusted nodular or flat lesions, it is important not to scrape the top, but to cut into it first and then to direct the blade into the cut parallel to the skin surface in order to sample the growing edge of the lesion [2].

Variants of this exfoliative technique include the use of swabs to obtain the material and imprint cytology [4].

FNA

Depending on the clinical situation, the cytopathologist or dermatologist may perform the FNA. The skin should be cleaned with an alcohol swab. A 25- or 23-gauge needle is used on a plastic disposable 10- or 20-ml syringe attached to a holder. The nodule is immobilised between the fingers and the needle tip is rapidly directed through the skin into the nodule. Once the needle enters the mass, the needle is continuously aspirated while the needle is rapidly moved in and out to obtain the sample. Suction is then relieved, and the needle is withdrawn and detached from the syringe. Air is aspirated, and the material is expelled on glass slides.

For superficial lesions, the trained cytopathologist is often the person best suited to perform the procedure. It has been repeatedly demonstrated that the best FNA result is obtained if the person who interprets the smears is the same person who has procured the aspirate material. On the other hand, good results can be obtained if the aspirator and interpreter are proficient but not the same person [5].

Specimen Preparation, Staining and Ancillary Studies

The simultaneous use of both wet-fixed and air-dried smears is recommended. The two methods of preparation complement each other, and their concomitant use facilitates interpretation. Air-dried smears are stained by Diff-Quick or May-Grünwald-Giemsa methods for immediate microscopic diagnosis. Wet-fixation is achieved by immediate immersion of slides in 95 % ethanol or by spray fixation. The former fixed smears are processed with Papanicolaou stain, which is excellent for nuclear detail.

Smeared large tissue fragments stain poorly and add little useful information. They should be picked up gently with a pipette or needle to avoid crush and placed directly in formalin for cell block preparation. To maximise cell recovery, the needle and the syringe may be rinsed into a container with formalin for adequate fixation of cell block material. A cell block enables the pathologist to examine the tissue similarly to a biopsy, and multiple sections can be obtained from paraffin-embedded material for special studies.

Standard histochemical and immunochemical techniques can be performed on cell blocks. A panel of antibodies and other ancillary special studies, including electron microscopy, flow cytometry, image analysis, cytogenetics and molecular diagnostics utilising polymerase chain reaction (PCR) and fluorescence in situ hybridisation (FISH), can all be performed on cytological material. These special tests should be used selectively.

Furthermore, a new method for preparing FNA specimens, known as liquid-based cytology, is used. This method provides a thinner layer of cells.

Indications, Contradictions and Complications

Virtually any palpable mass or any superficial lesion can be sampled by FNA or scrape method, respectively.

There are no absolute contraindications for FNA of superficial sites or scrape test. An uncooperative patient may not be suitable for cytological procedures.

The fine-needle technique and the direct scrape are minimally invasive. Both techniques are safer and less traumatic than a biopsy, and significant complications are usually rare, depending on the body site. Complications resulting from superficial aspiration are usually limited to an occasional small haematoma. Even in patients with haemostatic defects, bleeding can be controlled by applying pressure.

Fatalities from these procedures are almost nonexistent [5].

Advantages and Limitations

Advantages

Cytology has numerous advantages to offer the patient, the administrator and the dermatologist working in an outpatient setting. On the one hand, it gives the clinician the opportunity to have earlier diagnoses, thus decreasing the time between this and the final treatment. Second, it is probably the only conservative, non-scarring pretreatment diagnostic test available for basal cell carcinoma (BCC). This could be extremely beneficial in situations where even a simple 2-mm punch biopsy may be considered inappropriate, such as in a cosmetically sensitive site in a young person or in cases where a BCC might be treated without a previous diagnostic biopsy being taken, e.g. with cryosurgery, topical immunotherapy, photodynamic therapy or intralesional interferon alfa-2b.

Scrape cytology could also be very advantageous to patients. They do not need to return to an outpatient's minor procedure clinic, local anaesthetic is not required, and there is no resultant scarring. Very sick and debilitated patients, those taking anticoagulants, those allergic to local anaesthesia and patients with multiple suspected BCCs in whom multiple biopsies would be a major undertaking would especially benefit from exfoliative cytology.

Finally, this procedure is beneficial to the administrator. It is a cost-effective procedure requiring a minimum of equipment, medical and nursing time. Further, it requires less processing time than biopsy and can be performed at the first patient visit [4].

Limitations

Cytology diagnosis has certain limitations. First, adequate sampling is required. The smaller the lesion, the smaller the cytological specimen;

FNA specimens are harder to obtain when the lesions are too small. Although our department's pool rate of insufficient or indeterminate cytology specimens was low, it included significant malignant diagnoses. The user of this technique must therefore remember that an indeterminate specimen does not necessarily indicate a benign nature of disease. Moreover, cytology cannot differentiate between pleomorphic BCC with squamous differentiation and marked squamous cell atypia. In these cases an incisional biopsy should be recommended for diagnosis [6].

Finally, it has previously been shown in the literature that careful training of samplers and the ability of the practitioner to sample accurately are important factors. Further, either the dermatologist has to be specifically trained in reading cytological specimens or the pathologist needs to be on site in order to obtain the full benefit from this technique [4].

Cytological Findings of Skin Cancer

The cytologic features of malignancy are reflected in the nucleus and its relationship with the cytoplasm. The major criteria for cytologic malignancy include [1]:

- An increased nuclear cytoplasm ratio
- Irregularity of the nuclear membrane
- Irregularity of chromatin clumps
- Irregularity of nucleoli
- Nuclear moulding

The main cytological findings of the most frequent types of skin cancer are summarised as follows [2, 7].

Basal Cell Carcinoma (BCC)

- Cellular smear.
- Cohesive, sometimes anastomosing, usually flat sheets or clusters of various sizes composed of small hyperchromatic epithelial cells with scanty cytoplasm and indistinct cell borders (see Figs. 12.1 and 12.2).
- A somewhat elongated, sometimes columnar, peripheral cells usually forming a palisade.
- A slight nuclear pleomorphism.

Fig. 12.1 Basal cell carcinoma: cohesive clusters composed of small hyperchromatic epithelial cells

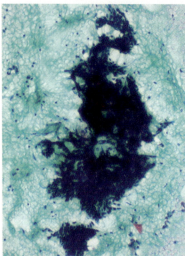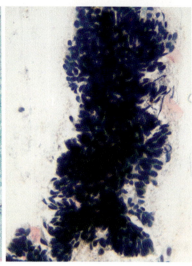

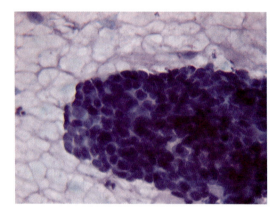

Fig. 12.2 Basal cell carcinoma: epithelial cells with scanty cytoplasm, indistinct cell borders and slight nuclear pleomorphism

- Occasional mitotic figures may be seen.
- Variants of basal cell carcinoma may show phagocytised melanin pigment (pigmented pattern), keratinised cell whorls within sheets of tumour cells (keratotic pattern) and elongated tumour cells or the presence of mucin. These findings reflect the histological variants of basal cell carcinoma and have no clinical significance. The differential diagnosis includes benign and malignant tumours of the sweat glands or of follicular apparatus.

BCC is the most common skin tumour and one which can be easily diagnosed by scrape specimen. Cytologic diagnosis has a high accuracy rate for margin control in BCC surgery. This application would especially be useful in areas with limited medical resources or in centres where Mohs micrographic surgery cannot be performed [8].

Squamous Cell Carcinoma (SCC)

- Single cells due to loss of cohesion although solid cohesive fragments of tumour may be present in the less well-differentiated tumours
- Bizarre cell shapes
- Large irregular hyperchromatic nuclei
- Necrosis
- The presence of numerous neutrophils and sometimes eosinophils

The cancer cells with smaller nuclei and abundant cytoplasm may mimic normal squamous cells. In poorly differentiated tumours the cancer cells are smaller.

Keratinisation is a common and useful feature in diagnosis, especially when Papanicolaou staining is used (see Fig. 12.3). Some of the cells appear highly orangeophilic. Single-cell keratinisation is the most reliable indicator of squamous differentiation.

The differential diagnosis includes:

- Basal cell carcinomas: Contrary to BCC, squamous cancers do not form cohesive clusters of small cells. The cancer cells are

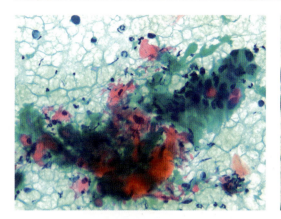

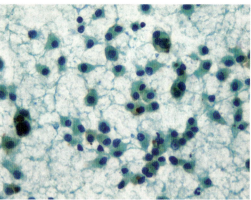

Fig. 12.3 Squamous cell carcinoma: small and loosely structured cluster composed of large keratinised (orangeo-philic) and non-keratinised epithelial cells with bizarre shapes and irregular nuclei

Fig. 12.4 Melanoma: cellular smear composed of a sin-gle-cell population with large nuclei, prominent nucleoli and occasional melanin pigment

much larger and dispersed and form only small, loosely structured clusters.

- Regenerative squamous epithelium at the edge of an ulcer: The regenerative squamous cells are usually cohesive and nuclear atypia is not generalised or severe.
- Solar keratosis and Bowen's disease have some similar features but lack the extremes of cytoplasmic and nuclear pleomorphism found in squamous cell carcinoma.

Malignant Melanoma

- Cellular smears.
- Single-cell population (aggregates of cells are rare).
- High nuclear/cytoplasmic ratio; large nuclei; prominent, often multiple large, irregularly shaped nucleoli and large intranuclear cyto-plasmic inclusions.
- Binucleated and multinucleated cells are frequent.
- Cytoplasmic pigment.

Malignant melanoma is notorious for the great variability of its presentation and may mimic almost any malignant tumour. The common denominator of most (but not all) tumours is the presence of melanin pigment in tumour cells (see Fig. 12.4). Still, the diagnosis must be based on malignant features of the cells, because the

melanin pigment phagocytised by macrophages may occur in a variety of skin disorders.

Merkel Cell Carcinoma (Primary Neuroendocrine Carcinoma of Skin)

- Cellular smears.
- Dispersed tumour cells or loosely structured clusters, sometimes forming rosettes.
- The cytoplasm is scanty and disintegrates easily with resulting debris and naked nuclei.
- Granular nuclei.
- Spherical, eosinophilic pink, cytoplasmic inclusions located near the nuclei or within nuclear indentations.

Paget's Disease

- Dispersed malignant cells
- Large hyperchromatic nuclei with prominent nucleoli

Sebaceous Carcinoma

- Moderately cellular smears
- Clusters of irregular cells with cytoplasmic vacuoles rich in lipidic material
- Central nuclei with prominent nucleoli
- Smaller basaloid cells [9]

Fig. 12.5 Cutaneous metastases from lung carcinoma (*left*) and cholangiocarcinoma (*right*): clusters of irregular epithelial cells with atypia

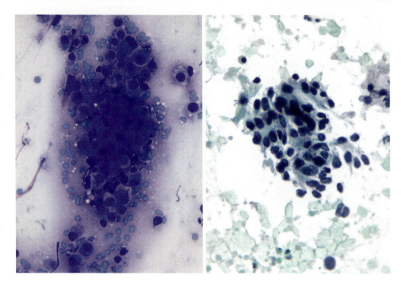

Dermatofibrosarcoma Protuberans

- Clusters and dispersed uniform or slightly atypical spindle cells
- Collagenous matrix
- Storiform pattern [10]

Other Malignant Primary Tumours

Cytological findings of skin tumours, such as ectopic meningioma [11], Ewing's sarcoma [12], malignant proliferating trichilemmal tumour [13], apocrine sweat gland carcinoma [14], Langerhans' cell histiocytosis [15] and other uncommon lesions, are described by other workers.

Metastatic Tumours

Although cutaneous metastases from tumours of internal organs do occur, they are uncommon.

Lung carcinoma was seen to metastasise most commonly to skin in males and breast carcinoma in females. The most common sites for a cutaneous/subcutaneous metastasis were chest wall, abdominal wall and scalp [16].

Occasionally, skin metastases are the first signs of an internal malignancy. The location of a metastatic deposit may give a clue to the site of the primary tumour; e.g. the so-called Sister Mary Joseph's nodule is a metastasis in the skin of the umbilicus from an intra-abdominal tumour mainly of ovary, stomach, colon or pancreas. Therefore, cytologic specimens may be a good method in the identification of unknown primary tumour.

Immunostaining can be useful in determining the site of origin of a metastatic tumour. The choice of immunostains can sometimes be determined by the cell pattern in the smear:

- In tumours with a dispersed cell pattern, the immunostain panel might include leucocyte common antigen for lymphoma, synaptophysin and chromogranin for neuroendocrine carcinoma, cytokeratin for carcinoma and S-100 for malignant melanoma.
- Smears with sheets or clusters of malignant cells are most likely to be epithelial in origin and generally cytokeratin positive (see Fig. 12.5).

Cytological findings of skin metastases from uncommon origin, such as renal cell carcinoma [17], follicular thyroid carcinoma [18], hepatocellular carcinoma [19], mesothelioma [20], transitional cell carcinoma [21] and cholangiocarcinoma [22], have been described by other authors.

Glossary

Diff-Quick Is a commercially available stain. It works as a fast variant of Giemsa

FISH Fluorescence in situ hybridization. It is a cytogenic technique used to detect presence or absence of specific DNA sequences on chromosomes

FNA Fine needle aspiration. It is a diagnostic procedure used to obtain cytologic sample from superficial tumours. A hollow needle is inserted in the mass and material is aspirated and later stained as a smear. It is safer and less traumatic than open surgical biopsies. For deep tumours, FNA requires US or CT guidance

Papanicolaou stain Is a multichromatic staining used principally on exfoliated cytological specimens

Tzanck test or smear Scraping of an ulcer base to look for multinucleated giant cells. It is used to diagnose It was named after Arnault Tzanck (1886–1954), a French dermatologist

References

1. Vega-Memije E, Martinez-de Larios N, Waxtein LM, et al. Cytodiagnosis of cutaneous basal and squamous cell carcinoma. Int J Dermatol. 2000;39:116–20.
2. Curling M, Oommen R. Chapter 38: Skin. In: Gray W, McKee GT, editors. Diagnostic cytopathology. 2nd ed. Oxford: Churchill Livingstone; 2003. p. 867–79.
3. Tzanck A. Le cytodiagnostic immediat en dermatologie. Ann de dermat et syph. 1948;8:205–18.
4. Bakis S, Irwing L, Wood G, et al. Exfoliative cytology as a diagnostic test for basal cell carcinoma: a meta-analysis. Br J Dermatol. 2004;150:829–36.
5. The Papanicolaou Society of Cytopathology Task Force on Standars of Practice. Guidelines of the Papanicolaou Society of Cytopathology for fine-needle aspiration procedure and reporting. Diagn Cytopathol. 1997;17:239–47.
6. Gordon LA, Orell SR. Evaluation of cytodiagnosis of cutaneous basal cell carcinoma. J Am Acad Dermatol. 1984;11:1082–6.
7. Koss LG. The skin. In: Koss LG, Melamed MR, editors. Koss' diagnostic cytology and its histopathologic bases. 5th ed. Philadelphia: Lippincott Williams and Wilkins; 2006.
8. Baba M, Durdu M, Seçkin D. A useful alternative approach for the treatment of well-demarcated basal cell carcinoma: surgical excision and margin control with Tzanck smear test. Dermatol Surg. 2010;36:659–64.
9. Atkins KA, Powers CN. Chapter 13: FNA cytology of skin lesions. In: Atkinson BF, editor. Atlas of diagnostic cytopathology. 2nd ed. Philadelphia: W.B. Saunders; 2004. p. 27–549.
10. Domanski HA. FNA diagnosis of dermatofibrosarcoma protuberans. Diagn Cytopathol. 2005;32:299–302.
11. Kolte SS, Lanjewar RA. Ectopic meningioma diagnosed on fine needle aspiration cytology. Acta Cytol. 2010;54:1075–6.
12. Kalra S, Gupta R, Singh S, et al. Primary cutaneous Ewing's sarcoma/primitive neuroectodermal tumor: report of the first case diagnosed on aspiration cytology. Acta Cytol. 2010;54:193–6.
13. Kini JR, Kini H. Fine-needle aspiration cytology in the diagnosis of malignant proliferating trichilemmal tumor: report of a case and review of the literature. Diagn Cytopathol. 2009;37:744–7.
14. Pai RR, Kini JR, Achar C, et al. Apocrine (cutaneous) sweat gland carcinoma of axilla with signet ring cells: a diagnostic dilemma on fine-needle aspiration cytology. Diagn Cytopahol. 2008;36:739–41.
15. Kini U, Bhat PI, Jayaseelan E. FNA diagnosis of primary adult onset lymphocutaneous Langerhans' cell histiocytosis masquerading as deep fungal mycosis. Diagn Cytopathol. 2005;32:292–5.
16. Sharma S, Kotru M, Yadav A, et al. Role of fine-needle aspiration cytology in evaluation of cutaneous metastases. Diagn Cytopathol. 2009;37:876–80.
17. Jilani G, Mohamed D, Wadia H, et al. Cutaneous metastasis of renal cell carcinoma through percutaneous fine needle aspiration biopsy: case report. Dermatol Online J. 2010;16:10.
18. Agarwal S, Rao S, Arya A, et al. Follicular thyroid carcinoma with metastasis to skin diagnosed by fine needle aspiration cytology. Indian J Pathol Microbiol. 2008;51:430–1.
19. De Agustin P, Conde E, Alberti N, et al. Cutaneous metastasis of occult hepatocellular carcinoma: a case report. Acta Cytol. 2007;51:214–6.
20. Pappa L, Machera M, Tsanou E, et al. Subcutaneous metastasis of peritoneal mesothelioma diagnosed by fine-needle aspiration. Pathol Oncol Res. 2006;12:247–50.
21. Dey P, Amir T, Jogai S, et al. Fine-needle aspiration cytology of metastatic transitional cell carcinoma. Diagn Cytopathol. 2005;32:226–8.
22. Pasquali P, Fortuño A, Casañas C, et al. Scalp and chest cutaneous metastasis of cholangiocarcinoma. Int J Dermatol. 2012. DOI: 10.1111/j.1365-4632.2011.05186.x

Dermoscopy

13

Susana Puig and Joseph Malvehy

Key Points

- It is an essential, noninvasive, simple-to-use method that allows the analysis of a large number of lesions with better sensitivity and specificity than naked-eye clinical examination.
- Its use in the evaluation of any skin tumor has a maximum level of evidence, and it is included as standard of care in clinical guidelines of melanoma.
- The inclusion of high-risk population in dermoscopy follow-up programs allows the detection of melanomas in early stages, with good prognosis even in the absence of clinical and dermoscopic features of melanoma.
- Dermoscopy in the screening of skin cancer performed by general practitioners (GPs) improves sensitivity without changing specificity.

S. Puig, MD, PhD (✉)
Melanoma Unit, Dermatology Department,
Hospital Clínic, Villarroel 170 & CIBER-ER,
Barcelona 08036, Spain
e-mail: susipuig@gmail.com

J. Malvehy, MD
Dermatology Department & CIBER-ER,
Melanoma Unit, Hospital Clínic,
Barcelona, Spain

Introduction

Dermoscopy (also known as dermatoscopy and epiluminescence microscopy) is a noninvasive, in vivo technique that has demonstrated to be an important aid in the early recognition of malignant melanoma [1, 2] and other skin tumors [3, 4]. Its use increases diagnostic accuracy of malignant melanoma between 5 and 30 % over clinical visual inspection depending on the type of skin lesion and the experience of the physician [3, 5–7]. At the present days, the use of dermoscopy in the evaluation of any skin tumor has a maximum level of evidence [1, 2, 5] and included as standard of care in clinical guidelines of melanoma [8].

It has been considered to be started in 1663 with Kolhaus who investigated the small vessels in the nail fold with the help of a microscope [9]. The term "dermatoscopy" was introduced in 1920 by the German dermatologist Johann Saphier who published a series of communications using a new diagnostic tool resembling a binocular microscope with a built-in light source for the examination of the skin [9]. Skin surface microscopy was further developed in the USA by Goldman in the 1950s using the name of "dermoscopy" and being the first dermatologist to use this new technique for the evaluation of pigmented skin lesions [9]. In 1971, Rona MacKie clearly identified, for the first time, the advantage of surface microscopy for the improvement of preoperative diagnosis of pigmented skin

A. Baldi et al. (eds.), *Skin Cancer*, Current Clinical Pathology,
DOI 10.1007/978-1-4614-7357-2_13, © Springer Science+Business Media New York 2014

lesions and for the differential diagnosis of benign versus malignant lesions [9]. These investigations were continued mainly in Europe by several Austrian and German groups and then spread worldwide [9].

Basic Principles

Physical Aspects and Material for Dermoscopy

Light is either reflected, dispersed, or absorbed by the stratum corneum because of its refraction index and its optical density, which is different from air. Thus, deeper underlying structures cannot be adequately visualized. However, when for the practice of contact dermoscopy an immersion liquid (immersion oil, alcohol, or ultrasonography gel) is used, the skin surface gets translucent and reduces the reflection, so that underlying structures are readily visible. Contact dermoscopy also uses a glass plate that flattens the skin surface and provides an even surface together with an optical magnification usually of 10× ([10, 11], and see videos in [12]).

Recently, newer handheld dermatoscopes use a polarized light and cross-polarization filter to significantly reduce irregular light reflection allowing underlying structures to be visualized without the need of applying an immersion liquid or a plate.

Photographic documentation can be performed with a dermoscopic attachment to a digital camera and then downloaded to a computer. This allows easy storage, retrieval, and follow-up of dermoscopic images of pigmented skin lesions. Photographic documentation of the dermoscopy image of a pigmented skin lesion allows also the practice of "teledermoscopy" ([10, 11], and see videos in [12]).

Digital dermoscopy equipments include a color video camera for total body photography and macro-clinical photos of the lesions and equipment for dermoscopy connected to a computer with specific software. The development of different types of software has facilitated image acquisition, storage, retrieval, and analysis. The fact that they allow digital total body photography ("body-mapping") and digital dermatoscopy to be performed makes them particularly useful in the follow-up of high-risk patients with multiple nevi for early melanoma detection [10–14].

By allowing visualization of submacroscopic pigmented structures that correlate with specific underlying histopathologic structures [15], dermoscopy provides a more powerful tool than the naked-eye examination for clinicians to determine the need to excise a lesion [1, 2]. This is main dermoscopic value that has made it an essential, noninvasive, simple-to-use method that allows the analysis of a large number of lesions with better sensitivity and specificity than naked-eye clinical examination in daily practice.

Dermoscopic Criteria

Colors
The use of dermoscopy allows the identification of many different structures and colors, not seen by the naked eye.

Colors play an important role in dermoscopy [16]. Commonly identified colors in dermoscopy include light brown, dark brown, black, blue, blue-gray, red, yellow, and white. The most important chromophores in dermoscopy are melanin and hemoglobin [10, 16]. We see melanin as black color when it is located in the stratum corneum and the upper epidermis. Light to dark brown color is produced by melanin in the epidermis. Gray to gray-blue color is consequence of the presence of melanin in the papillary dermis (usually inside melanophages). Blue color occurs when melanin is localized within the reticular dermis because of the Tyndall effect [10, 17, 18]. Hemoglobin may be seen as red, purple, blue, and even black according of the type of the vessel and the presence of thrombosis [11]. White color is often caused by regression, fibrosis, and/or scarring but may

Fig. 13.1 Clinical image (*left upper corner*) and dermoscopy of a nevus showing symmetry in the distribution of colors and structures and predominantly one color (*brown*). The predominant pattern is reticular with presence of some globules regularly distributed

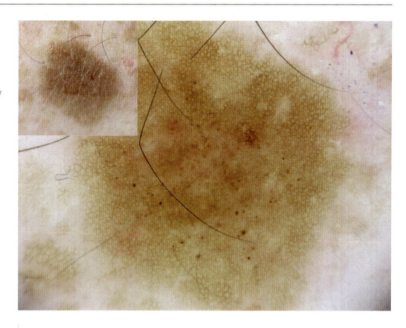

also be seen when keratin is compact as in milia-like cyst or scales [11]. Yellow color may also be associated to keratin but also to the presence of lipids (xantomized tumors) [19]. Green color is rarely seen but when present usually is consequence to the presence of hemosiderin in dermis [20].

Even the evaluation of color alone is insufficient to rule out melanoma, the basic principle "the more number of colors, the more suspicious" is useful for identifying atypical melanocytic proliferations [4].

Symmetry

The evaluation of symmetry in dermoscopy is extremely useful for the diagnosis of malignancy tending the benign lesions to be symmetric and malignant lesions to be asymmetric [4]. The evaluation of symmetry by dermoscopy includes the evaluation of the distribution of colors and structures but not the shape of the lesion.

All the algorithms developed for the diagnosis of melanoma include directly or indirectly the evaluation of the symmetry of the lesion. If a given lesion is symmetric and shows only one color, it could not be melanoma according to Menzies method [21] (Fig. 13.1).

Dermoscopy Features

Several dermoscopy structures with specific histopathological correlates have been described and used for the description of a given lesion. Some authors use more descriptive/geometrical terms, and others use the classical metaphorical description initiated with pattern analyses, but both describe the same structures with the same histopathological meanings. In this chapter the metaphoric terms will be used (see the definition, histopathological correlation, and diagnostic association of each feature in Table 13.1) [4, 10, 11]. The dermoscopy features associated with the presence of melanin in cutaneous structures are the pigment network, dots and globules, streaks, negative of pigment network, peppering, blue-white veil, blotches, and blue-gray-brown structures. The features associated to keratin are milia-like cyst, comedo-like opening, fissures, and crypts. The criteria associated to dermal component, mainly fibrosis, are crystalline structures or white shiny streaks, central white patch, and scar-like depigmentation. Features associated to the presence of hemoglobin are vessels (comma-like, dotted, polymorphous, corkscrew, arborizing, fine horizontal in focus, hairpin, crown, and glomerular), red-blue lagoons, and milky-red areas. Finally ulceration may also be seen.

Table 13.1 Definition of dermoscopy structures and their histopathological correlation

Structure	Definition	Histopathological correlation
Pigment network	Weblike structure consisting of brown or black lines and hypopigmented holes	Melanocytic pigmentation at the rete ridges
Typical network	Uniform, regular lines and holes, even color, fades in the periphery	Regular melanocytic pigmentation at the rete ridges in nevus
Atypical network	Nonuniform, darker, and/or broadened lines; heterogeneous holes in areas or shapes; abruptly ends at the perimeter	Disarranged melanocytic pigmentation at the rete ridges in atypical melanocytic lesions and melanoma
Pseudo-network	Because the face has absent or poorly developed rete ridges, diffuse pigmentation interrupted by the surface openings of the adnexal structures	Pigment at the epidermis or dermis interrupted by follicular openings of the face
Structureless (homogeneous) areas	Regions devoid of structures without signs of regression	
Dots	Black, brown, or blue-gray, small spherical structures less than 0.1 mm diameter	Aggregates of melanocytes or melanin granules at the dermis, epidermis, or stratum corneum
Globules	Brown, black, or red spherical or ovoid structures with diameters usually greater than 0.1 mm	Brown globules are nests of melanocytes at the upper dermis or dermoepidermal junction. Red globules are vessels
Cobblestone globules	Polygonal globules crowded together causing their deformation resulting in a cobblestone pattern	Large dermal nevus nests
Radial streaming	Linear extensions at the edge of the lesion	Aggregates of tumoral cells running parallel to the epidermis (Spitz/Reed nevi or radial growth phase of melanoma)
Pseudopods	Brown-black, fingerlike projections from the perimeter of the lesion. Variously shaped knobs are present at the termini of the projections	Aggregates of tumoral cells running parallel to the epidermis (Spitz/Reed nevi or radial growth phase of melanoma)
Streaks	Alternate term for radial streaming and/or pseudopods When symmetrically arranged around the entire edge of the lesion, the appellation "starburst pattern" is used	Aggregates of tumoral cells running parallel to the epidermis (Spitz/Reed nevi or radial growth phase of melanoma)
Blotches	Black, usually homogeneous, areas of pigment obscuring underlying structures	Aggregates of melanin in stratum corneum, epidermis, and upper dermis
Regression areas	White, scar-like depigmentation often combined with blue-gray peripheral zone and/ or peppering (speckled blue-gray granules)	Regression with melanophages, fibrosis, and neo-angiogenesis
Blue-white veil	Irregularly marginated, confluent blue pigmentation with overlying, white, ground-glass haze	Compact aggregation of heavily pigmented tumor cells in the superficial dermis in combination with compact orthokeratosis, acanthosis, and more or less pronounced hypergranulosis
Vascular structures	The primary structure of hemangiomas and vascular malformations are clusters of blood vessels called "lacunae" *or* "saccules" Various telangiectasias of multiple shapes and sizes including comma, pinpoint, arborizing, wreath-like, hairpin-like, irregular	Tumor vessels

Table 13.1 (continued)

Structure	Definition	Histopathological correlation
Maple leaflike areas	Brown to blue-gray, discrete structures resembling leaflike patterns	Nodules of pigmented epithelial cells located in the upper dermis
Spoke-wheel-like structures	Brown to gray-blue radial projections meeting at a darker brown or black central "hub"	Nests of basal cell tumor in the upper dermis
Large blue-gray ovoid nests	Circumscribed, blue-gray or brown, ovoid structures larger than globules	Nests of basal cell tumor in the upper dermis
Multiple blue-gray globules	Spherical, well-circumscribed structures which, in the absence of a pigment network, suggest basal cell carcinoma	Nests of basal cell tumor in the upper dermis
Milia-like cysts	Small, white, or yellow cystic structures resembling milia which often shine brightly ("stars in the sky") when viewed with the dermoscope. Pigmented milia-like cysts can resemble brown globules	Intraepidermal keratin cysts
Comedo-like openings	Blackhead-like plugs due to keratin-filled invaginations on the skin surface	Comedo-like openings containing keratin
Ridges and fissures	Cerebriform surface resulting in gyri and sulci. The latter can be filled with keratin producing irregular linear, pigmented bands	Tumoral masses with papillomatosis and acanthosis characteristics of seborrheic keratosis and papillomatous nevi
Fingerprint-like structures	Thin brown lines resulting in patterns that resemble fingerprints	Hyperkeratosis and acanthosis characteristics of seborrheic keratosis

Patterns

Pattern Analysis for the Diagnosis of Nevus

The presence of uniform and regularly distributed reticular, globular, starburst, and homogeneous blue patterns identifies a given lesion as a melanocytic nevus (i.e., per definition absence of melanoma-specific patterns) [4]. Each pattern corresponds to a specific underlying histopathologic correlate.

Based on the most common dermoscopic patterns associated with melanocytic nevi, a new classification has been recently proposed that includes four main categories: globular, reticular, starburst, and homogenous blue nevi [22, 23]. In this classification system, small congenital nevi, compound nevi, and dermal nevi are lumped together in the globular category based on their common dermoscopic-histopathologic features (globules correspond to predominantly dermal nests of melanocytes). The reticular pattern typically corresponds to junctional or lentiginous nevi, with the exception of congenital nevi in the

lower extremities [24, 25]. The starburst category includes both pigmented Spitz nevi and Reed nevi based on their striking dermoscopic features [26] (regular peripheral streaks). Homogenous structureless blue pigmentation without additional dermoscopic features is the pattern commonly observed in blue nevi [17]. Nevi with a homogeneous structureless brown pattern are not considered within the group of blue nevi because they reveal histopathologic correlates similar to reticular nevi [27, 28].

Based on the work of Kittler et al. [29, 30] in digital follow-up, growing nevi can be easily recognized by their striking dermoscopic hallmark of a peripheral rim of small brown globules frequent in adolescents and young adults (Fig. 13.2). The same pattern in individuals older than 60 years should raise suspicion and preferably be excised and studied to rule out malignancy.

Spitz and Reed nevi reveal different patterns, depending on the growth phase of the lesion [31–33]. After an initial globular pattern, Spitz and Reed nevi tend to show the classic starburst pattern, which represents an intermediate pattern

226   S. Puig and J. Malvehy

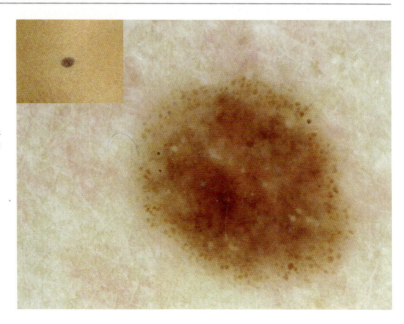

Fig. 13.2 Clinical image (*left upper corner*) and dermoscopy of a nevus showing symmetry in the distribution of colors and structures, with two colors (*brown* and *gray*) and globular-homogeneous pattern. The lesion presents a rim of globules characteristic of growth, in this case a nevus in young adult

of their evolution, showing finally a reticular or homogeneous pattern at the end. Since no single criterion allows differentiating such spitzoid-appearing melanomas from Spitz or Reed nevi with sufficient accuracy, excision of all spitzoid lesions, in adults, is always recommended [34, 35].

Conversely, homogeneous blue nevi seem to be highly stable lesions. This stability of blue nevi is an important, although subjective, clue for the diagnosis because blue color alone is a highly unspecific feature that may occur also in nodular melanoma, melanoma metastases, or pigmented basal cell carcinoma (4-17-23). Therefore, the diagnosis of blue nevi should always be based on the combination of the dermoscopic pattern and a convincing subjective history of no changes. When a reliable history is difficult to obtain, excision, not monitoring, must be performed.

Pattern Analyses for the Diagnosis of Melanoma

On the contrary, melanoma tends to show multiple colors and structures. A given melanocytic lesion with multiple colors, asymmetry, and multicomponent pattern (three or more structures) is highly suggestive of melanoma. For those lesions that we do not recognize at a first glance as

melanoma with global pattern analyses, various dermoscopic algorithms may be applied to differentiate nevi from melanoma [4, 36–38]. Pattern analyses consider the presence of some structures associated to melanoma as additional ten clues for the diagnosis of melanoma: the presence of atypical pigment network, atypical dots and globules, regression structures, crystalline structures, negative pigment network, irregular blotches, irregular pseudopods or streaks, blue-white veil, milky red areas, or polymorphous/dotted vessels (Figs. 13.3, 13.4, 13.5, 13.6, and 13.7).

According to the results of the Consensus Net Meeting on Dermoscopy, the sensitivity for melanoma of these algorithms (pattern analysis, the ABCD rule, 7-point checklist, or Menzies scoring method) was similar, but pattern analysis demonstrated a better specificity [4].

However, dermoscopy is not 100 % accurate, and a certain percentage of suspicious but benign lesions have to be excised in order not miss melanoma. It is worth highlighting again that malignant cutaneous melanoma may sometimes mimic benign melanocytic and non-melanocytic lesions. For this reason, it is important that a good clinical-dermoscopic correlation exists, and the presence of conflicting clinical-dermoscopic features should lead the clinician to perform a biopsy.

Fig. 13.3 Clinical image (*left upper corner*) and dermoscopy of a superficial spreading melanoma showing asymmetry in the distribution of colors and structures, multiple colors (*black*, *light brown*, *dark brown*, and *blue*), and multicomponent pattern. The lesion shows atypical network, atypical dots and globules, blotch and blue whitish veil

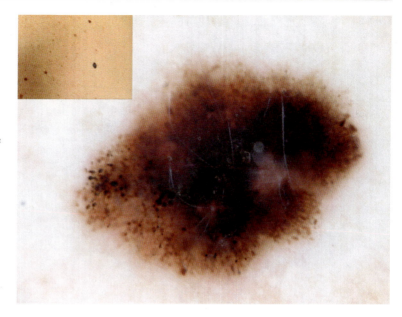

Fig. 13.4 Clinical image (*left upper corner*) and dermoscopy of a superficial spreading melanoma showing asymmetry in the distribution of colors and structures, multiple colors (*black*, *light brown*, *dark brown*, *red*, *white*, and *blue*), and multicomponent pattern. The lesion shows atypical network, atypical dots and globules, blue whitish veil, dotted vessels in milky red areas (*circle*), and crystalline white lines (chrysalides) (*square*)

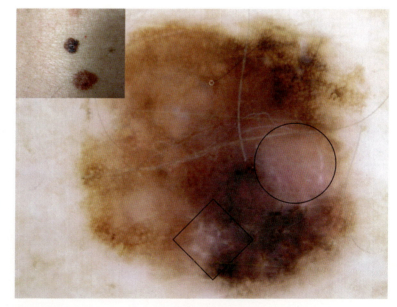

Pattern Analyses for the Diagnosis of Melanoma in Special Locations

On the contrary of what happen in other body sites, the application of dermoscopy in facial lesions increases the number of biopsies and in consequence the number of early melanomas identified.

Lesions on the face show specific dermoscopic patterns due to the anatomy of the region, being the classical pattern of melanocytic lesions the pseudo-network.

Early lentigo maligna melanomas (LMMs) may show annular granular pattern (with gray dots around hair follicles), irregular perifollicular pigmentation, short lines, and rhomboidal structures. When lentigo maligna progresses, occlusion of follicular openings and specific criteria of melanoma as blue whitish veil may appear [39].

The histopathological correlation of each dermoscopy criteria of LMM is also well known: the

Fig. 13.5 Clinical image (*left upper corner*) and dermoscopy of a superficial spreading melanoma showing asymmetry in the distribution of colors and structures, two colors (*dark brown* and *gray*), and reticular pattern. The lesion shows atypical network, atypical dots and globules, and peppering (*gray dots*) characteristic of melanophages in regression. It is a second melanoma diagnosed during follow-up of a patient carrier of the mutation G101W in *CDKN2A*

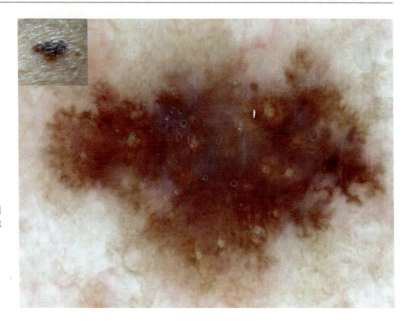

Fig. 13.6 Clinical image (*left upper corner*) and dermoscopy of an in situ melanoma showing asymmetry in the distribution of structures, three colors (*black*, *gray*, and *dark brown*), and reticular-homogeneous pattern. The lesion shows atypical network (*upper part*), atypical dots and globules, and a central black blotch

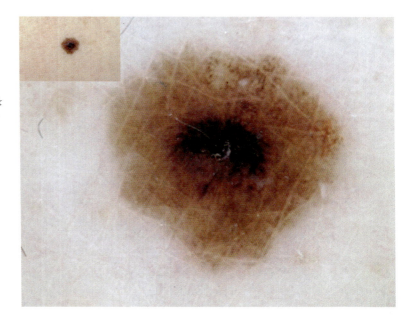

annular granular pattern corresponds to melanophages in papillary dermis and around hair follicles; perifollicular pigmentation corresponds to the proliferation/invasion of atypical melanocytes in the hair follicle; short lines and rhomboidal structures correspond to the proliferation of atypical melanocytes in the dermoepidermal junction; and finally, the occlusion of follicular openings corresponds to the progression of the

melanoma and complete invasion of the hair follicle.

Multiple gray dots (granularity) may also be seen in pigmented actinic keratosis and in liken planus-like keratosis (LPLK). Sometimes, in LPLK the granularity is coarser, but in other occasions the diagnosis is just performed after a biopsy. A difficult differential diagnosis with dermoscopy is between early LMM and pigmented

Fig. 13.7 Clinical image (*left upper corner*) and dermoscopy of a nodular melanoma showing asymmetry in the distribution of colors and structures, multiple colors (*black*, *light brown*, *dark brown*, *red*, *white*, and *blue*), and unspecific pattern. The lesion shows atypical dots and globules, blue whitish veil, atypical vessels, milky red areas, and ulceration with the sign of sticky fibers (textile fibers stick to the serum or blood in ulcerated tumors). In a nodular tumor the combination of black and blue and red and white is suggestive of malignancy

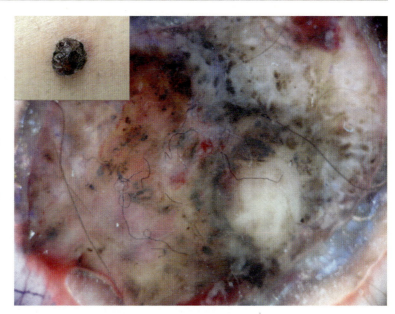

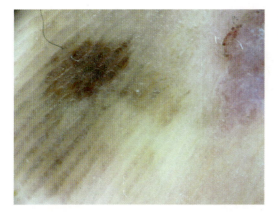

Fig. 13.8 Dermoscopy of a sole showing parallel ridge pattern in a lentiginous acral melanoma

actinic keratosis because both may show multiple gray dots, and again the diagnosis is performed by histopathology. Dermoscopy is useful not only to increase the index of suspicion in lesions on the face but also to select the best area to be biopsied to obtain a diagnosis.

For the diagnosis of melanoma in acral sites, the recognition of parallel ridge pattern [40] (Fig. 13.8) is highly specific, while benign patterns are also well characterized being the more frequent benign pattern the parallel furrow pattern [41]. Dermoscopy is very useful in the recognition of benign patterns and permits to avoid unnecessary excision.

Comparative Recognition for the Diagnosis of Melanoma

In clinical practice, physicians are dealing with patients with multiple lesions and not with isolated lesions. In these situations comparative recognition process is used. Most individuals have a predominant lesion's pattern; therefore, the examination of all lesions is an essential step in the recognition process because it allows the identification of lesions deviating from the individual's prevailing benign pattern (concept of the "ugly duckling sign") [42–45] (Fig. 13.9).

Digital Dermoscopy Follow-Up for the Diagnosis of Melanoma in High-Risk Patients

The importance of surveillance by digital dermoscopy follow-up programs to identify melanoma at an early stage in high-risk populations such as patients with hundreds of nevi, atypical mole syndrome (AMS), personal or family history of melanoma, and carriers of genetic mutations as in *CDKN2A* has been clearly demonstrated [14, 46] (Fig. 13.10). In a recent study comparing melanomas identified in patients included in digital dermoscopy follow up (DFU) program with melanomas diagnosed in patients referred to a melanoma unit, the multicomponent pattern (defined by the combination of three or more

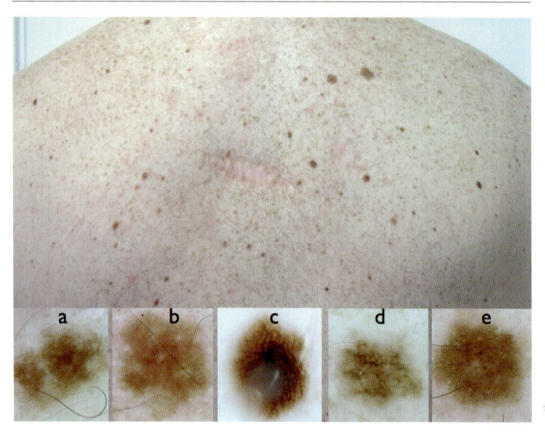

Fig. 13.9 Clinical image (*up*) of a patient with a previous melanoma. The "ugly duckling sign" of dermoscopy allows the identification of a second melanoma (**c**) compared with the predominant nevus pattern of the patient (**a, b, d, e**)

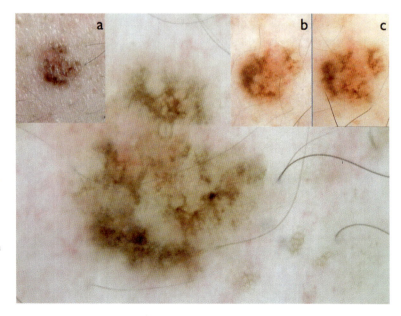

Fig. 13.10 Clinical image (**a**) of a melanoma diagnosed during digital follow-up (sequential dermoscopy images at 6 months, **b** and **c**) showing a focal change in the structure. High-resolution dermoscopy shows a lesion with atypical pigment network and peppering in less than 10 % of the lesion

Fig. 13.11 Clinical image (*left upper corner*) and dermoscopy of a basal cell carcinoma showing asymmetry in the distribution of structures and blue-white color (suggestive of malignancy in the 3-point checklist of dermoscopy algorithm). The lesion shows maple leaflike areas (*circle*), multiple blue-gray dots/globules (*square*), and crystalline white lines (chrysalides) in the central hypopigmented area

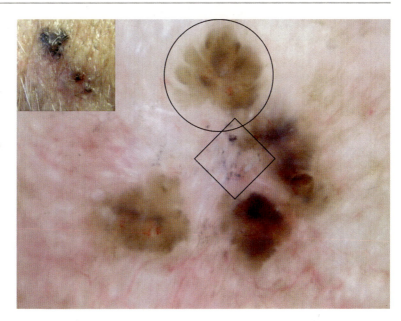

distinctive dermoscopic structures within a given lesion) was noted in 60 % of referred melanomas but in only 16 % of those identified in the DFU surveillance program. By contrast, the reticular pattern was the most frequent pattern observed in melanomas that appeared in patients included in the digital dermoscopic follow-up program [46]. This reticular pattern is the characteristic pattern of slow-growing melanomas described by Argenziano et al. [47] and that may be slow growing in a radial phase for years or decades being diagnosed when this pigment network is altered and a homogeneous structure appears [48] associated with a disruption of the dermoepidermal architecture or the occurrence of regression. The inclusion of high-risk population in follow-up programs allows the detection of melanomas in early stages, with good prognosis (mainly in situ, if not AJCC stage IA), even in the absence of clinical and dermoscopic features of melanoma. In a selected study population, with 90 % of the patients displaying AMS and almost 45 % having had a previous melanoma, one of eight developed melanoma during surveillance, which is more than 1,500 times higher than expected in the general population. According to these results, MM can be diagnosed at any time once a high-risk patient is included in the DFU

program. Thus, maintained surveillance is required in individuals at high risk, and the "two-step method of digital follow-up" allows detection of melanomas with few dermatoscopic criteria by digital dermoscopy follow-up (60 % of the new melanomas diagnosed in DFU) and also the detection of melanoma that present as a new lesion or arising from nevi not monitored by dermatoscopy (40 % of melanomas detected in digital follow-up) [14].

Pattern Analyses in the Diagnosis of Basal Cell Carcinoma
Classic Pattern

The dermatoscopic model for the diagnosis of the pigmented variant of BCC, initially described by Menzies and co-workers [49], is based on the absence of a pigmented network and the presence of at least one of six positive morphological features including ulceration (not associated with a recent history of trauma), multiple blue-gray globules, maple leaflike areas, large blue-gray ovoid nests, spoke-wheel areas, and arborizing (treelike) telangiectasia [49, 50] (Figs. 13.11 and 13.12). Several publications confirm the reproducibility and reliability of this method [50–52]. Arborizing vessels may also be seen in other conditions such as

Fig. 13.12 Clinical image (*left upper corner*) and dermoscopy of a basal cell carcinoma showing in-focus fine linear and branched vessels

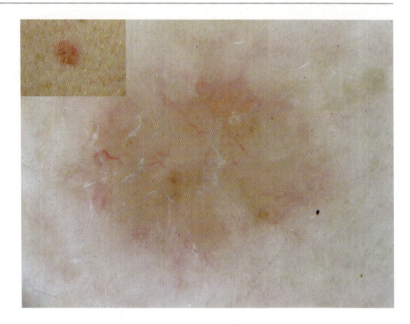

Fig. 13.13 Dermoscopy of a superficial basal cell carcinoma showing asymmetry in the distribution of structures and blue-white color (suggestive of malignancy in the 3-point checklist of dermoscopy algorithm). The lesion shows blue ovoid nests (*circles*) and multiple erosions (*arrows*) with pink areas and in-focus fine linear vessels

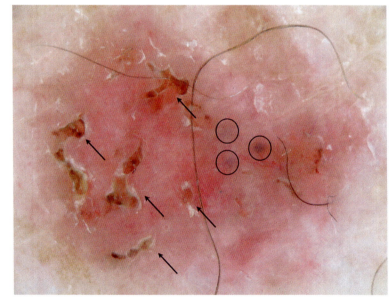

xanthogranuloma but in this case with a yellowish background [19].

Other Patterns of Basal Cell Carcinoma (BCC)
Altamura et al. reported four nonclassic BCC dermoscopic structures [50]: short fine superficial telangiectasia, multiple small erosions, concentric structures, and multiple in-focus blue-gray dots [50] (Figs. 13.13 and 13.14).

Other features described occasionally in BCCs are shiny pink-white areas in nonpigmented BCCs, blue-whitish veil in heavily pigmented BCC, and milia-like cysts in BCCs with trichilemmal differentiation.

In morpheaform basal cell carcinomas, the presence of fine small vessels in a whitish-pinkish area may be an important clue that also allows delimitating the primary lesion or diagnosing the relapse.

Fig. 13.14 Dermoscopy of a superficial basal cell carcinoma showing again asymmetry in the distribution of structures and blue-white color (suggestive of malignancy in the 3-point checklist of dermoscopy algorithm). The lesion shows multiple erosions and concentric structures (*arrows*) with pink areas

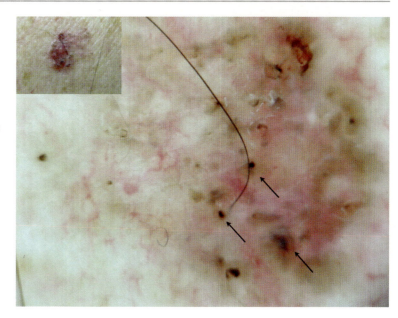

Dermoscopy of Superficial BCC

Superficial BCC is a generally nonpigmented type of BCC. The main dermoscopic criteria for its diagnosis are shiny white to red areas that appear translucent to opaque, correlating with the vascularized tumor, and tend to focally efface normal skin markings; short fine telangiectasia; and multiple small erosions [53–55] (Figs. 13.12, 13.13, and 13.14).

Dermoscopy of Fibroepithelioma of Pinkus

An uncommon variant of BCC is fibroepithelioma of Pinkus. This tumor exhibits repetitive dermoscopic characteristics including fine arborizing vessels sometimes combined with dotted vessels, white streaks, gray-brown structureless pigmentation with or without variable number of small gray-blue dots inside this area, and milia-like cysts (only seen as single units per lesion) [56, 57].

Dermoscopy Patterns of Actinic Keratosis and Squamous Cell Carcinoma

Nonpigmented actinic keratosis shows a pinkish structure also described as strawberry with yellow plugs in follicular openings surrounded by erythema [58]. Using polarized dermoscopy, an optical artifact may be seen in nonpigmented

keratosis as well as in relapsed BCC, "rosettas" that are described as white small dots distributed in a rhomboidal pattern [59]. Pigmented actinic keratoses usually present the granular annular pattern also characteristic of LMM [60]. In pigmented AK, this pattern may be associated to the presence of scaling and rosettas, but the diagnosis should be confirmed by histopathology.

Bowen's disease is dermatoscopically characterized by the presence of glomerular vessels in clusters associated to the presence of scaling (Fig. 13.15). Pigmented Bowen's disease is also a difficult differential diagnosis of melanoma, but there are some clues that may help in the diagnosis such as the presence of lineated pigmented globules or vessels at the periphery [61].

Invasive SCC usually is not pigmented and keratinizing [62]. On dermoscopy, hairpin vessels, clusters of glomerular vessels, keratin, and more recently described presence of white circles are clues for the diagnosis of SCC [61, 62].

Practical Considerations and Applications

In patients with multiple lesions, a comparative approach (the ugly duckling sign) (Fig. 13.9) would be much more useful than the analytical

Fig. 13.15 Clinical image (*left upper corner*) and dermoscopy of an in situ squamous cell carcinoma. The lesion shows clusters of glomerular vessels (*circles*) and multiple scales (*arrows*)

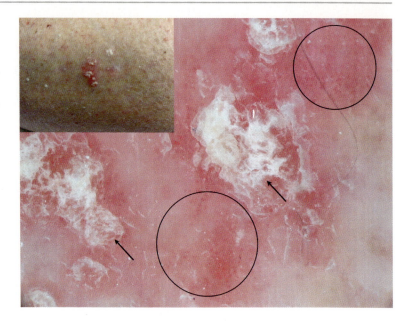

approach lesion by lesion [42, 43]. The key point in the examination of individuals with multiple nevi is therefore the identification of his or her predominant nevus pattern (defined as the pattern seen in more than 30 % of all nevi), which then permits the identification of atypical lesions that deviate from this pattern [42–45]. Patient-related factors as age, body site, and skin phototype influence the predominant nevus pattern [63].

The most common pattern in prepubertal children is globular nevi, mainly on the head and neck area and upper trunk [64]. Reticular nevi prevail in adults and are mostly located on the trunk.

Zalaudek et al. [63] observed significant skin-type-related differences in color and pigment distribution in an adult study population. Notably, the stereotypical nevus type in persons with skin type IV (also known as hypermelanotic or black nevus) is a small lesion with dark brown reticular pattern and central hyperpigmentation ("black lamella"). In phototype III lesions tend to be a smaller in diameter and homogeneous in pigmentation while in phototype I and II lesions are larger, light brown, and with central hypopigmentation.

Considering that in some cases malignant melanoma may be clinically and dermatoscopically indistinguishable from melanocytic nevi,

the "2-step approach" using total body photography (TBP) and digital dermatoscopy follow-up (DFU) [13] provides a comparative reference point that allows the identification of the appearance of subtle changes occurring over time in high-risk population. One of the basic rationales of this approach is based on the fact that benign lesions usually do not change, whereas melanomas significantly change over time. In high-risk populations, there is a double benefit to the DFU approach, to increasing the possibility that melanoma will not be missed and to minimize the excision of benign lesions.

Indications and Contraindications

Dermoscopy

Indications: Dermoscopy should be applied in the evaluation of any skin tumor supported with a maximum level of evidence.

All lesions should be evaluated with dermoscopy because if we use it just in clinically suspicious lesions, we will miss 20–30 % of melanomas (increase of the sensitivity of dermoscopy compared with clinical examination). But dermoscopy alone is also not enough for the evaluation of a given lesion. History, evolution, age, sex, location, clinical concern, and comparative analyses are also important.

Total Body Photography and Digital Dermoscopy Follow-Up

Indications: Patients at high risk to develop melanoma (familial melanoma with or without known mutation, multiple primary melanoma, previous melanoma, atypical mole syndrome) with multiple nevi. Lesions included in follow-up should not have a clear-cut dermoscopic diagnosis of melanoma and should be flat.

Contraindications: Patients with no good compliance, doctors without experience, and equipments that do not allow a correct comparison. Considering the type of lesions, nodular lesions and lesions with marked regression (more than 50 % of the lesion) should never be included in follow-up.

Future Considerations

Use of Dermoscopy for Preoperative Evaluation of Skin Tumors

Nowadays, clinical and dermoscopy information about the primary tumors is crucial for the correct interpretation of the histopathology of a given tumor and the final patient management. Documentation of the tumor before excision should be mandatory for any skin cancer, and dermoscopy together with the clinical image of the tumor should be in the patient's documentation.

Use of Dermoscopy in Gross Macroscopic Pathology

Correct orientation of the sample at the histopathology is crucial to obtain a correct sectioning. Dermoscopy can be applied to fixed tissues, with findings comparable to those of in vivo examination. Dermoscopy may be useful to guide tissue sectioning in gross pathology [65].

Use of Dermoscopy in Cancer Screening

Argenziano and coworkers [66] demonstrated in a prospective, randomized controlled trial that the introduction of dermoscopy in the screening of skin cancer performed by general practitioners (GPs) improves sensitivity without changing specificity. This increase in accuracy for the skin cancer screening is now starting to be implemented in Europe, the USA, Australia, and other countries. When patients have no direct access to dermatologist, dermoscopy should be used in the first step of skin evaluation. If just dermatologists are using dermoscopy but patients will be sent to dermatologists by GPs, 20–30 % of skin cancers will be missed at the first level of health assistance and never sent as suspicious for specific treatment.

Use of Dermoscopy in General Dermatology

Dermoscopy is not only useful in the diagnosis of skin tumors (i.e., melanoma, basal cell carcinoma, dermatofibroma) and in the differential diagnosis of skin tumors and non-tumors (i.e., between basal cell carcinoma in the face and molluscum contagiosum) but also in the diagnosis of inflammatory (i.e., lichen planus) or infectious diseases (i.e., scabies), called inflammoscopy [67]. Another growing field of dermoscopy is trichodermoscopy. The use of all of them will be growing in the future years but is not the aim of the present chapter.

Use of Dermoscopy in the Follow-Up of Noninvasive Treatments

With the implementation of nonsurgical treatments, as cryotherapy, imiquimod, 5-fluorouracil, ingenol mebutate, photodynamic therapy [68] for basal cell carcinoma and/or actinic keratosis and/or Bowen's disease and some of them even sometimes for lentigo maligna melanoma in elderly, dermoscopy showed their ability in the evaluation of the response to the treatment, allowing the documentation of responses and possible relapses.

Use of Dermoscopy in Self-Assessment for High-Risk Patients

In the new era of technology, patients may be aware of dermoscopy and also self-trained with the free information available in the Internet. Patients may use dermoscopy to identify suspicious lesions [69] or changing lesions before deciding to consult to their dermatologist or even doubtful dermoscopy images may be sent to their doctors by or using their cell phones. All these may seem unnecessary in developed countries but may be extremely useful in isolated areas. The final decision of the use of dermoscopy is not anymore in the hands of doctors dealing with skin cancer but in the net where patients may buy dermatoscopes as attachments for their cell phones and teaching activities or tutorials to learn how to recognize a suspicious lesion.

Glossary

Atypical Mole Syndrome (AMS) is the most important phenotypic risk factor for developing cutaneous melanoma. It is otherwise known as heritable melanoma syndrome; it refers to a group of patients who appear to inherit a tendency to develop dysplastic naevi. This inheritance appears to follow an autosomal dominant pattern

Cross-polarization filter in dermoscopy, is the system by which skin can be visualized through the stratum corneum without the need of applying immersion liquids. The scattered light from the deep tissue structures has altered its polarization and can pass through the filter for imaging. Cross-polarization cancels out the light that is being reflected by the skin surface, thus allowing a deep, glare-free view into the skin–without immersion fluids

Cyclin-dependent Kinase Inhibitor 2A (CD-KN2A) Acts as a tumor suppressor. In MM, disease susceptibility is associated with variations affecting this gene. In familial atypical

multiple mole melanoma-pancreatic carcinoma syndrome (FAMMMPC) mutation carriers within families may develop either or both types of cancer. In melanoma-astrocytoma syndrome (MASTS), disease is caused by mutations affecting this gene

DFU Digital dermatoscopy follow-up

GPs General practitioners

Non-polarized light dermoscopy requires oil or gel for contact. Gives brighter images. It allows a better visualization of milialike cysts and comedolike (more helpful for identification of seborrheic keratosis) and peppering, lighter colors, and blue-white areas are also more evident, facilitating recognition of regression areas. It is a complement to

Polarized light dermoscopy requires no contact. With PD, melanin appeared darker and blue nevi had more shades of blue; vessels and red areas are better visualized as well as shiny-white streaks

TBP Total body photography

Tyndall effect also known as Tyndall scattering, is light scattering by particles in a colloid or suspension. The preferential absorption of long light wavelengths by melanin and the scattering of shorter wavelengths, representing the blue end of the spectrum, by collagen bundles gives a blue color to those lesions where melanin is localized within the reticular dermis

References

1. Vestergaard ME, Macaskill P, Holt PE, Menzies SW. Dermoscopy compared with naked eye examination for the diagnosis of primary melanoma: a meta-analysis of studies performed in a clinical setting. Br J Dermatol. 2008;159:669–76.
2. Bafounta ML, Beauchet A, Aegerter P, Saiag P. Is dermoscopy (epiluminescence microscopy) useful for the diagnosis of melanoma? Results of a meta-analysis using techniques adapted to the evaluation of diagnostic tests. Arch Dermatol. 2001;137:1343–50.
3. Binder M, Schwarz M, Winkler A, Steiner A, Kaider A, Wolff K, et al. Epiluminescence microscopy. A useful tool for the diagnosis of pigmented skin lesions for formally trained dermatologists. Arch Dermatol. 1995;131:286–91.
4. Argenziano G, Soyer HP, Chimenti S, Talamini R, Corona R, Sera F, et al. Dermoscopy of pigmented skin lesions: results of a consensus meeting via the Internet. J Am Acad Dermatol. 2003;48:679–93.

5. Mayer J. Systematic review of the diagnostic accuracy of dermatoscopy in detecting malignant melanoma. Med J Aust. 1997;167:206–10.

6. Binder M, Puespoeck-Schwarz M, Steiner A, Kittler H, Muellner M, Wolff K, et al. Epiluminescence microscopy of small pigmented skin lesions: short-term formal training improves the diagnostic performance of dermatologists. J Am Acad Dermatol. 1997;36:197–202.

7. Westerhoff K, McCarthy WH, Menzies SW. Increase in the sensitivity for melanoma diagnosis by primary care physicians using skin surface microscopy. Br J Dermatol. 2000;143:1016–20.

8. http://www.nhmrc.gov.au/_files_nhmrc/publications/attachments/cp111.pdf

9. Braun RP, Rabinovitz HS, Oliviero M, Kopf AW, Saurat JH. Dermoscopy of pigmented skin lesions. J Am Acad Dermatol. 2005;52:109–21.

10. Malvehy J, Puig S. Principles of dermoscopy. Barcelona: CEGE; 2002.

11. Malvehy J, Puig S, Braun R, Marghoob A, Kopf A. Handbook of dermoscopy. Boca Ratón: Taylor & Francis; 2006. ISBN 0-415-384907 and 978-0-415-38490-2.

12. http://www.genomel.org/dermoscopy/ (see videos in learning how to use dermoscopy effectively).

13. Malvehy J, Puig S. Follow-up of melanocytic skin lesions with digital total-body photography and digital dermoscopy: a two-step method. Clin Dermatol. 2002;20:297–304.

14. Salerni G, Carrera C, Lovatto L, Puig-Butille JA, Badenas C, Plana E, Puig S, Malvehy J. Benefits of total body photography and digital dermatoscopy ("two-step method of digital follow-up") in the early diagnosis of melanoma in patients at high risk for melanoma. J Am Acad Dermatol. 2012;67(1):e17–27.

15. Zalaudek I, Leinweber B, Hofmann-Wellenhof R, Soyer HP. The impact of dermoscopic-pathologic correlates in the diagnosis and management of pigmented skin tumors. Exp Rev Dermatol. 2006;4:579–87.

16. Seidenari S, Pellacani G, Martella A. Acquired melanocytic lesions and the decision to excise: role of color variegation and distribution as assessed by dermoscopy. Dermatol Surg. 2005;31:184–9.

17. Ferrara G, Soyer HP, Malvehy J, et al. The many faces of blue nevus: a clinicopathologic study. J Cutan Pathol. 2007;34:543–51.

18. Zalaudek I, Argenziano G, Ferrara G, et al. Clinically equivocal melanocytic skin lesions with features of regression: a dermoscopic-pathological study. Br J Dermatol. 2004;150:64–71.

19. Lovato L, Salerni G, Puig S, Carrera C, Palou J, Malvehy J. Adult xanthogranuloma mimicking basal cell carcinoma: dermoscopy, reflectance confocal microscopy and pathological correlation. Dermatology. 2010;220(1):66–70.

20. Zaballos P, Llambrich A, Ara M, Olazaran Z, Malvehy J, Puig S. Dermoscopic findings of haemosiderotic and aneurysmal dermatofibroma: report of six patients. Br J Dermatol. 2006;154(2):244–50.

21. Menzies SW, Ingvar C, McCarthy WH. A sensitivity and specificity analysis of the surface microscopy features of invasive melanoma. Melanoma Res. 1996;6(1):55–62.

22. Argenziano G, Zalaudek I, Ferrara G, Hofmann-Wellenhof R, Soyer HP. Proposal of a new classification system for melanocytic naevi. Br J Dermatol. 2007;157:217–27.

23. Zalaudek I, Manzo M, Ferrara G, Argenziano G. A new classification of melanocytic nevi based on dermoscopy. Exp Rev Dermatol. 2008;3:477–89.

24. Seidenari S, Pellacani G, Martella A, et al. Instrument-, age- and site-dependent variations of dermoscopic patterns of congenital melanocytic naevi: a multicentre study. Br J Dermatol. 2006;155:56–61.

25. Changchien L, Dusza SW, Agero AL, et al. Age- and site-specific variation in the dermoscopic patterns of congenital melanocytic nevi: an aid to accurate classification and assessment of melanocytic nevi. Arch Dermatol. 2007;143:1007–14.

26. Ferrara G, Argenziano G, Soyer HP, et al. The spectrum of Spitz nevi: a clinicopathologic study of 83 cases. Arch Dermatol. 2005;141:1381–7.

27. Ahlgrimm-Siess V, Massone C, Koller S, et al. In vivo confocal scanning laser microscopy of common naevi with globular, homogeneous and reticular pattern in dermoscopy. Br J Dermatol. 2008;158:1000–7.

28. Teban L, Pehamberger H, Wolff K, Binder M, Kittler H. Clinical value of a dermatoscopic classification of Clark nevi. J Dtsch Dermatol Ges. 2003;1:292–6.

29. Kittler H, Pehamberger H, Wolff K, Binder M. Follow-up of melanocytic skin lesions with digital epiluminescence microscopy: patterns of modifications observed in early melanoma, atypical nevi, and common nevi. J Am Acad Dermatol. 2000;43:467–76.

30. Kittler H, Seltenheim M, Dawid M, Pehamberger H, Wolff K, Binder M. Frequency and characteristics of enlarging common melanocytic nevi. Arch Dermatol. 2000;136:316–20.

31. Nino M, Brunetti B, Delfino S, Brunetti B, Panariello L, Russo D. Spitz nevus: follow-up study of 8 cases of childhood starburst type and proposal for management. Dermatology. 2009;218:48–51.

32. Argenziano G, Zalaudek I, Ferrara G, Lorenzoni A, Soyer HP. Involution: the natural evolution of pigmented Spitz and Reed nevi? Arch Dermatol. 2007;143:549–51.

33. Pizzichetta MA, Argenziano G, Grandi G, de Giacomi C, Trevisan G, Soyer HP. Morphologic changes of a pigmented Spitz nevus assessed by dermoscopy. J Am Acad Dermatol. 2002;47:137–9.

34. Bowling J, Argenziano G, Azenha A, et al. Dermoscopy key points: recommendations from the international dermoscopy society. Dermatology. 2007;214:3–5.

35. Brunetti B, Nino M, Sammarco E, Scalvenzi M. Spitz naevus: a proposal for management. J Eur Acad Dermatol Venereol. 2005;19:391–3.

36. Zalaudek I, Argenziano G, Soyer HP, et al. The Dermoscopy Working Group. Three-point checklist

of dermoscopy: an open internet study. Br J Dermatol. 2006;154:431–7.

37. Henning JS, Dusza SW, Wang SQ, et al. The CASH (color, architecture, symmetry, and homogeneity) algorithm for dermoscopy. J Am Acad Dermatol. 2007;56:45–52.

38. Argenziano G, Fabbrocini G, Carli P, De Giorgi V, Sammarco E, Delfino M. Epiluminescence microscopy for the diagnosis of doubtful melanocytic skin lesions: comparison of the ABCD rule of dermatoscopy and a new 7-point checklist based on pattern analysis. Arch Dermatol. 1998;134:1563–70.

39. Schiffner R, Schiffner-Rohe J, Vogt T, Landthaler M, Wlotzke U, Cognetta AB, et al. Improvement of early recognition of lentigo maligna using dermatoscopy. J Am Acad Dermatol. 2000;42(1 Pt 1):25–32.

40. Saida T, Miyazaki A, Oguchi S, Ishihara Y, Yamazaki Y, Murase S, et al. Significance of dermoscopic patterns in detecting malignant melanoma on acral volar skin: results of a multicenter study in Japan. Arch Dermatol. 2004;140(10):1233–8.

41. Malvehy J, Puig S. Dermoscopic patterns of benign volar melanocytic lesions in patients with atypical mole syndrome. Arch Dermatol. 2004;140(5):538–44.

42. Gachon J, Beaulieu P, Sei JF, et al. First prospective study of the recognition process of melanoma in dermatological practice. Arch Dermatol. 2005;141:434–8.

43. Scope A, Dusza SW, Halpern AC, et al. The "ugly duckling" sign: agreement between observers. Arch Dermatol. 2008;144:58–64.

44. Scope A, Burroni M, Agero AL, et al. Predominant dermoscopic patterns observed among nevi. J Cutan Med Surg. 2006;10:170–4.

45. Blum A, Soyer HP, Garbe C, Kerl H, Rassner G, Hofmann-Wellenhof R. The dermoscopic classification of atypical melanocytic naevi (Clark naevi) is useful to discriminate benign from malignant melanocytic lesions. Br J Dermatol. 2003;149:1159–64.

46. Salerni G, Lovatto L, Carrera C, Puig S, Malvehy J. Melanomas Detected in a Follow-up Program Compared With Melanomas Referred to a Melanoma Unit. Arch Dermatol. 2011;147(5):549–55.

47. Argenziano G, Kittler H, Ferrara G, Rubegni P, Malvehy J, Puig S, et al. Slow-growing melanoma: a dermoscopy follow-up study. Br J Dermatol. 2010; 162:267–73.

48. Terushkin V, Dusza SW, Scope A, Argenziano G, Bahadoran P, Cowell L, et al. Changes observed in slow growing melanomas during long-term dermoscopic monitoring. Br J Dermatol. 2012;166:1213–20. doi:10.1111/j.1365-2133.2012.10846.x.

49. Menzies SW, Westerhoff K, Rabinovitz H, Kopf AW, McCarthy WH, Katz B. Surface microscopy of pigmented basal cell carcinoma. Arch Dermatol. 2000;136:1012–6.

50. Altamura D, Menzies SW, Argenziano G, et al. Dermatoscopy of basal cell carcinoma: morphologic variability of global and local features and accuracy of diagnosis. J Am Acad Dermatol. 2010;62:67–75.

51. Peris K, Altobelli E, Ferrari A, et al. Interobserver agreement on dermoscopic features of pigmented basal cell carcinoma. Dermatol Surg. 2002;28:643–5.

52. Demirtasoglu M, Ilknur T, Lebe B, Kusku E, Akarsu S, Ozkan S. Evaluation of dermoscopic and histopathologic features and their correlations in pigmented basal cell carcinomas. J Eur Acad Dermatol Venereol. 2006;20:916–20.

53. Scalvenzi M, Lembo S, Francia MG, Balato A. Dermoscopic patterns of superficial basal cell carcinoma. Int J Dermatol. 2008;47:1015–8.

54. Giacomel J, Zalaudek I. Dermoscopy of superficial basal cell carcinoma. Dermatol Surg. 2005;31:1710–3.

55. Micantonio T, Gulia A, Altobelli E, et al. Vascular patterns in basal cell carcinoma. J Eur Acad Dermatol Venereol. 2011;25:358–61.

56. Zalaudek I, Ferrara G, Broganelli P, et al. Dermoscopy patterns of fibroepithelioma of pinkus. Arch Dermatol. 2006;142:1318–22.

57. Zamberk-Majlis P, Velazquez-Tarjuelo D, Aviles-Izquierdo JA, Lazaro-Ochaita P. Dermoscopic characterization of 3 cases of fibroepithelioma of Pinkus. Actas Dermosifiliogr. 2009;100:899–902.

58. Zalaudek I, Giacomel J, Argenziano G, Hofmann-Wellenhof R, Micantonio T, Di Stefani A, et al. Dermoscopy of facial nonpigmented actinic keratosis. Br J Dermatol. 2006;155(5):951–6.

59. Cuellar F, Vilalta A, Puig S, Palou J, Salerni G, Malvehy J. New dermoscopic pattern in actinic keratosis and related conditions. Arch Dermatol. 2009; 145(6):732.

60. Zalaudek I, Ferrara G, Leinweber B, Mercogliano A, D'Ambrosio A, Argenziano G. Pitfalls in the clinical and dermoscopic diagnosis of pigmented actinic keratosis. J Am Acad Dermatol. 2005;53(6):1071–4.

61. Cameron A, Rosendahl C, Tschandl P, Riedl E, Kittler H. Dermatoscopy of pigmented Bowen's disease. J Am Acad Dermatol. 2010;62(4):597–604.

62. Segura S, Carrera C, Ferrando J, Mascaró Jr JM, Palou J, Malvehy J, et al. Dermoscopy in epidermodysplasia verruciformis. Dermatol Surg. 2006;32(1):103–6.

63. Zalaudek I, Argenziano G, Mordente I, et al. Nevus type in dermoscopy is related to skin type in white persons. Arch Dermatol. 2007;143:351–6.

64. Aguilera P, Puig S, Guilabert A, et al. Prevalence study of nevi in children from Barcelona: dermoscopy, constitutional and environmental factors. Dermatology. 2009;218:203–14.

65. Goulart JM, Malvehy J, Puig S, Martin G, Marghoob AA. Dermoscopy in skin self-examination: a useful tool for select patients. Arch Dermatol. 2011;147(1): 53–8.

66. Argenziano G, Puig S, Zalaudek I, Sera F, Corona RM, Alsina M, et al. Dermoscopy improves accuracy of primary care physicians to triage suspicious skin tumours. J Clin Oncol. 2006;24(12):1877–82.

67. Lallas A, Kyrgidis A, Tzellos TG, Apalla Z, Karakyriou E, Karatolias A, et al. Accuracy of dermoscopic criteria for the diagnosis of psoriasis,

dermatitis, lichen planus and pityriasis rosea. Br J Dermatol. 2012;166:1198–205. doi:10.1111/j.1365-2133.2012.10868.x.

68. Segura S, Puig S, Carrera C, Lecha M, Borges V, Malvehy J. Non-invasive management of non-melanoma skin cancer in patients with cancer predisposition genodermatosis: a role for confocal microscopy and photodynamic therapy. J Eur Acad Dermatol Venereol. 2011;25(7):819–27.

69. Scope A, Busam KJ, Malvehy J, Puig S, McClain SA, Braun RP, et al. Ex vivo dermoscopy of melanocytic tumors: time for dermatopathologists to learn dermoscopy. Arch Dermatol. 2007;143(12):1548–52.

Introduction to Ultrasonography in Skin Cancer

14

Ximena Wortsman

Key Points

- The primary lesions in skin cancer can be recognized on ultrasound.
- Ultrasound provides relevant anatomical data on extension in all axes, exact location, vascularity and deeper involvement.
- Locoregional staging of skin cancer can also be performed using ultrasound.

Skin cancers comprise the most frequent malignant condition among human beings. Even though NMSC (nonmelanoma skin cancer: basal cell and squamous cell carcinoma) is rarely a mortal disease and it rarely metastasizes, it can generate considerable disfigurement and usually affects highly exposed areas of the body such as the face. NMSC represents approximately 88 % of all malignant skin neoplasms [1]. Some authors report that up to 45.5 % of recurrent basal cell carcinomas are due to incomplete resections and up to 54.8 % have demonstrated at least partial aggressive-growth features [2].

Cutaneous malignant melanoma constitutes 4–11 % of all skin cancers but is responsible for more than 75 % of skin cancer-related deaths, producing more than 8,000 deaths per year in the United States [3, 4]. Thus, the assessment of depth in melanoma is a critical issue that may influence important clinical decisions such as the performance of a sentinel node procedure or the size of the excision [3].

In recent years, new ultrasound technology has been developed which has allowed a better definition of the sonographic images of the skin layers and deeper structures. These more sophisticated ultrasound machines have more channels and work with higher and variable frequency probes. Usually, their highest frequencies range between 15 and 22 MHz.

The main advantage of ultrasound is the provision of real-time images with a reasonable balance between resolution and penetration that allows the observation of tumors whose depth is between 0.1 and 60 mm, without changing the probe. The latter issue can be relevant since other imaging technologies used in dermatology, such as confocal microscopy (CFM) or optical coherence tomography (OCT), do not penetrate more than 0.5 mm (CFM) or 2 mm (OCT) which may leave critical information (deeper tumors) out of the medical treatment plan. This may be a potential source of recurrences. Another advantage of ultrasound is the assessment of the vascularization of the tumor by qualifying and quantifying in vivo the vessels within the tumor through the use of color Doppler and spectral curve analysis (showing the type of vessel and velocity of flow). Ultrasound also provides the anatomical location

X. Wortsman, MD
Department of Radiology and Dermatology,
Faculty of Medicine, Institute for Diagnostic Imaging and Research of the Skin and Soft Tissues,
Clinica Servet, University of Chile,
Almirante Pastene 150, Providencia, Santiago, Chile
e-mail: xwo@tie.cl, xworts@yahoo.com,
www.sonoskin.com

A. Baldi et al. (eds.), *Skin Cancer*, Current Clinical Pathology,
DOI 10.1007/978-1-4614-7357-2_14, © Springer Science+Business Media New York 2014

and extension of the tumors in all axes which may support one-time surgical planning [5].

The limitations of ultrasound are for lesions that measure less than 0.1 mm, the epidermal-only tumors, and the detection of pigments such as melanin [5]. However, the solid component of the primary tumor and its secondary lesions (nodal and extra-nodal) can be defined.

Thus, a very good correlation has been reported between the sonographic and histologic assessment of depth in basal cell carcinoma and melanoma [6, 7]. Furthermore, sonographic detection of subclinical basal cell carcinoma lesions has already been reported [6].

Also, ultrasonography may differentiate between melanomas that measure more or less than 1 mm depth and can assess the early anatomical changes in skin cancer, both in depth and vascularity, using a nonsurgical treatment [8].

Furthermore, the use of this noninvasive imaging technology can support the management of pleomorphic or asymmetric tumors that can show confusing histologic results due to partial samples of tissue. Also, this technique can provide a non-invasive follow-up in cases that are managed with nonsurgical treatments [9].

The objectives of ultrasonography are to provide additional and relevant information to that one already deduced by the naked eye of a well-trained physician [10]. Therefore, the assessment of anatomical sonographic patterns in the different types of skin cancer can support an early diagnosis and management and also may help to decrease the recurrence rates and improve the cosmetic prognosis of these patients [11].

Sonographic Signs in Primary Skin Cancer

Basal cell carcinoma usually appears on ultrasound as a well-defined, oval shape and hypoechoic lesion that commonly presents hyperechoic spots. Slow flow arterial and venous vessels are commonly detected at the bottom of the lesion. Occasionally, basal cell carcinoma shows pleomorphic presentations with asymmetric, bulging, lobulated or irregular appearances [12] (Figs. 14.1, 14.2 and 14.3).

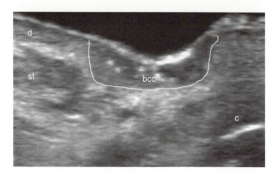

Fig. 14.1 Basal cell carcinoma gray-scale ultrasound (transverse view, tip of the nose). Hypoechoic lesion (*bcc* and *outlined*) that involves dermis and presents hyperechoic spots. The nasal cartilage is unremarkable. *Abbreviations*: *d* dermis, *st* subcutaneous tissue, *c* nasal cartilage

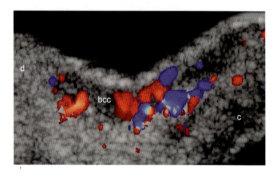

Fig. 14.2 Basal cell carcinoma color Doppler ultrasound (transverse view, tip of the nose) demonstrates increased vascularity (*colors*) within the lesion (*bcc*). *Abbreviations*: *d* dermis, *c* nasal cartilage

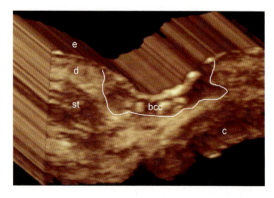

Fig. 14.3 Basal cell carcinoma 3D ultrasound reconstruction of the lesion (*bcc*, 5–8 s sweep, transverse view, tip of the nose). *Abbreviations*: *e* epidermis, *d* dermis, *st* subcutaneous tissue, *c* nasal cartilage, *bcc* basal cell carcinoma

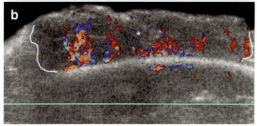

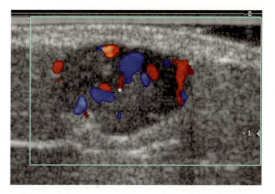

Fig. 14.5 Satellite metastasis in Melanoma. Color Doppler ultrasound (longitudinal view, left arm) demonstrates well-defined hypoechoic nodule (*asterisk*) in the hypodermis. Increased vascularity (*colors*) is detected within the nodule

Fig. 14.4 (**a**, **b**) Squamous cell carcinoma. (**a**) Grey scale ultrasound (longitudinal view, left cheek) demonstrates a 3.38 cm (long) × 1.25 cm (depth) well defined hypoechoic lesion (*asterisk*) affecting dermis and hypodermis. (**b**) Color Doppler ultrasound (transverse view, frontal region) shows ill-defined hypoechoic lesion (*asterisk* and *outlined*) that involves dermis and hypodermis. Notice the prominent blood flow within the mass (*colors*)

Squamous cell carcinoma tends to appear as a well or ill-defined hypoechoic lesion that commonly infiltrates deeper layers (for example cartilage or muscle). Importantly, intra-lesional hyperechoic spots have not been reported in squamous cell carcinoma. Vascularity is usually more prominent compared to basal cell carcinoma. On color Doppler squamous cell carcinoma usually presents slow flow arterial and venous vessels [11] (Fig. 14.4).

Melanoma, tend to show as a well-defined fusiform hypoechoic lesion that commonly present strong vascularity with slow flow vessels (arterial and venous). Hyperechoic spots have not been reported in melanoma. Ultrasound is also used to detect satellite (< 2 cm from the primary tumor), in–transit (≥ 2 cm from the primary tumor) or nodal metastases (Fig. 14.5). Locoregional sonographic staging of melanomas has allowed identification of the secondary involvement. The most common sonographic signs of malignant nodal infiltration are: balloon shape, nodular thickening of the cortex and loss of hyperechogenicity of the medullae. The anechoic areas frequently detected within the secondary lesions (extranodal or nodal) seem to be caused by the hypercellularity of the tumor rather than necrosis. Vascular density has been correlated with the metastatic potential in melanoma, and neovascularization has been described as a prognostic factor for metastasis equivalent to the Breslow index [3].

Conclusion

Ultrasound has proven to support the diagnosis of the skin cancer primary lesions and their locoregional staging. This non-invasive imaging technique can provide detailed anatomical data on extension in all axes, exact location, vascularity and deeper involvement.

Glossary

Color Doppler Ultrasound is a imaging technique which allows to visualize bloodflow. Using a Doppler effect, the US transducer detects pith changes found in vessels. A color value is assigned whether blood is moving forward or away from the transducer. In addition, color intensity will depend on the velocity of flow

HFUS High Frequency Ultrasound

Hyperechoic refers to an area that appears white. In skin malignant tumors, hyperechoic spots have been described inside basal cell carcinomas

Hypoechoic refers to an area that appears darker than the adjacent tissue. Skin malignant tumors (Basal and squamous cell carcinomas; melanomas) appear hipoechoic

Spectral curve analysis of blood flow is a tool that utilizes time, frequency, velocity and doppler signal power to give information on the blood flow. Vascular scattering can be represented as spectral wave velocity depending on time (velocity/time curve), or as dual-scale color mapping depending on the changes in average blood velocity. The flow-in is depicted in red and the flow-out in blue

References

1. Andrade P, Brites MM, Vieira R, Mariano A, Reis JP, Tellechea O, et al. Epidemiology of basal cell carcinomas and squamous cell carcinomas in a Department of Dermatology: a 5 year review. An Bras Dermatol. 2012;87:212–9.
2. Bartoš V, Pokorný D, Zacharová O, Haluska P, Doboszová J, Kullová M, et al. Recurrent basal cell carcinoma: a clinicopathological study and evaluation of histomorphological findings in primary and recurrent lesions. Acta Dermatovenerol Alp Panonica Adriat. 2011;20:67–75.
3. Wortsman X. Sonography of the primary cutaneous melanoma: a review. Radiol Res Pract. 2012;2012:814396.
4. Ekwueme DU, Guy G, Li C, Rim SH, Parelkar P, Chen SC. The health burden and economic costs of cutaneous melanoma mortality by race/ethnicity-United States, 2000 to 2006. J Am Acad Dermatol. 2011;65:S133–43.
5. Wortsman X, Wortsman J. Clinical usefulness of variable frequency ultrasound in localized lesions of the skin. J Am Acad Dermatol. 2010;62: 247–56.
6. Bobadilla F, Wortsman X, Muñoz C, Segovia L, Espinoza M, Jemec GBE. Pre-surgical high resolution ultrasound of facial basal cell carcinoma: correlation with histology. Cancer Imaging. 2008;22: 163–72.
7. Lassau N, Koscielny S, Avril MF, Margulis A, Duvillard P, De Baere T, et al. Prognostic value of angiogenesis evaluated with high-frequency and color Doppler sonography for preoperative assessment of melanomas. AJR Am J Roentgenol. 2002;178: 1547–51.
8. Music MM, Hertl K, Kadivec M, Pavlović MD, Hocevar M. Pre-operative ultrasound with a 12–15 MHz linear probe reliably differentiates between melanoma thicker and thinner than 1 mm. J Eur Acad Dermatol Venereol. 2010;24:1105–8.
9. Murchison AP, Walrath JD, Washington CV. Non-surgical treatments of primary, non-melanoma eyelid malignancies: a review. Clin Experiment Ophthalmol. 2011;39:65–83.
10. Wortsman X, Jemec G. Common inflammatory diseases of the skin: from the skin to the screen. Adv Psor Inflamm Skin Dis. 2010;2:9–15.
11. Wortsman X. Common applications of dermatologic sonography. J Ultrasound Med. 2012;31(1): 97–111.
12. Wortsman X. Sonography of facial cutaneous basal cell carcinoma: a first-line imaging technique. J Ultrasound Med. 2013;32:567–72.

Use of 22 MHz High-Frequency Ultrasound in the Management of Skin Cancer

15

Paola Pasquali, Elia Camacho,
and Angeles Fortuño-Mar

Key Points

- An underutilized noninvasive technique.
- It allows good discrimination of the skin layers.
- HFUS/HRUS provides surgeons with a preoperative information on shape and size of tumors.
- Ex vivo HFUS/HRUS lets surgeons know before histologic results whether the tumor has been completely excised.
- Trans- and post-cryosurgical procedure HFUS/HRUS allows a careful control of the freezing front.

P. Pasquali (✉)
Department of Dermatology,
Pius Hospital De Valls, Carrer Paul Cezanne 36C,
Cambrils, Tarragona 43850, Spain
e-mail: pasqualipaola@gmail.com

A. Fortuño-Mar, MD, PhD, MBA
Eldine Patologia Laboratory,
Valls, Tarragona, Spain
e-mail: af_mar@yahoo.es, afmar@comt.es

E. Camacho
Department of Dermatology,
Pius Hospital De Valls,
Pl. Sant Francesc, 1, Valls 43800, Spain

Introduction

Ultrasound provides a means of exploring the skin in a noninvasive way. It calculates different tissue parameters in vivo and gives information about skin tumors that are not available through clinical or dermoscopic examination. In normal skin, the dermis is markedly echogenic and sharply demarcated from hypoechogenic subcutaneous fat [3].

HFUS/HRUS can clearly separate lesional from extralesional areas, exogenous from endogenous components, and dermatologic from nondermatologic conditions [7]. It is a sensitive test that may add criteria for developing differential diagnoses of cutaneous lesions. It has proved to be particularly useful in outlining tumors.

BCC is the most frequent skin malignancies, rarely life-threatening, but capable of causing functional and aesthetic problems that can result from inadequate treatment, either for having used techniques too aggressive on thin tumors or for undertreating tumors that later do recurrences, hence the need for prior knowledge of the skin tumor.

The higher the frequency of the sound waves emitted by the transducer, the clearer the picture or resolution of tissues closer to the transducer [2]. The first 20 MHz ultrasound device for dermatology was developed in 1986 for commercial use (Taberna Pro Medicum). Their 22 MHz ultrasound equipment can reach a depth of 6–8 mm, with a bandwidth that goes up to 28 MHz, enabling to see the epidermis and dermis with a

A. Baldi et al. (eds.), *Skin Cancer*, Current Clinical Pathology,
DOI 10.1007/978-1-4614-7357-2_15, © Springer Science+Business Media New York 2014

resolution of over 72 μm. These devices are relatively inexpensive and easy to operate [1, 3].

Among the various uses for this equipment in dermato-oncology, we have:

- Diagnosis
- Determination of volume/depth/length of the tumor
- Control of freezing fronts in cryosurgery
- Excision margin guidance, pre- and postsurgery
- Monitoring noninvasive modalities of treatment like photodynamic therapy, radiotherapy, or topical treatments

Practical Considerations

Diagnosis

Cancerous skin tissue, chiefly basal cell carcinomas (BCC), has characteristic friability and possesses decreased signal penetration. They tend to appear more hypoechogenic than adjacent, normal dermis due to a medium change. This disturbance in acoustic impedance generates a clear, coherent image of BCC [3–5] (Fig. 15.1). The ultrasound image for BCC is that of an hypoechoic solid lesion, commonly with hyperechoic spots. A slight increase in the vascularity at the bottom of the lesion has been reported, visible with ecodoppler equipment. Squamous cell carcinoma (Fig. 15.2) is also hypoechoic, and melanoma (Fig. 15.3) appears as hypoechoic and sometimes fusiform lesions, commonly showing increased vascularity [6]. Wortsman [8] has reviewed the HFUS/HRUS findings in malignant melanoma showing its use in determining depth and vascularity as well as preoperative ultrasound-guided fine-needle aspiration cytology in nodal metastasis.

One limitation of the HFUS/HRUS is the lack of sensitivity to detect lesions localized to the epidermis or extremely thin (<0.1 mm) lesions.

HFUS/HRUS is not meant to replace histologic evaluation of BCC but may be a useful adjunct in surgical planning [3] since it allows knowing the exact measures of the lesion including the depth.

The previous knowledge of the tumor dimensions allow to choose the best treatment modality (surgical excision, cryosurgery, curettage, PDT, laser).

Determination of Volume/Depth/ Length of the Tumor

The first important consideration is to know if the image obtained with the HFUS equipment corresponds to the real tumor [9–12]. In a study done by the authors of this chapter (Pasquali P, Camacho E, Fortuny, A) and using a 22 MHz HFUS (Taberna Pro Medicum), it was determined that the length obtained by HFUS/HRUS in 57/60 BCC was larger than the one obtained by measuring the histological specimen, the average increase being 60.1 %. There was a strong correlation ($R^2 = 0.66$) among the length obtained by HFUS/HRUS and the one obtained by histology. For larger tumors, the percentage increase of the HFUS/HRUS length vs. histology length was smaller, with a medium correlation of $R^2 = 0.46$ (Fig. 15.4).

As far as the depth in 49/61 BCC, the depth obtained by HFUS/HRUS was larger than the one obtained by measuring the histological specimen, the average increase being 27 %. There was a strong correlation ($R^2 = 0.65$) among the depth obtained by HFUS/HRUS and the one obtained by histology. For larger tumors, the percentage increase of the HFUS/HRUS depth vs. histology depth was smaller, with a small correlation of $R^2 = 0.29$ (Fig. 15.5).

There is excellent correlation between dermoscopy, HFUS/HRUS, and histology of the BCCs. Dermoscopy is essential in achieving the diagnosis of a malignant tumor. It allows defining margins, and the length of the tumor obtained by dermoscopy correlates very closely with the HFUS/HRUS length. We compared the length obtained by dermoscopy (DMS), only for those cases with less than 12 mm (the largest length obtained through HFUS/HRUS). We found a strong correlation between the DMS length and the one from HFUS/HRUS ($R^2 = 0.66$) and also with the histology length ($R^2 = 0.75$) (Fig. 15.6).

From this information, the surgeon can feel confident to plan a treatment for a BCC knowing the information obtained from the dermoscopy and HFUS/HRUS.

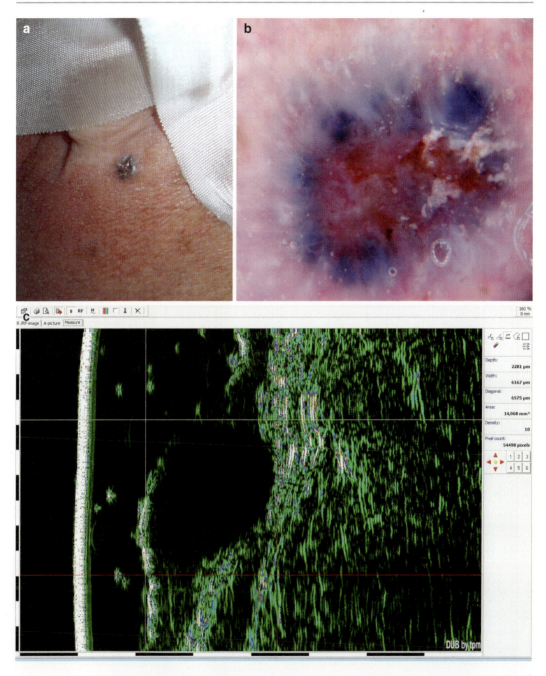

Fig. 15.1 Clinical (**a**), dermoscopic (**b**), and HFUS/HRUS (**c**) images of a retroauricular basal cell carcinoma (BCC)

Control of Freezing Fronts During a Cryosurgical Procedure

Monitoring the freezing front with HFUS/HRUS helps the cryosurgeon to visualize the extent of the freezing front and the development of the cryoinjury [13].

From the measurements mentioned above, we observed that the ratio between length and depth (L/D) for BCC was 4×1 mm (Fig. 15.7). In probe (close) cryosurgery, the iceball has an L/D ratio of 4×2 mm. In spray (open) cryosurgery, the ratio is 4×1.5 mm (Fig. 15.8). The radial distribution of the isotherms allows the surgeon to

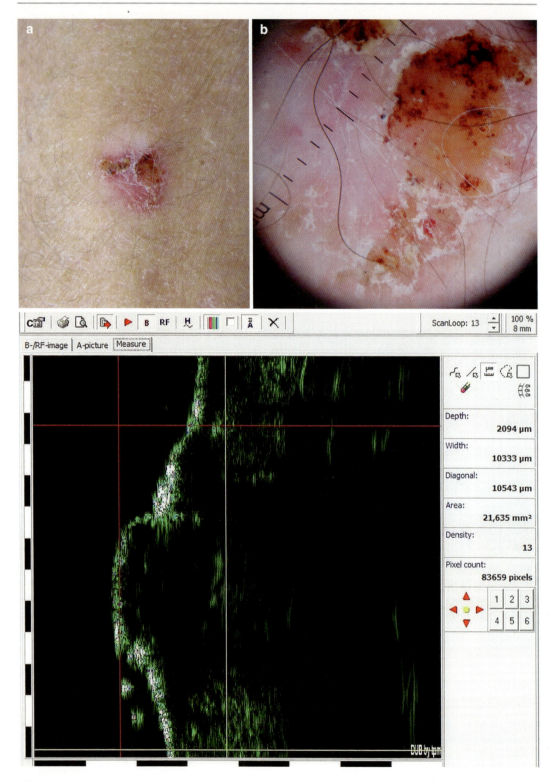

Fig. 15.2 Clinical (**a**), dermoscopic (**b**), and HFUS/HRUS (**c**) images of a squamous cell carcinoma (SCC) in the arm

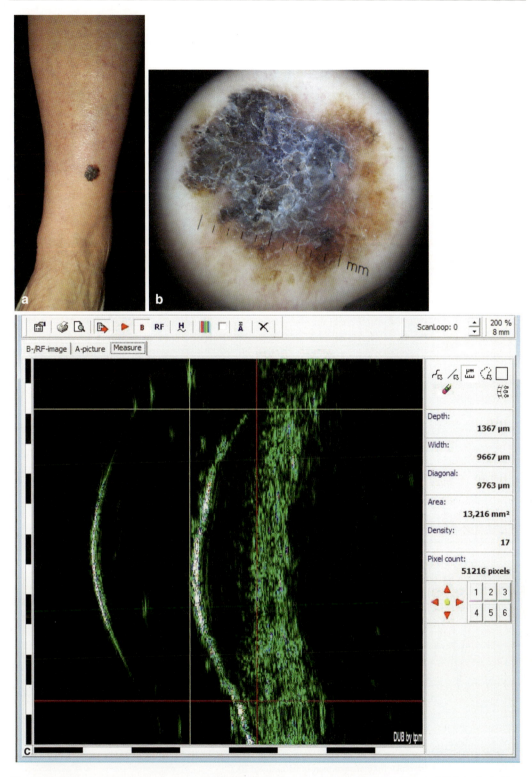

Fig. 15.3   Clinical (**a**), dermoscopic (**b**), and HFUS/HRUS (**c**) images of a malignant melanoma (MM) in the leg

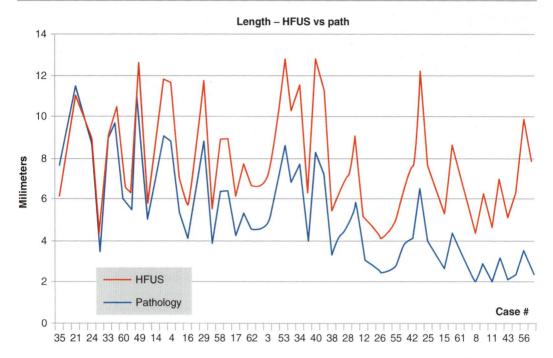

Fig. 15.4 Comparison between the length obtained by HFUS/HRUS (22 MHz Taberna Pro Medicum®) and the length obtained by measuring the histological specimen in 60 cases of BCC

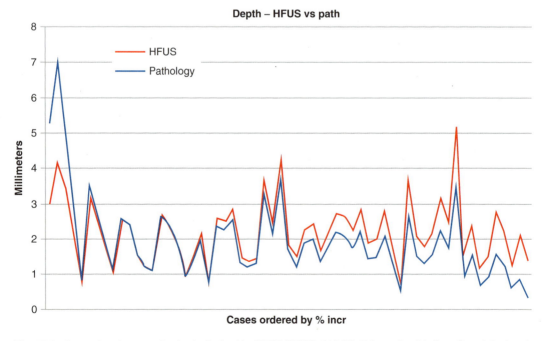

Fig. 15.5 Comparison between the depth obtained by HFUS/HRUS (22 MHz Taberna Pro Medicum®) and the length obtained by measuring the histological specimen in 61 cases of BCC

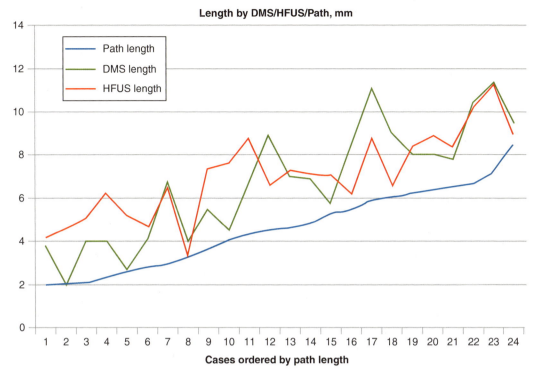

Fig. 15.6 Comparison of the length obtained from HFUS/HRUS and dermoscopy in relation to the length obtained by measuring the histological specimen in 24 cases of BCC

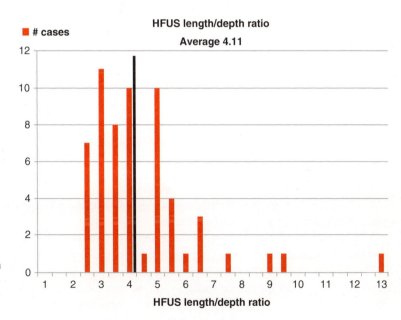

Fig. 15.7 The ratio between HFUS/HRUS length and depth from the measured BCC was 4 × 1

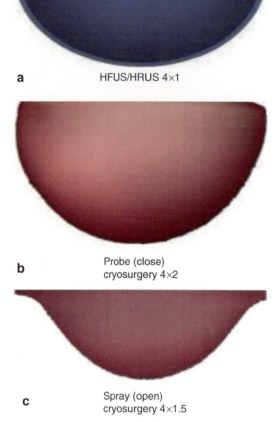

a   HFUS/HRUS 4×1

b   Probe (close)
cryosurgery 4×2

c   Spray (open)
cryosurgery 4×1.5

Fig. 15.8 Comparison between the HFUS/HRUS length/depth ratio (4 × 1) (**a**) and the iceball obtained in an experiment manner (gel) using a probe (**b**) and with a spraying tip (**c**)

know that the skin surface temperature at a given distance from the application point of LN (blue arrow in Fig. 15.9) will be the same at the depth of the tumor (Fig. 15.9).

Cancerous cells are destroyed at around −50 °C. In skin tumors, two freeze-thaw cycles are used in order to guarantee cell destruction.

HFUS/HRUS gives the cryosurgeon depth and length of the tumor as well as how far the freezing front has advanced. The latter is obtained by applying the HFUS probe immediately after freezing.

This gives the certainty that the complete and proper treatment has been done.

Immediately after freezing and with the tumor still frozen, the HFUS/HRUS shows a black area. The ultrasound images of the first and second cycle highlight the progression of the cryoinjury (Fig. 15.10).

Pre- and Postsurgical Excision Margin Guidance

An ex vivo HFUS/HRUS of skin tumors (Pasquali P, Camacho E, 2013) gives the surgeon the certainty of having removed the whole tumor, before receiving the histological confirmation (Fig. 15.11).

In vivo HFUS/HRUS locates and outlines cutaneous neoplasms [14, 15, 16] and these images correlate with ex vivo HFUS/HRUS of the same tumors.

Monitoring Noninvasive Modalities of Treatment like Photodynamic Therapy, Radiotherapy, Topical Treatments, or Cryosurgery

Monitoring noninvasive modalities with HFUS/HRUS avoids doing biopsies in areas with the clinical and/or dermoscopic suspicion of recurrence or persistence of tumor. Once a residual is identified by HFUS/HRUS, the dermatologist can proceed to indicate the most convenient treatment for the patient (Fig. 15.12). Although it does not substitute a histological confirmation, HFUS/HRUS is an extremely helpful tool in the management of patients with multiple BCC.

Conclusion and Future Considerations

HFUS/HRUS will hopefully become a more popular tool. Equipment are available nowadays with different probes (from 22 up to 100 MHz), giving the clinician a wide spectrum of possibilities. Additional clinical studies aimed to establish morphological differences between BCC subtypes as well as other malignant tumors are warranted.

Fig. 15.9 Iceball temperature can be visualized as isotherms. The temperature will be the same at both *blue arrows*. The required −50 °C should be measured at the periphery of the tumor, on the skin surface

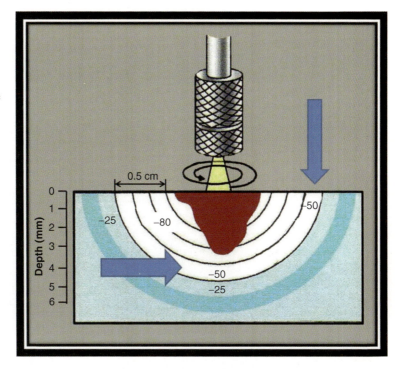

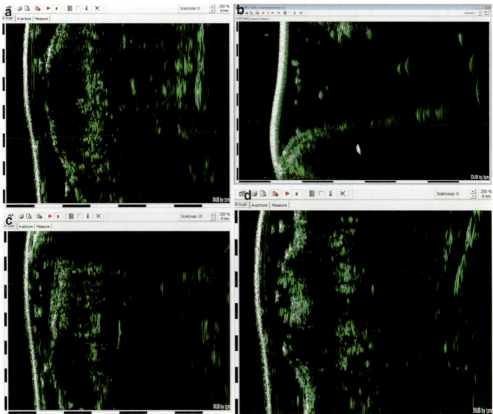

Fig. 15.10 HFUS/HRUS of (**a**) BCC (pretreatment), (**b**) with the probe applied over the frozen tumor, (**c**) after first cycle of close (probe) cryosurgery, (**d**) after second cycle of close (probe) cryosurgery

Fig. 15.11 HFUS/HRUS
of (**a**) BCC in the shoulder,
(**b**) ex vivo of the same lesion

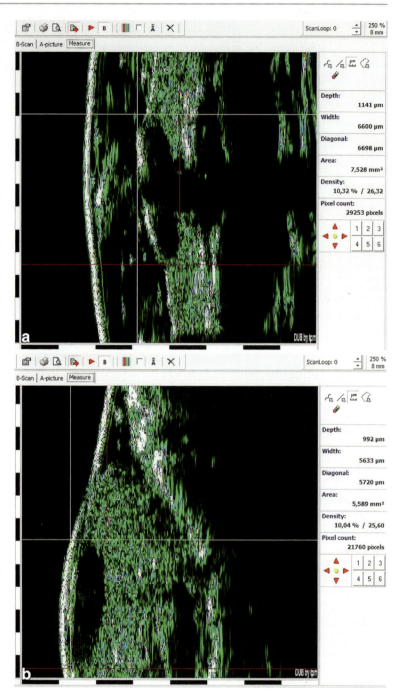

Fig. 15.12 HFUS/HRUS of residual superficial BCC lesion after topical treatment with imiquimod

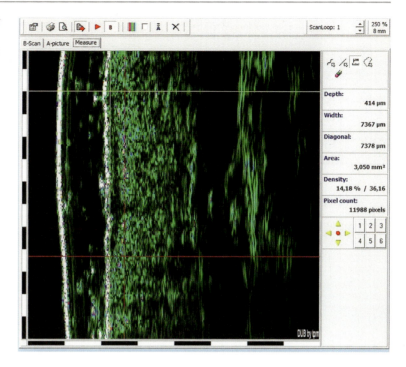

Glossary

HFUS/HRUS High Frequency Ultrasound/High Resolution Ultrasound are interchangeable terms

Isotherm line Refers to the line that connects points of equal temperature. In cryosurgery, the ice ball can be visualized by measuring isotherms

References

1. Wortsman X, Wortsman J. Clinical usefulness of variable-frequency ultrasound in localized lesions of the skin. J Am Acad Dermatol. 2010;62:247–56.
2. Kleinerman R, Whang TB, Bard RL, Marmur ES. Ultrasound in dermatology: principles and applications. J Am Acad Dermatol. 2012;67(3):478–87.
3. Hoffmann K, el Gammal S, Matthes U, Altmeyer P. Digital 20 mhz sonography of the skin in preoperative diagnosis. Z Hautkr. 1989;64(10):851–2, 855–8.
4. Hoffmann K, Stücker M, el-Gammal S, Altmeyer P. Digital 20 MHz sonography of basalioma in the B-scan. Hautarzt. 1990;41(6):333–9.
5. Machet L, Ossant F, Bleuzen A, Grégoire JM, Machet MC, Vaillant L. Léchographie cutanée haute resolution: utilité pour le diagnostic, le tratement et la surveillance des maladies dermatologiques diseases. J Radiol. 2006;87(12 Pt 2):1946–61.
6. Desai TD, Desai AD, Horowitz DC, Kartono F, Wahl T. The use of high-frequency ultrasound in the evaluation of superficial and nodular basal cell carcinomas. Dermatol Surg. 2007;33:1220–7.
7. Wortsman X. Common applications of dermatologic sonography. J Ultrasound Med. 2012;31:97–111.
8. Worstman X. Sonography of the primary cutaneous melanoma: a review. Radiol Res Pract. 2012. doi:10.1155/2012/814396.
9. Bobadilla F, Wortsman X, Muñoz C, Segovia L, Espinoza M, Jemec GBE. Pre-surgical high resolution ultrasound of facial basal cell carcinoma: correlation with histology. Cancer Imaging. 2008;8:163–72.
10. Hinz T, Ehler LK, Hornung T, Voth H, Fortmeier I, Maier T, Höller T, Schmid-Wendtner MH. Preoperative characterization of basal cell carcinoma comparing tumour thickness measurement by optical coherence tomography, 20-MHz ultrasound and histopathology. Acta Derm Venereol. 2012;92(2):132–7.
11. Nassiri-Kashani M, Sadr B, Fanian F, Kamyab K, Noormohammadpour P, Shahshahani MM, Zartab H, Naghizadeh MM, Sarraf-Yazdy M, Firooz A. Preoperative assessment of basal cell carcinoma dimensions using high frequency ultrasonography and its correlation with histopathology. Skin Res Technol. 2013;19(1):e132–8.
12. Crisan M, Crisan D, Sannino G, Lupsor M, Badea R, Amzica F. Ultrasonographic staging of cutaneous malignant tumors: an ultrasonographic depth index. Arch Dermatol Res. 2013;305(4):305–13.
13. Vaillant L, Grognard C, Machet L, Cochelin N, Callens A, Berson M, Aboumrad J, Patat F, Lorette G. Imagerie ultrasonore haute resolution: utilité pour le

tratement des carcinomas basocellualires part cryochirurgie. Ann Dermatol Venereol. 1998;125(8): 500–4.

14. Petrella LI, Valle HA, Issa PR, Martins CJ, Pereira WC, Machado JC. Study of cutaneous cell carcinomas ex vivo using ultrasound biomicroscopic images. Skin Res Technol. 2010;16(4):422–7.

15. Petrella LI, Pereira WC, Valle HA, Issa PR, Martins CJ, Machado JC. Study of superficial basal cell carcinomas and Bowen disease by qualitative and quantitative ultrasound biomicroscopy approach. Conf Proc IEEE Eng Med Biol Soc. 2010;2010: 5999–6002.

16. Petrella LI, de Azevedo Valle H, Issa PR, Martins CJ, Machado JC, Pereira WC. Statistical analysis of high frequency ultrasonic backscattered signals from basal cell carcinomas. Ultrasound Med Biol. 2012;38(10): 1811–9.

Optical Coherence Tomography

16

Mette Mogensen, Lotte Themstrup,
Christina Banzhaf, Sebastian Marschall,
Peter E. Andersen, and Gregor B.E. Jemec

Key Points

- It is an emerging non-invasive technique of relatively new application in dermatology, mostly for non-melanoma skin cancer.
- It has limited penetration but high resolution, filling the image gap between high-frequency ultrasound and confocal microscopy.
- It provides cross-sectional high-resolution skin images, thus making it possible to directly compare obtained images to standard histopathology images.

M. Mogensen, MD, PhD (✉)
Department of Dermatology,
Faculty of Health Sciences, Roskilde Hospital,
University of Copenhagen,
DK-4000 Roskilde, Denmark

Department of Dermatology, Bispebjerg Hospital,
University of Copenhagen,
Bispebjerg Bakke, Copenhagen, Denmark
e-mail: mogensen.mette@gmail.com

L. Themstrup • C. Banzhaf • G.B.E. Jemec
Department of Dermatology,
Faculty of Health Sciences, Roskilde Hospital,
University of Copenhagen,
DK-4000 Roskilde, Denmark

S. Marschall • P.E. Andersen
DTU Fotonik – Department of Photonics Engineering,
Technical University of Denmark,
Roskilde DK-4000, Denmark

Introduction

Optical coherence tomography (OCT) has developed rapidly since the first realisation in 1991 [1]. For several years, OCT has been commercially available and accepted as a clinical standard within ophthalmology diagnosing retinal diseases [1]. In dermatology, OCT has been studied in relation to photodamage, burns, nails and a variety of inflammatory and bullous diseases [2–5]. Most OCT research in dermatology has turned on non-melanoma skin cancer (NMSC) with respect to both diagnosis and non-invasive therapies. FDA-approved OCT systems are commercially available. Presently, there are more than 20 system manufacturers and many more suppliers of components and equipment [2]. Recently, the first commercial systems for intravascular imaging in cardiology were approved.

The development of various new in vivo imaging techniques in dermatology faces many challenges. Not only is skin very easily assessed by visual inspection, which for some Dermatologists rule out novel imaging techniques, but it is also a large area to scan compared the fx the retina [2]. In contrast to imaging of the eye, skin morphology provides an optical challenge to any imaging technique looking beyond the surface.

OCT has a limited penetration depth, but it provides a high resolution, which places OCT in the imaging gap between high-frequency ultrasound and confocal microscopy [2, 6, 7] (see Fig. 16.1). Studies have found good agreement between OCT images and histopathological

A. Baldi et al. (eds.), *Skin Cancer*, Current Clinical Pathology,
DOI 10.1007/978-1-4614-7357-2_16, © Springer Science+Business Media New York 2014

architecture of skin cancer, and OCT also allows non-invasive monitoring of morphological changes in skin diseases. This implies that OCT may have a particular role in the monitoring of medical treatment of, e.g. non-melanoma skin cancer, and therefore therapeutic monitoring has become the focus of some OCT studies [8].

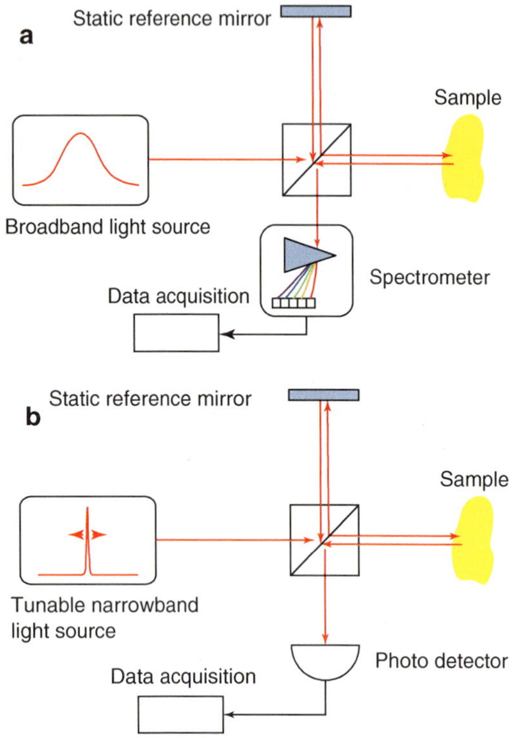

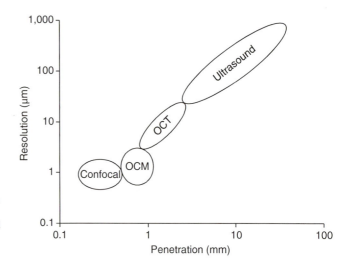

Fig. 16.1 In FD-OCT, each depth scan is performed by sampling the interference pattern in optical frequency space, either with a spectrometer and a broadband light source (**a**) or with a photo detector and a tunable narrow-band light source (**b**). In both cases, the reference mirror remains at a fixed position

Basic Principles

Optical coherence tomography is an interferometric technique that detects reflected or backscattered light from tissue. OCT probes the sample with a beam of light and lets the reflections interfere with a reference beam originating from the same light source. From the resulting interference signal, one can derive the reflectivity profile along the beam axis. This one-dimensional depth scan is called A-scan, in analogy to ultrasound imaging. OCT systems perform many adjacent A-scans in order to create two- or three-dimensional images of the sample. The scan speed allows video-rate imaging of three-dimensional volumes.

A-scans can be acquired either in the *time domain* (TD) or in the *frequency domain* (FD). TD-OCT systems (Fig. 16.2) were the first to be implemented [6]. These perform the depth scan based on low-coherence interferometry (LCI) which had previously been applied for one-dimensional length measurements of human eyes in vivo [9]. By using light with broad spectral bandwidth and thus low-coherence length, only backreflections from the sample with a round-trip path approximately equal to the reference path

Fig. 16.2 OCT and optical coherence microscopy (*OCM*) close the gap between high-resolution optical microscopy techniques (e.g. confocal microscopy) and techniques with long penetration depth (e.g. ultrasound imaging)

Fig. 16.3 Typically, an OCT system is based on a Michelson interferometer that directs a fraction of the light to the sample and the remaining part to a reference mirror. The backreflections from both arms interfere on a photo detector. In TD-OCT, the depth scan is performed by translating the reference mirror

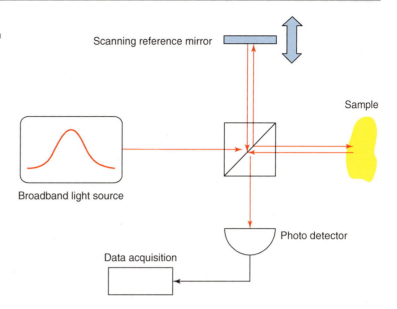

can interfere with the reference beam. This condition creates a spatial gate as wide as the coherence length of the light that selectively interrogates the backreflection from a certain depth within the sample. This *coherence gate* is shifted along the probing beam axis by changing the length of the reference path. Adjacent structures can be separated in a depth profile if they are further apart than the width of the coherence gate. Thus, the lower the temporal coherence of the probing light is, or the broader the bandwidth, respectively, the higher is the depth resolution.

An FD-OCT system acquires A-scans with a fixed reference path by measuring the spectral response of the interferometer [10]. The information is then encoded as an interferogram in optical frequency space, a sum of oscillations with different periods corresponding to reflections from different depths. A Fourier transform of this interferogram reveals the reflectivity profile of the sample. The same relation between bandwidth and depth resolution as in TD-OCT is also valid for FD-OCT.

Two basic approaches exist for implementing FD-OCT. One can illuminate the interferometer with broadband light and separate the spectral components with a spectrometer at the output [11, 12] (Fig. 16.3a). This method is termed *spectral domain-OCT* (SD-OCT). Alternatively, one can

probe with different optical frequencies sequentially and measure the power at the output with a single photo detector [13–15] (Fig. 16.3b). With a tunable narrowband light source, one performs a sweep over a broad range of optical frequencies, which led to the term *swept source-OCT* (SS-OCT).

Optical coherence tomography is often described as the optical analogue to ultrasound, as it probes the sample with light instead of sound and maps the reflectivity as a function of depth. The main strength of OCT is the depth resolution or *axial resolution* which is linked to the light source spectral shape. Typically, the axial resolution is around 5–10 μm in tissue, even though depth resolution down to 1 μm or less is possible [16–18].

Most optical microscopy techniques achieve high axial and transverse resolution with a high numerical aperture (NA) objective [19]. In contrast, OCT gains axial resolution from the coherence gate, and one uses typically a low NA objective that provides a long depth of focus covering the entire imaging depth range. Hence, the *transverse resolution* is usually moderate (several 10 μm). However, one can implement *optical coherence microscopy* (OCM), where so-called en face images are acquired in a plane transverse to the probing beam [20]. OCM combines the high spatial resolution of confocal microscopy

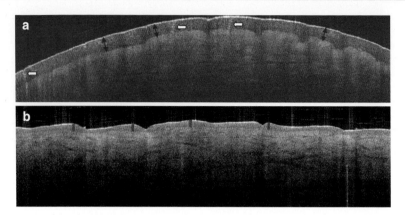

Fig. 16.4 Normal skin (**a**) demonstrates the OCT morphology of the normal fingertip skin. The stratum corneum is thick (*black double arrows*) and the spiral-shaped sweat ducts are seen penetrating the layer (*white arrows*). (**b**) OCT image of the skin of the lower arm – the stratum corneum is too thin to be imaged here, but the epidermis is easily delineated (*red lines*). OCT image recorded with an OCT system from Michelson Diagnostics

with the depth-selective coherence gate of OCT achieving high-resolution imaging transversely and longitudinally.

The penetration depth into scattering samples is limited, 2–3 μm typically for skin at 1.3 μm centre wavelength, which is nevertheless higher than what other high-resolution optical techniques, e.g. confocal microscopy [19], can achieve.

The choice between SD-OCT and SS-OCT depends mainly on the operating wavelength range [21]. For wavelengths below 1 μm, SD-OCT is favoured because silicon-based line cameras with sufficient pixel number and high read-out speed are readily available. Higher wavelengths require InGaAs-based cameras that are more expensive and not yet as technologically advanced. Therefore, above 1 μm SS-OCT is preferred, which is then the preferred choice for future systems applied in dermatological OCT. Operating at wavelengths in the range between 1 and 1.5 μm facilitates highest penetration into biological tissues [22]. Note, however, that operation at higher centre wavelengths might reduce the axial resolution due to increased demand for source bandwidth. In recent years, FD-OCT has become the preferred realisation due to its significantly higher imaging speed. FD-OCT allows for very high A-scan rates, because it requires no mechanical scanning of the reference path length. The scan speed allows video-rate imaging of three-dimensional volumes.

Practical Considerations and Applications

OCT Imaging of Normal Skin

The skin is unfortunately not an ideal optical medium. It is an optically complex, variable and multilayered optical structure that poses many problems to imaging. The penetration depth of OCT is highly tissue dependent and is typically limited to a maximum of 2 mm. OCT can reliably identify epidermis and the dermo-epidermal junction [23–25]. It is also able to identify the normal regional differences [24]. In glabrous skin, the stratum corneum presents as a thick hyporeflective granular-textured layer below a hyperreflective border of the skin surface. OCT images from glabrous skin show eccrine sweat gland ducts as hyperreflective coiling structures penetrating the stratum corneum (Fig. 16.4a). In comparison, follicular skin has distinct morphological differences. In follicular skin the stratum corneum layer is not defined and there are no identifiable eccrine sweat gland ducts. Furthermore, hair follicles and sebaceous glands tend to reduce the quality of the OCT images, and therefore, the follicular dermo-epidermal junction is not always as defined as in glabrous skin (Fig. 16.4b).

In general, structures that are anatomically well defined also produce well-defined OCT images, e.g. the nail [5]. Furthermore, quantitative

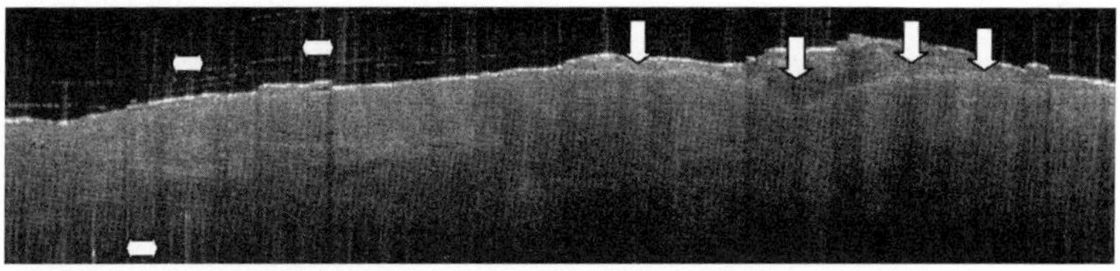

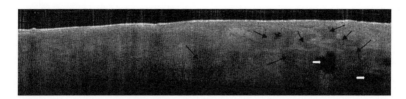

Fig. 16.5 An actinic keratosis lesion on the scalp. The thick dysplastic epidermis is shown (*vertical white arrowheads*) and the epidermis itself has lost the clear-cut layering. Hyperkeratosis tends to induce vertical white artefacts in the OCT image (*horizontal arrowheads*). OCT image recorded with an OCT system from Michelson Diagnostics

Fig. 16.6 Basal cell carcinoma on the forehead. The lobular pattern of basal cell carcinoma islands is recognised in the OCT image as grey rounded areas (*black arrowheads*). Necrosis is also seen as black well-defined areas (*white arrowheads*). OCT image recorded with an OCT system from Michelson Diagnostics

effects of age, gender, skin type and colour, anatomic site and external stimuli on the epidermal thickness have been described using OCT [23, 24, 26, 27].

OCT Imaging of Non-melanoma Skin Cancer

Non-melanoma skin cancer (NMSC) has been a natural focus for applied OCT research and it has been widely investigated [3, 25, 28–41]. The studies have mainly focused on actinic keratosis (AK) and basal cell carcinoma (BCC). Squamous cell carcinoma (SCC) has predominantly been examined on oral mucosal surfaces [42, 43], although a few SCC skin lesions have recently been examined with OCT [8, 44]. The changes described in SCC appear quite similar to those seen in BCC, but SCC tends to be more hyperkeratotic.

The studies on NMSC indicate that the characteristic layering of normal skin [23, 24, 26] found in OCT is lost in NMSC [3, 7, 29, 32, 35–37, 45]. Loss of normal OCT architecture may also be seen in various benign lesions [46]; however, other OCT characteristics of malignant lesions have been found. In AK lesions these include focal

thickening of epidermis [29, 47], hyperreflective streaks and also signal-poor irregular bands in the epidermis corresponding to keratin deposits [7, 44, 46, 47] (Fig. 16.5). OCT images of BCC lesions show dark rounded areas sometimes surrounded by white halo corresponding to islands of carcinoma basal cells and surrounding stromal tissue. In lesions with necrotic areas, the necrosis can be visualised as well-circumscribed black, i.e. signal poor, areas [7, 37, 44–46] (Fig. 16.6).

One advantage of OCT is that it provides cross-sectional high-resolution skin images, thus making it possible to directly compare obtained images to standard histopathology images. Several studies have suggested high correlation between OCT images and histopathology in BCC lesions [1, 30, 32, 33, 37, 45]; however, BCC subtypes could not be identified in OCT images [37, 40]. This also means that OCT may be of use in identifying residual tumour tissue in Mohs micrographic surgery [48].

In spite of the high correlation between OCT and histopathology, image quality of NMSC lesions does vary and some lesions appear blurred and poorly delineated. A study examined histological characteristics of BCC lesions associated with good OCT image quality [49]. The study finds that the presence of solar elastosis makes for

Fig. 16.7 Compound dysplastic naevus with atypical features. In (**a**), the well-defined elongation of rete ridges and melanocytes is marked by *black arrows*. In (**b**), the subtle variation in nuclear cytology and finely dispersed cytoplasmic melanin particles, arranged predominantly not only in nests but also as solitary units, along the dermo-epidermal junction, is seen. Some of the melanocytes contain enlarged and pleomorphic nuclei. Some intraepidermal nests are horizontally elongated with bridging of rete ridges (Courtesy of Professor Dan Siegel. OCT image recorded with an OCT system from Michelson Diagnostics)

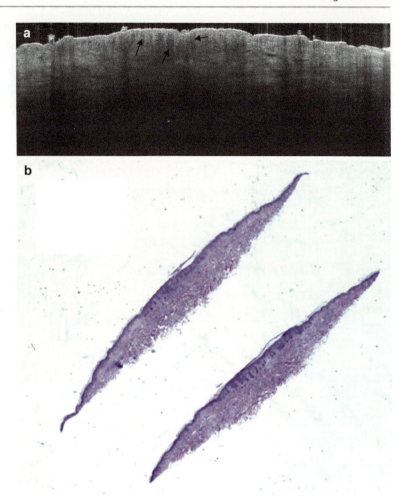

higher-quality OCT images, while inflammatory infiltrates significantly impair OCT imaging of BCC lesions. Reassuringly, neither ulceration nor hyperkeratoses seemed to impair OCT imaging of BCC significantly.

OCT Imaging of Malignant Melanomas (MM)

Because melanin is a strong scatterer of light and because malignant melanomas are usually pigmented neoplasms, MM imaging by techniques based on the penetration of light has proven more difficult to obtain. In ophthalmology, the use of OCT was studied in choroidal melanomas [50, 51], but only a few studies have investigated the use of OCT in melanocytic skin lesions [52–54].

Because cellular features cannot be visualised with OCT, disease diagnosis must rely on change in the skin morphology [1, 54]. In OCT images the most striking architectural feature of MM is the presence of vertical icicle-shaped structures, corresponding to dense infiltrates of tumour cells and lymphocytes [53]. In Fig. 16.7, a dysplastic compound naevus has been OCT imaged compared to histology. The dysplasia is however difficult to acknowledge in the OCT image.

Indications and Contraindications

OCT provides high accuracy in distinguishing lesions from normal skin [29, 46, 47, 55], which is of great importance in identifying tumour borders. In differentiating normal skin from lesions, a sensitivity of 79–94 % and specificity of 85–96 % were found for OCT. Discrimination of AK from BCC was not possible in this study [46]. Diagnosis of AK ranged in sensitivity from 73 to 100 % and the specificity from 65 to 70 % [29, 47].

Accurate measurements of tumour thickness may be more difficult to acquire in thick tumours that stretch beyond the 2 mm penetration of the OCT signal [56]. OCT measurements, however, seem more precise and less biased than high-frequency ultrasound thickness measurements of thin AK and BCC lesions [7]. Thin carcinomas and AK are of particular interest to non-invasive imaging as they are already amenable to treatment with non-invasive therapies such as photodynamic therapy (PDT), topical fluorouracil and topical imiquimod [57]. Also, OCT may be useful as a non-invasive monitoring tool during treatment. OCT-guided PDT is one of the promising approaches to discriminate tumour margins [8], and OCT could potentially allow for more precise individual adjustments of topical and nonsurgical therapies. This aspect of OCT is currently being studied.

In order to improve OCT image quality and expand the potential of OCT, technical developments are necessary. Several possibilities exist for developing OCT. Newer OCT modalities include the use of speckle reduction, polarisation-sensitive (PS) OCT, *en face* OCT, OCT elastography and wavelength-dependent OCT. Also, combining OCT with other functional information such as Raman spectroscopy, multimodal photoacoustic and optical coherence tomography PAT-OCT [58] or Doppler could make OCT images more informative [39, 45, 46, 58–63]. Finally, the introduction of image analysis as speckle reduction and machine learning algorithms may provide a more precise classification of AK and BCC lesions than relying on the human eye alone [2, 64].

In distinguishing MM from benign naevi, a general architectural disarray and unclear dermoepidermal junction have been suggested as important OCT features [53]. Sensitivity and specificity studies have not been performed, and the full potential of OCT in MM diagnosis therefore remains to be described.

OCT is capable of *real-time* imaging and, using nonionising near-infrared light, safe for repeated examinations. Hence, it is a valuable complement to other clinical tomography modalities like ultrasound imaging, magnetic resonance tomography or X-ray computed tomography (Fig. 16.1).

Many academic indications exist for using OCT as an investigative tool in scientific studies of pathogenic processes, and in addition, the OCT technology is rapidly maturing to achieve clinical utility in a more routine setting. It has been suggested that ex vivo or in vivo OCT may provide rapid and accurate histopathological diagnosis in conjunction with excisions or during Mohs surgery [65] or utilising the fact that staining of the tissue is not necessary in OCT [48].

The inherent safety of the technology allows for in vivo use of OCT in patients. It is suggested that the technology will be of particular interest to the routine follow-up of patients undergoing non-invasive therapy of malignant or premalignant keratinocyte tumours. The clinical decision to repeat or supplement therapy is generally based on the dichotomous question: Is there any abnormal tissue left? This is currently done clinically, but OCT carries the potential to adequately answer this question in high-risk patients better than clinical judgement alone.

Future Considerations

Skin imaging technologies in dermatology are in a tough competitive environment. The ease and tradition for clinical inspection of the skin coupled with the relative ease of biopsies have meant that the first step for any new imaging technique is very high. Nevertheless, there are at least three factors speaking in favour of the continued development of skin imaging techniques. Firstly, the non-invasive diagnostic methods allow for a more precise monitoring of therapeutic progress of all skin diseases; this potentially enables the treatment to be modified according to the response at an earlier point optimising treatment outcomes for patients. Hence, non-invasive monitoring of disease processes also allows for longitudinal studies of disease evolution and possibly patho-genesis. Secondly, in NMSC a number of non-invasive therapies are being increasingly used, e.g. photodynamic therapy and imiquimod. The advantages of a non-scarring nonsurgical treatment are to some degree reduced if the diagnosis depends on a biopsy. Thirdly, some patients, i.e. organ transplant recipient, display a great number of suspicious lesions, making individual biopsies very laborious and potentially disfiguring.

OCT is an emerging technology in the diagnosis of skin disease. The methodology provides an advantageous combination of resolution and penetration depth, but specific studies of diagnostic sensitivity and specificity are sparse [46, 47]. Because it is an emerging technology, such studies will however have to be repeated over time as the technology matures, in order to give a fair representation of its full potential. It is speculated that the continued technological development can propel the method to a greater level of dermatological use. Currently, dermatological OCT enthusiasts are working together to standardise the OCT vocabularium when describing skin morphology and pathology.

Glossary

TD-OCT Time domain OCT

FD-OTC Frequency domain OCT

LCI Low-coherence interferometry

OCT Optical coherence tomography. It is an interferometric technique that detects reflected or backscattered light from tissue

OCM Optical coherence microscopy

Michelson interferometer The principle of OCT is white light or low coherence interferometry. The optical setup typically consists of an interferometer, typically a Michelson type, with a low coherence, broad bandwidth light source

SD-OCT Spectral domain-OCT

SS-OCT Swept source-OCT

Axial resolution The axial and lateral resolutions of OCT are decoupled from one another; the former being an equivalent to the coherence length of the light source

Transverse resolution is defined as a function of the optics, as opposed to axial resolution

that matches the coherence length of the light source

InGaAs-based cameras Deep-cooled camera systems that employ indium gallium arsenide. These are cameras with focal plane arrays (FPAs) that can both amplify and broaden the utility of near infrared (NIR) and shortwave infrared (SWIR) regions of the spectrum

References

1. Marschall S, Sander B, Mogensen M, Jorgensen TM, Andersen PE. Optical coherence tomography-current technology and applications in clinical and biomedical research. Anal Bioanal Chem. 2011;400(9):2699–720.

2. Mogensen M, Thrane L, Jorgensen TM, Andersen PE, Jemec GB. OCT imaging of skin cancer and other dermatological diseases. J Biophotonics. 2009;2(6–7):442–51.

3. Steiner R, Kunzi-Rapp K, Scharffetter-Kochanek K. Optical coherence tomography: clinical applications in dermatology. Med Laser Appl. 2003;18(3):249–59.

4. Mogensen M, Morsy HA, Nurnberg BM, Jemec GB. Optical coherence tomography imaging of bullous diseases. J Eur Acad Dermatol Venereol. 2008;22(12):1458–64.

5. Mogensen M, Thomsen JB, Skovgaard LT, Jemec GB. Nail thickness measurements using optical coherence tomography and 20-MHz ultrasonography. Br J Dermatol. 2007;157(5):894–900.

6. Huang D, Swanson EA, Lin CP, Schuman JS, Stinson WG, Chang W, et al. Optical coherence tomography. Science. 1991;254(5035):1178–81.

7. Mogensen M, Nurnberg BM, Forman JL, Thomsen JB, Thrane L, Jemec GB. In vivo thickness measurement of basal cell carcinoma and actinic keratosis with optical coherence tomography and 20-MHz ultrasound. Br J Dermatol. 2009;160(5):1026–33.

8. Hamdoon Z, Jerjes W, Upile T, Hopper C. Optical coherence tomography-guided photodynamic therapy for skin cancer: case study. Photodiagnosis Photodyn Ther. 2011;8(1):49–52.

9. Fercher AF, Mengedoht K, Werner W. Eye-length measurement by interferometry with partially coherent light. Opt Lett. 1988;13(3):186–8.

10. Fercher AF, Hitzenberger CK, Kamp G, El-Zaiat SY. Measurement of intraocular distances by backscattering spectral interferometry. Opt Commun. 1995;117(1–2):43–8.

11. Bail MA, Häusler G, Herrmann JM, Lindner MW, Ringler R. Optical coherence tomography with the "spectral radar": fast optical analysis in volume scatterers by short-coherence interferometry. Proc SPIE. 1996;2925:298–303.

12. Häusler G, Lindner MW. 'Coherence radar' and 'spectral radar' – new tools for dermatological diagnosis. J Biomed Opt. 1998;3(1):21–31.

13. Chinn SR, Swanson EA, Fujimoto JG. Optical coherence tomography using a frequency-tunable optical source. Opt Lett. 1997;22(5):340–2.

14. Golubovic B, Bouma BE, Tearney GJ, Fujimoto JG. Optical frequency-domain reflectometry using rapid wavelength tuning of a Cr4+: forsterite laser. Opt Lett. 1997;22(22):1704–6.

15. Haberland U, Rütten W, Blazek V, Schmitt HJ. Investigation of highly scattering media using near-infrared continuous wave tunable semiconductor laser. Proc SPIE. 1995;2389:503–12.

16. Drexler W. Ultrahigh-resolution optical coherence tomography. J Biomed Opt. 2004;9(1):47–74.

17. Hartl I, Li XD, Chudoba C, Ghanta RK, Ko TH, Fujimoto JG, et al. Ultrahigh-resolution optical coherence tomography using continuum generation in an air-silica microstructure optical fiber. Opt Lett. 2001;26(9):608–10.

18. Považay B, Bizheva K, Unterhuber A, Hermann B, Sattmann H, Fercher AF, et al. Submicrometer axial resolution optical coherence tomography. Opt Lett. 2002;27(20):1800–2.

19. Inoué S. Foundations of confocal scanned imaging in light microscopy. In: Pawley JB, editor. Handbook of biological confocal microscopy. 3 ed. Springer: New York; 2006.

20. Izatt JA, Hee MR, Owen GM, Swanson EA, Fujimoto JG. Optical coherence microscopy in scattering media. Opt Lett. 1994;19(8):590–2.

21. Bouma BE, Yun S-H, Vakoc BJ, Suter MJ, Tearney GJ. Fourier-domain optical coherence tomography: recent advances toward clinical utility. Curr Opin Biotechnol. 2009;20(1):111–8.

22. Parrish JA. New concepts in therapeutic photomedicine; photochemistry, optical targeting and the therapeutic window. J Invest Dermatol. 1981;77(1):45–50.

23. Gambichler T, Matip R, Moussa G, Altmeyer P, Hoffmann K. In vivo data of epidermal thickness evaluated by optical coherence tomography: effects of age, gender, skin type, and anatomic site. J Dermatol Sci. 2006;44(3):145–52.

24. Mogensen M, Morsy HA, Thrane L, Jemec GB. Morphology and epidermal thickness of normal skin imaged by optical coherence tomography. Dermatology. 2008;217(1):14–20.

25. Welzel J, Lankenau E, Birngruber R, Engelhardt R. Optical coherence tomography of the human skin. J Am Acad Dermatol. 1997;37(6):958–63.

26. Welzel J, Reinhardt C, Lankenau E, Winter C, Wolff HH. Changes in function and morphology of normal human skin: evaluation using optical coherence tomography. Br J Dermatol. 2004;150(2):220–5.

27. Querleux B, Baldeweck T, Diridollou S, de Rigal J, Huguet E, Leroy F, et al. Skin from various ethnic origins and aging: an in vivo cross-sectional multimodality imaging study. Skin Res Technol. 2009;15(3):306–13.

28. Abuzahra F, Baron JM. Optical coherence tomography of the skin: a diagnostic light look. Hautarzt. 2006;57(7):646–7.

29. Barton JK, Gossage KW, Xu W, Ranger-Moore JR, Saboda K, Brooks CA, et al. Investigating sun-damaged skin and actinic keratosis with optical coherence tomography: a pilot study. Technol Cancer Res Treat. 2003;2(6):525–35.

30. Bechara FG, Gambichler T, Stucker M, Orlikov A, Rotterdam S, Altmeyer P, et al. Histomorphologic correlation with routine histology and optical coherence tomography. Skin Res Technol. 2004;10(3):169–73.

31. Gladkova ND, Petrova GA, Nikulin NK, Radenska-Lopovok SG, Snopova LB, Chumakov YP, et al. In vivo optical coherence tomography imaging of human skin: norm and pathology. Skin Res Technol. 2000;6(1):6–16.

32. Olmedo JM, Warschaw KE, Schmitt JM, Swanson DL. Optical coherence tomography for the characterization of basal cell carcinoma in vivo: a pilot study. J Am Acad Dermatol. 2006;55(3):408–12.

33. Olmedo JM, Warschaw KE, Schmitt JM, Swanson DL. Correlation of thickness of basal cell carcinoma by optical coherence tomography in vivo and routine histologic findings: a pilot study. Dermatol Surg. 2007;33(4):421–5; discussion 5–6.

34. Welzel J. Optical coherence tomography. Hautarzt. 2010;61(5):416–20.

35. Welzel J. Optical coherence tomography in dermatology: a review. Skin Res Technol. 2001;7(1):1–9.

36. Pierce MC, Strasswimmer J, Park BH, Cense B, de Boer JF. Advances in optical coherence tomography imaging for dermatology. J Invest Dermatol. 2004;123(3):458–63.

37. Gambichler T, Orlikov A, Vasa R, Moussa G, Hoffmann K, Stucker M, et al. In vivo optical coherence tomography of basal cell carcinoma. J Dermatol Sci. 2007;45(3):167–73.

38. Ulrich M, Stockfleth E, Roewert-Huber J, Astner S. Noninvasive diagnostic tools for nonmelanoma skin cancer. Br J Dermatol. 2007;157 Suppl 2:56–8.

39. Strasswimmer J, Pierce M, Park B, et al. Characterization of basal cell carcinoma by multifunctional optical coherence tomography. J Invest Dermatol. 2003;121:156.

40. Jensen L, Thrane L, Andersen P, et al. Optical coherence tomography in clinical examination of non-pigmented skin malignancies. Proc SPIE-OSA Biomed Opt SPIE. 2003;5140:160–7.

41. Andretzky P, Lindner M, Herrmann J, et al. Optical coherence tomography by spectral radar: dynamic range estimation and in vivo measurements of skin. Proc SPIE. 1998;3567:78–87.

42. Jerjes W, Upile T, Conn B, Hamdoon Z, Betz CS, McKenzie G, et al. In vitro examination of suspicious oral lesions using optical coherence tomography. Br J Oral Maxillofac Surg. 2010;48(1):18–25.

43. Wilder-Smith P, Jung WG, Brenner M, Osann K, Beydoun H, Messadi D, et al. In vivo optical coherence tomography for the diagnosis of oral malignancy. Lasers Surg Med. 2004;35(4):269–75.

44. Forsea AM, Carstea EM, Ghervase L, Giurcaneanu C, Pavelescu G. Clinical application of optical coherence tomography for the imaging of non-melanocytic cutaneous tumors: a pilot multi-modal study. J Med Life. 2010;3(4):381–9.

45. Khandwala M, Penmetsa BR, Dey S, Schofield JB, Jones CA, Podoleanu A. Imaging of periocular basal cell carcinoma using en face optical coherence tomography: a pilot study. Br J Ophthalmol. 2010;94(10): 1332–6.

46. Mogensen M, Joergensen TM, Nurnberg BM, Morsy HA, Thomsen JB, Thrane L, et al. Assessment of optical coherence tomography imaging in the diagnosis of non-melanoma skin cancer and benign lesions versus normal skin: observer-blinded evaluation by dermatologists and pathologists. Dermatol Surg. 2009;35(6): 965–72.

47. Korde VR, Bonnema GT, Xu W, Krishnamurthy C, Ranger-Moore J, Saboda K, et al. Using optical coherence tomography to evaluate skin sun damage and precancer. Lasers Surg Med. 2007;39(9):687–95.

48. Cunha D, Richardson T, Sheth N, Orchard G, Coleman A, Mallipeddi R. Comparison of ex vivo optical coherence tomography with conventional frozen-section histology for visualizing basal cell carcinoma during Mohs micrographic surgery. Br J Dermatol. 2011;165(3):576–80.

49. Mogensen M, Nurnberg BM, Thrane L, Jorgensen TM, Andersen PE, Jemec GB. How histological features of basal cell carcinomas influence image quality in optical coherence tomography. J Biophotonics. 2011;4(7–8):544–51.

50. Say EA, Shah SU, Ferenczy S, Shields CL. Optical coherence tomography of retinal and choroidal tumors. J Ophthalmol. 2011;2011:385058.

51. Bianciotto C, Shields CL, Guzman JM, Romanelli-Gobbi M, Mazzuca Jr D, Green WR, et al. Assessment of anterior segment tumors with ultrasound biomicroscopy versus anterior segment optical coherence tomography in 200 cases. Ophthalmology. 2011; 118(7):1297–302.

52. de Giorgi V, Stante M, Massi D, Mavilia L, Cappugi P, Carli P. Possible histopathologic correlates of dermoscopic features in pigmented melanocytic lesions identified by means of optical coherence tomography. Exp Dermatol. 2005;14(1):56–9.

53. Gambichler T, Regeniter P, Bechara FG, Orlikov A, Vasa R, Moussa G, et al. Characterization of benign and malignant melanocytic skin lesions using optical coherence tomography in vivo. J Am Acad Dermatol. 2007;57(4):629–37.

54. Smith L, Macneil S. State of the art in non-invasive imaging of cutaneous melanoma. Skin Res Technol. 2011;17:257–69.

55. Petrova G, Derpalyek E, Gladkova N, et al. Optical coherence tomography using tissue clearing for skin disease diagnosis. Proc SPIE. 2003;5140: 168–86.

56. Buchwald HJ, Muller A, Kampmeier J, Lang GK. Optical coherence tomography versus ultrasound biomicroscopy of conjunctival and eyelid lesions. Klin Monbl Augenheilkd. 2003;220(12): 822–9.

57. Wennberg AM. Basal cell carcinoma–new aspects of diagnosis and treatment. Acta Derm Venereol Suppl (Stockh). 2000;209:5–25.

58. Zhang EZ, Povazay B, Laufer J, Alex A, Hofer B, Pedley B, et al. Multimodal photoacoustic and optical coherence tomography scanner using an all optical detection scheme for 3D morphological skin imaging. Biomed Opt Express. 2011;2(8):2202–15.

59. Mogensen M, Jorgensen TM, Thrane L, Nurnberg BM, Jemec GB. Improved quality of optical coherence tomography imaging of basal cell carcinomas using speckle reduction. Exp Dermatol. 2010;19(8): e293–5.

60. Strasswimmer J, Pierce MC, Park BH, Neel V, de Boer JF. Polarization-sensitive optical coherence tomography of invasive basal cell carcinoma. J Biomed Opt. 2004;9(2):292–8.

61. Patil CA, Kirshnamoorthi H, Ellis DL, van Leeuwen TG, Mahadevan-Jansen A. A clinical instrument for combined Raman spectroscopy-optical coherence tomography of skin cancers. Lasers Surg Med. 2011;43(2):143–51.

62. Gambichler T, Moussa G, Sand M, Sand D, Altmeyer P, Hoffmann K. Applications of optical coherence tomography in dermatology. J Dermatol Sci. 2005; 40(2):85–94.

63. Patel JK, Konda S, Perez OA, Amini S, Elgart G, Berman B. Newer technologies/techniques and tools in the diagnosis of melanoma. Eur J Dermatol. 2008; 18(6):617–31.

64. Jorgensen TM, Tycho A, Mogensen M, Bjerring P, Jemec GB. Machine-learning classification of non-melanoma skin cancers from image features obtained by optical coherence tomography. Skin Res Technol. 2008;14(3):364–9.

65. Pomerantz R, Zell D, McKenzied G, Siegel DM. Optical coherence tomography used as a modality to delineate basal cell carcinoma prior to Mohs micrographic surgery. Case Rep Dermatol. 2011;3: 212–8.

Reflectance Confocal Microscopy in Skin Cancer   17

Salvador Gonzalez, Virginia Sanchez,
Susanne Lange-Asschenfeldt,
and Martina Ulrich

Key Points

- Reflectance confocal microscopy (RCM) is a novel in vivo, noninvasive imaging method and real-time examination of the skin.
- It consists of a low-power, near-infrared laser light source attached to a confocal microscope, which illuminates a small skin area with a resolution comparable to conventional histology.
- It provides in vivo real-time images of the skin in a horizontal bright gray scale.

S. Gonzalez (✉)
Dermatology Service,
Ramon y Cajal Hospital, Alcalá University,
Madrid, Spain

Dermatology Service,
Memorial Sloan-Kettering Cancer Center,
New York, NY, USA
e-mail: gonzals6@mskcc.org

V. Sanchez
Dermatology Service,
CEU University,
Madrid, Spain

S. Lange-Asschenfeldt • M. Ulrich
Department of Dermatology,
Charité – Universitätsmedizin,
Berlin, Germany

Introduction

Reflectance confocal microscopy (RCM) is a novel in vivo, noninvasive imaging method that has already demonstrated to be highly useful in diagnosis approach and therapeutic monitoring of skin cancer [1–3]. Validation of RCM for the diagnosis and prognosis of skin tumors, including melanocytic lesions, has been extensively correlated with dermoscopy and conventional histology [4, 5]. This technology is based on a low-power, near-infrared laser light source attached to a confocal microscope, which illuminates a small skin area. Backscattered light is sent through a pinhole, which only permits in-focus plane (confocal) light to reach the point detector and eliminates the light coming from out-of-focus planes. This results in a real-time transversal thin section image of the skin (XY-axis) with a resolution comparable to conventional histology (1 μm lateral and 3 μm of section thickness). Upward and downward movements of the lens change the depth of the confocal plane and permit the collection of sequential planes of the studied skin sample (Z-axis). Until now the maximum depth of cutaneous study obtained with this technology is 250 μm below the skin surface [6]. Light reflection depends on the refractive index of the different elements of the tissue, which is higher when the size of the illuminated structure is similar to the laser wavelength. At present, the most typical light utilized for RCM is a low-power (<20 mW) diode laser with 830 nm that maximizes reflection and prevents tissue damage. Consequently, confocal images are observed in a bright gray scale based on "endogenous contrasts" which are higher for structures containing melanin and keratin. Unlike traditional histology, RCM provides in vivo, real-time, in a bright gray scale horizontal images of the skin. The major disadvantages of confocal microscopy are the limited depth of imaging and the lack of exogenous contrast agents, even though current investigations are attempting to overcome these problems.

Normal Skin

Before using RCM for the diagnosis of skin tumors or other noncancer skin diseases, it is necessary to describe confocal imaging of normal skin. There are different factors that affect the real-time, in vivo visualization of the skin by confocal microscopy, mainly the area of study, the age, and the Fitzpatrick's phototype. Generally, confocal study starts in the outermost layer and progresses in depth. Stratum corneum appears as a variable refractive surface separated by dark linear valleys (dermatoglyphs) (Fig. 17.1a), which vary in depth depending on the skin area, the phototype of the patient, and the accumulated sun exposure. Corneocytes are observed as 25–50 μm in size, bright, polygonal, flattened, and anucleated cells. Granular and spinous layers are constituted by cells with dark central oval-shaped nuclei and bright cytoplasm. The borders of these keratinocytes are well demarcated and constitute a "honeycombed pattern" (Fig. 17.1b). Basal layer appears as one layer of small cuboid nucleated cells which are usually more brilliant due to the high content in melanin. Consequently, confocal image at the basal layer in dark phototypes is usually observed as a "cobblestone pattern" (Fig. 17.1c). Dermoepidermal junction is located at 60–120 μm in depth, and it appears as bright circular structures ("dermal papillary rings") made of basal cells that surround certain darker areas, which correspond to the dermal papillae (Fig. 17.1d). Within these dark spaces, we may observe refractive collagen bundles and blood vessels with inside rolling movement of erythrocytes and leukocytes.

Skin Cancer

Since RCM was first used to image live human skin in 1995 [7], numerous scientific studies have been carried out mainly focusing in keratinocytic and more recently in melanocytic and other skin tumors.

Malignant Keratinocytic Tumors

Basal Cell Carcinoma (BCC)

Maybe due to the reason that basal cell carcinoma (BCC) constitutes the most frequent malignancy of the skin, this is the cutaneous condition that has been more extensively analyzed by RCM [8, 9]. General confocal features of BCC include dense structures formed by homogeneous tumor cells that present elongated monomorphic nuclei along the same axis of orientation ("nuclear polarization") (Fig. 17.2b), which is often reflected as peripheral palisading when surrounding a tumor island in a perpendicular manner to the border (Fig. 17.2a, d). Frequently, a dark area, which is probably constituted by mucin depots surrounding the relatively refractive tumor aggregates, correlates with the "clefting" observed in traditional histology. Ulrich et al. reported 13 cases of nodular, nodulocystic, and superficial BCCs and found a good linear correlation between dark areas on RCM and thickness of peritumoral mucin [10]. Occasionally, the stroma reflectance is higher than the tumor islands, which are observed and consequently termed "dark silhouettes" (Fig. 17.2c). Also important are the frequently observed disarranged keratinocytes located above the tumor, probably caused by the chronic actinic damage that is usually associated to this type of tumor. The superficial dermal blood vessels are also affected, appearing numerous, dilated with the presence of intense leukocyte trafficking inside, and sometimes accompanied by a prominent

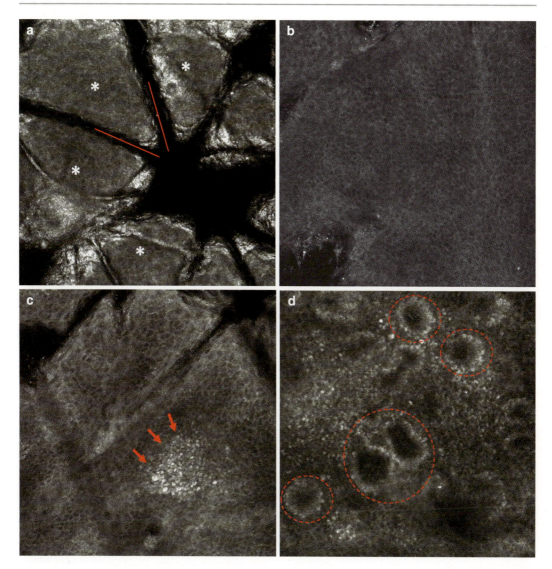

Fig. 17.1 Shows single RCM images (500×500 μm) of the different layers of normal skin. Panel (**a**) illustrates the morphology of the stratum corneum with the presence of a variable refractive surface (*white asterisk*) separated by dark linear valleys (*red lines*) representing skin folds, (**b**) shows typical honeycomb pattern of the epidermis at the spinous cell layer with regular appearance of polygonal keratinocytes, (**c**) shows small bright pigmented cells appearing as typical cobblestone pattern at the suprapapillary plate (*red arrows*), and (**d**) illustrates RCM morphology at the dermoepidermal junction (DEJ) with the presence of bright ring-like structures of pigmented basal cells (*dashed circle*)

perivascular inflammatory infiltrate [11, 12] (Fig. 17.2c). Besides, pigmented BCC presents highly refractive dendritic and granular structures inside the tumor islands correlating to dendritic melanocytes and melanosomes, respectively (Fig. 17.2d). Melanophages located in the stroma are frequently observed as bright and big, poorly demarcated structures [13, 14].

In 2004, a multicenter study was performed in a large cohort of patients to evaluate sensitivity and specificity of RCM for in vivo diagnosis of basal cell carcinoma [8]. Five major criteria were established: elongated monomorphic basaloid nuclei, polarization of these nuclei along the same axis of orientation, prominent inflammatory infiltrate, increased dermal vasculature, and

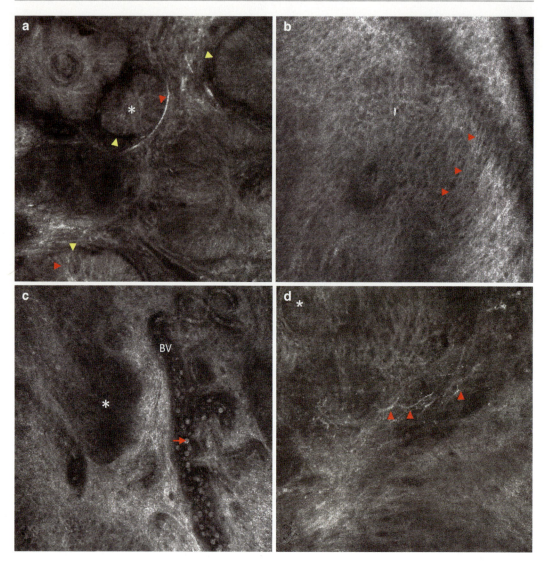

Fig. 17.2 Basal cell carcinoma. (**a**) Hyporefractile tumor islands of BCC (*white asterisk*) which are separated from the surrounding stroma by dark cleft-like spaces (*yellow arrowhead*). Within the tumor islands, peripheral palisading of the cells may be observed (*red arrowhead*). (**b**) Nuclear streaming and elongated and polarized basal keratinocytes (*red arrowheads*). (**c**) Dark silhouettes (*white asterisk*) and large caliber blood vessels (*BV*) with blood flow on in vivo examination. Within the BV single erythrocytes can be visualized (*red arrow*). (**d**) Tumor islands of médium refractility (*white asterisk*) surrounding by tumor stroma with collagen and inflammatory cells. Dendritic figures (*red arrowhead*) are seen

pleoamorphism of the overlying epidermis. The presence of two or more criteria was found to be 100 % sensitive and 53.6 % specific for the diagnosis of BCC, while four or more RCM criteria presented 95.7 % specificity and 82.9 % of sensitivity. As expected, specificity was directly proportional to the number of criteria observed by RCM and inversely proportional to the sensitivity of the criteria in the diagnosis of BCC.

RCM has been employed in different studies that describe the main features of different histological subtypes of BCC which is important in order to determine the therapeutics and prognosis of the tumor [15]. Infiltrative BCC is visualized as ill-defined invading structures composed of very polarized cells that penetrate and deform the dermis, while nodular BCC reveals well-defined tumor islands with peripheral palisading surrounded by dark areas.

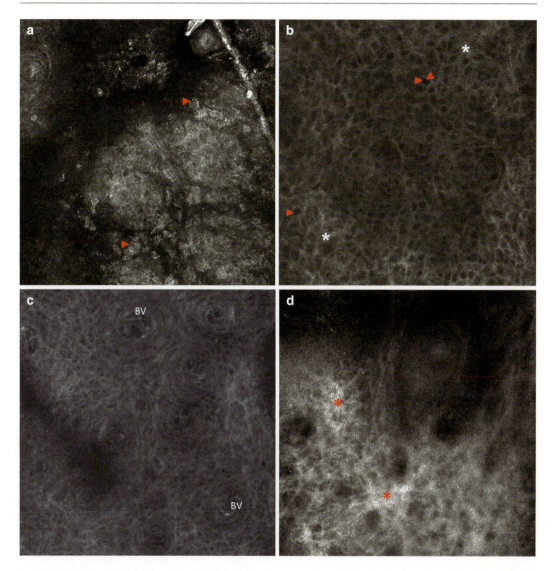

Fig. 17.3 Representative single RCM images (500 × 500 μm) of actinic keratoses. (**a**) Disruption of the stratum corneum with single detached keratinocytes (*red arrowheads*). (**b**) Atypical honeycomb pattern of granular-spinous layers with great variation of cells and nuclei (*red arrowhead*) as well as broadened and irregular cell borders (*white asterisk*). (**c**) Dilated blood vessels (*BV*) in the center of the dermal papillae. (**d**) Highly refractive reticulated thick fibers (*red asterisks*) which correlate to the altered collagen

Squamous Neoplasia

Squamous neoplasia derives from epidermal keratinocytes and is among the most common cutaneous malignancies. RCM features of invasive squamous cell carcinoma (SCC) and actinic keratosis (AK) have been previously described and have good correlation with histopathology [16–18]. At the corneum layer, some amorphous, variably refractive structures can be observed (Fig. 17.3a), which correspond to the scales of the lesion. At this level, some nucleated polygonal cells can be visualized as sharply delineated cells with a refractive thin outline surrounding a dark nucleus, corresponding to the parakeratotic cells of the histology. At the granular and spinous layers, the typical honeycombed pattern is altered and formed by pleomorphic cells with irregular size and shape (Fig. 17.3b). When there is severe atypia, the honeycombed pattern is replaced by a completely disarranged epidermal pattern. Dyskeratotic cells in the granular and spinous layers can also be seen with confocal microscopy as sharply delineated round structures surrounding a dark oval space (nucleus). Another characteristic feature is observed inside the dermal papillary rings as round dark spaces with infrequent leukocyte trafficking inside (Fig. 17.3c). These spaces correspond to the typical dotted and glomerular vessels seen in dermoscopy of SC [19]. Confocal imaging of the upper dermal layer generally reveals extensive highly refractive reticulated thick fibers which correlates to the altered collagen that constitutes the solar elastosis commonly found in this malignancy (Fig. 17.3d). An increasing number and frequency of all these abnormal RCM features can be visualized along the spectrum of squamous neoplasia. A recent study by Ulrich et al. evaluated ten cases of Bowen's disease (BD) by RCM and correlated the findings to routine histology [20]. The most prevalent features were stratum corneum disruption, atypical honeycomb pattern, presence of two types of targetoid cells, and round-to-oval dermal blood vessels. They also observed parakeratosis, inflammatory infiltrate, and multinucleated cells. The results of this study show that RCM can be used for rapid in vivo diagnosis of BD and its distinction from other non-melanocytic skin cancer and inflammatory simulators like psoriasis or eczema.

The detection of dermal RCM features of AK, BD, and SCC may be limited by the presence of significant hyperkeratosis which sometimes worsens its optical resolution in deeper areas. To solve this problem, some chemical or physical methods can be previously applied to remove the scales.

Melanoma

Melanoma is a malignant proliferation of melanocytes in which prognosis is related to depth of dermal invasion. This skin cancer is curable if diagnosed and excised at early stages which explains the importance of an early diagnosis [21]. Clinical diagnosis of melanoma is based on the ABCD criteria, but the accuracy of this method is as low as 64 % [22]. To avoid unnecessary surgical biopsies, which are painful and time-consuming and leave scars, noninvasive techniques for improving clinical diagnostic accuracy are being developed such as dermoscopy, high-frequency ultrasound, optical coherence tomography, magnetic resonance imaging, and RCM [6]. For its ability to explore at cellular level resolution skin structures up to 200 μm in depth, horizontal imaging, and noninvasiveness, RCM may be understood as a natural link between dermoscopy and histopathology, especially useful for diagnosis of early melanomas.

In the recent years, a good correlation between confocal aspects and specific dermoscopic features, such as pigment network, peripheral streaks, or pigment globules, has been demonstrated as well as the correspondence of confocal mosaics at dermoepidermal junction and global dermoscopic patterns [23–25]. Atypical pigment network, characteristic of atypical nevi and melanoma, corresponds to "non-edged papillae," while irregular pigment globules correspond to irregularly shaped clusters formed by atypical cells in melanomas or regular cytology in benign lesions. Pigment dots are clearly visualized by RCM as pagetoid melanocytes in melanoma that are easily distinguished from the melanin clumps typically found in common nevi [26]. Moreover, RCM is particularly useful for the interpretation of the bluish pigmentation and for differentiating the plump bright cells infiltrating the dermal papillae that correspond to melanophages from the malignant melanocytes that, singularly or in clusters, infiltrate the dermis in invasive melanomas [27, 28].

In a similar manner, the main histopathological features of melanoma have been identified with RCM showing high sensitivity and specificity values [5, 29]: altered epidermal architecture with pagetoid cells (Fig. 17.4a, b), ill-defined dermal papillae with cytological atypia at dermoepidermal junction (Fig. 17.4c), cerebriform clusters, and nucleated cells in superficial dermis (Fig. 17.4d). Furthermore, very high sensitivity and specificity values of some confocal aspects, such as melanocyte cytology, disarray of the

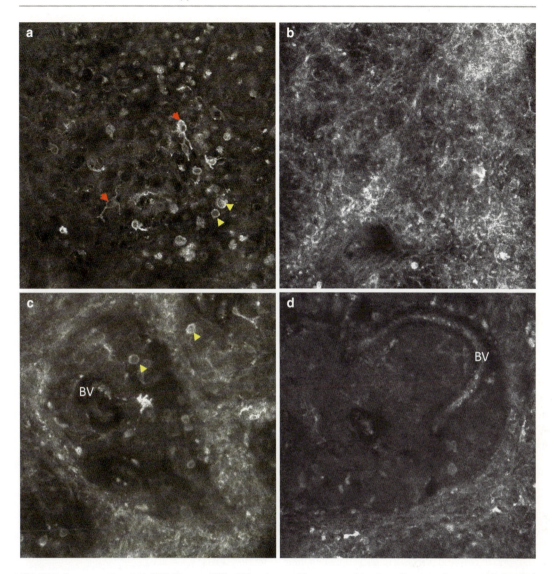

Fig. 17.4 Representative single RCM images (500×500 μm) of melanoma. (**a**) Presence of both dendritic (*red arrowhead*) and round (*yellow arrowhead*) pagetoid melanocytes in upper epidermal layers. (**b**) Complete disruption of the epidermal architecture resulting in a disarranged pattern. (**c**) Atypical melanocytes at the DEJ (*yellow arrowheads*) as well as in the dermal papillae containng blood vessels (BV). (**d**) Large dilated and elongated blood vessels (BV) in the upper dermis

architecture, and poorly defined keratinocyte cell borders, were identified by Gerger et al., comparing two preselected images per lesion from a database of 27 melanomas and 90 nevi, the majority of which corresponded to clearly benign lesions [30].

At present, two different confocal diagnosis algorithms for melanoma have been developed. Based on 102 melanocytic lesions, six criteria were identified as independently correlated with a melanoma diagnosis, and a diagnostic algorithm was developed [31]. Two major criteria were scored 2 points, corresponding to the cytological atypia at basal cell layers and non-edged papillae at dermoepidermal junction. Four minor criteria, represented by the presence of roundish cells in superficial layers spreading upwards in a pagetoid fashion, pagetoid cells widespread throughout the lesion, cerebriform clusters in the papillary dermis, and nucleated cells within dermal papilla, were scored 1 point. Considering a threshold score equal to or greater than 3, 97.3 % sensitivity and 72.3 % specificity were obtained, whereas increasing the threshold, specificity can be increased with a consequent decrement of sensitivity. Recently, the validity of the algorithm was blindly tested on a larger population of equivocal melanocytic lesions, showing in a reproducible clinical setting a 92 % sensitivity and 70 % specificity [5]. Segura et al. developed a two-step method for the diagnosis of melanoma by RCM [32]. In a preliminary study, they evaluated 154 skin tumors, including 100 melanocytic and 54 non-melanocytic lesions, by RCM before their excision. They observed four confocal features that differentiated melanocytic from non-melanocytic lesions: cobblestone pattern of epidermal layers, pagetoid spread, mesh appearance of the dermoepidermal junction, and the presence of dermal nests. Within melanocytic lesions, the presence of roundish suprabasal cells and atypical nucleated cells in the dermis was associated with melanoma, and the presence of edged papillae and typical basal cells was associated with nevi. Furthermore, a recent study [33] tried to determine whether specific histological features in dysplastic nevi had reliable correlates on confocal microscopy and developed an in vivo microscopic grading system, which consists in a simplified algorithm to distinguish dysplastic nevi from melanoma and non-dysplastic nevi. Sixty melanocytic lesions with equivocal dermatoscopic aspects were analyzed by RCM and histopathology, and they found good correlation between their features. As observed by RCM, dysplastic nevi were characterized by a ringed pattern, in association with a meshwork pattern in a large proportion of cases, along with atypical junctional cells in the center of the lesion and irregular junctional nests with short interconnections. The simultaneous presence of cytological atypia and of atypical junctional nests (irregular, with short interconnections, and/or with nonhomogeneous cellularity) was consistent with histological dysplasia, whereas widespread pagetoid infiltration, widespread cytological atypia at the junction, and non-edged papillae suggested melanoma diagnosis.

Interestingly, several confocal features for melanoma may be also identified in amelanotic melanomas. It is possible to detect melanocytes in a clinically amelanotic tumor due to the presence of some melanin inside the pre-melanosomes, which have similar size to the wavelength that we use for imaging. Considering that amelanotic tumors do not present a high refractivity as other heavily pigmented lesions, they may be more easily diagnosed with RCM than with dermoscopy, which suggests a better early diagnosis of certain clinically difficult pigmented lesions such as amelanotic melanoma [34].

Mycosis Fungoides

Mycosis fungoides (MF) represents the most common form of cutaneous T-cell lymphoma [29]. The clinical presentation may be diverse and, in the first stages, usually shows an indolent course with stable or slowly progressing lesions that may resemble chronic eczema of plaque psoriasis. Due to this reason, early diagnosis of the disease is frequently delayed. MF final diagnosis is based on histopathological evaluation in combination with immunohistochemistry and clonality studies.

In recent years, the main RCM features of MF have been published [35, 36]. RCM reveals the major features of MF such as exocytosis and Pautrier microabscesses, although early diagnosis of MF remains challenging. However, confocal microscopy may be useful to select highly suspicious lesions for biopsy and help to accelerate diagnosis.

At the patch stage of MF, the changes may be very subtle, and consequently the diagnosis at this early phase with confocal microscopy may be difficult. The most important confocal features include hyporefractivity of dermal papillary rings and small, weakly refractive round cells located in the spinous layer, which correlates to the interface changes and exocytosis process, respectively. In the plaque phase of MF, the visualization of typical confocal features of MF may be easier. Some small lightly refractive cells appear in the spinous layer correlating to epidermotropism of lymphocytes, which sometimes are grouped and located inside dark spaces within the epidermis corresponding to Pautrier microabscesses on histopathology. These vesicle-like spaces have to be distinguished from those seen in acute eczema by the absence of parakeratosis and spongiosis and the presence of other MF characteristic confocal features. In tumor-type MF, the hyporefractive papillary rings and the infiltration of small lightly refractive cells in the epidermis are frequently visualized in confocal images, while the vesicle-like spaces are rarely detected. Inside papillary dermis, highly refractive cells of small to medium size are observed and blood vessels may show a well-circumscribed thickened wall.

Clinical Applications Besides Diagnosis in Cutaneous Oncology

The high resolution obtained by RCM allows its utilization not only for diagnosis but also for surgery planning or evaluation of response to noninvasive therapies. The most important future applications are: guide for biopsy sample, preventing the "sampling error" so common in some situations like mycosis fungoides, malignant lentigo, or atypical nevus syndrome; tumor delimitation before excision in special areas, such as face or scalp, or ill-defined tumors such as malignant lentigo or amelanotic melanoma [3, 37–39]; monitoring the clinical response to noninvasive therapies for some keratinocytic tumors such as imiquimod cream or photodynamic therapy [40–43]; and for residual tumor detection after treatment [44].

Conclusion

RCM is an efficient tool for the study of the skin physiology and diseases. Its most important advantages are the noninvasiveness and the in vivo and real-time examination of the skin. Although it has been mostly utilized for cutaneous malignant tumors, some recent studies show its usefulness to diagnose other benign tumors and inflammatory skin diseases. Undoubtedly, confocal microscopy presents some technical and scientific limitations, which must be resolved before it becomes a tool of reference. It is necessary to improve imaging depth and, perhaps, to find contrast agents in order to recognize certain cell types

and subcellular structures. Furthermore, it is indispensable a training for dermatologists and dermatopathologists before they get used to horizontal sections of the skin and black and white colors. Although skin biopsy remains the gold standard in microscopic diagnosis, RCM offers an important approach for skin diagnosis.

Glossary

Cobblestone pattern is the pattern found in basal layer keratynocytes, which appears as one layer of small cuboid nucleated cells usually more brilliant due to the high content in melanin. It is the confocal pattern usually observed at the basal layer in dark phototypes.

Dark silhouettes found in BCC refer to those areas where the stroma reflectance is higher than the tumor islands.

Dermal papillary rings is the confocal pattern found at the dermoepidermal junction and it appears as bright circular structures made of basal cells that surround certain darker areas, which correspond to the dermal papillae.

Dermatoglyphs dark linear valleys

Honeycombed pattern is the pattern found in normal keratinocytes of the granular and spinous layers. These are cells with dark central oval-shaped nuclei and bright cytoplasm.

Nuclear polarization refers to the elongated monomorphic nuclei along the same axis of orientation and present as a general confocal feature of BCC (Basal cell carcinoma). It often reflects as peripheral palisading.

RCM Reflectance confocal microscopy.

References

1. Aghassi D, Anderson RR, González S. Confocal laser microscopic imaging of actinic keratoses in vivo: a preliminary report. J Am Acad Dermatol. 2000;43: 42–8.
2. Langley RG, Rajadhyaksha M, Dwyer PJ, Sober AJ, Flotte TJ, Anderson RR. Confocal scanning laser microscopy of benign and malignant melanocytic skin lesions in vivo. J Am Acad Dermatol. 2001;45: 365–76.

3. Busam KJ, Hester K, Charles C, et al. Detection of clinically amelanotic malignant melanoma and assessment of its margins by in vivo confocal scanning laser microscopy. Arch Dermatol. 2001;137:923–9.

4. Ulrich M, Stockfleth E, Roewert-Huber J, Astner S. Non invasive diagnostic tools for non-melanoma skin cancer. Br J Dermatol. 2007;157 Suppl 2:56–8.

5. Pellacani G, Guitera P, Longo C, Avramidis M, Seidenari S, Menzies S. The impact of in vivo reflectance confocal microscopy for the diagnostic accuracy of melanoma and equivocal melanocytic lesions. J Invest Dermatol. 2007;127:2759–65.

6. Rajadhyaksha M, González S, Zavislan JM, Anderson RR, Webb RH. In vivo confocal scanning laser microscopy of human skin II: advances in instrumentation and comparison with histology. J Invest Dermatol. 1999;113:293–303.

7. Rajadhyaksha M, Grossman M, Esterowitz D, Webb RH, Anderson RR. In vivo confocal scanning laser microscopy of human skin: melanin provides strong contrast. J Invest Dermatol. 1995;104: 946–52.

8. Nori S, Rius-Diaz F, Cuevas J, et al. Sensitivity and specificity of reflectance mode confocal microscopy for in vivo diagnosis of basal cell carcinoma: a multicenter study. J Am Acad Dermatol. 2004;51: 923–30.

9. González S, Tannous Z. Real-time, in vivo confocal reflectance microscopy of basal cell carcinoma. J Am Acad Dermatol. 2002;47:869–74.

10. Ulrich M, Roewert-Huber J, González S, Rius-Diaz F, Stockfleth E, Kanitakis J. Peritumoral clefting in basal cell carcinoma: correlation of in vivo reflectance confocal microscopy and routine histology. J Cutan Pathol. 2011;38:190–5.

11. González S, Sackstein R, Anderson RR, Rajadhyaksha M. Real-time evidence of in vivo leukocyte trafficking in human skin by reflectance confocal microscopy. J Invest Dermatol. 2001;117:384–6.

12. Ahlgrimm-Siess V, Cao T, Oliviero M, Hofmann-Wellenhof R, Rabinovitz HS, Scope A. The vasculature of non-melanocytic skin tumors in reflectance confocal microscopy: vascular features of basal cell carcinoma. Arch Dermatol. 2010;146:353–4.

13. Agero AL, Busam KJ, Benvenuto-Andrade C, et al. Reflectance confocal microscopy of pigmented basal cell carcinoma. J Am Acad Dermatol. 2006;54: 638–43.

14. Segura S, Puig S, Carrera C, Palou J, Malvehy J. Dendritic cells in pigmented basal cell carcinoma: a relevant finding by reflectance-mode confocal microscopy. Arch Dermatol. 2007;143:883–6.

15. González S, Gill M, Halpern AC, editors. Reflectance confocal microscopy of cutaneous tumors: an atlas with clinical, dermoscopic and histological correlations. London: Informa Healthcare; 2008.

16. Ulrich M, Maltusch A, Rius-Diaz F, Röwert-Huber J, González S, Sterry W, et al. Clinical applicability of in vivo reflectance confocal microscopy for the diagnosis of actinic keratoses. Dermatol Surg. 2008; 34(5):610–9.

17. Ulrich M, Krueger-Corcoran D, Roewert-Huber J, Sterry W, Stockfleth E, Astner S. Reflectance confocal microscopy for noninvasive monitoring of therapy and detection of subclinical actinic keratoses. Dermatology. 2010;220(1):15–24.

18. Rishpon A, Kim N, Scope A, Porges L, Oliviero MC, Braun RP, et al. Reflectance confocal microscopy criteria for squamous cell carcinomas and actinic keratoses. Arch Dermatol. 2009;145:766–72.

19. Zalaudek I, Giacomel J, Schmid K, Bondino S, Rosendahl C, Cavicchini S, et al. Dermatoscopy of facial actinic keratosis, intraepidermal carcinoma, and invasive squamous cell carcinoma: a progression model. J Am Acad Dermatol. 2012;66(4): 589–97.

20. Ulrich M, Kanitakis J, González S, Lange-Asschenfeldt S, Stockfleth E, Roewert-Huber J. Evaluation of Bowen disease by in vivo reflectance confocal microscopy. Br J Dermatol. 2012;166(2): 451–3.

21. Balch CM, Houghton AN, Sober AJ, Soong SJ, editors. Cutaneous melanoma. 3rd ed. St. Louis: Quality Medical Publishing; 1998.

22. Grin CM, Kopf AW, Welkovich B, Bart RS, Levenstein MJ. Accuracy in the clinical diagnosis of malignant melanoma. Arch Dermatol. 1990;126:763–6.

23. Scope A, Benvenuto-Andrade C, Agero AL, Halpern AC, González S, Marghoob AA. Correlation of dermoscopic structures of melanocytic lesions to reflectance confocal microscopy. Arch Dermatol. 2007;143:176–85.

24. Scope A, Gill M, Benveuto-Andrade C, Halpern AC, González S, Marghoob AA. Correlation of dermoscopy with in vivo reflectance confocal microscopy of streaks in melanocytic lesions. Arch Dermatol. 2007; 143:727–34.

25. Pellacani G, Longo C, Malvehy J, Puig S, Carrera C, Segura S, et al. In vivo confocal microscopic and histopathologic correlations of dermoscopic features in 202 melanocytic lesions. Arch Dermatol. 2008; 144(12):1597–608.

26. Pellacani G, Cesinaro AM, Seidenari S. Reflectance-mode confocal microscopy for the in vivo characterization of pagetoid melanocytosis in melanomas and nevi. J Invest Dermatol. 2005;125:532–7.

27. Pellacani G, Bassoli S, Longo C, Cesinaro AM, Seidenari S. Diving into the blue: in vivo microscopic characterization of the dermoscopic blue hue. J Am Acad Dermatol. 2007;57:96–104.

28. Segura S, Pellacani G, Puig S, Longo C, Bassoli S, Guitera P, et al. In vivo microscopic features of nodular melanomas: dermoscopy, confocal microscopy, and histopathologic correlates. Arch Dermatol. 2008; 144:1311–20.

29. Willemze R, Jaffe ES, Burg G, Cerroni L, Berti E, Swerdlow SH, et al. WHO-EORTC classification for cutaneous lymphomas. Blood. 2005;105:3768–85.

30. Gerger A, Koller S, Kern T, Massone C, Steiger K, Richtig E, et al. Diagnostic applicability of in vivo confocal laser scanning microscopy in melanocytic skin tumors. J Invest Dermatol. 2005;124:493–8.

31. Pellacani G, Cesinaro AM, Seidenari S. Reflectance-mode confocal microscopy of pigmented skin lesions – improvement in melanoma diagnostic specificity. J Am Acad Dermatol. 2005;53:979–85.

32. Segura S, Puig S, Carrera C, Palou J, Malvehy J. Development of a two-step method for the diagnosis of melanoma by reflectance confocal microscopy. J Am Acad Dermatol. 2009;61:216–29.

33. Pellacani G, Farnetani F, Gonzalez S, Longo C, Cesinaro AM, Casari A, et al. In vivo confocal micros-copy for detection and grading of dysplastic nevi: a pilot study. J Am Acad Dermatol. 2012;66(3):e109–21.

34. Guitera P, Pellacani G, Crotty KA, Scolyer RA, Li LX, Bassoli S, et al. The impact of in vivo reflectance confocal microscopy on the diagnostic accuracy of lentigo maligna and equivocal pigmented and nonpig-mented macules of the face. J Invest Dermatol. 2010; 130(8):2080–91.

35. Agero AL, Gill M, Ardigo M, Myskowski P, Halpern AC, González S. In vivo reflectance confocal micros-copy of mycosis fungoides: a preliminary study. J Am Acad Dermatol. 2007;57:435–41.

36. Gill M, Agero AL, Ardigo M, Myskowski P, González S. Mycosis fungoides. In: González S, Gill M, Halpern AC, editors. Reflectance confocal of cutaneous tumors. London: Informa Healthcare; 2008. p. 183–92.

37. Mihm MC, Flotte TJ, González S. In vivo examina-tion of lentigo maligna and malignant melanoma in situ, lentigo maligna type by near-infrared reflectance confocal microscopy: comparison of in vivo confocal images with histologic sections. J Am Acad Dermatol. 2002;46:260–3.

38. Curiel-Lewandrowski C, Williams CM, Swindells KJ, Tahan SR, Astner S, Frankenthaler RA, et al. Use of in vivo confocal microscopy in malignant melanoma: an aid in diagnosis and assessment of surgical and non surgical therapeutic approaches. Arch Dermatol. 2004;140:1127–32.

39. Chen CS, Elias M, Busam K, Rajadhyaksha M, Marghoob AA. Multimodal in vivo optical imaging, including confocal microscopy, facilitates presurgical margin mapping for clinically complex lentigo maligna melanoma. Br J Dermatol. 2005;153: 1031–6.

40. Trehan M, Swindells K, Taylor CR, Racette AL, González S. Confocal microscopy imaging of actinic keratoses post-photodynamic therapy with 5-ALA. Paper presented at: 20th World Congress of Dermatology, Paris, 2002.

41. Goldgeier M, Fox CA, Zavislan JM, Harris D, González S. Noninvasive imaging, treatment, and microscopic confirmation of clearance of basal cell carcinoma. Dermatol Surg. 2003;29:205–10.

42. Torres A, Niemeyer A, Berkes B, Marra D, Schanbacher C, González S, et al. 5% imiquimod cream and reflectance-mode confocal microscopy as adjunct modalities to Mohs micrographic surgery for treatment of basal cell carcinoma. Dermatol Surg. 2004;30:1462–9.

43. Astner S, González S, Stockfleth E, Lademann J. Confocal microscopy: innovative diagnostic tools for monitoring of noninvasive therapy in cutaneous malignancies. Drug Discov Today Dis Mech. 2008; 5(1):81–91.

44. Marra DE, Torres A, Schanbacher CF, González S. Detection of residual basal cell carcinoma by in vivo confocal microscopy. Dermatol Surg. 2005;31: 538–41.

Multiphoton Laser Microscopy with Fluorescence Lifetime Imaging and Skin Cancer

18

Stefania Seidenari, Federica Arginelli, and Marco Manfredini

Key Points

- In vivo MPT/FLIM is a non-invasive technique that can be repeated on the same site without restriction.
- The use of any other contrast agent or exogenous marker is unnecessary, simplifying both examination and patient preparation.
- MPT-FLIM is a promising device to study skin tumours, since it is able to define morphological and functional properties of cancer cells and of their associated stroma.
- The tissue sample can be studied three-dimensionally with a subcellular spatial resolution, thanks to the horizontal and vertical optical sections.
- Allows a deeper penetration than that of confocal microscopy, with a better discrimination of the various tissue components and a higher visualisation of the deep dermis.

S. Seidenari (✉) • F. Arginelli • M. Manfredini
Department of Dermatology,
University of Modena and Reggio Emilia,
Skin Center, via Zattera 130, Modena 41124, Italy
e-mail: stefania.seidenari@unimore.it

Introduction

Over the past decades a dramatic increase in the incidence of both melanocytic and non-melanocytic skin tumours has been reported [1–5]. The most dangerous tumour is malignant melanoma (MM), whose outcome and curability depends on diagnosis and excision at early stages of tumour progression. Despite extensive research investigating the physical and morphological characteristics of MM, diagnostic accuracy remains suboptimal, with values ranging from 56 to 81 % [6–8].

Basal cell carcinoma (BCC) is the most frequent skin cancer in humans and represents a major health concern especially in Caucasians [4, 5]. The tumour rarely gives rise to metastases; however, it frequently arises on the face leading to local tissue destruction. Surgery is the treatment of election, especially for invasive cancer, and has to be carried out possibly when the BCC is in an initial stage, sparing the surrounding healthy tissue as much as possible, though guaranteeing the total removal of the tumour [9]. The identification of tumour margins also represents a challenge since most BCCs have poorly defined boundaries. Thus, both early recognition of small lesions and identification of tumour borders during surgery are of great practical importance.

When facing a suspicious lesion on the skin, the usual course of action comprises visual inspection followed by a biopsy and subsequent histopathologic examination. This leads to a delayed definitive surgical treatment.

A. Baldi et al. (eds.), *Skin Cancer*, Current Clinical Pathology,
DOI 10.1007/978-1-4614-7357-2_18, © Springer Science+Business Media New York 2014

To circumvent these drawbacks, extensive research on new technologies has been carried out introducing real-time imaging methods such as dermoscopy, optical coherence tomography and confocal laser microscopy.

Dermoscopy, enabling the visualisation of subsurface anatomic structures of the epidermis and papillary dermis, has become a popular imaging method since it is reliable, cost-effective and non-invasive [10]. Confocal laser microscopy represents a 'third-level' technological aid further improving the diagnosis of skin tumours [11, 12]. In spite of the introduction of these techniques, there still remains a 'grey' zone constituted by a certain number of cutaneous lesions that are difficult to classify [13, 14]. Therefore, new technologies are needed aiming both at avoiding scars due to unnecessary biopsies and to provide a support for histopathology, which, in spite of remaining the Gold Standard for diagnosis, does not always show a satisfactory interobserver agreement [15].

Theoretical Background

One of the most promising imaging tools and fast-developing technologies in the field of optical sectioning, with high resolution, short acquisition time and good applicability, is multiphoton laser tomography (MPT) associated to fluorescence lifetime imaging (FLIM).

Although multiphoton excitation (MPE) was described theoretically in 1931 by Maria Goeppert-Mayer, Denk et al. were the first to introduce a functional instrument for biological applications and to demonstrate its utility as an alternative (and often advantageous) optical imaging technique [16].

Multiphoton microscopy is based on ultrafast laser physics and provides a harmless optical window for two-photon vital cell studies. The application of 80 MHz near infrared (NIR) femtosecond laser pulses to a scanning fluorescence microscope offers the unique possibility of safe autofluorescence imaging; in fact the required high transient light intensities for multiphoton processes can be achieved by tight focusing of ultrashort laser pulses within the sub-femtolitre focal volume of an objective of high numerical aperture. When using laser wavelengths between 700 and 1,100 nm and appropriate mean laser powers, the tissue absorption in out-of-focus regions is negligible and significant photobleaching and tissue damage can be avoided [17].

Fluorescence is a physical phenomenon that is observed when a fluorophore, excited to some higher vibrational level by single or multiple photon absorption, emits photons with a particular spectrum to return to its ground state [18]. Multiphoton microscopy relies on the simultaneous absorption of two or more photons of low energy in the near-infrared spectrum, avoiding biological tissue damage that occurs with higher laser powers. Moreover, with two-photon excitation, it is possible to avoid the oxidative damage induced by the shorter laser wavelength applied with single photon techniques.

With multiphoton microscopy, many endogenous fluorophores including NADH (reduced nicotinamide adenine dinucleotide), NADPH (reduced nicotinamide adenine dinucleotide phosphate), collagen, keratin, melanin, elastin, flavines, porphyrin, tryptophan, cholecalciferol and lipofuscin can be efficiently excited.

Besides autofluorescence, emission in the visible range, allowing the visualisation of images, also comprises second harmonic generation (SHG) signals. The SHG signal comes from non-centrosymmetric molecules such as collagen and myosin and is characterised by an emission wavelength corresponding to half of that of the incident photons; this particular signal allows the visualisation of dermal collagen bundles and their distinction from cellular components and elastin fibres [19].

Using the fluorescence emitted from endogenous molecules through fluorophores makes the use of any other contrast agent or exogenous marker unnecessary, simplifying both examination and patient preparation.

With MPT, bidimensional images are acquired and correspond to optical sectioning parallel to the tissue surface (reported to a defined xy plan). Pictures obtained at various depths, called z-stacks, can be acquired by sequentially modifying the depth of the focus plane in the tissue

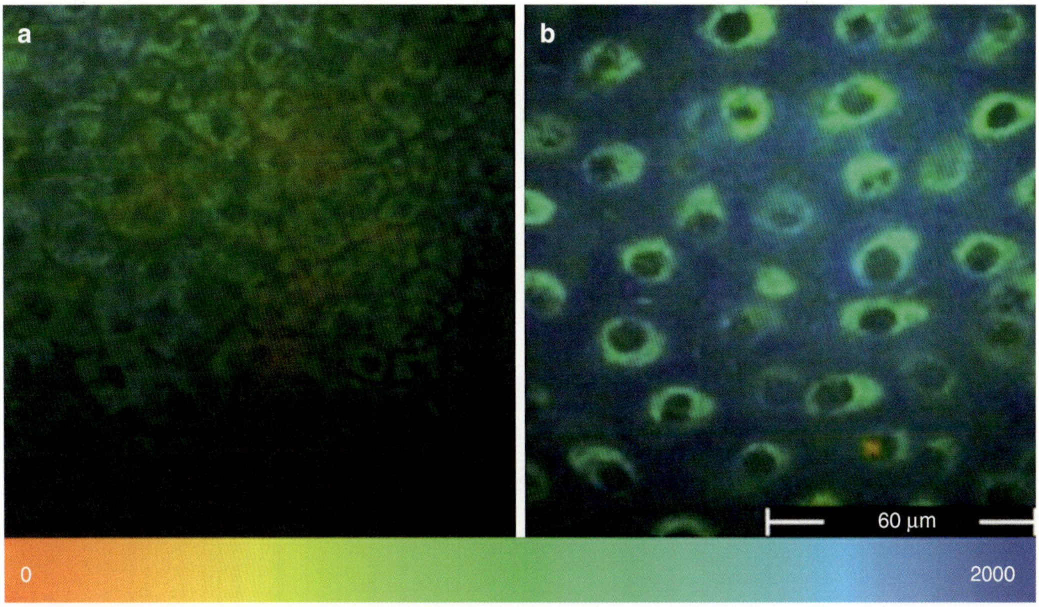

Fig. 18.1 FLIM images acquired at 760 nm excitation wavelength by the Imperial College FLIM system incorporated in the *DermaInspect*® and processed using the software SPC IMAGE (Becker & Hickl GmbH). (**a**) Healthy skin acquired in vivo at 20 μm depth: the keratinocytes appear as green cells tightly packed together. (**b**) Basal cell carcinoma acquired ex vivo: the keratinocytes are detached and appear blue-green, showing longer lifetimes compared to healthy skin

reaching levels of 200 μm measured from the departure point at the skin surface [20–22].

Greyscale images are generated, reproducing the fluorescence intensity in different tissue components (intensity images). The estimated resolution is 0.5 μm in the lateral direction and 1–2 μm in the axial direction [20–22].

Fluorescence Lifetime Imaging

Another possible imaging modality which can be obtained with MPT is based on fluorescence lifetime imaging (FLIM), which depicts the tissue under study based on the decay rate of fluorescence emission of endogenous fluorescent molecules in their surrounding medium. FLIM is most powerful in separating the different states of interaction of the fluorescent species with the local environment [23–25]. False colour coding (Fig. 18.1), where each colour corresponds to a certain fluorescent lifetime at each image pixel, permits the immediate visual identification of cellular, subcellular or extracellular structures according to their FLIM value, i.e. their colour. The distribution of fluorescence lifetimes within an image is visualised through a histogram that plots the fluorescence lifetime (x-axis) against the number of corresponding pixels at which that lifetime occurs (y-axis). The time-resolved analysis of the fluorescence signal generates four-dimensional images, where the tissue structure is not only studied according to its x-, y- or z-axis but also described according to the metabolic characteristics of its components.

FLIM acquisition has proved useful in the determination of parameters such as pH [26], ion concentrations [27, 28], oxygen saturation [29, 30], refractive index [31], conformation of proteins [32] and aggregation states [33]. FLIM is also used to distinguish DNA and RNA [34], to separate bound and unbound NADH or FAD [35] in autofluorescence images [36] and to separate interacting and noninteracting protein fractions in FRET (Förster resonance energy transfer) experiments [37, 38]. Importantly, two of the strongest sources of intrinsic fluorescence of cells are NADH and FAD, which are fundamental to metabolism and important regulators of cell behaviour as well as potential cancer biomarkers [39–41]. For these reasons, MPT-FLIM is a promising device to study skin tumours, since it is able to define morphological and functional properties of cancer cells and of their associated stroma.

Excitation Wavelength

Epidermal structures can be efficiently excited at a wavelength of 760 nm [16, 20–22, 42–47]. When the excitation wavelength is increased above 800 nm, most keratinocytes lose their excitability and progressively become invisible. Since melanin, compared with other organic fluorophores, has an absorption spectrum that decreases from the UV region to NIR, its selective excitation wavelength is 800 nm [23, 48]. Single cells visible in the basal layer, showing intense fluorescence at 800 nm, can be identified as melanocytes. This excitation wavelength can be used to study benign and malignant melanocytic lesions.

Collagen and elastin are the main dermal components, and their excitation takes place at a variable wavelength from 760 to 840 nm. To adequately visualise the fibrous structures of the dermis, an 800 nm wavelength is generally employed. At this wavelength, collagen fibres that generate the SHG signal are selectively excited, whereas at 760 nm, dermal autofluorescent components such as elastin are enhanced in the image.

Practical Considerations and Applications

Application Fields

The MPT/FLIM technique has numerous applications in dermatology, being suitable for the study of physiological and pathological conditions of the skin, in vivo, on ex vivo samples and on cultured cells [49, 50]. Mesenchymal stem cells undergoing various differentiation stimuli can be monitored in a non-invasive manner

evaluating morphology, metabolic activity and oxidative stress [49]. Fibroblast cultures are widely used as an experimental model to study the expression of specific genes or the effect of drugs, especially of new compounds with potential chemotherapeutic activity, and to check the mutagenicity and carcinogenicity of different substances. Using MPT and FLIM, a precise and rapid assessment of the morphologic and metabolic changes which fibroblasts undergo after exposure to various environmental factors can be achieved without the need of cell processing and staining [50].

When studying diseased states of the skin, knowledge about normal morphology is of utmost importance. As regards healthy epidermis, it has been shown that cell and nucleus diameters, cell density and fluorescence lifetime values vary not only according to epidermal cell depth but also depending on skin site [51]. Skin ageing is expressed by variations in shape, size, distribution and morphology of epidermal cells. Moreover, FLIM values at both the upper and lower layers increase, indicating a change in the metabolic activity of epidermal cells in the elderly [52]. These data can be used for the comparison with MPT/FLIM aspects of epidermal cells in pathological conditions.

The application of MPT/FLIM to the field of skin tumours appears promising [25, 35, 52–55].

Basal Cell Carcinoma

Employing MPT, a rapid and accurate tumour demarcation from the surrounding noninvolved skin can be achieved [25, 56]. Considering both autofluorescence images and fluorescence lifetime images Galletly NP et al. identified several alterations of cell metabolism and morphology, allowing the discrimination between healthy skin and the tumour region. On the basis of wide-field imaging lifetime information, they demonstrated that BCC exhibits longer fluorescence lifetime than surrounding healthy skin [25]. These observations were confirmed by another working group, which described a shift of the mean lifetime distribution of BCC towards longer values, especially in the intermediate epidermal layers [52].

Another feature revealed by MPT is the alteration of the extracellular matrix in the BCC stroma [46]. In BCC, dermal collagen is replaced by tumour nests of basaloid cells which destroy the surrounding environment by the collagenolytic activity of matrix metalloproteinases. The result consists in a disarrangement of the collagen molecule packing, thus altering the dermal distribution of the fluorophores and decreasing the SHG signal [46, 56, 57]. The increase in the autofluorescence signal in the cancer stroma, in comparison with that of normal dermal stroma, is unclear at this stage [56].

Lin et al. performed a quantitative analysis to discriminate normal dermal stroma from the tumour; in their approach, multiphoton fluorescence (MF) pixel number (a) and SHG pixel number (b) were determined within a region of interest, and the MF/SHG index was defined to be $(a-b)/(a+b)$. Consequently, MF/SHG reached the maximum value of 1 when only the MF signal was present (corresponding to the presence of only elastic fibres) and decreased with the growth of collagen content (which generates the SHG signal). Whereas in normal dermal stroma MF/SHG was very low, reflecting the high content of collagen bundles, in the cancer stroma it was significantly higher because of the low contribution of undamaged collagen [46].

The epidermis overlying the BCC may be thinned, thickened or ulcerated compared to normal skin [52]; conversely, all the ex vivo specimens investigated by Paoli et al. showed a marked increase in epidermal thickness compared to the corresponding normal perilesional skin [53, 55].

BCC is characterised by clumps of autofluorescent cells in the dermis [46] which show relatively large nuclei, little cytoplasm [55] and a higher nucleus to cytoplasm ratio [46, 56]. Peripheral basaloid cells palisading along the basement membrane [46, 56] are a distinctive histopathologic feature of basal cell carcinoma. They can also be observed in each cancer nest.

Paoli et al. described tumour cells which were monomorphous and palisading at the periphery, with nuclei polarisation corresponding to keratinocytes with elongated nuclei and cytoplasm oriented in the same direction in the X−Y plane [53, 55].

De Giorgi et al. analysed different surgical samples of BCC investigating cell shape and size:

compared with healthy skin cells, tumoural ones appeared smaller in dimensions and tightly packed together; they also exhibited a reduced fluorescent contrast between cytoplasm and nucleus [54].

Speckled perinuclear fluorescence was sometimes observed in subcorneal epidermis of superficial BCC but was also present in the corresponding normal perilesional skin [53].

In a study on 98 BCCs, Seidenari et al. identified three epidermal and seven tumour descriptors for BCC [58]. Compared to normal epidermal cells, those overlying the BCC exhibited irregular cellular contours, had lost the normal cohesion and were disposed in a random order; moreover, intercellular spaces were larger and irregular (Fig. 18.1). BCC cells appeared monomorphous with an elongated shape and nuclei; they were aligned along the same direction and tightly packed together (Fig. 18.2a); sometimes a double alignment was observable with divergent sheets of cells (Fig. 18.2b). At the edge of the nodule, a palisading phenomenon was often visible (Fig. 18.2c). By an excitation wavelength of 760 nm, basaloid nodules were observable as cell aggregates surrounded by fibres (Fig. 18.3). Whereas BCC cells exhibited a bluish colour corresponding to a high fluorescence decay time, the collagen fibres appeared in red due to very low fluorescence lifetimes (Fig. 18.3). When shifting the excitation wavelength to 800–820 nm, to explore the extracellular matrix, BCC cells disappeared and only red fibres surrounding black spaces were visible (phantom islands) (Fig. 18.4). Finally, BCC cells showed mean fluorescence lifetime values which were significantly higher with respect to normal epidermal cells, indicating that FLIM may also provide quantitative data for the identification of single tumour cells.

The diagnostic aid provided by MPT can sometimes be limited by the deep location of the tumour nests, especially in the nodular BCC type [47] or by epidermal thickening and hyperkeratosis [55] which makes the exploration of the tumour mass difficult.

MPT can also be very useful for the investigation of surgically removed samples before pathologist's examination on ex vivo specimens [47] or as an alternative to Mohs' surgery.

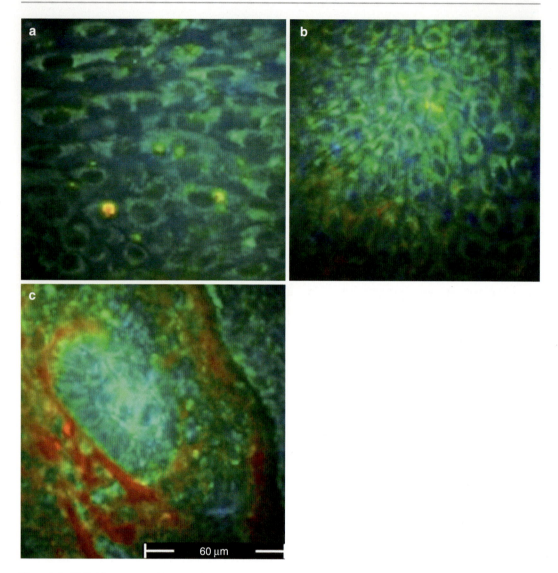

Fig. 18.2 FLIM images acquired at 760 nm excitation wavelength by the Imperial College FLIM system incorporated in the *DermaInspect®* and processed using the software SPC IMAGE (Becker & Hickl GmbH). (**a**) Basal cell carcinoma. FLIM image acquired at 40 μm depth that shows elongated and aligned blue cells. The alignment occurs at one direction. (**b**) Basal cell carcinoma. FLIM image acquired at 100 μm depth that shows elongated blue-green cells aligned in two different directions. (**c**) Basal cell carcinoma. FLIM image acquired at 100 μm depth. It is possible to see the upper part of a basaloid nest which shows a palisade of blue cells tightly packed. A vessel, which appears linear and red, circumscribes the left edge of the nest

Epithelial Precancers

Skala and colleagues investigated low- and high-grade epithelial precancers compared with normal epithelial tissues. A significant decrease in the contribution of protein-bound NADH and a significantly increased variability in the redox ratio and NADH fluorescence lifetime were observed in precancerous cells [35]. Precancerous and cancerous samples generally show increased keratin thickness, increased epithelial thickness, decreased nuclear density ratio and decreased keratin layer fluorescence [59]. Moreover, cellular fluorescence becomes progressively weaker and more perinuclear in precancerous and cancerous tissue when compared with normal tissue [60].

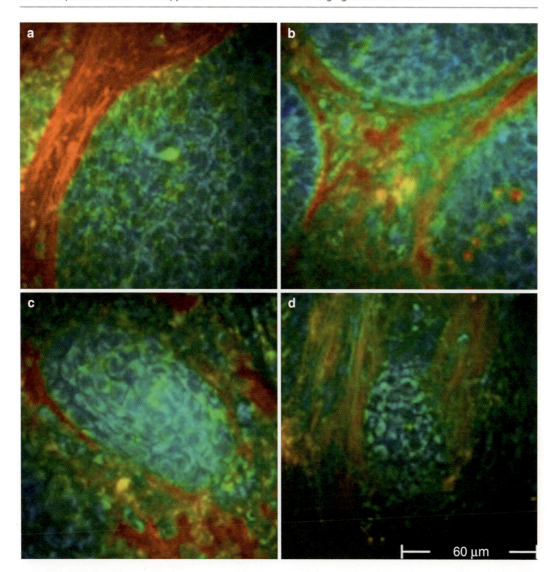

Fig. 18.3 FLIM images acquired at 760 nm excitation wavelength by the Imperial College FLIM system incorporated in the *DermaInspect*® and processed using the software SPC IMAGE (Becker & Hickl GmbH). (**a**) Basal cell carcinoma. FLIM image acquired at 40 µm depth that shows elongated and aligned blue cells. The alignment occurs at one direction. The figure shows four examples of basaloid nests (FLIM images) acquired from different patients at a 760 nm wavelength. (**a**) 110 µm depth: a basaloid island surrounded by a network of red collagen fibres. (**b**) 120 µm depth: bundles of collagen fibres which separate three basaloid blue nests. (**c**) 70 µm depth: a tumoural nest in the upper dermis. (**d**) 80 µm depth: poorly defined tumoural islands, intermingled with collagen fibres

Squamous Cell Carcinoma

Paoli et al. investigated five squamous cell carcinoma specimens. In these samples the stratum corneum was abnormally thick compared to the corresponding perilesional skin. In the same specimens, fluorescent nuclei compartments within the corneocytes were observed. This morphological and fluorescent feature had been described earlier in the presence of hyperkeratosis [20]. In two hyperkeratotic lesions, large, rounded bundles of keratin were observed within the SC, corresponding to the so-called keratin pearls.

In all but one lesion, the keratinocytes within the SG, the SS and the SB were irregularly distributed, reflecting a loss of cell polarity. Dimly fluorescent and widened intercellular spaces were present in three of these four lesions. Signs

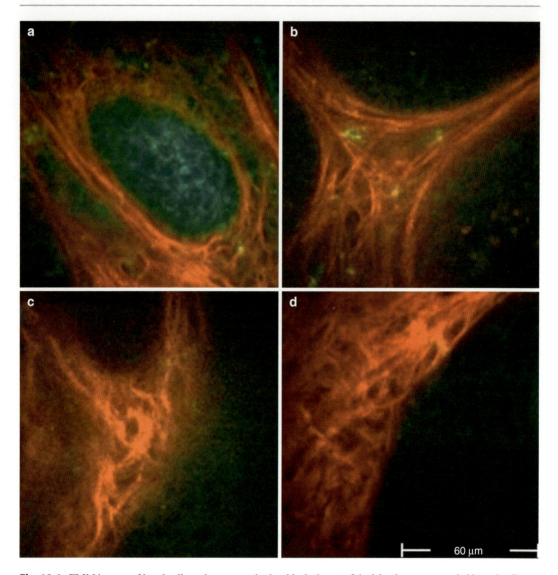

Fig. 18.4 FLIM images of basal cell carcinoma acquired at 800–820 nm excitation wavelength by the Imperial College FLIM system incorporated in the *DermaInspect®* and processed using the software SPC IMAGE (Becker & Hickl GmbH). Increasing the wavelength, the blue keratinocytes become less visible, appearing as dark spaces; the black shapes of the islands are surrounded by red collagen fibres. (**a**) FLIM image at an 800 nm excitation wavelength, 90 μm depth. (**b**) FLIM image at an 820 nm excitation wavelength, 140 μm depth. (**c**) FLIM image at an 820 nm excitation wavelength, 120 μm depth. (**d**) FLIM image at an 820 nm excitation wavelength, 105 μm depth

of bowenoid dysplasia, including pleomorphism and substantial variation of nuclei size, were observed within the epidermis of four lesions. Large, multinucleated cells were noticed in all five lesions. Keratinocytes with brighter cytoplasmic fluorescence compared to surrounding cells in the SG and the SS were discerned in two lesions, possibly corresponding to dyskeratosis. Four lesions presented speckled perinuclear fluorescence in the SG and/or the SS, whereas

this feature was only observed in one corresponding normal perilesional skin sample.

Malignant Melanoma (MM)

Melanocytic lesions are easily investigated when considering that melanin is a fluorophore characterised by emission lifetimes different from those of other endogenous fluorophores.

Dimitrow et al. investigated some procedures of selective melanin imaging and spectral fluorescence lifetime imaging in combination with high-resolution multiphoton laser tomography by analysing 46 melanocytic lesions of human skin [23]. Remarkable differences in lifetime behaviour of keratinocytes in contrast to melanocytes were observed. The fluorescence lifetime distribution was found in correlation with the intracellular amount of melanin. Examining the unique light absorption behaviour of melanin, they found a selective fluorescence of melanin-containing cells at an excitation wavelength of 800 nm. Their results revealed that keratinocyte lifetime values correspond to NAD(P)H and melanocyte lifetime values to the endogenous fluorophore melanin. Thus, whereas FLIM on single data points allowed a clear separation of different melanised cell types (e.g. keratinocytes, melanocytes), it seemed to be unsuitable for a classification of benign versus malignant melanocytic skin lesions. Both melanocytic nevi and MM were characterised by enhanced cell density of melanocytes primarily in the basal epidermal layer. Being the alteration of the upper epidermal layers a unique characteristic of malignant proliferation, the crucial point of differentiation was identified in the presence of ascending melanocytes. Spectral analysis of MM revealed a main fluorescence peak around 470 nm in combination with an additional peak close to 550 nm throughout all epidermal layers. From this they concluded that morphological alterations, in combination with a selective excitability at 800 nm, a short medium lifetime and a distinct peak around 550 nm in suprabasal epidermal layers, are highly suggestive of MM.

Advantages, Disadvantages and Future Objectives of MPT/FLIM

The results obtained with MPT are extremely coherent with those of the histopathologic analysis, which suggests that this new technique, once fully developed, may replace histology [22].

Autofluorescence images are immediately visualised during the examination process in real time. FLIM images require a further elaboration to produce a pseudocolor image and to allow the operational system to develop a diagram of the fluorescence decay time [25, 51]. Images generated by MPT/FLIM can be analysed either on a morphological basis, comparing the architecture of the tumour and cell shape, size and morphology, or on a functional one, studying the kinetics of the fluorescence decline and the differences produced by the excitation of a sample with various wavelengths [24, 25]. In pseudocolor images, colours correspond to different fluorescence decay values, which are characteristic of different types of cells or extracellular matrix components. When employing an established colour scale, for example, 0–2,000 ps from red to blue, the contrasted image provides further information with respect to the autofluorescence one, since a determined colour marks specific structures. Thus, red filamentous structures are immediately recognisable as collagen fibres, whereas blue ones correspond to elastic fibres; red cells match with melanin-containing cells, contrasting with green keratinocytes; etc.

Regarding the technique as non-invasive and the laser illumination harmless, in vivo examination by MPT/FLIM can be repeated on the same site without restrictions, allowing long-term studies of skin diseases [22]. Thanks to the possibility of obtaining horizontal and vertical optical sections, the tissue sample can be studied three-dimensionally with a subcellular spatial resolution. Moreover, the nonlinear excitation produced by the NIR radiation allows a deeper penetration than that of confocal microscopy, with a better discrimination of the various tissue components and a higher visualisation of the deep dermis [22].

On the other hand, the use of the MPT/FLIM technique presents some drawbacks. Image acquisition time is longer compared to traditional fluorescent microscopy and confocal microscopy, and this implies that the patient is forced to keep still for the entire duration of the examination in order to obtain good-quality images. Therefore, one goal is to reduce the acquisition time to avoid imaging deformities caused by involuntary movements, to cardiac pulsations or muscular thrills. Another important aim is to make the instrument probe more flexible and manageable by introducing a specific device to explore difficult body sites or irregular surfaces [22]. Finally, since at present only a very small area of investigation of the tissue is feasible, the risk of missing diagnostic parts of a lesion cannot be ruled out. It is therefore necessary to increase the exploration surface implementing the possibility to make lateral movements and acquire contiguous images, which could be automatically assembled through specific software generating an overview of the entire lesion.

Glossary

FAD Flavin adenine dinucleotide.
FLIM Fluorescence lifetime imaging.
FRET Förster resonance energy transfer, is a mechanism describing energy transfer between two chromophores.
MPE Multiphoton excitation.
MPT Multiphoton laser tomography
MPT/FLIM Multiphoton laser microscopy with Fluorescence lifetime imaging.
Multiphoton microscopy is a specialized optical microscope that relies on the simultaneous absorption of two or more photons of low energy in the near-infrared spectrum, avoiding biological tissue damage that occurs with higher laser powers.
NADH Nicotinamide adenine dinucleotide.
SHG (second harmonic generation) is a method for probing interfaces in atomic and molecular systems.

References

1. Garbe C, Blum A. Epidemiology of cutaneous melanoma in Germany and worldwide. Skin Pharmacol Appl Skin Physiol. 2001;14(5):280–90.
2. Welch H, Woloshin S, Schwartz L. Skin biopsy rates and incidence of melanoma: population based ecological study. BMJ. 2005;331(7515):481.
3. Stang A, Ziegler S, Buchner U, et al. Malignant melanoma and nonmelanoma skin cancers in Northrhine-Westphalia. Germany: a patient-vs. diagnosis-based incidence approach. Int J Dermatol. 2007;46(6):564–70.
4. Roewert-Huber J, Lange-Aschenfeldt B, Stockfleth E, et al. Epidemiology and etiology of basal cell carcinoma. Br J Dermatol. 2007;157(Suppl):47–51.
5. Leiter U, Garbe C. Epidemiology of melanoma and nonmelanoma skin cancer: the role of sunlight. Adv Exp Med Biol. 2008;624:89–103.
6. Morton CA, Mackie RM. Clinical accuracy of the diagnosis of cutaneous malignant melanoma. Br J Dermatol. 1998;138:283–7.
7. Dolianitis C, Kelly J, Wolfe R, et al. Comparative performance of 4 dermoscopic algorithms by nonexperts for the diagnosis of melanocytic lesions. Arch Dermatol. 2005;141:1008–14.
8. Annessi G, Bono R, Sampogna F, et al. Sensitivity, specificity, and diagnostic accuracy of three dermoscopic algorithmic methods in the diagnosis of doubtful melanocytic lesions: the importance of light brown structureless areas in differentiating atypical melanocytic nevi from thin melanomas. J Am Acad Dermatol. 2007;56:759–67.
9. Telfer NR, Colver GB, Morton CA. Guidelines for management of basal cell carcinoma. Br J Dermatol. 2008;159:35–48.
10. Argenziano G, Soyer HP, Chimenti S, et al. Dermoscopy of pigmented skin lesions: results of a consensus meeting via the Internet. J Am Acad Dermatol. 2003;48:679–93.
11. González S, Tannus Z. Real-time in vivo confocal reflectance microscopy of basal cell carcinoma. J Am Acad Dermatol. 2002;47(6):869–74.
12. Pellacani G, Cesinaro AM, Seidenari S. Reflectance-mode confocal microscopy of pigmented skin lesions – improvement in melanoma diagnostic specificity. J Am Acad Dermatol. 2005;53(6):979–85.
13. Guitera P, Pellacani G, Longo C, et al. In vivo reflectance confocal microscopy enhances secondary evaluation of melanocytic lesions. J Invest Dermatol. 2009;129(1):131–8.
14. Vestergaard ME, Macaskill P, Holt PE, et al. Dermoscopy compared with naked eye examination for the diagnosis of primary melanoma: a meta-analysis of studies performed in a clinical setting. Br J Dermatol. 2008;159:669–76.
15. Bauer J, Leinweber B, Metzler G, et al. Correlation with digital dermoscopic images can help dermatopathologists to diagnose equivocal skin tumours. Br J Dermatol. 2006;155(3):546–51.
16. Denk W, Strickler JH, Webb WW. Two-photon laser scanning fluorescence microscopy. Science. 1990;248:73–6.
17. König K, Schenke-Layland K, Riemann I, et al. Multiphoton autofluorescence imaging of intratissue elastic fibers. Biomaterials. 2005;26(5):495–500.
18. Lakowicz JR. Principles of fluorescence spectroscopy. New York: Springer; 2006.
19. Zhao J, Chen J, Yang Y, et al. Jadassohn-Pellizzari anetoderma: study of multiphoton microscopy based on two-photon excited fluorescence and second harmonic generation. Eur J Dermatol. 2009;19(6):570–5.
20. König K, Riemann I. High-resolution multiphoton tomography of human skin with subcellular spatial resolution and picoseconds time resolution. J Biomed Opt. 2003;8(3):432–9.
21. Riemann I, Dimitrow E, Fischer P, Reif A, Kaatz M, Elsner P, et al. High resolution multiphoton tomography of human skin in vivo and in vitro. SPIE-Proceeding. 2004;5312:21–8.

22. König K. Clinical multiphoton tomography. J Biophotonics. 2008;1(1):13–23. Review.
23. Dimitrow E, Riemann I, Ehlers A, et al. Spectral fluorescence lifetime detection and selective melanin imaging by multiphoton laser tomography for melanoma diagnosis. Exp Dermatol. 2009; 18(6):509–15.
24. Elson D, Requejo-Isidro J, Munro I, et al. Time-domain fluorescence lifetime imaging applied to biological tissue. Photochem Photobiol Sci. 2004;3: 795–801.
25. Galletly NP, McGinty J, Dunsby C, et al. Fluorescence lifetime imaging distinguishes basal cell carcinoma from surrounding uninvolved skin. Br J Dermatol. 2008;159:152–61.
26. Hanson KM, Behne MJ, Barry NP, et al. Two-photon fluorescence imaging of the skin stratum corneum pH gradient. Biophys J. 2002;83:1682–90.
27. Kaneko H, Putzier I, Frings S, et al. Chloride accumulation in mammalian olfactory sensory neurons. J Neurosci. 2004;24:7931–8.
28. Lakowicz JR, Szmacinski H. Fluorescence-lifetime based sensing of pH, Ca2þ, and glucose. Sens Actuator Chem. 1993;11:133–4.
29. Gerritsen HC, Sanders R, Draaijer A, et al. Fluorescence lifetime imaging of oxygen in cells. J Fluoresc. 1997;7:11–6.
30. Schweitzer D, Hammer M, Schweitzer F, et al. In vivo measurement of time-resolved autofluorescence at the human fundus. J Biomed Opt. 2004;9:1214–22.
31. Treanor B, Lanigan PMP, Suhling K, et al. Imaging fluorescence lifetime heterogeneity applied to GFP-tagged MHC protein at an immunological synapse. J Microsc. 2005;217:36–43.
32. Calleja V, Ameer-Beg S, Vojnovic B, et al. Monitoring conformational changes of proteins in cells by fluorescence lifetime imaging microscopy. Biochem J. 2003;372:33–40.
33. Kelbauskas L, Dietel W. Internalization of aggregated photosensitizers by tumor cells: subcellular time-resolved fluorescence spectroscopy on derivates of pyropheophorbide-a ethers and chlorine6 under femtosecond one- and two-photon excitation. Photochem Photobiol. 2002;76:686–94.
34. Van Zandvoort MAMJ, de Grauw CJ, Gerritsen HC, et al. Discrimination of DNA and RNA in cells by a vital fluorescent probe: lifetime imaging of SYTO13 in healthy and apoptotic cells. Cytometry. 2002;47: 226–35.
35. Skala MC, Riching KM, Gendron-Fitzpatrick A, et al. In vivo multiphoton microscopy of NADH and FAD redox states, fluorescence lifetimes, and cellular morphology in precancerous epithelia. Proc Natl Acad Sci U S A. 2007;104(49):19495.
36. Lakowicz JR, Szmacinski H, Nowaczyk K, et al. Fluorescence lifetime imaging of free and protein-bound NADH. Proc Natl Acad Sci U S A. 1992; 89:1271–5.
37. Becker W, Bergmann A, Hink MA, et al. Fluorescence lifetime imaging by time-correlated single photon counting. Microsc Res Tech. 2004;63: 58–66.
38. Peter M, Ameer-Beg SM, Hughes MKY, et al. Multiphoton-FLIM quantification of the EGFP-mRFP1 FRET pair for localization of membrane receptor-kinase interactions. Biophys J. 2005;88: 1224–37.
39. Pitts JD, Sloboda RD, Dragnev KH, et al. Autofluorescence characteristics of immortalized and carcinogen-transformed human bronchial epithelial cells. J Biomed Opt. 2001;6:31–40.
40. Galeotti T, van Rossum GD, Mayer DH, et al. On the fluorescence of NAD(P)H in whole-cell preparations of tumours and normal tissues. Eur J Biochem. 1970;17:485–96.
41. Palmer GM, Keely PJ, Breslin TM, et al. Autofluorescence spectroscopy of normal and malignant human breast cell lines. Photochem Photobiol. 2003;78:462–9.
42. Kollias N, Zonios G, Stamatas GN. Fluorescence spectroscopy of skin. Vib Spectrosc. 2002;28(1): 17–23.
43. Zipfel WR, Williams RM, Christie R, et al. Live tissue intrinsic emission microscopy using multiphoton-excited native fluorescence and second harmonic generation. Proc Natl Acad Sci U S A. 2003;100(12): 7075–80.
44. Schenke-Layland K, Riemann I, Damour O, et al. Two-photon microscopes and in vivo multiphoton tomographs-powerful diagnostic tools for tissue engineering and drug delivery. Adv Drug Deliv Rev. 2006;58(7):878–96.
45. Becker W, Bergmann A, Biskup C. Multispectral fluorescence lifetime imaging by TCSPC. Microsc Res Tech. 2007;70(5):403–9.
46. Lin SJ et al. Multiphoton microscopy: a new paradigm in dermatological imaging. Eur J Dermatol. 2007; 17(5):361–6.
47. Tsai TH, Jee SH, Dong CY, et al. Multiphoton microscopy in dermatological imaging. J Dermatol Sci. 2009;56(1):1–8.
48. Teuchner K, Ehlert J, Freyer W, et al. Fluorescence studies of melanin by stepwise two-photon femtosecond laser excitation. J Fluoresc. 2000;10:275–81.
49. Rice WL, Kaplan DL, Georgakoudi I. Two-photon microscopy for non-invasive, quantitative monitoring of stem cell differentiation. PLoS One. 2010;5(4): e10075.
50. Seidenari S, Schianchi S, Azzoni P, et al. High-resolution multiphoton tomography and fluorescence lifetime imaging of UVB-induced cellular damage on cultured fibroblasts producing fibres. Skin Res Technol. 2013. [Epub ahead of print].
51. Benati E, Bellini V, Borsari S, et al. Quantitative evaluation of healthy epidermis by means of Multiphoton microscopy and FLIM. Skin Res Technol. 2011;17(3): 295–303.
52. Cicchi R, Massi D, Sestini S, et al. Multidimensional non-linear laser imaging of basal cell carcinoma. Opt Express. 2007;15(16):10135–48.
53. Paoli J, Smedh M, Wennberg AM, et al. Multiphoton laser scanning microscopy on non-melanoma skin cancer: morphologic features for future non-invasive diagnostics. J Invest Dermatol. 2008;128(5):1248–55.

54. De Giorgi V, Massi D, Sestini S, et al. Combined nonlinear laser imaging (two-photon excitation fluorescence microscopy, fluorescence lifetime imaging microscopy, multispectral multiphoton microscopy) in cutaneous tumours: first experiences. J Eur Acad DermatolVenereol. 2009;23(3):314–6.

55. Paoli J, Smedh M, Ericson MB. Multiphoton laser scanning microscopy-a novel diagnostic method for superficial skin cancers. Semin Cutan Med Surg. 2009;28(3):190–5. Review.

56. Lin SJ, Jee SH, Kuo CJ, et al. Discrimination of basal cell carcinoma from normal dermal stroma by quantitative multiphoton imaging. Opt Lett. 2006;31:2756–8.

57. Brancaleon L, Durkin AJ, Tu JH, et al. In vivo fluorescence spectroscopy of nonmelanoma skin cancer. Photochem Photobiol. 2001;73:178–83.

58. Seidenari S, Arginelli F, Dunsby C, French P, König K, Magnoni C, Manfredini M, Talbot C, Ponti G. Multiphoton laser tomography and fluorescence lifetime imaging of basal cell carcinoma: morphologic features for non-invasive diagnostics. Exp Dermatol. 2012;21(11):831–6.

59. Skala MC, Squirrell JM, Vrotsos KM, et al. Multiphoton microscopy of endogenous fluorescence differentiates normal, precancerous, and cancerous squamous epithelial tissue. Cancer Res. 2005;65:1180–6.

60. White FH, Gohari K, Smith CJ. Histological and ultrastructural morphology of 7,12 dimethylbenz(a)-anthracene carcinogenesis in hamster cheek pouch epithelium. Diagn Histopathol. 1981;4:307–33.

Paola Pasquali

Key Points
- Essential tool to complement the patient's electronic medical history. Useful for treatment control (before and after pictures) and follow-up of disease
- Educational tool for the clinician, peers, and other health personnel involved in the patient's care, when a second opinion is required (by email) and for teledermatology/teledermoscopy
- Indispensable for academic purposes (lectures, publications)

Introduction

Registry of skin ailments has been always in the mind of those who treat dermatological conditions. With the advent of digital photography, taking clinical pictures has become a low cost and simple matter. The price of a good camera is sufficiently low to make it accessible to everyone, making it almost unjustifiable not to have one. In oncology, the use of photography is even more important since it allows to locate the lesion, compare before and after treatment images, send the image for second opinion, rethink the diagnosis once the pathologist has given his/her diagnosis, compare clinical vs. dermoscopy appearance of a lesion, and do follow-up to lesions for possible changes (pigmented lesions), recurrences, and early diagnosis of photodamage (UV photography).

Despite the above statements, there is plenty of room for improvement as far as number of images taken by dermatologists, the quality and the use of these records.

A clinical picture freezes in time an instant where a patient had an ailment, and follow-up pictures create a historical record of the disease progress or the response to treatment. A picture is worth a 1,000 words.

From the times when dermatology departments had a professional photographer as part of the staff, it's all water under the bridge. For those who do feel the need to create a photographic record, digital photography has shortened the gap between professional and amateurs.

Why, How, and When of Clinical Photography

Why?

Clinicians take pictures for numerous reasons, among them:

P. Pasquali
Department of Dermatology,
Pius Hospital De Valls, Carrer Paul Cezanne 36C,
Cambrils, Tarragona 43850, Spain
e-mail: pasqualipaola@gmail.com

A. Baldi et al. (eds.), *Skin Cancer*, Current Clinical Pathology,
DOI 10.1007/978-1-4614-7357-2_19, © Springer Science+Business Media New York 2014

1. To leave a record of the disease in the patient's history for future references.
2. Educational tool:
   To teach themselves about the patient's condition once the complete diagnosis is achieved
   To teach others (students, colleagues)
   For publications
3. To get a second opinion (in teledermatology, teledermoscopy, person-to-doctor consultation, doctor to doctor).
4. To show the patient the effect of treatment on the skin condition.
5. To assess changes in lesions (as in digital dermoscopy follow-up).
6. For scientific purposes. Proper photographic records allow researchers to determine patterns present in lesions and compare different presentations of disease. It is difficult to imagine the advances in noninvasive tools for dermatological diagnosis without photography.

How?

Conventional reflex cameras focus light onto a piece of film to create an image. The quality of the images of those cameras was excellent. However, the quality depended heavily on the operator since they did not have many automatic features. In addition, they have become expensive and difficult to find and filmmakers have disappeared from the market (Kodak, one of the main manufacturers of film photography, went bankrupt as of January 2012), there was no way of knowing the output of a picture until the 35 mm was developed, storage of pictures is laborious and difficult, and, last but not least, cartridges were delicate to manipulate and expensive and film cellulose was perishable and easily contaminated by fungi.

Digital reflex cameras have come to substitute conventional reflex film cameras. The option of digital cameras available in the market is so enormous that clinicians are spoilt for choice.

In digital cameras, the light is focused into a semiconductor device that records light electronically. A computer then breaks this electronic information down into digital data [1].

Good quality cameras are also incorporated into PDA (personal digital assistant) and smart mobile phones. Images taken with a mobile phone through a dermoscope (which includes its own light source) can be of excellent quality.

Cameras [2]

Generally speaking, cameras can be:

1. Basic compact or point-and-shoot cameras:
   Advantages: they are small, low weight, low cost, and easily manageable; LCD (liquid crystal display) present.
   Disadvantages: no lens exchange, low storage capacity, lower quality pictures. No optical viewfinder present. Most point-and-shot cameras do not allow for flash regulation.
2. Compact bridge cameras:
   Advantages: small body, though bigger than compact ones; good to excellent pictures; manual control. Incorporated macro feature is sufficiently powerful to get excellent images. LCD (liquid crystal display) included and also optical viewfinder. Ring flash can be adapted.
   Disadvantages: fixed and not interchangeable lenses.
3. Interchangeable-lens mirrorless camera:
   Advantages: interchangeable-lens camera with body similar to compact bridge camera.
   Disadvantages: does not have a mirror-based optical viewfinder. As expensive as SRL camera.
4. SRL camera:
   Advantages: has through-the-lens (TTL) metering, which allows the camera to measure the actual light levels and use the information to select exposure and thus control the amount of light from the flash. Optical viewfinder included. Highest digital quality. Lens exchange possible with wide range of choice. Ring flash available.
   Disadvantages: Bigger cameras, heavier and bulky, and more expensive.

Image Size

The size of the image sensor is directly related to the image quality. Larger sensors mean that more details are captured under low light. The number of photosites or sensels of the image sensor corresponds with the number of pixels of the image

Table 19.1 Pictures required for the different types of lesions

		Type of lesion		
		Single lesion (e.g., a small tumor)	Localized lesion (e.g.. metameric lesion)	Generalized lesions (e.g., multiple skin metastasis)
Pictures required	Close-up	✓	✓	✓
	Medium view	✓	✓	✓ (not essential)
	Distant view	✗	✓ (helps to determine symmetry/asymmetry)	✓

generated by that sensor [2], i.e., a ten million sensor generates 10 MP pictures.

Although the presence of a larger number of pixels translates into more detailed images, the initial race for pixels that occurred in the first years of digital photography is now over and most of today's cameras can fulfill the requirements for good dermatological pictures.

The macro feature is of outmost importance for the dermatologist because it allows to capture close-up pictures with details that will help clinicians to make diagnosis. In close-up photography, the image obtained is similar to the original size. It reproduces in a 1:1 or larger scale. For most automatic compact cameras, the macro feature is indicated by a small flower on the dial.

Backdrop

The presence of the flat backdrop will be determinant in the quality of the picture. In order to avoid pictures out of focus, the lens has to be able to focus only on the subject/lesion area. In automatic focusing, the presence of objects in the background will result in an average focusing between the subject and the background, which will leave your point of interest out of focus. The most common backgrounds are blue or green cotton sheets. Black velvet can work very nicely too. It is important to have at hand a bib made out of the same material. This will allow taking pictures of the head, without including in the picture other details of the body.

Picture Format (Table 19.1)

Since visual clues are fundamental for diagnosis, pictures should be able to show such clues as well. Distribution, configuration, and close-up look are important elements to evaluate when looking at a skin ailment [3].

Distribution

It is important to show the location of the lesion(s) in an anatomical area. Lesions can be generalized (i.e., generalized herpes zoster in an immunosuppressed cancer patient) [4], segmental, sun-exposed area, etc.

Pictures should include some noninvolved area; for unilateral lesions, a far view involving the contralateral side should be taken to give information on symmetry (i.e., the lineal distribution of a metastasis in one arm should be capturing the contralateral arm, for comparison).

For multiple small lesions (like nevi or multiple carcinomas), it is convenient to capture a far view of the area, taking care to previously mark them with a number or a circle (Fig. 19.1).

For these far views, no macro is needed and the user of a backdrop is fundamental to avoid distractions.

The perception of depth that perspective gives is an important attribute. For 35 mm film, a lens of around 100 mm focal length allows distortion-free images in most clinical situations, but a shorter focal length of around 50–60 mm will be needed for full-length photographs or when working in a confined space [5].

Configuration

It refers to the arrangement of the lesions with respect to one another. In oncology, for example, metastasis can have linear, zosteriform (Fig. 19.2), or perilesional distribution and paraneoplastic manifestations can mimic inflammatory diseases [6].

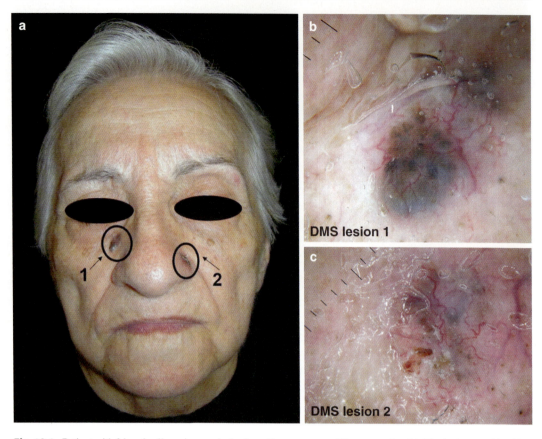

Fig. 19.1 Patient with 2 basal cell carcinomas in the face. Eyes are covered for convention (**a**). The lesions are identified in the clinical picture in order to associate its relative dermoscopic (DMS) image (**b**, **c**)

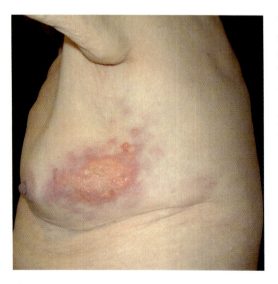

Fig. 19.2 Zosteriform distribution of metastatic prostate cancer

Medium-distance views are required usually with macro. The presence of a backdrop is usually required. Always try to capture distinctive elements like typical representative lesions, particular configuration, or distribution patterns. (Always include a recognizable body landmark so that the location is obvious. For example, for lesions on the abdomen, include the umbilicus in the medium-distance shot.)

Primary lesion is a close-up view that requires macro. In this case, the use of backdrop is unnecessary. It requires though a perfect balance of the flash, in order to avoid shadows and bright spots in the center. Pictures are usually taken perpendicularly to the skin. Oblique views might be required to show the trimensional aspects of a tumor. For lesions with a crust, it is better to take the picture with and without, to put in evidence, the hidden elements (Fig. 19.3). The presence of a ruler leaves evidence of the size.

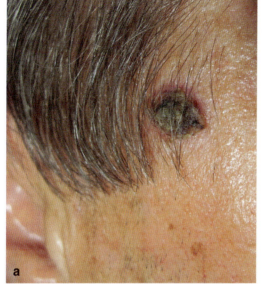

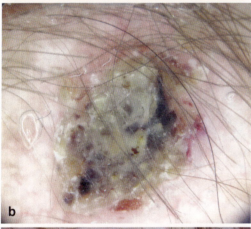

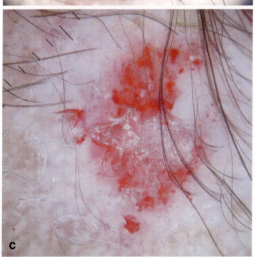

Fig. 19.3 Lesion with crust (**a**). The dermoscopic image with the crust gives little information (**b**). Once the crust is taken out (**c**), abnormal vessels suggest a squamous cell carcinoma, later confirmed by excisional biopsy

Use macro feature at distances within the 30–60 cm range.

For dermoscopy registry, two views should be taken: a far view (leaving under focus the ruler incorporated in the dermoscope) and close-up. If the clinician wants to take both polarized and immersion fluid dermoscopy, it is best to take the polarized first (with no immersion fluid) and later the second (to avoid the need to remove the fluid in between pictures).

For single lesions, take a medium view to identify location (Fig. 19.4). New photographic softwares include body location features that allow framing images by location thus making this medium view unnecessary. It would be advisable to take close-up shots from more than one angle and also to include oblique shots. Shots with and without flash may be taken and the best shot selected for filing.

Consistency

Take pictures following the same frame of reference. This will allow you to have comparable pictures even when they are taken in different time periods. There are photographic equipments (Canfield, Microcaya) useful for face photography that allow to take before and after pictures that can be later superimposed with digital softwares. This is a feature that can be useful to measure the extent of improvement of photodamaged areas.

Have the patient close his/her eyes when taking a face picture in order to have eyes always shut (Fig. 19.5). Try to keep the same distance from the patient, same background and same anatomical position. If you get into the routinary and systematic way of working, pictures will be comparable in follow-ups.

Use the same backdrop every time. Blue, green, or black are the most commonly used. They have to be made of nonreflecting material.

Remove jewelry or cloth whenever interfering with the area that is to be photographed.

Take several pictures in order to choose the best one.

Ideally, pictures should be taken under the same light conditions. Although ideal, this is not always possible. Adjust the white balance at the beginning of the day or whenever we feel that

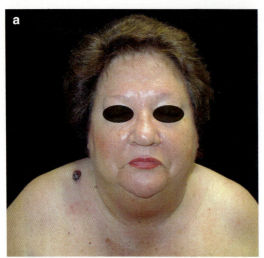

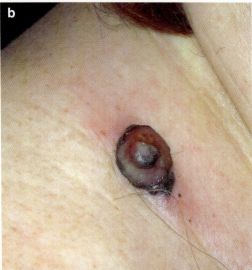

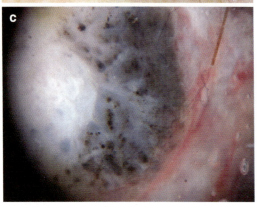

Fig. 19.4 (a) Far, (b) medium, and (c) dermoscopy view of a lesion in the right shoulder of a 61-year-old woman with a malignant melanoma

light conditions have changed. White balance (present in bridge cameras and above) is essential to warranty the correct skin color. We have to adjust this balance prior to taking the picture. Cameras like the Canon G11 include auto-adjustment, daylight, cloudy day tungsten, fluorescent, and fluorescent H. White balance adjustment prepares the camera for the particular color of the light source illuminating the subject.

Avoid the use of flash too close to the lesion in order to avoid whiteout. It is best to take the picture with flash at a certain distance and zoom in the subject or even enlarging the picture later on. Digital cameras include a control over the flash intensity. In addition, the built in flash can be diffused by applying over it a white tape. External flashes and ring flashes can help avoiding central whiteout, peripheral darkening, and undesirable shadows.

Use a tripod whenever possible.

Always take high-resolution images. It will always leave you with images for future use in conferences and publications. A picture's weight can always be lowered if necessary.

Consent Form

Get consent form signed for pictures taken and use chaperons when appropriate. Include in it multiple uses: clinical record, academic purposes, publications, second opinion, and teledermatology.

Packing and Storing

Digitalization has simplified the tracking of images. At the time of slides, each picture had to be handled with care (using cotton gloves), identified on the frame, saved in appropriate envelops, kept away from humidity or excess heat, and so on. However, the number of images taken nowadays has increased exponentially, thanks to the relatively simplicity in taking a picture and its low cost.

Every time you take a picture, make sure you leave a record of which this picture belongs to. One practical way is to photograph the patients file which includes name, last name, and number of clinical record. This will be later indispensable when downloading the images from the camera.

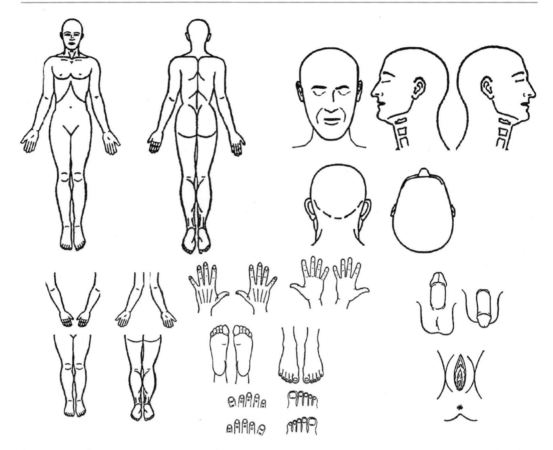

Fig. 19.5 Suggested standardized positions

Download daily (or as frequent as you find convenient, depending on the number of shots taken). The sooner it is done, the easier to track back any missing information.

Make sure to frequently make safety copies of your patient's photographs in order to avoid irreparable losses. It is advisable to have a backup at a different location in case of fire, flooding, or any other disaster.

For hospital/private practice settings, a DICOM (Digital Imaging and Communications in Medicine) is a standard for handling, storing, printing, and transmitting information in medical imaging. It includes a file format definition and a network communications protocol.

A picture archiving and communication system (PACS) is a storage system of electronic images and reports that has substituted manual filing, retrieving, and transporting of film jackets. The format for PACS image storage and transfer is DICOM (Digital Imaging and Communications in Medicine). Each DICOM file includes tags with administrative patient's information plus the image itself in JPEG/TIFF/RAW format [7]. To integrate the patient's images into the file, they first have to be "dichotomized." There are special softwares, like MIO (Medical Images Organizer), that turn images into DICOM format and send them to the PACS.

Total Body Photography/UV Photography/IR Photography/Other Filters

One of the consequences of digitalization has been the opportunity to observe changes over time. Total body photography aids physicians to identify the appearance of new pigmentary lesions or changes in existing ones in follow-up of patients at high risk of malignant melanoma.

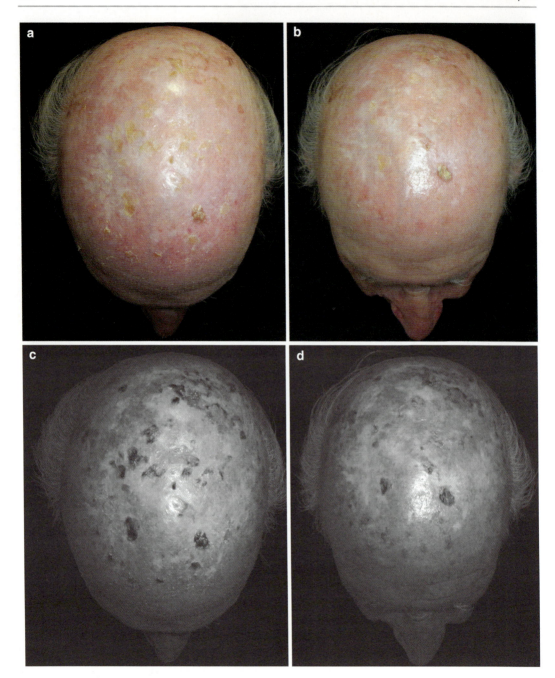

Fig. 19.6 (a) Scalp on a patient with severe photodam-aged skin. (b) After 3-month treatment with Solaraze® (topical diclofenac). (c) Same image as (a), passed through a blue filter to highlight sun damage. (d) After treatment blue filtered picture. Filtering the pre- and post treatment pictures has better put into evidence the improvement

Computer-assisted diagnostic devices have the capacity to identify individual lesions (dermoscopic pictures) either benign or malignant. They are becoming more precise with time, and they are very helpful in decision making once faced with a suspicious pigmented lesion.

UV photography [8] is an underutilized technique helpful to highlight sun-damaged skin. UV-damaged skin has increased amounts of melanin as well as hemoglobin. UV photography can be done by either removing UV filters found in the camera or applying filters that block other [9] wavelengths.

Another option is to apply filters to pre- and posttreated images taken to sun-damaged skin in order to measure changes in the skin's vascular, melanic, and keratin content (Fig. 19.6).

Future Considerations

With the arrival of extremely high-pixel photography (over 300 MP) and the use of new filtering techniques and new analyzing softwares, dermatological photography will soon turn into a non-invasive tool for diagnosis.

Glossary

DICOM Digital Imaging and Communications in Medicine. It is a standard for handling, storing, printing, and transmitting information in medical imaging.

JPEG format Joint Photographers Experts Group format. It is the most common format for storing and transmitting photographic images.

LCD Liquid crystal display. It is a flat panel that uses the light modulating properties of liquid crystals.

Medical Images Organizer (MIO) It is a group of software tools developed to incorporate digital medical imaging into medical records. It integrates medical images in a centralized manner, facilitating access to it. It turns into DICOM a medical image or video, among other features.

PACS Picture archiving and communication system. It is a medical imaging technology which provides economical storage of, and convenient access to, images from multiple modalities.

PDA Personal digital assistant, also know as palmtop computer or personal data assistant is a mobile device that functions as a personal information manager and nowadays mostly substituted by smartphones.

RAW format Sometimes called digital negatives, as they fulfill the same role as negatives in film photography. They are intended to capture as closely as possible the radiometric characteristics of the scene, that is, physical

information about the light intensity and color of the scene.

SRL camera (Single-lens Reflex Camera) is a camera that uses a mirror and prism system that permits to view through the lens and see what exactly what will be captured.

Total Body Photography (TBP) is a diagnostic technique used to track changes in the skin, helping to identify new moles and melanomas.

TIFF format (Tagged Image File Format) It is a file format for storing images. As of 2009, it is under the control of Adobe Systems.

TTL metering (Through-The-Lens Metering) Often associated to SRL cameras, is a photographic term describing the capability of measuring light levels is a scene through their taking lenses.

References

1. Kaliyadan F, Manoj J, Venkitakrishnan S, Dharmaratnam AD. Basic digital photography in dermatology. Indian J Dermatol Venereol Leprol. 2008;74:532–6.
2. Barco L, Ribera M, Casanova JM. Guide to buying a camera for dermatological photography. Actas Dermosifiliogr. 2012;103(6):502–10.
3. Major Hon S. Basic guide to dermatologic photography. 1999. http://www.americantelemed.org/files/public/membergroups/teledermatology/telederm_DermatologicPhotography.pdf.
4. Hata S, Tamaki T. Unusual varicella zoster virus infection in a patient with colon carcinoma and Evans syndrome – delayed virus shedding generalized recurrent necrotic herpes zoster. J Dermatol. 1990;17(5):326–8.
5. Nayler JR. Clinical photography: a guide for the clinician. J Postgrad Med. 2003;49:256–62.
6. Ravić-Nikolić A, Milicić V, Jovović-Dagović B, Ristić G. Gyrate erythema associated with metastatic tumor of gastrointestinal tract. Dermatol Online J. 2006; 12(6):11.
7. Taberner R, Contestí T. Digital photograph storage systems in clinical dermatology. Actas Dermosifiliogr. 2010;101(4):307–14.
8. Gamble RG, Asdigian NL, Aalborg J, Gonzalez V, Box NF, Huff LS, et al. Sun damage in ultraviolet photographs correlates with phenotypic melanoma risk factors in 12-year-old children. J Am Acad Dermatol. 2012;67:587–97.
9. Demirli R, Otto P, Viswanathan R, Patwardhan S, Larkey J. RBX™ technology overview. Technical paper from Canfield Imaging Systems. Fairfield. Available at: http://www.canfieldsci.com/FileLibrary/RBX%20tech%20overview-LoRz1.pdf. Accessed 4 Mar 2011.

Topical Treatment

20

Miguel Alejandro López

Key Points

- Alternative treatment to physical methods of treatment of premalignant and malignant skin lesions.
- First line of treatment of field cancerization.
- It is an excellent alternative treatment in single or multiple low-risk cancers and for patients that refuse surgery.
- It includes treatments with topical 5-fluorouracil (5-FU), imiquimod, mechlorethamine hydrochloride (nitrogen mustard), carmustine, alitretinoin (9-cis retinoic acid), bexarotene, diclofenac, miltefosine, bleomycin, retinoids, colchicine, T4 endonuclease, resiquimod, and ingenol mebutate.

Introduction

There are several therapeutic modalities to treat various types of skin cancer. In general, in the early stages of most common skin cancers, the

M.A. López
Dermatologic Surgery and Cutaneous Oncology Section,
Department of Dermatology,
Hospital Militar "Dr. Carlos Arvelo",
Caracas, Venezuela
e-mail: miguelalejandrolb@yahoo.com

surgical option by removing the tumor and leaving an adequate oncologic margin is usually the best and most used option; in addition, surgery generally offers the best chance of cure with the advantage of having histopathologic evaluation of the excised margins. In other less frequent malignant neoplastic diseases such as mycosis fungoides and Kaposi's sarcoma, topical treatment is an option and even a choice option in the early stages of the disease [1, 2].

There are patients who have personal and/or clinical characteristics that allow us to consider the use of nonsurgical treatment options. These features are:

- Patients with high surgical risk
- Patients with tumors with a low risk of recurrence and/or low risk of local regional or distant metastases
- Patients with advanced cancer in whom surgery would not guarantee a cure
- Patients in whom the disease is incurable and so the possibility of using a palliative treatment raises as an option
- Patients who do not want to have surgery
- Patients with a type of skin cancer in which there is enough scientific evidence that topical treatment is a valid and effective option [1–3]

These modalities beyond conventional cancer surgery include:

- Physical methods with which the tumor tissue is destroyed and normal tissue is included in the oncologic surgical margins. This category includes cryosurgery and curettage with electrodesiccation.

A. Baldi et al. (eds.), *Skin Cancer*, Current Clinical Pathology,
DOI 10.1007/978-1-4614-7357-2_20, © Springer Science+Business Media New York 2014

- Physical-chemical methods: in this mode photodynamic therapy is included; a topical medication is used to sensitize the tumor tissue to a physical medium such as light with certain physical characteristics.
- Chemotherapy: using chemicals or drugs that act directly on the tumor. These drugs can be given systemically (intravenous, oral, subcutaneous, etc.), intralesionally, or topically.
- Immune response modifiers: these are drugs that act on the patient's immune system by increasing their ability to defend against the tumor.
- Biological therapy: using drugs that are obtained by high tech and modify significantly the biological behavior of the immune system, with improvement of the patient's response to the tumor. Biological drugs are used in cases of patients with advanced diseases.

In this chapter we will focus on various topical modalities used to treat primary or metastatic skin cancer, with emphasis on indications, usage, dosage, contraindications, side effects, advantages, and disadvantages. We included treatment options for actinic keratosis; for didactic reasons we considered them as starting malignancies.

5-Fluorouracil

It is a powerful antimetabolite that has been useful in the treatment of various dermatological conditions including various types of skin cancer [3–5].

Pharmacology: Irreversibly inhibits the enzyme thymidylate synthase, preventing methylation of deoxyuridylic acid, which inhibits the formation of thymidylic acid, therefore interfering with the formation of thymidine, an essential nucleotide component of DNA and RNA. 5-Fluorouracil arrests the cell cycle in S phase. This action on the formation of DNA and RNA has a greater effect on rapidly growing and proliferating cells such as malignant cancer cells. Its bioavailability is not well known, its metabolism is mainly hepatic, and excretion occurs mainly in urine and the lungs [3–5].

Formula: $C_4H_3N_2FO_2$

Bioavailability: Unpredictable and incomplete [4].

Metabolism: Hepatic

Average Half-Life Time: 8–20 min

Excretion: Lungs and urine

Uses:

Squamous cell carcinoma in situ (Bowen's disease)

Actinic cheilitis

Leukoplakia

Basal cell carcinomas with a low risk of recurrence or in patients that are not able or willing to undergo surgical treatment

Actinic keratosis

Kaposi's sarcoma

Dosage (Topical)

Squamous Cell Carcinoma In Situ (Bowen's Disease): 1–2 daily applications for 4–6 weeks. Bargman et al. reported a 92.4 % cure rate after 10 years of follow-up in 26 patients with Bowen's disease treated with 5-fluorouracil [6].

Basal Cell Carcinoma: 2 applications a day for 6–12 weeks.

Gross et al. reported a 90 % histopathologic cure rate in 29 patients with 31 superficial basal cell carcinomas treated with 5 % 5-fluorouracil cream used 2 times a day for 12 weeks, most patients presented only mild erythema; local cosmetic satisfaction was high [7].

Epstein reported a recurrence rate of 6 % after 5 years in patients with basal cell carcinomas treated with a 25 % 5-fluorouracil paste [8].

Orenberg et al. reported an 80 % effectiveness using an intralesional 5-fluorouracil implant once a week for 6 weeks [9].

In general, topical treatment with 5-fluorouracil is indicated for the treatment of superficial basal cell carcinomas that are small in size and are located in low-risk anatomical regions [10].

Actinic Keratosis: 1–2 applications a day for 3–5 weeks (Fig. 20.1).

Askew et al. found in a review which systematically evaluated the topical use of 5-fluorouracil for the treatment of actinic keratosis in 29 studies that in general a complete clearance of lesions in half of the patients and a decrease between 80 and 90 % in the number of lesions should be expected; approximately 2/3 of patients require retreatment after 1 year, and although only a few patients discontinued treatment due to side

Fig. 20.1 Before (*left*) and after treatment with 5 % 5 FU, three times a week for 4 weeks

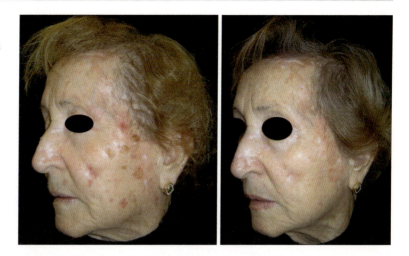

effects, only half of them completed a full course of treatment. The authors felt that the level of evidence to evaluate the use of 5-fluorouracil in actinic keratosis was poor, taking into account the quality of the studies; also considered as poor is the level of evidence that exists for other therapeutic options available for treatment of actinic keratosis [11]. 0.5 % 5-fluorouracil cream preparations seem to have similar effectiveness when compared with the 5 % cream preparation in its ability to reduce the number of lesions, but their action depends more on the treatment time, which can be a problem because many patients stop treatment because of local adverse effects [12].

Actinic Cheilitis: Once a day for 7–14 days, a lot of swelling and inflammation is to be expected (kiss of fire); some authors recommend the use of topical corticosteroids after the treatment to help resolve the inflammation. Epstein reported good experience in 12 patients with recurrences in only 2 patients; there was inflammation with cracking and scabbing, but they report a good cosmetic result [13].

Bowenoid Papulosis: 1–2 daily applications for 4–6 weeks. This treatment should be considered if surgery is not possible [14].

Patients treated with 5-fluorouracil usually develop scaling, erythema with vesicles and blisters formation, pain, and burning, and patients should be warned in advance. Sometimes the frequency of drug application must be decreased to a daily and even a one another day schema depending on the severity of the reaction. The process of re-epithelialization and healing takes place between 1 and 2 months [5, 8].

5-Fluorouracil has been used systemically for the treatment of metastatic breast and gastrointestinal carcinomas as well as ovary, cervix, prostate, bladder, pancreatic, and pharyngeal carcinomas [4].

Available Forms: 0.5, 1, 2, and 5 % cream and lotion. Most reports of topical treatment of skin cancer have been with the 5 % cream.

Safety in Pregnancy (See Table 20.1 *for Category Definitions*): Category D (IV), Category X (topical).

Adverse Effects: Erythema, peeling, blistering, contact dermatitis, photosensitivity, phototoxicity, burning sensation, angioedema, erythema multiforme, rash, folliculitis, necrosis, pigmentation, pruritus, seborrheic dermatitis, lupus-like syndrome, xerosis, alopecia, onycholysis, nail pigmentation, dysgeusia, ectropion, mucositis, paresthesia, stomatitis, and tongue pigmentation [15].

Imiquimod

Imiquimod is an imidazoquinoline amide which acts by stimulating the immune response both innate and acquired. It has antiviral, antitumor, and immunoregulatory activity [3, 5].

Pharmacology: It works by stimulating toll-like receptor 7 on dendritic cells and induces the production of various cytokines such as tumor necrosis

Table 20.1 United States Food and Drug Administration (FDA) pregnancy categories

Category	Description
A	*Controlled studies show no risk* – adequate, well-controlled studies in pregnant women have failed to demonstrate a risk to the fetus in any trimester of pregnancy
B	*No evidence of risk in humans* – adequate, well-controlled studies in pregnant women have not shown increased risk of fetal abnormalities despite adverse findings in animals, *or* in the absence of adequate human studies, animal studies show no fetal risk. The chance of fetal harm is remote but remains a possibility
C	*Risk cannot be ruled out* – adequate, well-controlled human studies are lacking, and animal studies have shown a risk to the fetus or are lacking as well. There is a chance of fetal harm if the drug is administered during pregnancy, but the potential benefits may outweigh the potential risk
D	*Positive evidence of risk* – studies in humans or investigational or post-marketing data have demonstrated fetal risk. Nevertheless, potential benefits from the use of the drug may outweigh the potential risk. For example, the drug may be acceptable if needed in a life-threatening situation or serious disease for which safer drugs cannot be used or are ineffective
X	*Contraindicated in pregnancy* – studies in animals or humans or investigational or post-marketing reports have demonstrated positive evidence of fetal abnormalities or risk which clearly outweigh any possible benefit to the patient

http://edocket.access.gpo.gov/2008/pdf/E8-11806.pdf

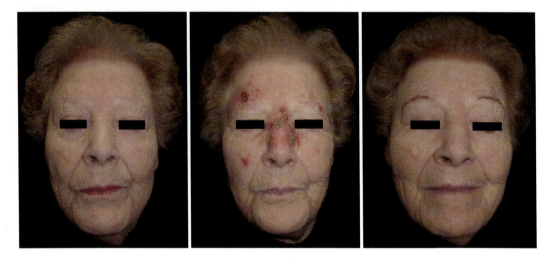

Fig. 20.2 Pretreatment (*extreme left*), immediately posttreatment, and after 1 month posttreatment with imiquimod for three weeks

factor alpha, interferon alpha, and interleukins 1, 6, 8, and 12. Interferon alpha produced by a dendritic cell interacts with the FAS-FAS ligand complex of the tumor cell, leading to apoptosis. Interleukin-12 induces production of interferon gamma by CD4 lymphocytes activating cytotoxic T lymphocytes to act directly against tumor cells [3, 5].

Formula: $C_{14}H_{16}N_4$

Half-Life Time: 30 h (topical dose), 2 h (subcutaneous dose)

Uses:

Squamous cell carcinoma in situ (Bowen's disease)

Actinic cheilitis

Basal cell carcinomas with a low risk of recurrence or in patients who are not able or willing to undergo surgical treatment

Actinic keratosis (Fig. 20.2)

Cutaneous T-cell lymphoma (mycosis fungoides)

Malignant melanoma in situ, in patients that are not candidates for surgical treatment

Metastatic malignant melanoma as an adjunct therapy to chemotherapy and as a palliative treatment that helps to control local skin metastases

Dosage:

Squamous Cell Carcinoma In Situ (Bowen's disease): 1 application per day for 9–16 weeks

Mackenzie-Wood et al. in 2001 reported clinical and histopathologic cure in 15 of 16 patients treated: there was no relapse or recurrence in a follow-up period of 6 months. This effectiveness has been confirmed by other case reports [16–18].

Superficial Basal Cell Carcinoma:

2 daily applications for 12 weeks (effectiveness of 100 %) [19]

1 daily application for 12 weeks (effectiveness of 87 %) [19]

1 daily application, 5 times a week for 12 weeks (effectiveness of 81 %) [19]

1 daily application, 3 times a week for 12 weeks (effectiveness of 52 %) [19]

2 daily applications for 6 weeks (effectiveness of 100 %) [20]

1 daily application for 6 weeks (effectiveness of 88 %) [20]

2 daily applications, 3 times a week for 6 weeks (effectiveness of 73 %) [20]

1 daily application, 3 times a week for 6 weeks (effectiveness of 67 %) [20]

Nodular Basal Cell Carcinoma:

1 daily application for 12 weeks (effectiveness of 78 %) [21]

1 daily application, 5 times a week for 12 weeks (effectiveness of 70 %) [21]

1 daily application, 3 times a week for 12 weeks (effectiveness of 60 %) [21]

1 daily application for 6 weeks (effectiveness of 71 %) [21]

2 daily applications, 3 times a week for 6 weeks (effectiveness of 42 %) [21]

1 daily application, 3 times a week for 6 weeks (effectiveness of 59 %) [21]

In basal cell carcinoma, the dosing regimen and tumor histopathologic variety seem to directly influence the effectiveness of treatment. The higher the frequency of daily and weekly application, the higher is the effectiveness. It is more effective in the superficial histopathologic variety than in the nodular variety and is more effective in lowering the risk of recurrence in anatomic locations such as trunk and limbs. The problem is that the higher the frequency of application, the

higher are also the side effects like inflammation, crusting, edema, and pain. These side effects can significantly affect adherence to treatment [20–22].

Geisse et al. reported an 82 % cure rate in treating small superficial basal cell carcinomas with a 5 times a week for 12 weeks course of treatment and 79 % cure rate in a 7 times per week for 12 weeks scheme compared with the vehicle results that were close to 2 % [22].

Schulze et al. reported an 80 % histopathologic cure rate in treating superficial subtypes using a 1 application a day for 7 days a week for 6 weeks schema; the cure rate with the vehicle was 6 % [23].

Gollnick et al. conducted a prospective study in 182 patients with superficial basal cell carcinomas treated with 5 % imiquimod cream, 5 times per week for 6 weeks, resulting in a cure rate of 69 % at 5 years; apparently the effectiveness of treatment decreases the longer the follow-up periods are [24].

Eigentler et al. reported a clinical and histopathologic response of 72 and 64 %, respectively, in a phase 3 study that evaluated the effectiveness of imiquimod 5 % cream for the treatment of nodular basal cell carcinoma in 102 patients using a regimen of one application 3 times a week for 8 and 12 weeks [25].

Actinic Keratosis: 2 applications a week for 4–16 weeks [3–5].

Edwards et al. reported a 75 % reduction in the number of actinic keratosis using imiquimod 5 % cream 3 times a week for 16 weeks in 40 patients [26].

Salasche et al. conducted a study in 25 patients that used imiquimod 5 % cream, 3 applications per week for 4 weeks followed by a 4-week rest period; if at that time lesions persisted, another course of 4 weeks of treatment was indicated, with a maximum of 3 cycles (12 weeks of treatment and 12 off). Complete response in 82 % of lesions was obtained including subclinical lesions that become evident with treatment; this is a good way to maximize the effectiveness of treatment by decreasing adverse effects [27].

A similar scheme was tested in a phase 3 study conducted by Stockfleth et al. in 829 patients using 2 cycles of 3 times a week for 4 weeks schema, getting total clearance of lesions in 68.9 % and partial clearance in 80.2 % [28].

In a randomized, multicenter, double-blind, placebo study conducted by Szeimies et al. in 286 patients, the use of imiquimod 5 % cream 3 times per week for 16 weeks compared with placebo cream was evaluated; complete response was observed in 57.1 % of lesions in subjects treated with imiquimod compared with 2.2 % in those patients treated with placebo [29].

In a meta-analysis conducted by Gupta et al., imiquimod 5 % cream and 5-fluorouracil 5 % cream were compared for topical treatment of actinic keratosis on the face and scalp, and they concluded that imiquimod was more effective than 5-fluorouracil (70 ± 12 % vs. 52 ± 18 %, respectively) [30].

Actinic Cheilitis: 1 application 3 times a week for 4–6 weeks.

Smith et al. reported total clinical response in 100 % of the 15 patients with diagnosis of actinic cheilitis treated with imiquimod; the result was maintained for 4 weeks of follow-up. No histopathologic control was made. Use of oral valacyclovir as a preventive measure in patients with a personal history of herpes in the facial region was recommended (1 g/day) [31].

Lentigo Maligna: 1–2 applications per day for 5–7 days a week. Treatment time varies depending on the series (12 weeks to 1 year).

Ahmed et al. reported its use for the first time in lentigo maligna in 2000 in an elderly patient who refused to undergo surgery; they used it for a total period of 7 months with frequent rest periods due to local inflammatory reactions and ulcerations and found no evidence of recurrence or relapse 9 months later [32].

Naylor et al. reported histopathologic cure in 26 of 28 (93 %) patients treated with a regimen of one application per day for 12 weeks and no recurrences or relapses during a follow-up period of 1 year [33].

Van Meurs et al. reported in 2010 a 100 % histopathologic cure rate in ten patients with lentigo maligna; the average follow-up was 36 months [34].

Imiquimod is recommended in patients who are not candidates for surgery, which remains the treatment of choice, treatment should be prolonged, and a close and long follow-up period is advised. Cure rates ranging from 60 to 100 % have been reported. Effectiveness of topical imiquimod treatment is not well established in cases of invasive lentigo malignant melanomas and is not recommended due to the risk of local, regional, and distant organ metastases [33, 35].

Narayan et al. reported in a small pilot study an increased number of T cells in local and regional skin and in sentinel lymph nodes in patients with primary invasive malignant melanoma treated with imiquimod; further studies are needed in this type of tumor to clarify the meaning of these findings [36].

Metastatic Malignant Melanoma: 3–5 times a week and extends to periods that vary depending on the series 10–28 weeks. Treatment regimens vary and have been used alone and in combination with dacarbazine, interleukin-2, interferon alpha-2b, and 5-fluorouracil. Most authors report its use under occlusion. Good response rates for local disease control were reported [37, 38].

Available Forms: 3.75 and 5 % cream

Safety in Pregnancy: Category C

Adverse Effects: Inflammation can become severe, crusting, blistering, flu-like malaise, lupus-like reactions, psoriasis, edema, erosions, erythema, abrasions, fungal infections, pigmentation, itching, pain, ulceration pigmentation of hair, aphthous stomatitis, depression, induration, and myalgias [4, 15].

Mechlorethamine Hydrochloride (Nitrogen Mustard)

Is an alkylating agent that acts mainly through alkylation of DNA, generating a cytotoxic effect [3, 4].

Pharmacology: The most important pharmacological effect is that it interferes with DNA synthesis and cell division. The capacity of alkylating agents to affect the function and integrity of DNA in tissues that reproduce quickly and fast is what gives this drug its clinical utility and is also what accounts for their toxicity when used systemically. The cytotoxicity of these agents is enhanced in proliferating tissues in which most cells are actively dividing and their action is even greater in those cells with DNA damage and that are in the process of actively dividing. If the cellular mechanisms of DNA repair in cells are intact and are able to repair target DNA before the next division, the effect of these agents is not lethal. The seventh nitrogen atom of guanine is the most likely position where covalent bonding with the alkylating agent occurs. This also applies to other atoms of the purine and pyrimidine bases in DNA, such as the first and third nitrogen atoms of adenine, the third nitrogen atom of cytosine, and the sixth oxygen atom of guanine. It is a very unstable drug that is rapidly degraded. It can only be used intravenously and topically. It undergoes rapid chemical transformation on contact with water and tissues. Within minutes after administration, it is not possible to detect the drug in its active form [3, 4].

Formula: $C_5H_{11}Cl_2N$

Metabolism: Rapid plasma hydrolysis, demethylation in plasma

Half-Life Time: <1 min

Excretion: Urine (50 % as metabolites, <0.01 % as unchanged drug)

Uses:

Cutaneous T-cell lymphoma (mycosis fungoides) in stages IA and IB. Therapeutic schemes usually start with daily applications over the entire affected area, decreasing the dosage to one another day application after winning control of the disease, depending on patient response and severity of local adverse effects. Two types of preparations have been used, the aqueous formulation for which a solution is prepared at a concentration of 10 mg/50 ml; this solution is applied with a brush on the affected areas and must be prepared daily, and this drug preparation is rapidly degraded on contact with water. The other way to prepare it is by using petrolatum as a vehicle in a concentration of 10 mg per 50 g of petrolatum; this has the advantage of producing less irritation and being more stable, does not require daily preparation, and should be applied with hand protected by latex or rubber gloves.

Some authors recommend concomitant treatment with high-potency topical steroids, which reduces or attenuates the contact dermatitis caused by treatment and enhances the antineoplastic effect.

Treatment should be extended until 2–3 years after disease control is achieved.

Nondermatological Uses: Hodgkin's disease (stages III and IV), lymphosarcoma, acute myelocytic or chronic lymphocytic leukemia, polycythemia vera, and bronchogenic carcinoma

Dosage

Mycosis Fungoides: Start with everyday applications and then decrease the frequency of application according to the therapeutic response and side effects. Treatment should be extended until 2–3 years after disease control is achieved.

de Quatrebarbes et al. reported 61 % of complete response in patients with stage IA mycosis fungoides, 58 % of complete response in patients with stage IB, and 40 % of complete response in patients with stage IIA, after a treatment period of $3,6 \pm 2,5$ months. Twenty-eight percent of patients discontinued treatment due to local adverse effects, and 46 % of patients relapsed after a disease-free interval of 7.7 ± 6.5 months [39]. Others have reported complete response rates of 76–80 % for stage IA and 35 to 68 % for stage IB patients. Response rates are similar for both preparations used (aqueous and ointment) [40].

Available Forms: 10 mg mechlorethamine hydrochloride powder vial

Safety in Pregnancy: Category D. May cause fetal harm if the drug is absorbed during pregnancy.

Adverse Effects: Delayed hypersensitivity reactions (contact dermatitis), hyperpigmentation, hypopigmentation, other skin malignancies (spindle cell carcinoma), angioedema, herpes zoster, erythema multiforme, pruritus, purpura, xerosis, rash, alopecia, anaphylactoid reactions, dysgeusia, and tinnitus [4, 15].

Carmustine

Is an alkylating agent of the nitrosoureas group [4].

Pharmacology: Its therapeutic effect is done through DNA alkylation at the O^6 position of guanine. Cell death occurs in all phases of the cell cycle. It is unstable in aqueous solutions and body fluids. The half-life ranges from 15 to 90 min and its excretion occurs in urine, 80 % as degradation by-products 24 h later [4].

Formula: $C_5H_9Cl_2N_3O_2$
Bioavailability: 5–28 % (oral)
Protein Binding: 80 %
Metabolism: Hepatic
Half-Life Time: 15–30 min
Uses:
Cutaneous T-cell lymphoma (mycosis fungoides). It is the option of choice in patients allergic to mechlorethamine. Therapeutic schemes usually start with one another day applications over the entire affected area, space dosages depending on patient response and severity of local and systemic adverse effects. Two types of preparations, the aqueous formulation and petrolatum ointment, have been used.

Dosage: 10 mg once daily for 7–14 weeks (maximum 17 weeks). If the response is poor, give a second course of topical treatment with 20 mg once a day for 4–8 weeks according to tolerance after a rest period of 6 weeks.

It has been reported a partial or a complete remission in 92 % of stage IA patients and in 64 % of stage IB patients treated with carmustine after a follow-up period of 36 months [41, 42].

Available Forms: Vials of 100 mg powder
Safety in Pregnancy: Category D. May cause fetal harm if the drug is absorbed during pregnancy
Adverse Effects: Dermatitis in up to 50 % of cases, telangiectasias, erythema, bone marrow suppression, eccrine syringometaplasia, rash, flushing, cutaneous pain, alopecia, gynecomastia, oral mucositis, and stomatitis. It is recommended to control blood cells in lab tests. It has been reported an increased risk of pulmonary fibrosis when combined use with bleomycin or radiotherapy [4, 15].

Alitretinoin (9-cis Retinoic Acid)

It is a first-generation retinoid that has been used to treat HIV-associated Kaposi's sarcoma.

Pharmacology: It binds to and activates all substrates of intracellular retinoid receptors. Once these receptors are activated, they act as transcription factors that regulate the expression of genes that control the differentiation and proliferation of both normal and neoplastic cells.

Formula: $C_{20}H_{28}O_2$
Uses:
Topical: Treatment of Kaposi's sarcoma lesions associated with AIDS should not be used when systemic treatment for Kaposi's sarcoma is indicated.
Oral: Chronic eczema of the hands in patients who have not responded to conventional therapy.
Dosage:
Topical: 2–4 applications daily for 12 weeks
Response rates of 35–37 % in patients with epidemic Kaposi's sarcoma have been reported; most were partial responses [43]. There is anecdotal evidence on case reports that it is less effective for the treatment of classic Kaposi's sarcoma [44].

Available Forms: 0.1 % Gel
Safety in Pregnancy: Category D. May cause fetal harm if the drug is absorbed during pregnancy
Adverse Effects: Pain, paresthesia, pruritus, exfoliative dermatitis, edema, and crusting [15].

Bexarotene

It is a synthetic retinoid that acts through the activation of retinoid X receptors (RXR) [3, 4].

Pharmacology: It binds selectively to retinoid X receptors in the nucleus of the cell, generating a ligand-receptor complex that acts as a transcription factor, and through the regulation of gene expression modulates differentiation, proliferation, and cell apoptosis. Its metabolism occurs mainly in the liver via cytochrome P450 (CYP450 3A4); four metabolites of bexarotene have been identified in plasma and are active in vitro, but their clinical significance is not known [3, 4].

Formula: $C_{24}H_{28}O_2$
Metabolism: Hepatic via cytochrome P450
Protein Binding: 99 %
Half-Life Time: 7 h
Elimination: Hepatobiliary system, less than 1 % via the urine
Uses: Cutaneous T-cell lymphoma (mycosis fungoides), stage IA and IB. It is generally used in patients who have not tolerated or not responded to at least one of the other topical treatments such as mechlorethamine or carmustine [4].
Dosage: Treatment should be initiated with application of the gel once every 2 days during the first week, and then increase the dose weekly to one another day, once a day, twice a day, three times a day, and finally four times a day as tolerated. Most patients are able to tolerate doses of two to four times a day. The duration of treatment is variable and schemes ranging from 6 to 52 weeks and even up to 687 days have been described. This varies according to the therapeutic response and tolerability.

Breneman et al. reported an overall response of 63 % in patients treated with bexarotene; only 21 % of patients had complete response. The percentage of responders increased to 75 % in cases where bexarotene was the first treatment used [45].

Heald et al. reported in a phase 3 study response rates of 64 % in stage IA patients and of 50 % in stage IB patients; no response was observed in two stage IIA and in one stage IIB patients [46].

Available Forms: 1 % Gel
Safety in Pregnancy: Category X. Causes defects in the embryo, fetus, or unborn child if applied topically. Pregnancy test should be negative a week before the start of treatment and should be repeated once a month until the end of the treatment.
Side effects: Acne, bacterial infections, exfoliative dermatitis, cheilitis, chills, flu-like symptoms, peripheral edema, pruritus, rash, pustular rash, cold sensation in hands and feet, facial edema, skin ulcers, xerosis, rash, vesicular-bullous eruption, gingivitis, hyperesthesia, hypoesthesia, breast pain, myalgia, pain, and xerostomia [3, 4, 15].
Recommendations: Use of adequate contraception in women of childbearing age. Limit the

use of vitamin A orally; do not apply insect repellent containing DEET (N,N-diethyl-m-toluamide) during treatment.

Diclofenac

It is a nonsteroidal anti-inflammatory drug, with anti-inflammatory, antipyretic, and analgesic effects [4, 5].

Pharmacology: Is absorbed rapidly and almost completely after oral administration. It inhibits prostaglandin synthesis through inhibition of cyclooxygenase (COX); there is also evidence that it has inhibitory activity on the lipoxygenase which would limit the production of leukotrienes [4, 5].

Formula: $C_{14}H_{11}Cl_2NO_2$
Protein binding: >99 %
Half-Life Time: 1.2–2 h
Metabolism: Hepatic via the enzyme cytochrome P450 CYP2C (not known active metabolites)
Excretion: Bile (<1 % in urine)
Uses:
Topic: Actinic keratosis (3 % gel), topical anti-inflammatory (gel 1 %)
Systemic: As an anti-inflammatory in a large number of musculoskeletal, immunological, degenerative, and traumatic diseases, migraine, pain, posttraumatic and postoperative pain, and pain management in kidney and gallstones
Dosage:
Actinic Keratosis: 0.5 g for each 5 cm² of the skin to be treated, two times a day for 60–90 days

Nelson et al. reported a 75 % clearance of treated lesions (target lesions) in 91 % of patients 1 year after use of diclofenac gel two times daily for 90 days [47].

In a phase 3 study, a 100 % clearance of treated lesions (target lesions) in 47 % of patients was reported [48].

In an open phase 4 study, an average clearance in 83 % of treated lesions (target lesions) at the end of 90 days of treatment was reported; this effectiveness rate increased to 90 % when patients were evaluated 30 days after the end of the treatment [49] (Fig. 20.3).

Fig. 20.3 Before (*left*) and after treatment with Solaraze®, two times a day for 12 weeks

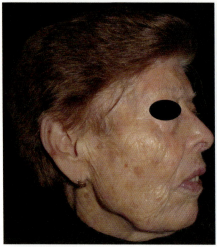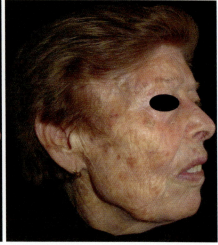

Inflammatory Musculoskeletal and Pain Management (Systemic)

Daily dose of 100–200 mg, divided into 3 or 4 doses

Available Forms:

For Topical Use: 1 and 3 % Gel

For Systemic Use: 50 and 75 mg tablets. There are also combined presentations with misoprostol to reduce the risk of gastric erosions and ulcers, maintaining the anti-inflammatory effect.

There are also parenteral use presentations.

Safety in Pregnancy: Category B

Adverse Effects: Allergic reactions, blistering, angioedema, contact dermatitis, eczema, edema, erythema, erythema multiforme, erythema nodosum, exfoliative dermatitis, fixed eruption, lichenoid eruption, lupus erythematosus, photosensitivity, pruritus, purpura, pustular reaction, Stevens-Johnson syndrome, toxic epidermal necrolysis, toxic shock syndrome, urticaria, vasculitis, alopecia, stomatitis, aphthous stomatitis, dysgeusia, oral ulcers, pseudolymphoma, tinnitus, xerostomia [15].

Miltefosine

It is a phospholipid-derived molecule that exerts its cytotoxic action by interfering with enzymatic processes in the cell membrane. It has antineoplastic, immunomodulatory, antiviral, and antiprotozoal properties [50].

Formula: $C_{21}H_{46}NO_4P$

Pharmacology: The active ingredient in miltefosine is called hexadecylphosphocholine and is very similar to the membrane phospholipids; this allows its incorporation into cell membranes and exerts its main action which is to inhibit the protein kinase C and interfere with the normal signaling and function of the cell membrane. Protein kinase C plays an important role in the cellular differentiation [50].

Uses:

Topical: Skin metastases from breast cancer and cutaneous T-cell lymphomas

Oral: Visceral leishmaniasis, American cutaneous leishmaniasis

Dosage:

Skin Metastases of Skin Cancer: Apply two drops of a 6 % solution per each 10 cm² of affected skin; it should be applied in an area of 3 cm around the affected zone as an oncologic margin in areas where clinical lymphocytic infiltration is evident. Do not apply more than 5 ml/day. Use it once a day during the first week then two times a day. The duration of treatment should be extended from 5 to 15 months [50].

Terwogt et al. reported an overall response rate of approximately 43 % (23 % complete response and 20 % partial response). The average duration of response was 18 weeks; no systemic toxicity was observed [51].

Cutaneous Lymphomas: Apply two drops of 6 % solution per each 10 cm² of affected skin once a day for a week and then twice a day for 7–11 weeks.

Leishmaniasis: 100 to 150 mg/day orally for 28 days, children can use a dose of 2.5 mg/kg/day for 28 days.

Available Forms: 6 % solution.

Adverse Effects:

Topical: Pruritus, xerosis, desquamation, numbness, pain, and ulcers. These effects are more frequent at baseline decreasing to the end of treatment. Systemic effects have been described as nausea, vomiting, and anorexia; these effects increase in proportion in the treated skin area and are believed to occur as a result of absorption of the drug through the skin. Raised values of laboratory tests, including creatinine, platelets, white cells, and enzymes, have also been described.

Oral: Motion sickness has been reported in up to 40 % of patients with oral use, gastrointestinal effects such as nausea, vomiting, diarrhea and constipation, neurotoxicity, hepatic toxicity, and ocular disturbances. Impaired renal function, liver, and hematologic laboratory tests [50, 51].

Safety in Pregnancy: Category X. Cause defects in the embryo, fetus, or unborn child if applied topically. Its use is contraindicated in pregnancy.

Recommendations: The use of adequate contraception during treatment and up to 6 months after the end of the treatment is recommended. Avoid contact with healthy skin and mucous membranes as it is a very irritating agent. Should be applied using latex or rubber gloves. If contact with eyes occurs, washing with plenty of eye saline solution or clean water is advised; if contact with healthy skin, should wash the area with mild soap and clean water.

Other Therapies

Bleomycin

Bleomycin is generated as a product of fermentation of *Streptococcus verticillus*; it belongs to a group of antibiotics that act by cleaving DNA. Its pharmacologic action occurs by oxidative damage to the deoxyribose of thymidylate among other nucleotides, which generates simple breakdowns

in the chain of double-stranded DNA and stops the cell cycle at G2 phase. Topically, it has been used with some success in the treatment of dysplastic leukoplakia of the oral mucosa, using a 1 % solution in a dimethyl sulfoxide vehicle, obtaining a partial response in up to 94 % and a total response in 31.6 % of patients, and seems to have an effect on slowing the progression of these lesions to carcinomas [52, 53]. Watring et al. successfully used topical bleomycin treatment in a case of vulvar Paget's disease [54]. Poignonec and colleagues in 1995 used a solution containing bleomycin 15 mg, lidocaine 1 g, and epinephrine 1 mg for intralesional treatment of epidemic Kaposi's sarcoma in 134 patients in France, obtaining regression in 43 % of tumors; relapses were not reported [55].

Retinoids

Retinoids are vitamin A-related drugs that are widely used in dermatology. While there are retinoids such as bexarotene and alitretinoin known to have specific antitumor activity against certain kinds of skin cancer, the role of the most commonly used topical retinoids such as retinoic acid and adapalene in the prevention and treatment of skin cancer is not clear. Retinoids have been used to treat actinic keratosis, obtaining modest results in reducing the number of lesions. Its use may be more as a complement to other topical or systemic treatments in the management of malignant skin neoplasms [3, 56–58].

Colchicine

It is an alkaloid extracted from the seed and the bulb of the saffron. It has been used topically for the treatment of actinic keratosis, Paget's disease, and psoriasis, among other skin diseases. It has been used as a 1 % gel, applied two times a day for 2 months on the affected areas. It can generate an intense inflammatory reaction that is limited to the skin where actinic keratoses are located; this reaction may interfere with the adherence to treatment. Responses were obtained in up to 70 % with a recurrence-free follow-up of 2 months [3, 59–61].

T4 Endonuclease V

It is an enzyme involved in repairing DNA obtained from a bacteria. It apparently acts by reversing DNA mutations before the formation of actinic keratosis and prevents the ultraviolet radiation-stimulated elevation of the levels of suppressor interleukins (IL-10) and of TNF-α. This product has been used with a liposomal vehicle that has proved to be useful in releasing the enzyme to the keratinocytes. It has shown to be effective in the prevention and reduction of the number of actinic keratosis in patients with xeroderma pigmentoso [62, 63].

Resiquimod

It is an agonist of toll-like receptors 7 and 8, which has an imiquimod-similar effect but on monocytes. It is considered 10–100 times more potent than imiquimod. In addition to its action on the toll-like receptors, it also induces the activity of several factors such as the IL-1 receptor antagonist, granulocyte colony-stimulating factor, the granulocyte and macrophage colony-stimulating factor, the alpha and beta inflammatory protein of macrophages, and the monocyte chemotactic protein. Szeimies et al. conducted a phase 2 study in 32 patients with actinic keratosis on the face and/or scalp; different concentrations of resiquimod were applied once a day 3 times a week for 4 weeks. Response rates ranged from 40 to 74.2 %. There was no difference in the response to the different concentrations of resiquimod used, but the formulations were better tolerated with the less concentrated preparation [3, 64].

Ingenol Mebutate

This medication is an extract of the plant *Euphorbia peplus* known as milkweed. It acts by causing cell membrane disruption and affecting the respiratory cell mechanism through the alteration of mitochondrial structure and function. This drug acts more quickly and intensely on dysplastic and neoplastic keratinocytes and generates necrosis. Rapid clinical and histopathologic healing of the affected area has been reported. It also stimulates neutrophil chemotaxis and humoral immunity, generating an antibody-mediated immune damage to the tumor tissues. Siller et al. reported a clinical reduction of 67–71 % in the number of actinic keratosis with very short treatment regimens using different concentrations of the product (0.0025, 0.01, and 0.05). It is currently undergoing phase 3 trials to evaluate its efficacy in the treatment of actinic keratosis [65, 66] (Table 20.1).

Glossary

Alitretinoin 9-cis Retinoic Acid
Nitrogen Mustard Mechlorethamine hydrochloride
5-FU 5-Fluorouracil

References

1. Miller SJ, Moresi JM, et al. Actinic keratosis, basal cell carcinoma and squamous cell carcinoma. In: Bolognia JL, editor. Dermatology. 1st ed. Philadelphia: Elsevier Mosby; 2003.
2. Greenway HT, Maggio KL, et al. Mohs micrographic surgery and cutaneous oncology. In: Robinson JK, editor. Surgery of the skin. Procedural Dermatology. Philadelphia: Elsevier Mosby; 2005.
3. Ceilley RI, Del Rosso JQ. Topical chemotherapy for the treatment of skin cancer. In: Rigel DS, editor. Cancer of the skin. Madrid: 1st ed. Elsevier; 2004.
4. Wyatt EL, Sutter SH, Drake LA. Dermatological pharmacology. In: Hardman JG, Limbird LE, editors. Goodman & Gilman's the pharmaceutical basis of therapeutics. 10th ed. New York: McGraw Hill; 2001.
5. Amini S, Viera MH, Valins W, Berman B. Nonsurgical innovations in the treatment of nonmelanoma skin cancer. J Clin Aesthet Dermatol. 2010;3(6):20–34.
6. Bargman H, Hochman J. Topical treatment of Bowen's disease with 5-fluorouracil. J Cutan Med Surg. 2003; 7(2):101–5.
7. Gross K, Kircik L, Kricorian G. 5 % 5-fluorouracil cream for the treatment of small superficial basal cell carcinoma: efficacy, tolerability, cosmetic outcome, and patient satisfaction. Dermatol Surg. 2007;33:433–40.
8. Epstein E. Fluorouracil paste treatment of thin basal cell carcinoma. Arch Dermatol. 1985;121:207–13.

9. Orenberg EK, Miller BH, Greenway HT, Koperski JA, Lowe N, Rosen T, et al. The effect of intralesional 5-fluorouracil therapeutic implant (MPI 5003) for treatment of basal cell carcinoma. J Am Acad Dermatol. 1992;27:723–8.

10. Love WE, Bernhard JD, Bordeaux JS. Topical imiquimod or fluorouracil therapy for basal and squamous cell carcinoma: a systematic review. Arch Dermatol. 2009;145:1431–8.

11. Askew DA, Mickan SM, Soyer HP, Wilkinson D. Effectiveness of 5-fluorouracil treatment for actinic keratosis-a systematic review of randomized controlled trials. Int J Dermatol. 2009;48(5):453–63.

12. Dinehart SM. The treatment of actinic keratoses. J Am Acad Dermatol. 2000;42(1 Pt 2):25–8.

13. Epstein E. Treatment of lip keratoses (actinic cheilitis) with topical fluorouracil. Arch Dermatol. 1977;113(7):906–8.

14. Kossow AS, Cotelingam JD, MacFarland F. Bowenoid papulosis of the penis. J Urol. 1981;125(1):124–6.

15. Litt JZ. Pocketbook of drug eruptions and interactions. New York: Parthenon Publishing; 2004.

16. Mackenzie-Wood A, Kossard S, de Launey J, Wilkinson B, Owens ML. Imiquimod 5 % cream in the treatment of Bowen's disease. J Am Acad Dermatol. 2001;44(3):462–70.

17. Wu JK, Siller G, Whitehead K. Treatment of Bowen' disease and basal cell carcinoma of the nose with imiquimod 5 % cream. Australas J Dermatol. 2003;44(2):123–5.

18. Schroeder TL, Sengelmann RD. Squamous cell carcinoma in situ of the penis successfully treated with imiquimod 5 % cream. J Am Acad Dermatol. 2002;46(4):545–8.

19. Beutner KR, Geisse JK, Helman D, et al. Therapeutic response of basal cell carcinoma to the immune response modifier imiquimod 5 % cream. J Am Acad Dermatol. 1999;41:1002–7.

20. Geisse J, Rich P, Pandya A, et al. Imiquimod 5 % cream for the treatment of superficial basal cell carcinoma: a double blind randomized, vehicle controlled study. J Am Acad Dermatol. 2002;47:390–8.

21. Berman B, Villa A. Moduladores inmunitarios en el tratamiento del cancer de piel. In: Rigel DS, editor. Cancer de piel. 1st ed. Madrid: Elsevier; 2006.

22. Geisse J, Caro I, Lindholm J, Golitz L, Stampone P, Owens M. Imiquimod 5 % cream for the treatment of superficial basal cell carcinoma: results from two phase III, randomized, vehicle-controlled studies. J Am Acad Dermatol. 2004;50(5):722–33.

23. Schulze HJ, Cribier B, Requena L, et al. Imiquimod 5 % cream for the treatment of superficial basal cell carcinoma: results from a randomized vehicle-controlled phase III study in Europe. Br J Dermatol. 2005; 152(5):939–47.

24. Gollnick H, Barona CG, Frank RGJ, et al. Recurrence rate of superficial basal cell carcinoma following successful treatment with imiquimod 5 % cream: interim 2-year results from an ongoing 5-year follow-up study in Europe. Eur J Dermatol. 2005;15(5):374–81.

25. Eigentler TK, Kamin A, Weide BM, et al. A phase III, randomized, open label study to evaluate the safety and efficacy of imiquimod 5 % cream applied thrice weekly for 8 and 12 weeks in the treatment of low-risk nodular basal cell carcinoma. J Am Acad Dermatol. 2007;57(4):616–21.

26. Edwards L, Owens ML, Andres KL, et al. A pilot study evaluating imiquimod 5 % cream versus vehicle in the treatment of actinic keratoses. Poster presented at the 58th annual meeting of the American Academy of Dermatology, San Francisco, 10–15 Mar 2000.

27. Salasche SJ, Levine N, Morrison L. Cycle therapy of actinic keratoses of the face and scalp with 5 % topical imiquimod cream: an open-label trial. J Am Acad Dermatol. 2002;47(4):571–7.

28. Stockfleth E, Sterry W, Carey-Yard M, Bichel J. Multicentre, open-label study using imiquimod 5 % cream in one or two 4-week courses of treatment for multiple actinic keratoses on the head. Br J Dermatol. 2007;157 Suppl 2:41–6.

29. Szeimies RM, Gerritsen MJ, Gupta G, et al. Imiquimod 5 % cream for the treatment of actinic keratosis: results from a phase III, randomized, double-blind, vehicle-controlled, clinical trial with histology. J Am Acad Dermatol. 2004;51(4):547–55.

30. Gupta AK, Davey V, McPhail H. Evaluation of the effectiveness of imiquimod and 5-fluorouracil for the treatment of actinic keratosis: critical review and meta-analysis of efficacy studies. J Cutan Med Surg. 2005;9(5):209–14.

31. Smith KJ, Germain M, Yeager J, Skelton H. Topical 5 % imiquimod for the therapy of actinic cheilitis. J Am Acad Dermatol. 2002;47(4):497–501.

32. Ahmed I, Berth-Jones J. Imiquimod: a novel treatment for lentigo maligna. Br J Dermatol. 2000;143(4):843–5.

33. Naylor MF, Crowson N, Kuwahara R, Teague K, Garcia C, Mackinnis C, et al. Treatment of lentigo maligna with topical imiquimod. Br J Dermatol. 2003;149 Suppl 66:66–70.

34. Van Meurs T, Van Doorn R, Kirtschig G. Treatment of lentigo maligna with imiquimod cream: a long-term follow-up study of 10 patients. Dermatol Surg. 2010;36(6):853–8.

35. Demirci H, Shields CL, Bianciotto CG, Shields JA. Topical imiquimod for periocular lentigo maligna. Ophthalmology. 2010;117(12):2424–9.

36. Narayan R, Nguyen H, Bentow JJ, et al. Immunomodulation by imiquimod in patients with high-risk primary melanoma. J Invest Dermatol. 2012; 132:163–9. doi:10.1038/jid.2011.247.

37. Sigüenza M, Pizarro A, Mayor M, et al. Tratamiento tópico de las metástasis cutáneas de melanoma con imiquimod. Actas Dermosifiliogr. 2005;96(2):111–5.

38. Turza K, Dengel LT, Harris RC, et al. Effectiveness of imiquimod limited to dermal melanoma metastases, with simultaneous resistance of subcutaneous metastasis. J Cutan Pathol. 2010;37(1):94–8.

39. de Quatrebarbes J, Estève E, Bagot M, et al. Treatment of early-stage mycosis fungoides with twice-weekly

applications of mechlorethamine and topical corticosteroids: a prospective study. Arch Dermatol. 2005; 141(9):1117–20.

40. Kim YH. Management with topical nitrogen mustard in mycosis fungoides. Dermatol Ther. 2003;16(4):288–98.

41. Zackheim HS. Topical carmustine (BCNU) for patch/plaque mycosis fungoides. Semin Dermatol. 1994; 13(3):202–6.

42. Zackheim HS, Epstein Jr EH, McNutt NS, et al. Topical carmustine (BCNU) for mycosis fungoides and related disorders: a 10-year experience. J Am Acad Dermatol. 1983;9(3):363–74.

43. González-de-Arriba A, Pérez-Gala S, Goiriz-Valdés R, Ríos-Buceta L, García-Díez A. Sarcoma de Kaposi clásico tratado con alitretinoína tópica. Actas Dermosifiliogr. 2007;98(1):50–3.

44. Bodsworth NJ, Bloch M, Bower M, et al. Phase III vehicle-controlled, multi-centered study of topical alitretinoin gel 0.1 % in cutaneous AIDS-related Kaposi's sarcoma. Am J Clin Dermatol. 2001;2(2):77–87.

45. Breneman D, Duvic M, Kuzel T, et al. Phase 1 and 2 trial of bexarotene gel for skin-directed treatment of patients with cutaneous T-cell lymphoma. Arch Dermatol. 2002;138(3):325–32.

46. Heald P, Mehlmauer M, Martin AG, et al. Topical bexarotene therapy for patients with refractory or persistent early-stage cutaneous T-cell lymphoma: results of the phase III clinical trial. J Am Acad Dermatol. 2003;49(5):801–15.

47. Nelson C, Rigel D. Long-term follow up of diclofenac sodium 3 % in 2.5 % hyaluronic acid gel for actinic keratosis: One-year evaluation. J Clin Aesthet Dermatol. 2009;2(7):20–5.

48. Wolf Jr JE, Taylor JR, Tschen E, Kang S. Topical 3.0 % diclofenac in 2.5 % hyaluronan gel in the treatment of actinic keratoses. Int J Dermatol. 2001;40: 709–13.

49. Nelson C, Rigel D, Smith S, Swanson N, Wolf J. Phase IV, open-label assessment of the treatment of actinic keratosis with 3.0 % diclofenac sodium topical gel (Solaraze™). J Drugs Dermatol. 2004;3(4):401–7.

50. Clive S, Leonard RCF. Miltefosine in recurrent cutaneous breast cancer. Lancet. 1997;349:621–2.

51. Terwogt JMM, Mandjes IAM, Sindermann H, Beijnen JH, BokkelHuinink WW. Phase II trial of topically applied miltefosine solution in patients with skin-metastasized breast cancer. Br J Cancer. 1999;79(7/8): 1158–11613.

52. Epstein JB, Wong FL, Millner A, Le ND. Topical bleomycin treatment of oral leukoplakia: a randomized double-blind clinical trial. Head Neck. 1994; 16:539–44.

53. Epstein JB, Gorsky M, Wong FL, Millner A. Topical bleomycin for the treatment of dysplastic oral leukoplakia. Cancer. 1998;83:629–34.

54. Watring WG, Roberts JA, Lagasse LD, Berman ML, Ballon SC, Moore JG, et al. Treatment of recurrent Paget's disease of the vulva with topical bleomycin. Cancer. 1978;41:10–1.

55. Poignonec S, Lachiver LD, Lamas G, et al. Intralesional bleomycin for acquired inmunodeficiency syndrome-associated cutaneous Kaposi's sarcoma. Arch Dermatol. 1995;131:228.

56. Jorizzo J, Carney P, Ko W. Treatment options in the management of actinic keratosis. Cutis. 2004;74:9–17.

57. Barrera MV, Herrera E. Tratamiento quimioterápico tópico de la queratosis actínica y el cáncer cutáneo no melanoma: situación actual y perspectivas. Actas Dermosifiliogr. 2007;98(8):556–62.

58. Graaf YGL, Euvrard S, Bavinck JNB. Systemic and topical retinoids in the management of skin cancer in organ transplant recipients. Dermatol Surg. 2004;30: 656–61.

59. Marshall J. Treatment of solar keratoses with topically applied cytostatic agents. Br J Dermatol. 1968; 80:540–2.

60. Grimaitre M, Etienne A, Fathi M, Piletta PA, Saurat JH. Topical colchicine therapy for actinic keratoses. Dermatology. 2000;200:346–8.

61. Akar A, BulentTastan H, Erbil H, Arca E, Kurumlu Z, Gur AR. Efficacy and safety assessment of 0.5 % and 1 % colchicine cream in the treatment of actinic keratoses. J Dermatolog Treat. 2001;12:199–203.

62. Wolf P, Maier H, Müllegger R, Chadwick CA, Hofmann-Wellenhof R, Soyer HP, et al. Topical treatment with liposomes containing T4 endonuclease V protects human skin in vivo from ultraviolet-induced upregulation of interleukin-10 and tumor necrosis factor-α. J Invest Dermatol. 2000;114:149–56.

63. Zahid S, Brownell I. Repairing DNA damage in xeroderma pigmentosum: T4N5 lotion and gene therapy. J Drugs Dermatol. 2008;7(4):405–8.

64. Szeimies RM, Bichel J, Ortonne JP, et al. A phase II dose-ranging study of topical resiquimod to treat actinic keratosis. Br J Dermatol. 2008;159(1):205–10.

65. Ogbourne SM, Suhrbier A, Jones B, et al. Antitumor activity of 3-ingenyl angelate: plasma membrane and mitochondrial disruption and necrotic cell death. Cancer Res. 2004;64(8):2833–9.

66. Siller G, Gebauer K, Welburn P, et al. PEP005 (ingenol mebutate) gel, a novel agent for the treatment of actinic keratosis: results of a randomized, double-blind, vehicle-controlled, multicentre, phase IIa study. Australas J Dermatol. 2009;50(1):16–22.

Mohs Micrographic Surgery

21

Joan Ramon Garcés

Key Points
- Mohs micrographic surgery
- Fresh frozen tissue
- Mohs surgery office
- Mohs histopathology laboratory

Introduction

Mohs micrographic surgery (MMS) provides the highest cure rate for skin cancer while maximally sparing surrounding healthy tissue. False negatives and false positives are avoided by histologic studies of 100 % of the tumour margins and by sophisticated processing of horizontal sections during surgery, respectively. By sparing noncancerous tissue, MMS offers a solution to the dilemma of removing a tumour in its entirety while preserving as much tissue as possible intact. Since interactive microscopic control of removed tissue means that the neoplasm can be eliminated in stages, cure is theoretically confirmed by the end of surgery, depending on the type and characteristics of the removed tumour [1].

J.R. Garcés, MD
Department of Dermatology,
Universitat Autònoma de Barcelona,
Hospital de la Santa Creu i Sant Pau,
Sant Antoni Maria Claret, 167, Barcelona, Spain
e-mail: jrgarces@telefonica.net

MMS success mainly depends on correctly performing a number of steps between removing the cancerous tissue and obtaining samples for histologic study. Studies have demonstrated that errors in technique and microscopic interpretation are particularly relevant to cases of tumour recurrence after MMS [2]. Therefore, in addition to mastering the basic principles of surgical dermatology, the Mohs surgeon needs to be trained in advanced MMS.

Basic Principles

MMS is underpinned by two basic principles. The first principle is that microscopic confirmation of tumour-free surgical margins immediately on removing the tumour is far more specific than any visual inspection [3]. The intraoperative process therefore aims to microscopically view 100 % of the tumour margins. Since the surgeon needs to be able to identify tumour cells and their exact location and distribution to be able to perform excision precisely where the residual tumour is located, a diagram representing the excised area is made for orientation purposes. This map launches successive MMS stages, as necessary, until the tumour is removed in its entirety. As its name indicates, MMS is indeed micrographic.

The second principle concerns the need for coordination, as MMS is a single procedure performed in stages. Since a number of disciplines are involved, successful MMS requires one person—the Mohs surgeon—to assume responsibility for

A. Baldi et al. (eds.), *Skin Cancer*, Current Clinical Pathology,
DOI 10.1007/978-1-4614-7357-2_21, © Springer Science+Business Media New York 2014

organising the procedure and ensuring effective communication when different tasks are carried out by different professionals. The Mohs surgeon thus needs to be knowledgeable about all the steps so as to oversee them and intervene interactively when necessary; the surgeon also makes decisions about how and where excisions are to be performed at each stage and, once the MMS is concluded, about the most suitable approach to reconstruction. Thus, even if not directly involved in all the stages, the Mohs surgeon is ultimately responsible for the procedure from beginning to end [4].

Equipment

As well as the basic dermatological surgical equipment required for standard cutaneous surgical procedures, performing MMS requires a cryostat, a microscope and a staining device. The cryostat, which can have a motorised or manual object head, requires the following additional supplies: microtome lubricating oil, microtome tools, antiroll brushes, disposable blades, 25- and 30-mm specimen chucks, forceps and scalpel.

The microscope should be equipped with ×4, ×10 and ×40 objective lens and should also be equipped with a low-power ×2 objective lens that allows the entire histologic section to be scanned in a single power field. A dual-view side-by-side adapter or dual-view face-to-face adapter may be preferred for teaching purposes [5].

Staining equipment can be automatic or manual, depending primarily on the volume of staining carried out. An automatic stainer can considerably reduce reagent waste and processing time. The reagents used will vary depending on the preferred staining formula. The most popular stains are toluidine blue and haematoxylin and eosin (H&E), but 95 % alcohol, 100 % alcohol and xylene are also frequently necessary.

Other necessary laboratory supplies include Petri dishes, marking dyes, cryospray, optimal cutting temperature (OCT) compound, mounting medium, cover slipping glue, slides, cover glasses, charge slides and slide folders. Also useful are a fire extinguisher, a storage cabinet for flammable materials and a slide storage system (slides should be saved for at least 10 years) [6].

Surgery layout is very important. In view of the importance of effectively coordinating all the MMS stages, the Mohs laboratory in our practice is located next to the operating room. To avoid error, specimens are grossed and inked in the operating room by the surgeon working together with the histotechnician. The microscope is located next to the cryostat so that the histotechnician can, if necessary, rapidly check the histologic sections before staining. In our view, this distribution is ideal; nonetheless, certain principles must be respected. The cryostat should not be placed directly under an air vent, as exposure to air currents could lead to frosting. Adequate ventilation is also important and a fume hood should be installed if hazardous chemicals are used for histologic staining.

Effective layout ultimately facilitates feedback between all team members and so enhances the effectiveness of MMS [5].

Techniques

Since Frederic Mohs invented, in the early 1930s, what was originally known as chemosurgery, based on using a 20 % zinc chloride paste, a number of variations in the technique have been experimented with, all aimed at fully analysing surgical margins (100 %) without sacrificing surrounding healthy tissue [3, 7]. The Mohs fresh-tissue technique as used by Tromovitch and Stegman—occasionally with minor variations—is the most widely used approach, especially for the treatment of non-melanoma skin cancer (NMSC) [8]. Frozen sections of fresh-tissue specimens are sectioned horizontally so as to include all the tissue in a single section. The surgery is interactive and takes place in stages, each consisting of three main steps: collection of tumour tissue; processing of the tissue and orientation for histologic sectioning; and histologic reading of the sections. If cancer cells are observed in the margins, the procedure is repeated until the entire tumour is removed (Fig. 21.1).

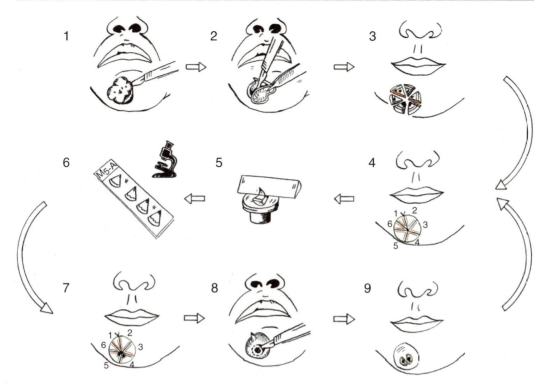

Fig. 21.1 MMS technique (*1*). Debulking. The visible tumour is debulked with scalpel (*2*). Excision of 1–2 mm of healthy tissue surrounding the wound resulting from debulking (*3*). The specimen is sectioned and marked with ink on its cut edges. Each section is individually marked in its entire perimeter (*4*). Mapping. The segments are numbered and the tissue is oriented according to a map or diagram representing the anatomical area from where the tissue is excised (*5*). The tissue sample is flattened and sliced in the microtome. Proper flattening makes it easier to obtain sections that enable the epidermis to the deep dermis in a single specimen (*6*). Histopathological interpretation (*7*). Mapping of residual tumour. The location of the residual tumour revealed under the microscope should be drawn on the Mohs map (*8*). Subsequent Mohs stages. A next layer should be taken from where the residual tumour resides (*9*). Sectioning and inking as in number 3. Repeat steps 4, 5 and 6, until tumour-free margins are histologically confirmed

Frozen-section study is both more immediate and more interactive than microscopic readings of paraffin-embedded tissue. It also allows for immediate reconstruction, if required, in full confidence that there is no residual tumour. Horizontal sectioning compared to vertical sectioning saves time and also minimises the possibility of false negatives, as it requires fewer specimens for a comprehensive view of tumour margins from the epidermis to the deep dermis [9].

When doubts arise over fresh-tissue readings, MMS is performed in paraffin-embedded sections. This approach, called slow Mohs, requires more time; however, although it loses in interactivity, it gains in terms of enhanced margin control [10]. Some tumours require special immunohistochemical staining to identify tumour cells in Mohs surgery margins. Different immunostains have proved useful in detecting tumour cells in a number of malignancies, including melanoma. Furthermore, it is now possible to use rapid stains for certain melanoma antigens in frozen sections with the same reliability as permanent paraffin-embedded sections [11]. Below we review each of the MMS stages in more detail.

First MMS Stage

Harvesting

MMS commences when the Mohs surgeon removes tumour tissue. It is important to first delimit the area well, however, bearing in mind the subsequent steps until a histologic section is obtained. Tissue removed en bloc with a bevel angle of 45 % will be easier to process later. It is also important that the histotechnician is present when the tissue is excised. Many surgeons debulk the tumour before commencing MMS, as debulking enables more accurate definition of the clinical margins, eliminates the possibility of false positives and facilitates the teasing down of the peripheral margins so that complete sections can be obtained without loss of epidermis [4, 12]. The first Mohs stage involves excision of 1–2 mm of healthy tissue surrounding the clinically visible tumour or the wound resulting from debulking. On excision, the surgeon makes a notch as a reference point for the tissue, typically at 12 o'clock. For specimens measuring more than 2 cm, another reference notch is made at 3 o'clock or coinciding with a specific anatomical fold or crease.

Processing

The tissue is oriented according to a map or diagram representing the anatomical area from where the tissue is excised. The surgeon places the tissue on the map and makes a drawing that matches the resected specimen in size and location. A photograph can also be used for this purpose. Working with the histotechnician, the surgeon cuts a minimum number of segments that are small enough to fit on the slides and be cut by the cryostat in a single section. The segments are numbered and the borders of each section are inked. Different colours are used to represent the epidermis to the deep dermis, with the result that each section is individually marked in its entire perimeter. The colours used should correspond to those used in the diagram.

The tissue is next prepared for sectioning in the cryostat. Different methods have been described to obtain histologic sections that can be observed across the entire margin of specimen previously in contact with the patient. The best-known approaches include the heat extractor technique with an OCT embedding medium, microscopic glass slides and mechanical flattening techniques with liquid nitrogen [13, 14]. This sectioning step is crucial, and irrespective of the system used, success depends greatly on the experience of the histotechnician. Proper flattening makes it easier to obtain sections that enable the epidermis to the deep dermis of a single specimen to be viewed.

The obtained sections are then stained, most commonly with H&E; toluidine blue is sometimes preferred for basal cell carcinoma (BCC), as it highlights the mucopolysaccharide stroma in metachromatic pink [15].

Histopathologic Interpretation

Even if an experienced pathologist makes the histologic readings, the Mohs surgeon needs to view each and every slide. The Mohs surgeon first scans the slides to make sure that the sections are fully represented and to check that inking is complete, the epidermis is completely visible, the notches correspond to the map, the colour of the stain is appropriate and that there is no loss of tissue that could result in false negatives [16]. Magnification with a ×2 objective lens is usually sufficient for this purpose. If any of the sections are observed to be defective, recuts should be made to obtain a suitable specimen. The Mohs surgeon next looks for evidence of residual tumour in the margins. Failure to find cancer cells means that MMS is complete. If tumour cells are identified, they are carefully drawn on the diagram, which is used to guide the next MMS stage.

Subsequent MMS Stages

As in the first stage, the Mohs surgeon proceeds to remove 1–2 mm of margin coinciding with the map drawing. Cancer foci located in the epidermis or dermis require the defect to be extended laterally, whereas persistent neoplasms in subcutaneous fat or underlying structures may only require extending the excision in a deeper plane [4]. It is therefore important for the Mohs surgeon to view the histologic sections under the microscope to know the exact distribution and location of residual tumour involvement. Once histology readings confirm negativity, the type of reconstruction can be decided and MMS is complete.

Practical Considerations and Applications

Although MMS in some cases is performed under general anaesthesia in hospital, the vast majority of surgeries are performed in outpatient settings under local or locoregional anaesthesia with sedation. The dermatological oncological surgeon specially trained in the Mohs discipline usually has a team of assistants (trained nurses, histotechnicians, etc.) to hand, including, as necessary, specialists such as pathologists, plastic surgeons, otolaryngologists and ophthalmologists. The success or failure of MMS depends on effective coordination of each step in the procedure. Some practical considerations based on our own experience are described below, all aimed at maintaining cure rates while saving time and as much healthy tissue as possible.

Preoperative Evaluation

The patient should be an appropriate candidate for MMS. In the initial screening visit, it is advisable to ensure that the patient understands MMS and is aware of the medical, functional and aesthetic outcomes. It is also desirable, depending on the location and extent of the tumour, to perform imaging and other studies and to consult with other specialists if they are to be called on during the procedure.

First MMS Stage

The ideal MMS is performed in a single stage, as maximum efficiency is achieved when the first stage is the last and the tumour is accurately delimited so that no more tissue than necessary is removed. As mentioned above, it is important to debulk the tumour prior to implementing the first stage, as this minimises the number of stages, reduces false positives and helps flatten the specimen [13]. Mohs surgeons typically use curettage for tumour debulking; in our department, however, we have a preference for using a scalpel for several reasons. The scalpel is cleaner than the

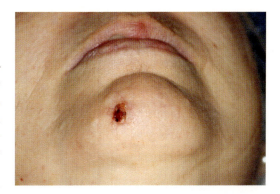

Fig. 21.2 Morpheaform basal cell carcinoma on the chin. The lesion is very ill defined

curette as it leaves no impurities that can sometimes cause floaters [17]. It can also be used in locations where curettage is difficult, for example, the free edge of the eyelids and the mucosa of the lips. However, the most important reason is that the scalpel, unlike the curette, preserves the debulked tissue for histologic processing together with first-stage tissue. In our laboratory, vertical cuts of debulked tissue are processed together with sections obtained in first-stage Mohs, resulting in biopsies of tumour tissue with the same stain as the Mohs specimen. Thus, if we have any doubt regarding the existence of residual tumour in a Mohs specimen, we can check whether the suspect cells have the same configuration, layout, colour and cellularity as those in the biopsied debulked tissue. This comparison is more reliable than comparison with a previous paraffin-embedded biopsy that uses a different stain. It also means that we can send tumour tissue for paraffin-embedded study if in doubt or if a previous biopsy is unavailable (Figs. 21.2, 21.3, 21.4, 21.5 and 21.6).

Although debulking is aimed at removal, delineating the actual tumour is clinically difficult. A number of studies have described different approaches to delineating tumour boundaries prior to MMS, including Doppler ultrasound, confocal microscopy and, more recently, aminolevulinic acid-induced fluorescence in photodynamic diagnosis; [18–20] these approaches, however, do not represent any advance over clinical judgement.

Delimiting the tumour may be problematic yet it is clinically the most important step in terms of saving time during MMS. The tumour

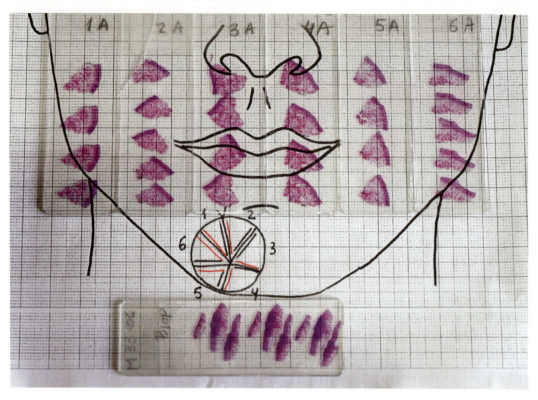

Fig. 21.3 First stage of Mohs surgery for lesion in Fig. 21.2. Note the biopsies (vertical cuts) of the debulked tumour together with all sections obtained in first Mohs stage

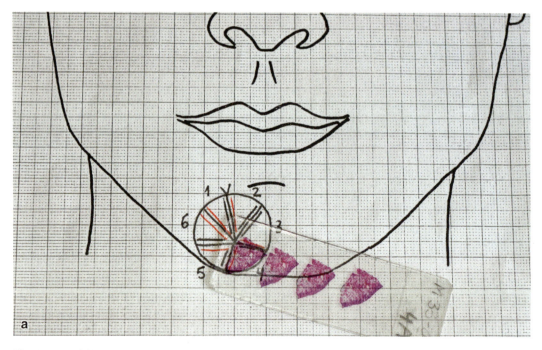

Fig. 21.4 (**a**) Slide corresponding to number 4. The slide is on the map. The sections match in size and location. (**b**) Residual basal cell carcinoma persists at the deeper margin. Section of Fig. 21.4a (haematoxylin and eosin, original magnification ×2)

Fig. 21.4 (continued)

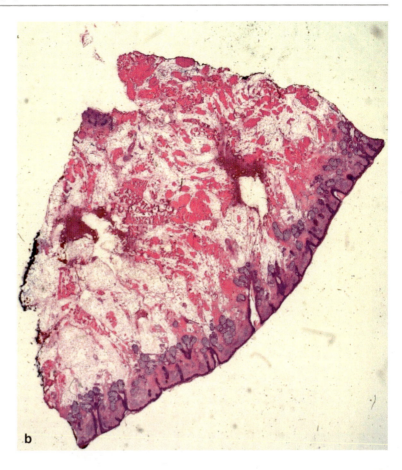

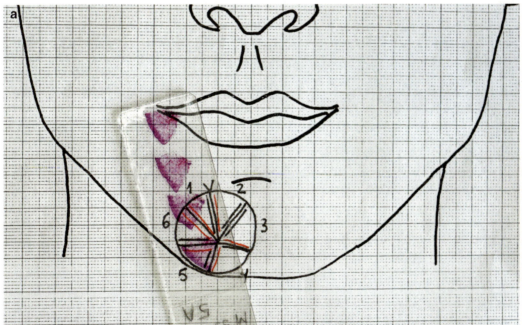

Fig. 21.5 (**a**) Slide corresponding to number 5. (**b**) Remaining basal cell carcinoma is observed on examination of the histopathology deep in the corner close to the previous section (haematoxylin and eosin, original magnification ×2)

Fig. 21.5 (continued)

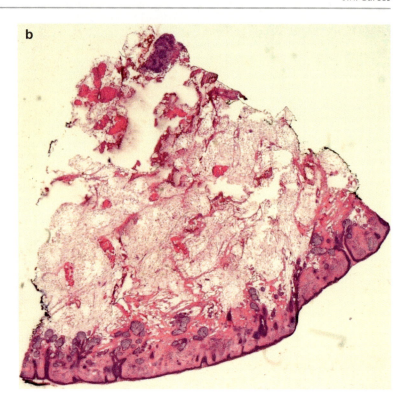

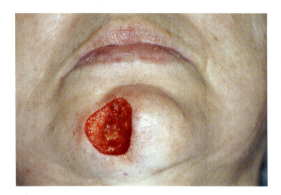

Fig. 21.6 Patient in Fig. 21.2. Postoperative photograph at completion of Mohs surgery

to be removed often persists after previous treatments failed to eradicate the tumour in its entirety. In such cases, as well as excising the tumour, the scar must also be removed, as it may contain contiguous tumour remains. Scars resulting from previous treatments (surgery, radiotherapy, curettage, cryotherapy, imiquimod, etc.)

should also be removed as they may conceal residual tumour beyond the unaffected tumour margins. In the interest of ensuring a cure, we cannot run the risk of tumour recurrence due to remains excluded by MMS.

In the remaining histologic sectioning steps in our department, the Mohs surgeon and histotechnician work together, with the surgeon responsible for preparing, grossing and inking the tissue, map drawing and specimen orientation, and the histotechnician responsible for sectioning, embedding, cutting and staining. This close collaboration enhances efficiency and minimises the possibility of the most common errors.

In the cryostat, cutting temperature should be between −24° and −26°, although fatty specimens cut better at lower temperatures, which can be obtained using cryospray or liquid nitrogen. The histotechnician should review the sections under the microscope prior to staining to ensure completeness and so avoid the need for additional cuts [21].

Subsequent MMS Stages

If massive tumour positivity is evident in the histology readings, the corresponding margins should be checked for indirect clinical signs of tumour involvement. If tumour involvement is very evident, it is advisable to debulk again to facilitate subsequent interventions and to avoid false positives and floaters. Successively debulked tissue can be processed in conjunction with the specimens obtained in each stage to confirm positivity and to detect any histologic change in tumour morphology.

Final MMS Stage

Whether MMS can be considered to be complete is uncertain if residual tumour is suspected despite negative results. As a matter of routine, for squamous cell carcinoma (SCC) with granulomatous inflammation, we make an additional cut for paraffin-embedded study purposes, as studies have demonstrated that such granulomas can conceal tumour cells [22]. We do the same for lentigo maligna, sebaceous carcinoma, Paget disease, Merkel cell carcinoma and other tumours in which cellular detail is important [23]. For dermatofibrosarcoma protuberans (DFSP), given the difficulty in obtaining fresh-tissue readings, we perform slow Mohs with paraffin-embedded sections that frequently require CD34 staining to assess tumour infiltration. [24]

Indications and Contraindications

Bearing in mind the patient's age and health status, MMS indications are based on the type and characteristics of the tumour, although the main prerequisite for MMS is that the tumour is intact. This concept is fundamental to MMS, as surgery concludes once healthy tissue is encountered. Tumour invasion, despite negative histologic sections for malignancy, would inevitably represent failure of MMS.

But is Mohs surgery recommended for all contiguous skin neoplasms and is contiguity the only requirement? The answer is that although this is a necessary condition, in itself it is insufficient.

Tumour characteristics and circumstances ultimately determine the indication for MMS. Aggressive histology, poorly defined clinical margins, size and location are major issues. Tumours located in high-risk areas (the embryonic fusion planes), for example, are usually more aggressive, have poorly defined margins and also tend to persist after previous treatments [25].

Tumour persistence is, in fact, the most common indication for MMS, which has come to be regarded as the treatment of choice for 'long-haul' skin malignancies that are inadequately treated by other means. A tumour that has not been removed in its entirety becomes chopped and fragmented and is converted into a discontiguous tumour, composed of one or more residual tumours—in short, a new multiple tumour.

Among the NMSC, BCC and SCC have traditionally been the tumours targeted for treatment with MMS, although the technique is indicated for any single, intact skin cancer. The list of single cutaneous neoplasms other than BCC and SCC that can be treated with MMS is long, yet limited use is often made of the technique, whether due to the low frequency of occurrence of neoplasms suitable for treatment with MMS or due to the difficulty of interpreting histologic sections during surgery [26]. Relatively recent developments in immunohistochemical staining have facilitated diagnosis, with specific staining of paramount importance in reaffirming the MMS indication for neoplasms such as atypical fibroxanthoma, microcystic adnexal carcinoma, DFSP, sebaceous carcinoma and extramammary Paget disease, to name just a few cancers [27].

The use of MMS for malignant melanoma merits separate discussion. Malignant melanoma is a potentially metastatic tumour, and satellitosis and in-transit metastases are both likely. Use of MMS to treat malignant melanoma is the subject of controversy [28], as numerous studies have yielded conflicting results—so much so that MMS is not a protocolary indication in our setting, or at least not generally.

Confusion is partly due to the different presentations of malignant melanomas, although essentially they can be considered in terms of two groups: in situ malignant melanomas and invasive malignant melanomas. In situ malignant melanomas are characterised by the proliferation of atypical melanocytes, whether solitary or nested and distributed throughout the epidermis. Although these cells can invade adnexal structures, they usually do not do so beyond the dermoepidermal junction; tumour lesions are therefore contiguous. The effectiveness of MMS compared to wide surgical resection or other therapeutic techniques has been repeatedly demonstrated for these melanomas [29]. Furthermore, the melanoma antigen recognised by T-cells (MART-1) is now as reliable for frozen sections as for paraffin-embedded sections [30, 31].

MMS has a number of limitations. The large, extensive, primary or persistent tumours for which MMS is broadly indicated are actually complex to treat with conventional MMS [32, 33]. The processing of the histologic sections necessary to study the tumour perimeter may be excessively time consuming, thereby effectively rendering MMS unworkable. Furthermore, certain structures (such as the eyeball) cannot be sectioned or laminated when invaded by cancer cells. Other structures (bone tissue, glandular tissue, etc.) present difficulties in terms of the orientation and study of histologic sections. In such cases, MMS can be used to peripherally delimit the tumour, but definitive tumour removal requires en bloc resection of the underlying tissue (orbital exenteration, excision of the bone plate, etc.).

At the other extreme are metastatic skin tumours of any kind, unsuitable for treatment with MMS. MMS can only remove intact tumours, so once the disease has metastasised, even if only locally, it can no longer be used as a treatment.

Future Considerations

Several fronts are open in an attempt to expand the boundaries of MMS, all seeking to save time and enhance efficiency. MMS is more viable for larger tumours if histologic section size can be increased. Fewer cuts mean faster surgery and fewer false negatives. Several articles describe improvements to equipment that enable histologic section size to be increased significantly [34, 35]. This both reduces intervention times and renders MMS more suitable for currently nonviable large tumours.

More specific stains for frozen processing would also increase efficiency by reducing histologic interpretation errors. Recently published studies referring to different substances indicate that it is not beyond our wildest dreams to imagine having at our disposal a battery of reagents suitable for different tumour types [36].

Also being studied are treatments with different mechanisms of action that act synergistically with MMS to enhance its efficacy. Certain destructive treatments prior to MMS, such as the application of topical imiquimod to reduce the treatment area and, consequently, postsurgical morbidity [37], may not necessarily be wise because if the malignancy is not completely removed, the remains after topical therapy may not necessarily be arranged as a single, smaller tumour and the outcome would be a new multiple tumour whose treatment with MMS may be difficult. Very different, however, is the case of imatinib used for DFSP prior to MMS, as it achieves a reported reduction of over a third in tumour size. Imatinib can be considered to be a genuine adjunctive treatment, as it produces the kind of persistent, reduced-size intact tumour [38] for which MMS is ideally indicated.

Glossary

Cryostat is a device used to maintain low temperatures of samples
MART-1 Melanoma antigen recognised by T-cells
MMS Mohs micrographic surgery
NMSC Non-melanoma skin cancer
OCT Optimal cutting temperature

References

1. Swanson NA, Taylor WB, Tromovitch TA. The evolution of Mohs surgery. J Dermatol Surg Oncol. 1982;8: 650–4.
2. Hruza GJ. Mohs micrographic surgery local recurrences. J Dermatol Surg Oncol. 1994;20:573–7.
3. Brodland DG, Amonette R, Hanke CW, Robbins P. The history and evolution of Mohs micrographic surgery. Dermatol Surg. 2000;26(4):303–7.
4. Benedetto PX, Poblete-Lopez C. Mohs micrographic surgery technique. Dermatol Clin. 2011;29(2):141–51,vii. Review.

5. Thornton SL, Beck B. Setting up the Mohs surgery laboratory. Dermatol Clin. 2011;29(2):331–40, xi. Review.

6. Hetzer MR. The Mohs laboratory. In: Snow SN, Mikhail GR, editors. Mohs micrographic surgery. 2nd ed. Madison: University of Wisconsin Press; 2004. p. 329–37.

7. Trost LB, Bailin PL. History of Mohs surgery. Dermatol Clin. 2011;29(2):135–9, vii.

8. Tromovitch T, Stegman S. Microscopically controlled excision of skin tumors: chemosurgery (Mohs) fresh tissue technique. Arch Dermatol. 1974; 110:231–2.

9. Morgan M, Bowland T. Mohs and frozen section overview. In: Morgan MB, Hamill JR, Spencer JM, editors. Atlas of Mohs and frozen section cutaneous pathology. New York: Springer; 2009. p. 3–8.

10. Otley C, Roenigk R. Mohs surgery. In: Bolognia J, Jorizzo J, Rapini R, editors. Dermatology. 2nd ed. St Louis: Mosby; 2008. p. 2269–79.

11. Stranahan D, Cherpelis BS, Glass LF, Ladd S, Fenske NA. Immunohistochemical stains in Mohs surgery: a review. Dermatol Surg. 2009;35:1023–34.

12. Chung VQ, Bernardo L, Jiang SB. Presurgical curettage appropriately reduces the number of Mohs stages by better delineating the subclinical extensions of tumor margins. Dermatol Surg. 2005;31(9 Pt 1):1094–9 [discussion: 1100].

13. Miller LJ, Argenyi ZB, Whitaker DC. The preparation of frozen sections for micrographic surgery. J Dermatol Surg Oncol. 1993;19:1023–9.

14. Silapunt S, Peterson SR, Alcalay J, et al. Mohs tissue mapping and processing: a survey study. Dermatol Surg. 2004;30(6):961.

15. Humphreys TR, Nemeth A, McCrevey S, et al. A pilot study comparing toluidine blue and hematoxylin and eosin staining of basal cell and squamous cell carcinoma during Mohs surgery. Dermatol Surg. 1996; 22:693–7.

16. Bouzari N, Olbricht S. Histologic pitfalls in the Mohs technique. Dermatol Clin. 2011;29(2):261–72, ix. Review.

17. Walling HW, Swick BL. Identifying a tissue floater on Mohs frozen sections. Dermatol Surg. 2009;35: 1009–10.

18. Mogensen M, Jemec GB. Diagnosis of nonmelanoma skin cancer/keratinocyte carcinoma: a review of diagnostic accuracy of nonmelanoma skin cancer diagnostic tests and technologies. Dermatol Surg. 2007;33(10): 1158–74.

19. Bobadilla F, Wortsman X, Munoz C, et al. Presurgical high resolution ultrasound of facial basal cell carcinoma: correlation with histology. Cancer Imaging. 2008;8:163–72.

20. Redondo P, Marquina M, Pretel M, et al. Methyl-ALA-induced fluorescence in photodynamic diagnosis of basal cell carcinoma prior to Mohs micrographic surgery. Arch Dermatol. 2008;144(1):115–7.

21. Nguyen DH, Siegel DM, Zell D, et al. Quality assurance. In: Morgan MB, Hamill JR, Spencer JM, editors. Atlas of Mohs and frozen section cutaneous pathology. New York: Springer; 2009. p. 9–14.

22. Leshin B, Prichard EH, White WL. Dermal granulomatous inflammation to cornified cells. Significance near cutaneous squamous cell carcinoma. Arch Dermatol. 1992;128(5):649–52.

23. Requena C et al. Dermatofibrosarcoma protuberans: clinical, pathological, and genetic (COL1A1-PDGFB) study with therapeutic implications. Histopathology. 2009;54(7):860–72.

24. Rapini RP. Pitfalls of Mohs micrographic surgery. J Am Acad Dermatol. 1990;22:681–6.

25. Swanson NA. Mohs surgery. Technique, indications, applications, and the future. Arch Dermatol. 1983; 119(9):761–73.

26. Siegel DM. Mohs surgery for large and difficult tumors and in special clinical situations. In: Gross KG, Steinmann HK, Rapini RP, editors. Mohs surgery fundamentals and techniques. St Louis: Mosby; 1999. p. 231–8.

27. El Tal AK, Abrou AE, Stiff MA, et al. Immunostaining in Mohs micrographic surgery: a review. Dermatol Surg. 2010;36(3):275–90.

28. Whalen J, Leone D. Mohs micrographic surgery for the treatment of malignant melanoma. Clin Dermatol. 2009;27(6):597–602.

29. Temple CL, Arlette JP. Mohs micrographic surgery in the treatment of lentigo maligna and melanoma. J Surg Oncol. 2006;94:287–92.

30. Zalla MJ, Lim KK, Dicaudo DJ, et al. Mohs micrographic excision of melanoma using immunostains. Dermatol Surg. 2000;26(8):771–84.

31. Chang KH, Finn DT, Lee D, Bhawan J, Dallal GE, Rogers GS. Novel 16-minute technique for evaluating melanoma resection margins during Mohs surgery. J Am Acad Dermatol. 2011;64(1):107–12.

32. Levine H, Bailin P, Wood B, et al. Tissue conservation in treatment of cutaneous neoplasms of the head and neck. Combined use of Mohs' chemosurgical and conventional surgical techniques. Arch Otolaryngol. 1979;105(3):140–4.

33. Ducic Y, Marra DE, Kennard C. Initial Mohs surgery followed by planned surgical resection of massive cutaneous carcinomas of the head and neck. Laryngoscope. 2009;119(4):774–7.

34. Bakhtar O, Close A, Davidson TM, Baird SM. Tissue preparation for MOHS' frozen sections: a comparison of three techniques. Virchows Arch. 2007;450(5): 513–8.

35. Hanke CW, Leonard AL, Reed AJ. Rapid preparation of high-quality frozen sections using a membrane and vacuum system embedding machine. Dermatol Surg. 2009;34(1):20–5.

36. Miller CJ, Sobanko JF, Zhu X, Nunnciato T, Urban CR. Special stains in Mohs surgery. Dermatol Clin. 2011;29(2):273–86, ix. Review.

37. Butler DF, Parekh PK, Lenis A. Imiquimod 5 % cream as adjunctive therapy for primary, solitary, nodular nasal basal cell carcinomas before Mohs micrographic surgery: a randomized, double blind, vehicle-controlled study. Dermatol Surg. 2009;35(1):24–9.

38. Han A, Chen EH, Niedt G, Sherman W, Ratner D. Neoadjuvant Imatinib therapy for dermatofibrosarcoma protuberans. Arch Dermatol. 2009;145(7):792–6.

Skin Cancer Surgery

22

Michele de Nuntiis, Enrico Baldessari,
and Riccardo Garcea

Key Points
- This chapter deals with generality under which treatments of the different dermatological lesions undergo, with special emphasis on surgical techniques in view of current medical credited for their treatment.
- The most used techniques and widely approved principles in plastic and reconstructive surgery of the skin, with special emphasis on reconstruction after cancer excisions are described.

Benign lesions such as warts, keratosis, cysts, and nevi represent most cancerous lesions usually encountered in dermatological practice [1, 2]. However, in recent years has been reported an increase in the percentage of precancerous and frankly malignant lesions [3]. Never as before the treatment has a necessity to be accompanied by histopathological examination of the excided tissues and to be supplied by a careful medical history and study of their nature [4, 5].

This chapter deals with all the generality under which treatments of the different dermatological lesions undergo, with special emphasis on surgical techniques and keeping an eye on current medical treatment.

Introduction

Plastic surgery is a branch of surgery that aims to correct and repair morphological defects or functional losses of substance of different tissues that make up the human body (skin, subcutaneous tissue, fascia, muscle, bones, etc.) either congenital or acquired as a result of trauma, cancer, or degenerative diseases [6]. The basic techniques are the most reliable today which provide primary closure of the breach, the use of grafts, and/or use of skin flaps.

The reason for the development of these solutions is the need of closure of an area in which substance is lost from surgical excision or traumatic event. In the present chapter will be considered only the first, surgical, case, without defining or assessing the issues resulting from a trauma.

The plastic surgeon is a surgeon able to perform proper surgical techniques connecting sensitivity to handling and accuracy to performance, precision to incision, thoroughness to hemostasis, and inventiveness to medication, in order to reduce the appearance of residual scars. In addition he or

M. de Nuntiis (✉) • E. Baldessari
Plastic Surgery, Casa di Cura Addominale EUR,
Viale Africa, 32, Rome 00144, Italy

Fondazione Futura-onlus,
Rome, Italy
e-mail: michele@micheledenuntiis.it

R. Garcea
Plastic Surgery, Casa di Cura Addominale EUR,
Viale Africa, 32, Rome 00144, Italy

A. Baldi et al. (eds.), *Skin Cancer*, Current Clinical Pathology,
DOI 10.1007/978-1-4614-7357-2_22, © Springer Science+Business Media New York 2014

she must be fully aware of the processes of wound healing and of the precautions needed to avoid infection [7].

Skin Excisions

Generality

The excision of a skin tumor can involve the loss of an extensive portion of skin, subcutaneous tissue, adnexal structures, etc. The dilemma that often the surgeon has to face is the feasibility of a direct closing of the margins of the defect with respect to coverage using skin grafts and/or flaps [8]. In all cases where possible, the surgeon must always follow the "golden rule," corollary to good sense, of removing the skin or mucosal pathological lesions by simple excision, even in the case of the deeper lesions, so to manage a direct closure of the defect created [9, 10]. The application of this "golden rule" appears to be a necessary condition especially if the diagnosis of the lesion tends toward malignancy, as could be the case of a cutaneous melanoma. This suspicion must necessarily be confirmed histologically [11], especially to undertake the proper therapeutic procedure, or if a second a lesion with macroscopic features similar to those excised in the same anatomical region is found [12–15]. The key issue is the differential diagnosis of these tumors, which could be extremely difficult if the repair of the defect has been accomplished through grafting of tissue taken from areas more or less distant from the region affected by the histological study [16]. With tissue transplantation, all the cells, benign and malignant, that assemble the graft are conveyed to the recipient site, with the consequent possibility not of a repetition of the lesion removed but of the transfer of a new malignancy in the excision site. Increasing the possibilities of misdiagnosis, management difficulties and the risk of subsequent over demolishing and invasive therapeutic treatment [17].

Key focus for a good functional and aesthetic result should be placed to the perpendicularity of all the incisions and to the study of the direction of the relaxed skin tension lines the engraving involves. The direction in which to proceed in

order to correctly make the incisions is often limited by the maximum diameter of the lesion itself, which should be carefully evaluated and properly marked during the study phase that precedes the operation. Even the equipment available to the surgeon plays an important role in the decision making of directing the surgery. Still, it is a good idea if the surgeon follows some basic principles in order to get to the desired result. The lines of engraving that will lead to a closure of the defect without or with reduced tension forces are those that run parallel to "relaxed skin tension lines," according to Borges, defined for all the anatomical subunits of the body, and which in to the face region almost always run parallel to the course of expression or age wrinkles [14] (Fig. 22.1).

In the end, the surgeon must keep in mind, during planning of the surgical technique chosen, the respect of the integrity of tissues, opting for delicate surgical instruments and which most suite his work and limiting the hemostasis to "needed" (avoiding "the hunt for the red blood cell") with an adequate intensity that will prevent postoperative hematoma.

Choice for Margins' Incisions

The surgeon must not under any circumstances choose direct closing of the excision area at the expense of the removal of the entire tumor [18], although there are suspicions of benignity, with adequate margins of safety as prescribed by international oncology protocols [19–24].

The ways in which a plastic surgeon can operate for removal of abnormal growths, malignant or benign, are nowadays numerous. Depending on the anatomical site, the extent of the lesion, and the surgery chosen, the surgeon will have to address and resolve issues concerning the direction of the engraving lines and/or the type of repair to be performed in accordance with the basic principles of plastic surgery. In the following pages, the authors will first describe the basic surgical techniques, then will describe the set of techniques that encompasses advanced surgical procedures as complex as the microsurgical or pedicled flaps, and finally will describe some methods for dressing procedures.

Fig. 22.1 Relaxed skin tension lines and biopsy notes

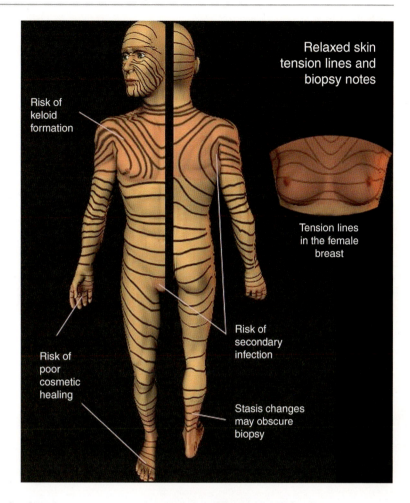

Punch or Circular Scalpel [25]

The use of punch should be relegated to small skin lesions, i.e., not exceeding the maximum size of 8 mm. The resulting gap will have a "round" shape and will be difficult to close through direct suturing. The transition from circular to the oval shape, easier to suture, can be obtained by applying a technical shrewdness during the execution of the incision: the skin incision site should be stretched with two fingers applying forces perpendicularly to relaxed skin tension lines. Once the stretching force exerted is released, the elastic forces of the skin will change the round shape of the punch excision to an oval shape, easier to close and with axis parallel to these skin tension lines. The breach produced by the use of punch can, in alternative and if necessary, be left to heal by secondary intention, as it could result in an acceptable aesthetic result.

Lozenge or Wedge Incision [25]

The lozenge excision is nowadays the most widely used incision to remove skin tumors in all areas of the human body. This surgical practice requires, for all the tension forces involved, matching of the direction of the incision lines to axes coincident or parallel to the course of the relaxed skin tension lines, with dimensions that comply with the ratio of 3–1, i.e., the major axis of the lozenge should be three times the size of the minor axis. The use of this form of excision is necessary for facilitating closure of the breach, free from or almost devoid of tension.

Wedge excisions are generally used if the lesion to be removed is on or adjacent to the free margin of anatomical structures such as eyelids, lips, and ears, allowing for an easy and aesthetically acceptable rebuilding of structures approaching and matching the different tissue planes.

Fig. 22.2 "Dog ear" removal technique

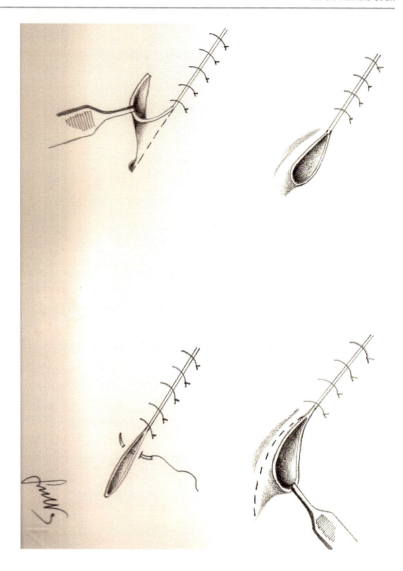

Some rules must be followed in carrying out this method with respect to anatomical site: i.e., wedge excision involving the lower lip should never exceed more than 1/3 of the length of the lip itself; moreover, if the excision involves the eyelid, it should never exceed a length equal to 1/4 of the total length of the eyelid; etc.

In order to further reduce tension along the edges of the suture, the surgeon may and sometimes should mobilize widely the margins of the breach itself. The mobilization will be carried out, with few exceptions, within the subcutaneous layer and with respect of the anatomical area: by means of delicate dissecting scissors, mobilization forceps, using scissors stronger than the above but with blunt tips, or even with the use of a finger of a hand.

Then a subcutaneous suture is placed, preferably with braided absorbable suture, which will favor the approach of the edges of the breach so as to minimize possible tension that the skin closure should fight to bring together the margins of resection.

In case of the need of dealing with very large lozenge excisions or excisions located in convex regions of the body that normally generate higher tension forces with respect to flat areas, it is common the formation of "pockets" of exuberant skin and subcutaneous tissue taking triangular shape defined "dog ear." Usually those pockets are located at the end of the suture, at the prongs of the breach in correspondence of the points in which the rotation axis converge, in case of rotation or transposition flaps, in the area of the mobilization

Fig. 22.3 (a–c) Incision line and shapes

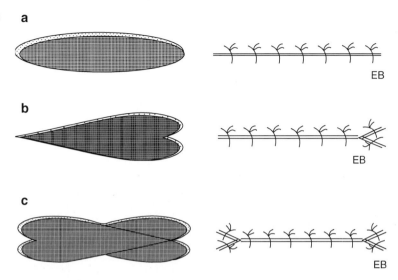

for plain flaps. This tissue should be removed in order to obtain a linear suture (Fig. 22.2).

The use of lozenge excision lends itself to numerous variations that can be adapted to the needs for size of the available skin, to the configuration of the lesion to be removed, etc. Still, the need to orient the major axis of the incision parallel to relaxed skin tension lines remains, changing the shape of the lines of incision in order to draw an "M," a "Y," a double "M," a star, and other shapes (Fig. 22.3a–c).

Direct closure of the excision is not always possible and feasible because of excessive skin tension that would be generated, and that will increase the risk of diastase of the suture itself. In these cases, the surgeon will choose for an alternative solution such as seriate excision (multiple excisions spaced in time) or the use of skin expanders that create an tissue exuberance, following a slow but progressive tissue distension, which is necessary to cover the residual defect.

The use of grafts and/or flaps for the coverage of the surgical breach remains a valid alternative.

Seriate Excisions [25]

In general, seriate excisions are used to treat spindle-like damages or whose smaller diameter is in size too large to allow direct closure without the risk of diastase due to excessive tension generated, i.e., giant congenital nevus (Fig. 22.4).

The technique involves at first an intralesional excision and in the end an extralesional one, through several sessions that should be at least 1 month apart. The procedure is to be repeated up to the point in which the complete removal of the skin formation is achieved. As mentioned before, the excision is carried out at the beginning without crossing the margins of the lesion that is to be surgically removed, using an incision shaped as a lozenge, as a double "M," as an "M," as a "Y," etc. according to the most suited needs for shape, position, and extent of the breach.

Since this type of excision involves the development of a great amount of strain on the margins of suture, the surgeon must pay particular attention in obtaining a good matching of the skin edges of the wound, in order to not let them diastase until the next surgical session. As a result, the matching of the skin layers should be made through a careful approach of all the subcutaneous tissues, using absorbable suture, before skin closure. Especially during the last surgical round, the surgeon is required to pay accurate respect to aesthetics, having to remove during the entire process the scar tissue formed after the previous excision.

Hemostasis

Last of the surgical procedures to be performed during an operation, it still remains a procedure

Fig. 22.4 Seriate excision

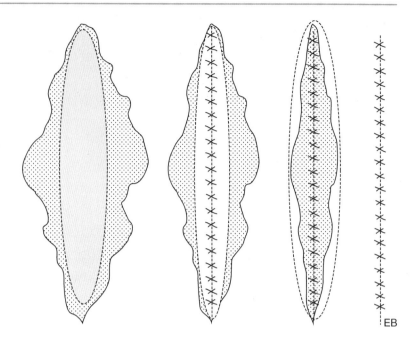

EB

in surgery. Failure to comply with the accuracy in performing hemostasis involves unequivocally the formation of a hematoma in the context of the wound. This can delay or even prevent the physiological processes leading to the healing of the wound, resulting in a dehiscence of the suture and representing a perfect breeding ground for the development of pathogens and subsequent local or even systemic infection.

Careful hemostasis of small- and medium-diameter vessels can be accomplished in several ways: compression, plugging with H_2O_2, and suturing the vessels; the methodology that is more efficient, easier, and more rapidly put into practice is diathermocoagulation. This procedure uses the heat produced by the passage of electrical current through biological tissues. The procedure can be made more precise through the use of a bipolar forceps, which provides the current to flow only through the tips of the forceps, thus avoiding to cross the tissues that separate the positive from the negative pole. The bipolar forceps also allows the surgeon to limit the damage of burning the tissues surrounding the area of application of the current.

In the case where there are large caliber vessels or if it is not possible to apply electric current, for example, due to the presence of pacemakers, it is preferable to perform a ligation of these vessels with absorbable or nonabsorbable suture.

Whether doubts about the effectiveness of the hemostasis exist or in cases where bleeding may still be possible, as can occur in the face district, where vessels are subjected to an average blood pressure higher than other districts, the authors recommend the use of a drain to prevent the formation of a hematoma.

Medication

The quality of the scar, in cosmetic surgery, is considered a fundamental part of the action unlike other surgical specialties. It turns out to be one of the more visible consequences of the intervention. The authors are not asserting that when the surgery does not involve plastic surgery, the operator is permitted not to pay attention to the surgical suture of the breach; on the contrary, any surgeon should devote time and attention to the last note of an operation, which will be the one the patient will refer after surgery and after he or she had become sufficiently accustomed to the new body appearance.

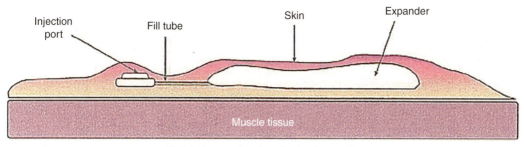

Deflated expander placed subcutaneously

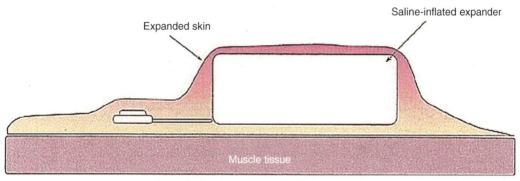

Inflated expander demonstrating expanded skin

Fig. 22.5 Skin expander

Skin Expanders [25]

The use of skin expanders is now a viable alternative to seriate excision of large skin lesions. A skin expander is essentially a bag of silicone of various shapes and sizes, which is gradually filled through transcutaneous injections of sodium chloride solution. The filling is done through a valve integrated in the expander or positioned at a distance and connected through a tiny tube (Fig. 22.5). The valve is always placed subcutaneously and is palpable and detectable by means of magnets.

The result of skin expansion is the formation exuberance of tissue, which can be used to surgically repair the breach. Of central importance is the identification of the area where the expander is placed, along with its shape and size. A placement in an location far apart from the excised area would result in difficulty using the obtained tissue, while, on the contrary, implant placement in an area immediately below the area to be excised would increase the amount of tissue excision. Incorrect positioning is also in the area immediately below the incision made for insertion of the expander, because it may lead to insufficient coverage or risk of rupture. Not to mention that incorrect placement may result in the presence of additional and unnecessary scarring.

To be evaluated when choosing to use skin expanders is the rate of the expansion, which must be adequate to avoid tissue damage from hypoperfusion, resulting in necrosis. The surgeon must remember that skin expansion necessarily involves pain in the affected area as a consequence of pressure. The period of expansion varies depending on the circumstances and the anatomical region but generally lasts a period of time ranging from 1 to 3 months.

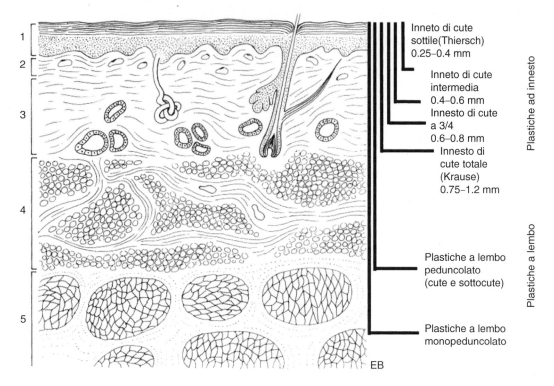

Fig. 22.6 Skin thickness versus graft and flaps

As the sufficient skin expansion needed is reached, the expander is removed through a skin incision, while the fibrotic capsule that is formed as a result of skin reaction to the foreign body may be left in place.

Skin expansion is indicated especially in the correction of extensive burn scars or posttraumatic removal of giant congenital nevi, in which skin needs to be expanded to reach a more acceptable cosmetic result. The main complications of this technique are represented by the ever-present possibility of infection, which will be necessarily followed by the removal of the expander, and the possibility of skin necrosis and pain during the expansion process. At any time the expander can undergo leaking, the result is the leakage of saline solution of NaCl in the same pocket where the expander is hosted, but makes it impossible to continue the expansion because the expander no longer is capable of exercise and maintain the necessary pressure. All this is associated with the disadvantage of a broad time necessary to achieve the required volume and defacement of body shape and appearance of the patient, especially if the expander is to be placed in exposed areas.

Recent scientific studies have established that the maximum percentage of tissue expansion obtainable never exceeds 130 %.

Practical Surgery

Although numerous techniques exist for the reconstruction of a tissue loss, it is possible to develop a scale for decision-making process that the surgeon should always keep in mind in working the choice of reconstructive method:

⬧Direct closure
⬧ Skin grafts
⬧ Local flaps
⬧ Distant flaps
⬧ Microsurgical free flap

Whenever a direct closure is not possible, i.e., the suture of the margins of the wound, the surgeon would resort to use one of the following large sets:
1. Grafts
2. Flaps

According to the needs and complexity of the case (Fig. 22.6).

Grafts

A skin graft is a segment of one or more tissues that have lost all connection with the donor area, does not contain a network of blood vessels of its own, and can be transferred from a donor site to a receiving area of substance loss (deficit), for reconstructive purposes, resulting from trauma or tumor excision.

There is considerable confusion about the classification and definition of key elements such as grafts, plasty, and flaps. Many authors use the term "skin graft" to refer to the transfer of tissue from a donor site to the recipient site, assuming the only differentiation into two main groups: grafts and flaps. For those authors the term grafting involves transplanting a portion of skin variable in thickness and other measurements which, totally separate from the donor seat, is capable of fully nourishing itself at the expense of the new seat, unlike the flap that retains a vascular link with the origin site [26].

On the contrary, other authors (e.g. Kirschner) consider part of the definition of "flap" the whole part, either referring to open and/or closed (tube) flaps or to simple grafts. There even are authors who use the term "local grafts" to indicate local skin plasty (sliding, rotational flaps, etc.) [27].

The differences are significant and cause a confusion of terms and ideas, if some simple basic concepts are defined and can be enough to thin out the haze: the authors consider a skin graft including all the skin grafted which is required to survive entirely in the new site. The definition does not exclude the vessel disconnection from the donor site to take place in a less abrupt and more gradual way, allowing the new site to ensure the survival of the transplanted tissue. Exactly this is the difference between free and pedicled graft, and it is on this difference that the classification of direct engagement (or free) and mediated (or pedunculated) flap relies. Besides, the term *flap* may not be comparable to graft, since the latter is something concrete and definite (with its own personality and character), while the former is a surgical technique used to make plasty correction by means of local transfer of neighboring tissues (feed, slip), pedicled or remote (microsurgery) flaps [28].

Reverdin in 1869 presented a paper that refers to the method of free transfer of small segments of epidermis. Since then, the number of classifications and names proposed for this surgical technique, adopted by authors from different schools, was so large, diverse, and sometimes contradictory that it would be essentially impossible to make a really complete list. From a strictly anatomical point of view, it is possible to distinguish grafts as epidermal, dermoepidermal, dermal, and full thickness, depending on the depth. However, if, we consider the evidence that the latter (epidermal) are not feasible in practice, because it is impossible to get them from any donor area, with the exception of those taken at the plantar region as demonstrated by J.S. Davis that studied seriate sections of the skin, that there is an obstacle distinguishing the different layers, identifying the real plane of dissection of the graft itself, in this chapter the authors propose to simply adopt the anatomical classification. To demonstrate the desirability of this classification, we can mention a few emblematic examples from the best known classifications: Thiersch grafts (the thinner dermoepidermal) are called "split" grafts, fine section grafts (Blair Brown), epidermal grafts (Barsty), fine grafts extracted with razor (Gillies), Ollier-Thiersch surface grafts (Sanchez Arbid), etc.; dermoepidermal grafts of intermediate thickness are called "split" grafts (Blair Brown), roughly split graft (Harkins), large grafts extracted with razor (Gillies), Ollier-Thiersch deep grafts (Sanchez Arbid), intermediate depth grafts (Padgett), etc.; and dermoepidermal large grafts are called calibrated grafts (Harkins), grafts intermediate depth (Padget), big "split" grafts (Blair Brown), etc. In addition, Kirschner believes that while the classic Reverdin graft includes all the layers of the skin, the majority of authors use the name of Reverdin grafts for small dermoepidermal superficial grafts and there are those who distinguish the two types (superficial and deep) as Reverdin graft (Sanchez Arbid) [6].

Island Grafts [25]

The present array includes two different major groups:

1. Reverdin, or superficial, which includes the epidermis and upper layers of the papillary dermis

2. Davis or deep, described by S.J. Davis in 1914, embracing all the skin layers (epidermis, papillary dermis, corium, and hypodermis) in the shape of an inverted cone

Among the variants of the island grafts, we can consider the so-called Wagenstein "sprouts" grafts, which in truth are nothing more than the Reverdin-type grafts placed deeply in the granulation tissue.

Laminar Grafts [25]

They match, as we said before, the "split" grafts of Anglo-Saxon source and include all large dermoepidermal grafts regardless of thickness, but do not include all skin layers. There are three types of laminar grafts:

1. Thiersch (or thin), described in 1874, which is equivalent to the laminar Reverdin island graft, one third of the total skin (from 0.2 to 0.25 mm) depth, containing part of the epidermis and papillary dermis.
2. Blair Brown (of intermediate thickness), described in 1929, is about half the thickness of the skin in depth (which includes a thickness selected among 1/3 and 2/3 of the total skin section), whose size varies from 0.3 to 0.4 mm. It is the most widely used to treat early deep burns.
3. Padgett (or thick), subject to precise specified measures by the author techniques in 1939 (Harkins calibrated grafts), otherwise known as "trocar graft" because it includes more than 2/3 of the skin section, it is harvested at about 0.5–0.6 mm deep and includes the epidermis, the papillary dermis, and most of the deep dermis or corium.
4. Brown "implant" grafts and Goode-Gabarra "matrix" grafts are technical variations to the application of either type of laminar graft mentioned.

Total Skin Grafts [14, 25]

They are made including all the skin layers. Used by Wolfe in 1875 to reconstruct the lower eyelid, they were introduced and described in detail by Fedor Krause in 1893. Although the success of the application is tied to a lot of attention, needed more than for other types of grafting, the aesthetic and functional results are much higher than those of any other type of free skin graft (because

the morphology and physiology are exactly the same as those of normal skin). The Douglas grafts or "sieve" like and those "tunnel" like or Keller are Wolfer-Krause grafts, with slight technical variations.

Dermal Grafts [14, 25]

Introduced by Loewe in 1913 for the treatment of hernias and reinforcement of the abdominal wall, dermal grafts find multiple indications in surgical practice, successfully used for the repair of tendons, meninx, ligaments, etc. and especially as autologous material for sutures. Cannady deems dermal grafts as the autoplastic material of choice, superior even to the fascia lata. Plastic surgery is currently dominated by two applications of the dermal grafts:

- As filler for the correction of craniofacial defects (Eitner, 1920).
- To repair skin losses just like dermoepidermal grafts, through the lamination process (Zintel technique) of a thick Padgett laminar graft, previously obtained with the dermatome, in this way it can be completely divided through its cross section so as to double the surface of the obtained graft. The dermal graft obtained in this way is suitable to cover the receiving site surface and plays to perfection the task of repairing the skin like any other laminar graft. The application of these dermal grafts is extremely useful in the treatment of extensive burns, where donor areas are reduced in number and extension. It therefore opens new possibilities thanks to the "laminated grafts," a name that indicates the origin and clearly distinguishes them from the laminar grafts (dermoepidermal) to avoid possible confusion in interpretation and nomenclature.

Pedicle or Mediated Grafts [29]

Include all those skin grafts or transplants that are temporarily maintaining vascular connections with the donor area, up to the time in which nutrition of the tissue transplanted is actually at the expense of the new site. Mediated or pedicled grafts can be applied directly, where the dissected flap is applied directly on the area to repair, or indirectly, where the transfer of tissue takes place by successive steps, through an area or region that is intermediate (temporary host). Either direct or indirect mediated flaps can be prepared in an open or closed shape, depending on whether or not they are isolated from the outside of the cruented side. The "closure" of a flap can be done through three different procedures:

- The process of tubular flaps by Gillies-Filatov
- Covering the cruented surface of the flap by applying a laminar graft
- Through the juxtaposition of another similar pedicle flap but of opposite base, taken from the receiving or intermediate area depending on whether it is a direct or indirect pedicle graft.

Direct Pedicled Grafts

Include grafts made directly from the donor site to the one intended for repair. They can be distinguished as follows:

- Near flap, taken from regions adjacent or close to the defect. They are used mainly for the repair of craniofacial loss of substance; flaps can be based on a single vessel (e.g., the classic Indian flap nasal reconstruction based on a front flap) or double-pedicle flaps, such as the flap called "a helmet," mainly used to repair areas of the chin at the expense of the hairy scalp;
- Direct remote flaps, where the transplant takes place between regions anatomically distant from each other but can be approached and kept in this last position (e.g., using a cast) for the time necessary to make the flap root in the new site; these types of flaps include the so-called direct distance flap crossing arms and legs of the patient ("cross-arm flaps" and "cross-leg flap" according to the Anglo-Saxon authors), used to repair the upper and lower limbs.

Indirect Pedicled Grafts

They are made via an intermediate zone or "temporary" host. It is worth quoting "larva" flaps or "seriate jumps" flaps Hahn's "migrant" flaps, in which the approach to the skin defect is done by means of subsequent steps, alternatively dissecting either one of the pedicles of the bridge that forms the tubular flap and then replanting it each time closer to the receiving site.

Among indirect pedicle grafts, the transported flaps (with intermediate Schrody's carrier), in which the transplant is done at the expense of a host area. The flap can be rolled in a tubular shape, usually using the wrist as the intermediate zone, or in the form of wide transported flap (the Anglo-Saxon "closed carried flap") with the juxtaposition of two very broad-based pedicle flaps in the abdomen and in the forearm. The abdominal flap will be placed permanently in the area to be repaired, while the forearm (which served as a nutrient base to another provisional) will be retrieved to the original site.

The skin graft is a graft that must live at the total expense of the new recipient area. It is defined as free graft (or immediate) when the nutritional gap is abrupt, occurring in a single operative time, and it is called pedicle graft (or mediated) if the transfer takes place keeping those connections that ensure temporary nutrition through the vascular pedicle which joins the donor area, until it has completed the formation of the vascular network that ensures the survival of the graft at the expense of the new site.

A simplified classification is based on grafts' [14, 17, 25]:

1. Antigenicity
2. Seat
3. Composition
1. Antigenicity (increasing)
   (a) *Autologous*: Donor and recipient are the same individual.
   (b) *Homologous*: Donor and recipient are different individuals but belong to the same species. In the event that it presents the same antigenic structure, such as identical twins, it is defined as "isografts"; otherwise, it is defined as "allografts."
   (c) *Heterologous*: Donor and recipient belong to different species.
2. Location
   (a) *Isotopic*: tissue transplants with identical characteristics to the tissue of the receiving area
   (b) *Heterotopic*: tissue transplants with different characteristics from those of the recipient
3. Histological composition
   (a) *Simple*: consisting of a single tissue
   (b) *Compound*: made up of several tissues

For simplicity and quickness of execution and the multiplicity of applications, skin grafts are widely used and have broad indication in surgical practice today. The class of grafts which are used most frequently is that of autologous grafts, in which the individual donor and recipient match. Even because a proper packaging and placement are rarely followed by complications, still easy to manage. On the other hand, the use of homologous and heterologous grafting is now largely reduced compared to the past, because of the strong immunogenicity which results in significant compatibility issues, which are followed by complete digestion and subsequent rejection of the transplanted tissue. Their main indication is the management of large burned as a biological dressing.

Special surgical instruments called dermatome, manually or electrically operated and adjustable in thickness, are used for the harvesting of the desired graft. The use of electric dermatome is usually associated with a higher precision in thickness and greater uniformity with respect to harvesting made with a hand dermatome.

Autologous skin grafts (or autografts) can be further divided into the following:
1. Partial-thickness skin grafts
2. Full-thickness skin grafts

Partial-Thickness Grafts [14, 17, 25]

The partial-thickness grafts are mostly used as a cover in losses of substance of wide portion of the skin surface. Their thickness includes the epidermis and the dermis, even if the total thickness varies according to the usage meant, being differentiable as partial-thickness thin, average, and total skin grafts.

This set of grafts is characterized by a much faster revascularization with respect to the one that includes full-thickness grafts, but more frequently presents complications such as higher percentage of retraction, higher frequency of color alteration in the sense of hyper- or hypopigmentation, and poor coverage of deeper tissues. The shrinkage occurs mainly after engraftment and is due to the physiological contraction of scar tissue that is interposed between the graft and the recipient site (secondary retraction). This phenomenon, which can last several months, may result in the reduction of the surface of the grafts up to 50 % of the total. The color alteration that may occur as a complication of partial-thickness graft is a consequence of the action of hormones and ultraviolet light on the melanophores present in the grafted dermis.

The donor area for a partial-thickness graft heals by second intention; in other words, reepithelialization starts from the remaining skin appendages, with almost complete restitutio ad integrum. As logic dictates, the thinner the graft, the greater the amount of adnexal residual are left in the donor area and much quicker the donor site heals: in the case of a thin graft, healing time is about 7–9 days, while if the same area undergoes intermediate-thickness harvesting, it will heal within 10–14 days; finally, if it is harvested, a full-thickness graft reepithelialization time can stretch to nearly 3 weeks. The extension of the healing time is due to the gradual reduction of adnexal residual, which is directly proportional to the thickness of the graft. Healing will progress forming granulations in the area of the harvesting beginning from the edges of the wound, with a slower process and a greater probability of hypertrophic scars formation. In this case, average and full-thickness harvests must then be covered with a thin graft.

To increase the surface of the skin grafts, thin or full-thickness, an instrument called a Mesher is used: the procedure involves the passage of the graft through the rolls of the instruments that are capable of cutting full thickness of the sheet of skin in a regularly seriate cutting, changing the solid layer into a net (mesh graft) which will heal starting from the edges of the mesh. The size of the net is adjustable, changing the expansion ratio as surgery demands. The mesh graft has the advantage of allowing the coverage of extensive loss of substance even when they have limited amount of tissue harvested; thus, the presence of fenestrations (mesh) promotes the drainage of any collected blood and serous, reducing complications such as hematoma and seromas.

Full-Thickness Grafts [14, 17, 25]

A full-thickness graft is a graft in which the harvesting is deepened to include the whole skin, i.e., epidermis and dermis. This harvesting is performed with a scalpel and not with the dermatome; any remaining fat residuals of the subcutaneous tissue is carefully removed using sharp instruments, such as scissors, because it may prevent implantation of the graft itself. As a consequence of the important thickness of the graft, the timing of revascularization will be longer than any other thinner graft. Precisely, it is the thickness that reduces the frequency of complications such as retraction, which in this case is primary; in fact it is the result of the presence of elastic fibers into the skin, which will contract immediately after harvesting. Even color alteration, greater resistance, and coverage of deep layers are consequences of the greater thickness. Unlike partial-thickness graft, the donor area needs to be sutured, as of any subsequent breach of a surgical excision, to approach the edges. This detail limits the harvesting areas for full-thickness grafts to those in which the tissue elasticity allows a good distension of the skin, it allows to efficiently conceal the residual scar and limits the extent of the possible harvesting. The main indication for use of full-thickness grafts is for limited coverage areas, small and medium sized, and whose bed is normo-vascularized. As with any thickness grafts, it is necessary that infection is not present in the recipient area. The end result is usually aesthetically more desirable with respect to a partial-thickness graft.

Virtually the entire body surface can be considered as a donor area for partial-thickness grafts; much more limited appears to be the body surface that can serve as a donor area for full-thickness grafts. The face is still excluded from this count. Common sense has it that the search of the donor site should begin in the immediate vicinity of the recipient site, in order to ensure an effective residual scar concealment, and only subsequently other donor sites will be considered for harvesting such as the one on the medial thighs, arms, or buttocks. In case of a need for full-thickness graft, areas that can be taken into consideration with the before-mentioned requirements are far less extensive than in previous and are limited to the retroauricular region, the inguinal fold, the base of the neck, and the lower fold of the buttock. The rule stands

as in preferring harvesting in areas where the tissue is most similar to the one present around the receiving site, for a more acceptable cosmetic result.

The complications associated with skin graft surgery are substantially comparable to those of any other surgical procedure; these must be added to those that we can define as "proper" of the surgical method in question and which are represented by the possibility of shrinkage and alteration of the skin color, which, respectively, are directly and inversely proportional to the thickness of the skin graft.

Surgical Technique [30]

To allow revascularization of a graft, exact conditions must be met. The graft must have a regular thickness and be totally free from residues of the subcutaneous fat, and the recipient site must be cleaned, free of necrotic debris and foreign bodies, and well vascularized to allow for immediate survival. The contact between graft and recipient area must be secured by a moderate pressure and a strict immobilization.

The harvesting of a skin graft is performed with a scalpel when a full-thickness graft is needed and in other cases using special devices called dermatomes (Fig. 22.7).

Several types exist:

- Adjustable blade knife: It is quick and easy to use but requires good manual experience.
- Drum dermatome: It is of a more complex use but allows very precise and regular graft harvesting, nowadays fell into disuse.
- Electric and pneumatic dermatome: Easier to control; they can be used even by inexperienced surgeons and in harvesting in areas with uneven surface.

The areas generally considered more suitable for harvesting a graft of thin or medium thickness are the thighs, the buttocks, and the abdomen, being large, relatively flat areas, allowing large skin harvesting. In these areas, scars are also easily concealed beneath clothing, thus reducing the patient's discomfort for possible cosmetic damage. For the harvesting of a full-thickness skin graft, preferred areas are with soft, thick, and colorful evenness, such as the retroauricular

Fig. 22.7 Dermatome

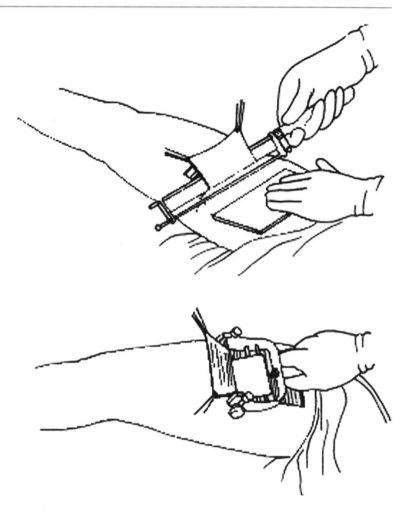

region, supraclavicular region, the elbow fold, the groin, and the inner surface of the arm.

The healing period of the donor area varies depending on the thickness of the graft harvested. Sure enough, in the case of skin harvesting of thin or average thickness, the donor area tends to heal spontaneously by reepithelialization, beginning from the bottom of the bed of the wound and will include the skin adnexal. The healing will be complete within 15–21 days. After the time interval, if necessary, harvesting in the same area can be repeated.

In the case of harvesting three quarters of or full-thickness graft, spontaneous healing can occur only by secondary intention. Margins should be approached if the donor is narrow; when surfaces are larger, a thin graft harvested from an adjacent area can be used to cover the first donor site. The repair by secondary intention

leads to a rather slow recovery, with formation of scars in general exuberant and hyperpigmented.

Mode of Engraftment [30]

Graft harvesting disconnects all vascular and nervous connections with the donor area, and the appearance of the tissue immediately after is intensely pale. The contact between graft and recipient area is initially established through a weave of fibrin, while the survival of the graft cells, during the period of time elapsed from the harvesting moment to the complete recovery of vascular connections, is ensured by the fluid exuding in the recipient region. This process, previously mistakenly referred to as plasma circulation, is today more properly defined as serum imbibition and is capable of providing a valuable contribution for the nutrition to grafted tissues throughout a 2-day time period. Relatively recent scientific studies have led us to believe that the role of the vascular network, the grafted tissues, is only transitory and that these vessels act as a guide for the reorganization of the local vascular network. Sure enough, only 5 h after surgery, in the bed of the receiving area, several endothelial mitoses can be observed beginning from the bottom and the margins of the wound, finally establishing vascular connections to the recipient site vessels. The first vascular anastomoses between the graft and the host area are documentable 24–72 h after surgery. A real blood flow in the graft is evident already starting on the third day after surgery, and revascularization is completed between the sixth and the seventh day, with the differentiation between arterioles and venules which is completed on the eighth day. The blood flow in the graft stabilized itself to normal within 20 days from surgery. These statistics give us the reason why it is strictly necessary to immobilize the graft during the first 5–7 days post-surgery and the problems thicker grafts have to take root, considering the more complex skin structure and the increased effort needed to complete the formation of the vascular network. Within 3 months after the operation, reinnervations is completed but is often accompanied by subjective disorders such as paresthesia and hyperesthesia with spatial dissociation. With regard to skin adnexal, the sweating function is kept limitedly to a slight recovery only in the full-thickness grafts, while sebum-secreting function may also be present in the thinner grafts.

The graft revascularization follows three different mechanisms:

1. Inoculation: Direct reconnection of the vessels of the graft to the vessels of the recipient area.
2. Vessel growth: Host vessels grow to from anastomosis with the graft vessels.
3. New formation: A new vascular network is formed beginning from the host vessels.

Flaps [26]

A flap is defined as a transfer of one or more tissues from a donor site to a receiving site while maintaining integrity in the vascular network.

Same as, transferring vascular connections to supply the tissue. This blood supply can be maintained in connection with the original one, as in the case of local tissue flaps, or reconnected to the vascular network of the recipient site, as in the case of the distance flaps. As with any surgery, the planning phase is of fundamental importance for the indication, the study of the vascular anatomy of the areas, and the preoperative drawings.

Flaps can be classified considering the following:

Anatomical relationships	Local	Sliding
		Rotational
		Transpositional
		Z, M, trident, W, etc.
	Distant	Direct
		Tubular
		Free or microvascular
Composition	Simple	Cutaneous
		Fascial
		Muscular
		Osseous
	Composite	Fasciocutaneous
		Myocutaneous
		Osteocutaneous
		Adipose-fascial
		Myofascial
Vascularization	Axial	Direct flow
		Reverse flow
	Random	

Local Flaps

The indication of local flaps is the closure of defects adjacent to the donor site. To get the best aesthetic and functional results in the coverage of a defect is recommended the use of the skin adjacent of the defect itself. These flaps are composed of skin and subcutaneous tissue, and their transfer to cover the surgical breach is carried out through surgical procedures that can be classified as sliding, rotation, and transposition. Obviously, the procedure to be adopted is related to the size of excision, the anatomical site in which the excision occurs, and the orientation with respect to the relaxed skin tension lines, in other words, to the skin tension that is generated as a result of excision.

As the general surgical approach should be to make the excision with the specific intention of

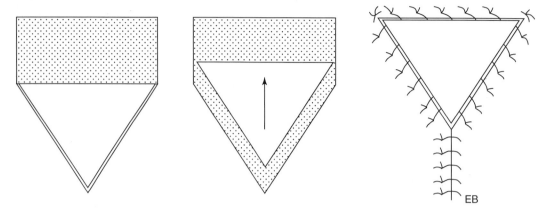

Fig. 22.8 "V-Y" sliding flap

direct closing the wound suturing, not always easy, likewise when choosing for the use of flaps, the surgeon should aim for direct closure of the secondary defect. Surgical practice has pointed out that even this approach will not always be easy; in these cases it would be necessary to close the secondary defect by means of skin grafting to preserve the underlying tissues and anatomical structures. Of central importance is the accurate per-operatory planning, dedicating time to the careful measurement and delimitation of excision areas, to evaluating the size and scope of harvesting and to the study of relaxed skin tension lines as they appear before and after the flaps are transferred, as well as to the perfusion topography of the areas involved. The same careful attention must be paid in respecting local conditions existing in the area before surgery. As for the lozenge excisions, the mobilization of margins is followed by a reduction of the tension exerting on them, as well, in a reduction of the most frequent complication that might happen: necrosis. Sometimes it will be necessary and appropriate to leave in place a fall drainage, which must be maintained during the first 2–3 postoperative days. The medication applied should always be moderately compressive, in order to avoid hypoperfusion for the vascular pedicle of the flap from excessive compression.

Sliding Flaps

The result of excision and removal of skin area is the formation of a breach in the outer envelope of the human body. The repair of the breach usually is carried out with direct suturing, even after loosening the margins of the breach itself and stretching of the adjacent skin. The tension exerted to dislodge the mobilized skin will be directly exerted on the margins of the wound itself and precisely where the suture maintains those margins adjacent. If the traction is excessive, it may expose the suture to risk of diastases; the tension can be dissipated engraving one or more "V" incisions, both superiorly and inferiorly. The suture is performed so to change the "V" shape to a "Y" shape, "V-Y" plasty, increasing the mobilization of the tissue of the area, thereby reducing the tension on the margins of the wound. This simple method can be applied whenever it is necessary to unload the excessive traction as can result, for example, from plastic elongation of retracting scars.

Today, flap surgery offers more than proven solutions that supply remarkable plasticity and adaptability to surgical needs. The patterns of etching techniques are shown in Fig. 22.8.

Advancement Flaps

The transfer of this flap type occurs following a linear path from the donor to the receiving site, along its longitudinal axis. The shape varies considerably depending on the defect to be repaired and the anatomical region; even if most often are rectangular in shape, they can be shaped as V's, U's, and H's, usually with a length/width ratio of

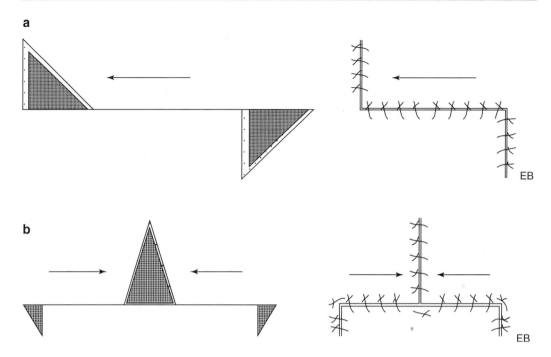

Fig. 22.9 Advancement flaps. (**a**) Lateral advancement. (**b**) Bilateral advancement

2.5–3:1 cm. Close to the proximal end of the flap, a triangular incision should be made to exceed the exuberant tissue present. The indication for the use of this set of flaps is the repair of a small skin defect, up to a maximum of 2 cm in length (Fig. 22.9).

Rotational Flaps

Similar to the previous set of flaps for what concerns the surgical technique, it differs for the incisions, distinguished by having a semicircular or arched shape, which rotate along an arc in the direction of the defect until the skin defect is completely covered. Also in this case, to reduce the tension mounting in the area, an incision can be made or a triangle of skin can be removed near the base of the flap (Burow's triangle). Depending on the needs, flaps can be of various shapes but retaining the intrinsic property to rotate sideways. The donor site is closed either through redistribution of tissue and direct suture of the breach or by skin grafting if the residual defect is particularly large or is located in body areas where the tissues are adherent to the underlying bony structures such as the scalp.

Transposition Flaps

A transposition flap is defined as a flap in which the tissues used to repair the defect "leap over healthy tissue," turning and covering all or part of the primary defect. These flaps are of different shapes, arcuate, angular, sharp, "V" shaped, "W" shaped, "trident" shaped, and "Z" shaped, and are generally carved at one edge of the defect. The donor site is then closed by direct suture, skin graft, or a secondary flap, such as the bilobed flap.

Peculiar and widely used is the Limberg flap, described for the first time in 1946. It is a diamond-shaped transposition flap. The area to be excised is inscribed in a rhomb with angles of 60° and 120°, planned in close relation to the amount of tissue available to cover the resulting defect. The uniqueness comes from the ability to choose one of the four sides of the diamond that will serve as the pedicle of the flap. When transportation direction is chosen, the incisions will be oriented according to the relaxed skin tension lines, prolonging the minor diagonal throughout its length. At the end of the extension, a line parallel to the side of the diamond and of equal length is

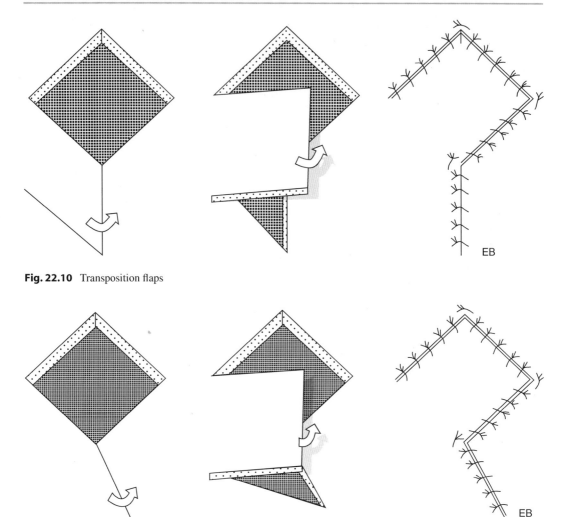

Fig. 22.10 Transposition flaps

Fig. 22.11 Dufourmentel transposition flap

incised. The outcome is a flap whose three sides and whose bases are of equal length, whose corners coincide with those of the breach. After the transposition, the donor site is sutured directly. The association of more than one Limberg flap is possible if the skin defect is of wide proportions (Fig. 22.10).

Variant of the previous flap is the flap of Dufourmentel, described for the first time in 1962. In this case the defect is inscribed into a rhomb, whose angles are 30° and 150°. The first side is drawn along the bisector of the angle opposite to the one formed by one of the sides and the minor diagonal, and the second side is parallel to the major diagonal and of equal length.

The advantages over a Limberg flap are the following: less tension acting on the suture of the donor site and greater availability of the tissue to cover the defect (Fig. 22.11).

Differently addressed is the "Z" plasty, which is useful in stretching a surgical incision or to reorient the direction of a scar, resulting in lengthening of the tissues present, in the redistribution of tension exerted over the surrounding areas and the disruption of the major axis of the scar. The technique involves the exchange of opposing skin flaps, the side incisions will be long as the lateral axis, and the angle of incision can have values between 30° and 60° with respect to the direction of the scar, remembering that a smaller angle

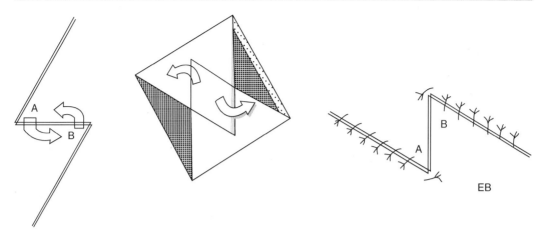

Fig. 22.12 "Z" plasty flaps. A: superior flap. B: inferior flap

increases the risk of necrosis of the tip of the flap, while any larger angle makes it difficult to rotate the flap itself. The length of the central axis determines the value of the final gain, while the amplitude of the corners determines the amount of lengthening achieved. With 30° angle, the resulting increase in the length would be around 25 %; with angle of 45°, the percentage rises to 50 %; and with amplitudes of 60°, resulting gain reaches of about 75 %. From practical experience, the authors have noted that the amplitude of the most useful angle is 60°, because more acute angles determine insufficient elongation, while more obtuse angles result in an excessive increase in the tension of the adjacent tissues, making it difficult to transpose the flaps. This kind of technique can be applied as seriate surgery, multiple Z plasty, if the amount of skin available is not sufficient or in case of injury of large dimensions. The "Z" variant is used primarily in flexor regions (Fig. 22.12).

Distant Flaps [26]

When near the repair area is not possible to find enough tissues, flaps must be moved from distant donor sites. This can be achieved with the flap temporarily joining two nonanatomically contiguous areas. The transplant performed can be separated from the donor site only after a period of at least 3 weeks, because it needs to establish vascular connections to the vascular network of the recipient site, so to allow disconnection of the pedicle without damaging the viability of the flap. This method has, compared to proximity flap, some negative aspects for the two anatomical regions, joined by the transplant, must be kept in strict immobility and the posture is often not comfortable for patients. In particular in elderly patients, it may result in joint ankylosis not easily solvable. Thus, being necessary more than one operation, the patient is exposed even to risks deriving from repeated anesthesia and contamination, along with the problem of prolonged hospitalization.

Depending on the anatomical regions involved, different types of flaps are characterized:

- Direct
- Tubular
- Free or microvascular

Direct Flaps

The term "cross leg" refers to the repair of a loss of substance of a lower limb using a direct, distance flap from the contralateral limb; the flap is usually obtained from the sural region or from the thigh. The indication for this flap is the repair of lesions with exposed tendons and bones, osteomyelitis, skin fistulas, or necrosis deriving from exposed fractures with metal plates and screws system.

"Cross arm": The flap is drawn on the inner surface of the arm and used to repair injuries of the contralateral limb, in particular of the hand.

"Cross finger": Repair the volar surface of a finger using a strip obtained from the interdigital surface of an adjacent finger. To repair losses of substance of the fingertips, a similar flap harvested from the thenar region can be used [31].

A historical example of a flap harvested from the inner face of the arm used to repair a loss of substance of the face, in particular the nose, is known as the Italian method. The thorax and abdomen can also provide plenty of skin for the repair of losses of substance of the upper limbs, which are easily approached and kept in contact with them.

Tubular Flaps

Nowadays rarely used, a tubular flap is bipedicle, plan flap, sutured to itself along the two long sides to form a canal with on the outer surface the skin and subcutaneous part on the inside. The flap can have a considerable length because it is sufficiently fed by the two pedicles.

Its main indication is the need to transfer a lot of skin at a great distance.

The tubular flap is harvested in preferential areas such as the base of the anterior cervical region, the abdomen, the pectoral region, and the inside face of the arm. After 3 weeks of its harvesting, the transfer can take place; it can be direct if the donor and the receiving site are close or can be brought together or indirect through a first transfer to a carrier region, normally represented by the wrist. Once the flap has reached, its final location is unfolded along the ventral scar and set in place.

In the early stages of the tubular flap transfer, it can be set autonomous to increase possible grafting. Down aspects of these flaps are the large number of operations needed to reach the repair and the extremely long hospitalization period; is also consistent the risk of large losses of substance for ischemic necrosis, which is present at each step.

Tubular flaps, which for decades have been a mainstay of reconstructive surgery, have become obsolete, because the problem of transferring from a distance of copious amounts of skin is now electively dealt with other techniques (skin expansion and free flaps).

Free Flaps

Free flaps are based on the isolation and division of the vascular pedicle, then anastomosed with the previously isolated pedicle in the recipient site: it is a microsurgical technique.

The indications for these flaps are the cases that require a distance flap, avoiding the time required by other intermediate operators such as tubular flaps.

The gradual spread of manual skills in the field of microsurgery and the ever-higher quality of the technology and materials available today make the use, with reasonable safety, of the procedures based on these reconstructive flaps feasible. In addition to elective surgery, the free flaps are now also used for treatment in hospital emergency care of severe trauma, in association with revascularization of a limb.

Simple Flaps [26]
Skin Flaps

Treated in the section: skin grafts

Fascial Flaps

The fascial flaps are meant to convey their adherent vascular network, thereby improving the circulatory condition of the recipient region. They must be covered with a skin flap or skin grafting.

They are indicated in those clinical situations in which requested coverage with perfused, vital tissue is associated with the need for thinness and/or flexibility of the tissue. Their clinical use is expanding, particularly in reconstructive techniques following trauma.

Muscle Flaps

The isolated muscle can be used as transplant, mainly to fill serious loss of skin substance and subcutaneous tissue; on top of the muscle, repair can be done with a proximity skin flap or with a simple graft. An example is the filling of the orbital cavity after exenteratio orbitae with the use of the temporalis muscle appropriately rotated. The reanimation of the facial muscles to correct the deficits resulting from the VII cranial nerve palsy (facial paralysis) is achieved by means of a microsurgical transplant revascularization and reinnervation of muscle units.

Bone Flaps

Bone flaps are microsurgical transfers of portions of bone. The main indication is in the reconstruction and repair of the jaw, limb, or bone segments in general.

Composite Flaps [26]

The study of the vascular anatomy of the skin, seen not in a merely descriptive way but aimed to perform skin grafts, has led, since the 1970s, to the formulation of the concept of "angiosomes," multi-tissular anatomical units, based on a precise vascular tree. This allowed the creation of new reconstructive units, including tissues different from the skin. Knowledge of the vascular anatomy of all the tissues that constitute an angiosome provides the doctrinal basis for the transfer of composite skin, muscles, nerves, tendons, and bone units, all supplied by a single, arteriovenous system.

In a composite flap, the presence of different tissues has sometimes the only means to adequately support the skin but is more often aimed at the realization of a complex multi-tissular reconstructive project; finally, sometimes flaps are harvested so that skin is completely absent (e.g., fascial flaps and muscle flaps).

In this type of transplantation, empiricism, which is at the base of the harvesting of random skin flaps, is completely lost because blood supply is always exactly identified, as well as the size of the tissues that can be transferred.

Composite flaps
Fasciocutaneous flaps
Myocutaneous flaps
Osteocutaneous flaps
Prefabricated flaps
Neurocutaneous flaps

Nowadays the search is still open for the identification of new, safe reconstructive units.

Fasciocutaneous Flaps

They consist of skin, subcutaneous tissue, and fascia and represent a variant of the classic plain flaps.

The inclusion of deep fascia in the flap structure is necessary to preserve and convey the dominant cutaneous vessels, which shall run in the context of the fascia; the skin is nourished through the vascular plexus located just above the fascia.

The classification most used is the one proposed in 1984 by Cormack and Lamberty:
- *Type A*: multiple perforans vessels running parallel to the pedicle
- *Type B*: single perforans vessel nourishing the fascial plexus
- *Type C*: a series of multiple perforans vessels that detach from an artery deep and contained in a fascial septum

The surgeon must be aware that the harvesting of these flaps may lead to the formation of hernias in the muscle present in the donor site. Fasciocutaneous flaps are frequently used to repair losses of substance of the limbs, where the longitudinal fascial vascular structure allows harvesting of different flaps along the major axis of the limbs.

Myocutaneous Flaps

These are reconstructive units, whose design dates back to Tansini, in the early twentieth century, which were taken up, studied, and used in large scale only since the late 1970s.

These flaps are set on the principle of preservation of perforans vessels that connect the skin to underlying muscles. Preserving the vascular pedicle of a muscle can also ensure the viability of a given island of overlying skin. With this in mind, the different muscles are classified into five different categories, based on the characteristics of the different vascular pedicles. Initially only used to transplant large amounts of skin in one surgical time, soon these flaps have been proved valuable to fill the deepest loss of substance and improve the circulatory function of the recipient region. The myocutaneous flap can be used as arterialized flaps leaving intact the vascular pedicle of the muscle or as free flaps.

In 1981, Mathes and Naha have highlighted the following types:
- *Type I*: single vascular pedicle (*TFL*)
- *Type II*: a dominant pedicle and minor pedicles various (*gracilis*)
- *Type III*: two dominant pedicles (*rectoabdominal*)
- *Type IV*: multiple segmental pedicles (*sartorius*)

- *Type V*: a dominant pedicle and various segmental pedicles (*latissimus dorsi*)

Their indication is made up of lesions with wide and deep loss of substance and conditions that require surgical repair in a single time.

Every muscle is potentially used to harvest a flap.

The only limitation is the considerable aesthetic and functional deficits that can residuate in the donor area.

Osteocutaneous Flaps

They are characterized by two major nourishing methods: a dominant vascular pedicle and a series of segmental pedicles that nourish the portion of bone or by direct blood supply through the periosteum. Used almost exclusively as a free flap, these flaps allow the reconstruction of entire anatomical structures (e.g., osteocutaneous of fibula flap for reconstruction of the entire region of the mandible). Recent anatomical studies concerning the perforans vessels have demonstrated how the vessels' network of skin islands connected to bone segments is capable of maintaining a good and safe blood flow, allowing an expansion of their clinical applications in reconstructive surgery.

Adipofascial Flaps

They are special flaps harvested below the skin environment, specifically in the adipose layer, and mainly used in cases where it is necessary to restore volume in a poorly perfused area. The donor site does not present difficulties for direct suture.

Musculofascial Flaps

This type of flap is harvested from a subcutaneous environment, especially in cases where reconstruction needs resistant and highly vascularized tissue.

Neurocutaneous Flaps

Flaps proving the possibility of transferring skin on top of the course of a sensory nerve, which acts as a carrier for its concomitant vessels, since such vessels are able to ensure the viability of the flap.

In harvesting these flaps, it is important to include a protective sheath of nerve surrounding tissue, because in that nervous sheath run both the vasa nervorum and the concomitant vessels, which partially contribute to perfusion of the flap itself.

Axial Vascularization Flaps [29, 32]

Axial flaps are defined as flaps that have their own arterial and venous vascular pedicle. The first classification was organized in 1972 by McGregor and Jackson, even though since 1869 many authors have used those flaps. In 1977, McCraw and Dibbel were the first who really comprehended the enormous potential of the richly represented vasculature identifiable within the fascia as a support to large skin islands, followed by Elliot and Hartrampf whom in 1983 demonstrated the feasibility of large musculocutaneous rectoabdominal flap.

Time was ripe for the next step, particularly through the development of surgical instruments and the introduction of the operating microscope, the free transfer of tissues with an immediate revascularization using microvascular anastomosis. After several attempts on animals, Komatsu and Tamai in 1968 transferred successfully a human thumb. Only in 1971, Kaplan and Buncke used a groin free flap (groin flap) for reconstruction of the oral cavity. Since then, studies on the anatomical structure of compound flaps and on the vascular structure of the territories of the body, the so-called angiosomes, made possible to widen the use and identification of these flaps and increase the use in reconstructive surgery of axial flaps, offering new and unimagined possibilities for reestablishment of morpho-functional properties so far impossible.

In this type of tissue transplant, the length of the flap tissue can cover the entire extent of the vascular pedicle, to which can be added a distal extension of the skin nourished by the subcutaneous vascular network. In fact, the blood supply occurs through septo-fascial vessels and perforans vessels that anastomosed to the vascular network under the skin (Fig. 22.13).

As for any surgical procedure, preoperative planning appears to be of fundamental importance, carefully considering the position of the

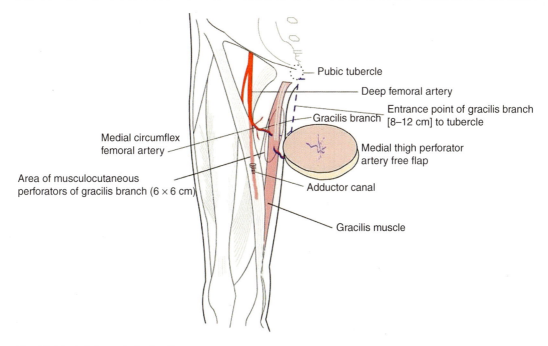

Fig. 22.13 Axial vascularization flap

pedicle and the size and shape of the flap. The skin incision should start from the distal portion of the flap and carefully following the lines, deepening to reach the tissue that you want to include in the structure (fascia, muscle, bone). The flap must be handled with extreme care to avoid any damage to the vascular pedicle. The surgeon should suture to the muscle, to the fascia, and the skin so as to include all the tissues adequately in the flap.

The axial vascularization flaps, by definition, are characterized by the existence of a vascular pedicle easily identifiable and always present; this feature also defines their method of harvesting:

1. *Transpositional flaps*: maintaining a skin bridge at the base that includes the vascular pedicle.
2. *Island flaps*: maintaining only the vascular pedicle at the base, which in this case must be identified and isolated, this flap has greater mobility compared to the previous one.
3. *Free flaps*: where the flap is completely isolated, after identifying and isolating the vascular pedicle, and then anastomosed to the vascular network of the receiving area.

Arterial Flaps (Direct Flow)

An arterialized flap is a skin graft, which includes, in its pedicle, artery and vein with the satellite cutaneous lymphatic vessels.

It can be carved either as a plain pedicle skin flap or as a subcutaneous pedicle island flap. In the first case, the vascular pedicle is maintained for the entire length of the flap and the graft is not bound to particular dimensional relationship between the width and length of the pedicle of the flap because, since it includes the artery, the blood supply is guaranteed for all its extension.

In the second case, however, the subcutaneous vascular pedicle is isolated and the resulting island of skin is nourished only from a central position: the form and extent of the flap will vary depending on the anatomical region involved.

The arteries which are based on the most common arterialized flaps are:

- *Arteria temporalis superficialis*: a flap that can fill the whole forehead and is used in the reconstruction of the nose, mouth, and cheek
- The first four perforans branches of the *arteria mammaria internae*: for a deltopectoral flap used to reconstruct the cervical esophagus, the pharyngostomes, and the nuchal region

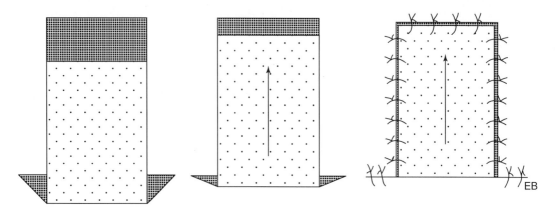

Fig. 22.14 Plain monopedicle flap

- The superficial branch of *arteria epigastrica inferior*: hypogastric flap for repair of the surrounding areas or at distance as for the lower limb
- The superficial branch of the *circumflex iliac artery*: for a flap that corresponds to the groin area and that is used to repair perineal and pubic region or as distance flap
- *Dorsal pedal artery*: a dorsal flap of the foot
- *Arteria labialis*: used to transfer a portion of the upper lip to repair the lower lip or from entrusting the entire thickness of a lip flap with a thin stalk of pink border inside which runs this artery

Reverse Flow Flaps

Although the principle of reverse flow flaps has probably been in use for many years (the inverted superficial temporal artery scalp flap of Orticochea), the axiality of these flaps has only recently been appreciated.

The essential feature of this sort of flap is the reverse flow of blood produced by the flap design. Pinal and Taylor performed cadaveric, surgical, and hemodynamic studies in humans and dogs to investigate the arteriovenous system and the contribution that venous valves have in the survival of distally based reverse flow (e.g., radial) flaps. The capability for survival of these flaps is explained by two systems of venous arcades which facilitate bypass of blood in a reverse fashion.

Macrovenous connections are defined as interconnecting veins, devoid of valves, which range from 1 to 3 mm in diameter and which skip the valves of the venae comitantes. The macrovenous connections are insufficient to bypass all the valves unless the pedicle length is 2.5 cm or less.

Microvenous connections are a plexus of tiny veins, also free of valves, which surround the artery as the vena arteriosa and also provide a connection to the venae. The microvenous connections, because of their small size, require a relatively high pressure and reasonable period of time for blood to flow through them, hence the cyanosis seen in these flaps for 12–24 h after transfer. Contraction of smooth muscle in the valve cusps could result in incompetence, in addition to extrinsic pressure on the valve which may produce distortion.

Random Vascularization Flaps [29]

The random vascularization flaps (random flaps) are more commonly used in the repair of deficits resulting from surgical excisions of skin lesions of considerable size. The blood supply can be guaranteed by a single or a double pedicle. Moreover, flaps can also be harvested as plain or tubular and used in the vicinity or at a distance.

Classification of random flaps vascularization:

Plain monopedicle	Local and distant
Plain bipedicle	
Island flaps	Only local
Tubular flaps	Only distant

Plain Monopedicle Flaps

The flaps have plain, monopedicle, elongated, roughly rectangular, or oval in shape (Fig. 22.14):

one of the smaller sides is not cut into, constituting the vascular and nervous pedicle of the flap. A general rule defines the maximum size of the flap with regard to the width of the pedicle, which should never exceed half the length of the flap itself, to avoid an insufficient blood supply resulting in partial or even total necrosis of the flap itself. In the transfer of a flap from the donor to the recipient site, attention should be paid to avoid an excessive stretching or twisting of the pedicle that could cause strangulation of the vessels.

The flaps should never be harvested in areas of not perfectly intact skin, as, for example, those affected by a scar or affected by radiodermatitis resulting from treatment with ionizing radiation, which could have rendered insufficient blood supply to the area.

Using a random vascularization flap, the surgeon must follow certain rules that are different depending on the region where the harvesting of the flap is necessary: in the trunk region the midline should never be crossed, and the vascular pedicle of the limbs must be located necessarily proximal to the receiving area. However, there is a region where all these rules can be violated: in the face there is a rich vascular network that can substantially allow the survival of any type of flap, even those apparently very bold.

The most common complications that can occur even a few hours after surgery are in most cases represented by the following: suffering from ischemia (where the artery nourishment is insufficient, the flap will appear pale in color) and suffering from stagnation (in the event that there is insufficient venous drainage, the flap will change color, gradually becoming cyanotic).

The surgeon, in addition to the need to repair a loss of substance, whichever it may be, must also address the repair of the donor area of a flap in one of two ways: by "direct suture," a simple approximation of the margins, if this is allowed by the size of the substance loss and by the elasticity of the region skin, or by applying a thin skin grafting. Grafting can be carried out in the same surgical time of flap rotation or even at later time, which can be done 8 or more days after,

allow the formation granulation tissue, which will facilitate engraftment and survival.

In the anatomical regions where blood supply is at risk, as in the lower limbs, or when harvesting flaps particularly large in size, a preliminary procedure called autonomization should be performed. The procedure consists in harvesting the desired flap, but instead of rotating or sliding it toward the recipient site, it is left temporarily in the donor site. This allows to verify, before the final transfer, if the flap is sufficiently vascularized; otherwise, after a few days, a suffering portion of the flap can be eliminated using only the remainder.

Moreover, in doing so, the flap gets used to living in conditions of reduced blood supply: it is demonstrated that a reduction of nourishment stimulates vascular growth in size and number of vessels in the pedicle, thus improving the chances of survival of the flap when transferred. The surgery for the permanent transfer in the recipient site can be performed 8 days after the autonomization. In special cases it is also possible to split the autonomization process in different steps, in order to make it even less risky.

A plain flap can be transferred close to the receiving site by means of sliding or rotating movements depending on the particular needs of wound repair.

Plain Bipedicled Flaps

A particular category of flaps is the plain bipedicled flaps, which could also be defined bridge flaps. In fact, they have two pedicles and can therefore be very long, even with a length to width ratio of 4–1. They can be used as proximity flap to use, for example, scalp tissue in the reconstruction of a hairy upper lip, or at distance to repair, for example, an injured hand with a flap of abdominal skin. These are flaps not frequently used.

Island Flaps

The island flap (Fig. 22.15) is a particular type of plain flap: its pedicle is in fact constituted only by subcutaneous tissue, and the skin is incised and completely isolated from the surrounding skin. The added value of these flaps is their versatility

Fig. 22.15 The island flap

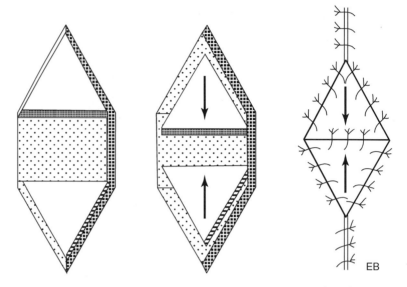

because the subcutaneous pedicle allows twisting, stretching, and much more agile movement than allowed by a skin pedicle.

The island flap with random subcutaneous vascularization is almost only used to repair face defects, where the extreme richness of the vascular network allows safe usage.

Tubular Flaps

Tubular Flaps argument was treated in the distance flaps paragraph.

Prefabricated Flaps

A recent innovation in composite flaps is discovery of prefabricated flaps. In these flaps, tissue composition is not directly borrowed from a naturally existing anatomical scheme but surgically produced by one or more operations. Such transactions, called "preparation," are used to prefabricate reconstructive unit, which will hereafter be transferred with microsurgical technique.

They allow the repair of complex multi-tissular lesions, as, for example, the reconstruction of the entire nasal pyramid with bones and cartilage components using a skin flap prefabricated on the surface of a forearm, in which the constituent parts of the nasal pyramid reconstruction have been properly assembled during one or more previous surgeries.

Mohs Surgery in Skin Cancer [33–36]

Mohs surgery is a seriate surgical technique for progressive removal of tumor tissue using immediate microscope histological controls to determine the extent of the tumor. This procedure ensures the radical operation and at the same time allows to better preserve the surrounding healthy tissue. Most people think that a tumor will grow in almost spherical shape, and if this were true, its removal with a healthy margin of a few millimeters from the edge of the lesion would give security of absolute radicalism. The reality, unfortunately, is different: the peripheral rim of the lesion is often indistinct or non-determinable, and deep zones of the lesion almost never have a regular expansion. The tumor in its growth, in fact, is affected by several factors (density of the substrate, the fusion of embryonic leaflets, cleavage planes, the presence of different anatomical structures, scar tissue, etc.) that cause irregular, random, and bizarre anatomical architecture.

The histological appearance of a newly arisen skin cancer is the so called 'iceberg like' appearance (the tumor overflows from the wound edges evident on the skin surface) or the dendritic (they originate from the tumor and girders cellular cords that infiltrate the surrounding tissues with root development). These configurations involve, for radical surgery, always the removal of very large and considerably more extensive lesion than the clinically evident, even with sacrifice of presumably harmless tissue. Since in oncological surgery the goal must be radicalism of removal, the dismantling concept is accepted relatively easily, although in recent years all over the world, surgical oncology, with an eye to quality of life of the work and his psychology, seeks to combine radical, safety, and minimal trauma. In dermatological oncology surgery, particularly if extensive scarring or loss of substance is accepted on the trunk or limbs because they are easily masked, this concept is more difficult to implement on the face or other cosmetically or functionally important areas. And we must not forget that more than 2/3 of skin cancer occurs on exposed areas!

Another problem of dermatological oncology is the fact that the histological examination of the specimen is always a few days posterior or, at best, follows the surgical suture of the breach. If, as sometimes happens, the response shows a histological incomplete excision of the lesion, the patient must undergo a second surgery to enlarge the removal. It is however also possible that multiple histological sections, as normally occurs in traditional histology, give false negatives. All these drawbacks can be overcome using a technique widely used in the United States (about 65 % of all dermatologic oncology surgery) called Mohs surgery. This surgery was designed in the 1930s by F. Mohs, a professor of surgery at Wisconsin University, and named in his honor; it can be defined as a progressive seriate removal of all and only the tumor tissue either in its solid mass or in its possible ramifications.

It is a super-specialist treatment using microscopic histological controls to determine the extent of the tumor, its location, and its architecture. The technique is schematically simple, the advantages are many, security is virtually complete, but the organization affects a wide amount of relatively complex procedure. The action takes place in stages. On the skin surface of the cancer, acetic acid is brushed which allows the elicitation of the margins of the lesion; if the tumor involves the mucosa, it is advisable to use methylene blue. After local infiltration of anesthetic, the lesion is removed en bloc, tumor clinically evident with a border of about 3 mm of tissue, presumably healthy. First, a map of the excised tissue oriented according to its anatomical location is drawn, after which it is divided into subsections of about 2×2 cm, which are carefully numbered and marked with colored landmarks to facilitate orientation during the preparation and reading of the slide. Each of the subsections is immediately attached to the cryostat where, however, it is placed upside down, in order for the first section to be place at the bottom of the lesion. The slides thus prepared are read under a microscope. If the entire bottom and all edges of the subsections are considered, free of tumor cells means that the lesion is completely included in the piece and you can be assured of absolute radical surgery. If, however, tumor tissue is found in the bottom or edges of the excision, the histology will be able to specify the exact location and, according to the mapping done previously, indicate exactly where in the skin or subcutaneous unsuspected residual tumor lurks. The surgeon removes, in this case, an additional layer of tissue only in the positive areas of the map; the process described above is repeated until the histologist does not confirm that the entire base and all the edges gradually removed of tissue are free of cancer debris. It is obvious that this method allows the complete removal of the tumor definitely, better preserving surrounding healthy tissue.

As easily imagined, the method is time consuming: the removal of each layer of tissue takes approximately thirty to forty minutes, of which only ten are of actual surgery, while more than twenty are used to organize all the steps. Since surgery can take up to two or three stages, it commits the patient for about 2 h, but during the needed time necessary to prepare and read the slides, the patient can move around, walk, read and so on. Another advantage of the method is experienced in the rare cases of very large or invasive tumors. If it takes several stages, to be easy on the patient or overload of anesthetic, the surgery can even be divided into several days.

Graphical representation of Mohs surgery:
- *Stage I*: Margins elicitation
- *Stage II*: En block excision
  - Subsections splitting
  - Mapping
  - Histological examination of the sub-reversed
  - Positivity of subsections
- *Stage III*: Area ablation
  - Subsections splitting and mapping
  - Histological exam
  - Positivity of subsection
- *Stage IV*: Section ablation
  - Subsections splitting and mapping
  - Histological exam
  - Negativity of the subunits

The complexity of the process explains why the Mohs surgery requires a team (surgeon, nurses, lab technician, histopathologist) that is well coordinated to minimize the inevitable time-consuming processes. In view of these disadvantages, the percentage of cures is over 99 % even in ineffective cases. In addition, the Mohs technique, defining the areas affected by the tumor microscopically and selectively removing them, saves the best healthy tissue and minimizes the residual scars and provides better immediate cosmetic results. Another great advantage of this method is its running under local anesthesia; the procedure in stages allows the use of small doses of anesthetic repeated at intervals. You realize that narcosis is not advisable for an operation whose actual surgical times are reduced. Although it would be desirable that all skin cancers could be treated with Mohs surgery, it is particularly indicated in recurrent tumors, in basal dermatosclerosis or the intermediary, and in very large tumors. Other indications are the preferential areas in tumors of early deep infiltration (eye-hand inside, nasolabial folds, furrows, and pre- or retroauricular) or functional areas such as noble eyelids, nose, lips, ears, genitals, and hands.

Indications for Mohs surgery:
- Recurrent basal cell carcinoma
- Spinocellular carcinoma
- Primary tumors:
  - Developing on "at risk" areas (nose, orbit, ear, forehead)
  - Developing on scars
  - Developing on mucous membranes (genital or lips)
- Basal cell carcinoma:
  - Dermatosclerosis
  - Multicentric
  - Intermediate
- Malignancies in areas of high aesthetic value

In conclusion, the Mohs surgery has no downside compared to traditional surgery, and the latter has many advantages that can be schematically listed as follows:
- It allows an immediate diagnostic feedback.
- It avoids radical reoperation.
- It is conservative and minimizes the loss of reparative tissue unscathed with minor problems.
- It is favorable as outpatient.
- It is convenient because it can be divided into several times.
- It is safe even in elderly and in patients at risk as it is performed under local anesthesia.
- It is suitable even for very large lesions.

Basic Suturing Techniques

In dermatologic cancer surgery, full- or partial-thickness excision repair involving the fascia has the following objectives:
1. Skin (and fascia) layer reconstruction
2. Granting low tension on tissues layers on all levels
3. Improve hemostasis
4. Prevent complications (diastase, infection, seromas, etc.)
5. Provide a final result aesthetically acceptable

According to those objectives, a wound resulting from skin surgery due to cancer must be closed paying attention to anatomical structure of the skin layers, which is, performing different sutures following those layers: fascia, hypodermis, and dermis.

The Fascia

Excisions of this tissue can be reconstructed with direct suture using permanent or absorbable material, in areas where good coverage of the subcutaneous tissue is available in order to prevent the sutures to be felt under the skin.

Intact fascia may also be used to reduce skin tension, if sutured with a particular crossed knot. Thus, suturing the fascia will drag along the above skin layers and will allow for easier closure and reduction of tension on the wound margins. The surgeon must pay attention to the final placement of the knot, which should be deep beneath the margin of the fascia folding, in order to reduce the possibility for the patient to feel the knot under the skin, even in case of an atrophic scar. The technique requires the use of permanent or slowly reabsorbable sutures.

Small fascia damages occurred during the surgical demolitive phase can be sutured directly, using reabsorbable material.

The Subcutaneous Tissue

Subcutaneous tissue layers should be approached using either continuous or interrupted suture in order to avoid formation of gaps in the tissue's continuum (which would be eventually live space for seromas), hemostasis is accurate, tension is sufficiently reduced along the margins on the skin breach, healing results would be as aesthetic as possible, and complications, such as wound diastase, skin necrosis, or aesthetic scars, are reduced to minimum.

The surgeon should always prefer interrupted suture to close surgical wounds, since it can eventually allow accessibility to a small area in which complication could have arisen, without having to reopen the whole suture length. This can be achieved by simply removing one or two suture points, and the surgeon is able to easily manage margin approaching, even if surgical removal of small imperfections is needed.

The suture can be interrupted or with self-tightening suture, as shown in figure. This surgical option offers the advantage of being more resistant to traction; in the same time it can also cause tissue ischemia, increasing the risk of suffering from blood reduction of the overlying tissues.

If the surgeon's choice is to close using intradermal suture, it should not only involve subcutaneous tissue but also the deeper dermis, so to improve adhesion and achieve a more effective reduction of the skin traction on the margins' tissues.

In case of different margin thickness, the choice is between balancing the thickness and, if not possible for aesthetic reasons, placing a thin layer of subcutaneous tissue of the thicker margin under the thinner one so to equalize the depths.

In patients with a tendency to form cheloid scars, it is advisable to limit the number of suture points to a minimum, in order to avoid stimulation of collagen genesis by suturing material.

The Dermis and Epidermis

Generally the superficial dermis and epidermis are approached using continuous intradermal suture, while wounds which suture does not involve the deep dermis are closed with interrupted sutures.

The choice of which suture to use depends on several factors:

- Experience of the surgeon
- Skin tension lines
- Healing processes of the patient (visible on other scars)
- Bleeding tendency (patients in therapy with anticoagulants, suffering from hemostatic disorders, etc.)

Interrupted suture has the advantage of being faster and easier to place but results in less aesthetic scar quality with respect to a continuous intradermal suture. It can also be useful as hemostatic means.

The ligature should preferably be nonabsorbable, so as to avoid a foreign-body inflammatory reaction, which can degrade the quality of the scar and increases the tendency to form cheloid scars. The use of absorbable ligatures, even for a short period of time, may be indicated in areas such as the mucosa or the genitals (in order to avoid embarrassment to the patient for removal) or in rare cases of people "in transit," who could not return for removal of the sutures.

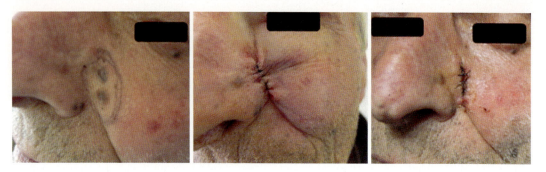

Fig. 22.16 Note the uneven appearance after 1 and 2 weeks; the appearance will improve by the time of suture removal

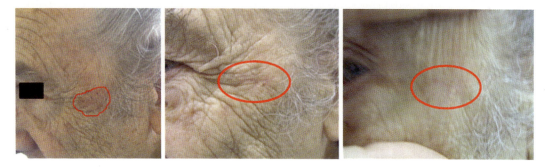

Fig. 22.17 Outcomes after 6 months of the excision, *dotted in red*

Stitches can be simple or "U" shaped (also known as mattress or "Donati's" suture); the latter can be applied either horizontally or vertically. Vertical suturing is preferable as it allows greater adhesion of the dermis, is more effective on the hemostatic side, and offers better aesthetic results if compared to the horizontal one.

A continuous suture can be performed, as explained before for the fascia, letting the knot rest on the skin (using simple or self-tightening points) or completely within the dermis: "intradermal" suture.

If the surgeon were to use an absorbable ligature to perform intradermal suture, the end knot must run deeper than the rest of the suture, so as to avoid outbreak of the knot itself.

Other Sutures

In areas of the face where the skin is loose due to wrinkles and where a circular excision is performed [37], surgeons can run "purse-string" suture even

known as "tobacco pouch" suture, described by Peled for the first time in 1985 [38]. Purse-string suture offers the advantage of significantly reducing the removal area, allowing closure of major injury using surrounding tissue, without the need for skin flaps, as well as offering a high-quality hemostasis and being less expensive [39].

The disadvantage of this type of suture is that the wound will appear for the first few weeks aesthetically non-satisfactory and irregular, being surrounded by wrinkles, even compared to the surrounding ones (Fig. 22.16). The aesthetical quality of the final scar will be less than the one following the use of a flap but will affect a much smaller area, and in some cases, after few weeks, it will result in a less visible scar compared to the results obtained with other techniques (Fig. 22.17).

This suture can also be used for a partial closure, to be associated to a skin flap and/or graft, which will be of smaller dimensions.

This suture is preferably performed after dissection of surrounding tissue and only in the

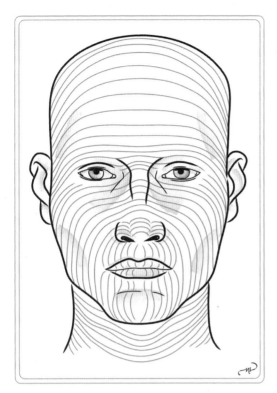

Fig. 22.18 Langer's lines for the face

subcutaneous plane, closing the overlying skin with an interrupted nonabsorbable ligature. It should be absolutely avoided in patients prone to cheloids scaring.

Cancer Surgery of the Face [40]

Any removal of facial skin cancer should follow, whenever possible, skin tension lines proposed by Langer in 1861 (Fig. 22.18).

In addition, it is almost 50 years [41] that facial aesthetic subunits have been identified: face skin changes from area to area in terms of histological origin; thus, reconstruction of subunits utilizing skin originating from the same area (and therefore similar) grants better aesthetic results.

A first paper was written in 1956 and was followed by many others, whose only merit is to have narrowed down the extension, increasing the number and basically just dividing the subunits into smaller one, always inspired by histological considerations (Fig. 22.19).

The reconstruction of the face after a cancer excision should be performed with a technique that does not cause skin tension, choosing, where possible, direct closure or flap grafting [42]. The use of grafts or closure by secondary intention is an option to be used rarely and only if there are no alternatives, due to the poor cosmetic results. A wound should not be left open or sutured after days (awaiting for histological result), neither other peculiar solutions at times proposed in literature should be granted credit [43–46].

Forehead

A tumor resection in the frontal region is normally dealt with a direct suture using skinfolds as tissue donor sites.

For larger excisions, surgeons can turn their attention to flap rotation: this option is thought to be a difficult answer to the problem and can scare an unskilled surgeon, since the length of the flap should never exceed a 4:1 ratio with respect to the excision area. Actually it is but a simple technique, which follows tissue planes easily detachable and requires some anatomy knowledge along with attention to hemostasis. Whenever flap dissection involves the scalp, particular care is to be spent when rebuilding the hairline.

Rotation or Limberg's flaps are feasible but offer worse cosmetic results.

Temporal Region

The anatomical knowledge of the temporal region is important since the surgeon faces high risk of neurological or vascular injury.

When a direct suture is not possible, the breach of this area can easily be closed using rotational or Limberg's flaps.

Zitelli's bilobed flap offers discrete aesthetic results and is a viable reconstruction alternative for defects larger than the abovementioned.

Minor and circular injuries in elderly patients with very loose skin can be sutured using purse-string technique.

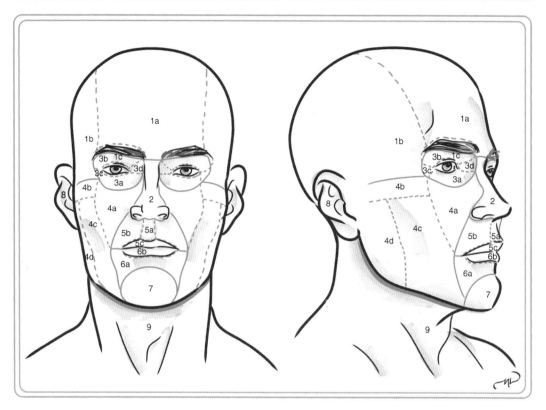

Fig. 22.19 Aesthetic units and subunits of the face. Source: TT Fattah. *1* Forehead unit (*1a* the first central subunit, *1b* lateral subunit, *1c* eyebrow subunit). *2* Nasal unit. *3* Eye lid units (*3a* lower lid, *3b* upper lid unit, *3c* lateral canthal subunit, *3d* medial canthal subunit). *4* Cheek unit (*4a* medial subunit, *4b* zygomatic subunit, *4c* lateral subunit, *4d* buccal subunit). *5* Upper lip unit (*5a* subunit philtrum, *5b* lateral subunit, *5c* mucosal subunit). *6* Lower lip unit (*6a* central subunit, *6b* subunit mucosal). *7* Chin unit. *8* Auricular unit. *9* Neck unit

Scalp

Excision of tissue in the scalp area should follow the hair follicles' angle, in order to damage as few as possible of those and result in hardly visible scars. Usage of skin expansion in the scalp region is possible, but it is a slow process and is reported to be extremely uncomfortable by patients.

After excision of the tumor, the breach is usually closed utilizing a double opposed sliding flap or by grafting. A microsurgical reconstruction is a viable alternative but has drawbacks such as longer operating times, more complex, and suitable for large excisions only.

The use of a rotation flap to close the loss of substance, associated with grafting of the donor site, when even the periosteum is removed is a technique rarely used, when there are no other solutions.

A hair transplant done 6–12 months postoperative may reduce the imperfection of the scaring outcome in the recipient area.

Eyebrows

Eyebrow reconstruction is done, primarily, using the contralateral eyebrow as donor site for hair follicles (if of appropriate dimensions). Otherwise, similar hair follicles can be transplanted from other body areas, with similar characteristics, to the eyebrow that has to be reconstructed.

Another option for small dimension reconstruction of the eyebrow is the so-called buried flap. This flap consists of part of the contralateral eyebrow hair and skin, grafted in the subcutaneous tissue of the eyebrow to be reconstructed and left buried under the sutured skin for 3 weeks, in

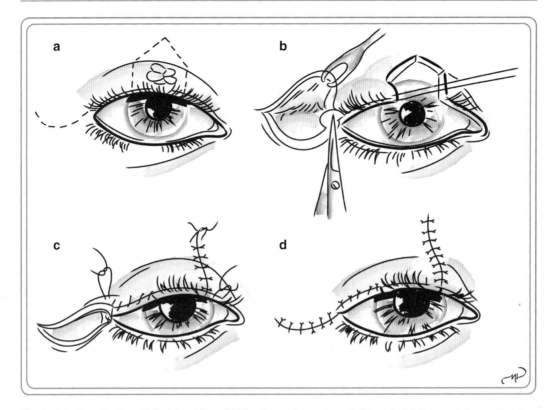

Fig. 22.20 Tenzel's flap. (**a**) Incisions' line. (**b**) Flap harvesting and surgical breach. (**c**) Suture of the scrolled flap. (**d**) Final aspect

order to obtain a revascularization. Elapsed the 3-week period, the skin is incised and the buried tissue is dug up in place.

Utilizing hair should be considered as a last chance, since it would mean for the patient the need of shorting the growing hair from time to time.

Upper Eyelid

Basic goal for any eyelid reconstruction is the perfect coverage of the conjunctiva.

Cancer excision as wide as 1/3 of the dimension of the eyelid (or even wider in case of elderly patients, with skin laxity and little or no tarsal conjunctiva involvement) can be directly sutured or reconstructed or with small local flaps, with minimal aesthetical damage.

Excisions involving less than half of the eyelid can benefit from local flap (Tenzel's flap), which allows the rest of the eyelid to scroll sideways so to close the defect (Fig. 22.20).

For larger excisions, not interesting areas larger that 2/3 of the dimensions of the eyelid, tissue can be transposed from the lower eyelid. This flap is harvested using tarsal conjunctiva tissues (Cutler-Beard flap or bridge flap); it is left attached to the donor site for at least 3 weeks and then excised, changing it into a simple graft (Fig. 22.21).

If the entire eyelid is to be demolished, reconstruction can be obtained with an arterialized flap, harvested from the temporal region, which can provide coverage of the eye but leaves poor-quality aesthetic results.

Lateral Canthus

Either direct suture or purse-string suture technique is a useful answer for closing small-diameter excisions, while local rotation flap is often enough for the reconstruction of larger loss of substance in this area.

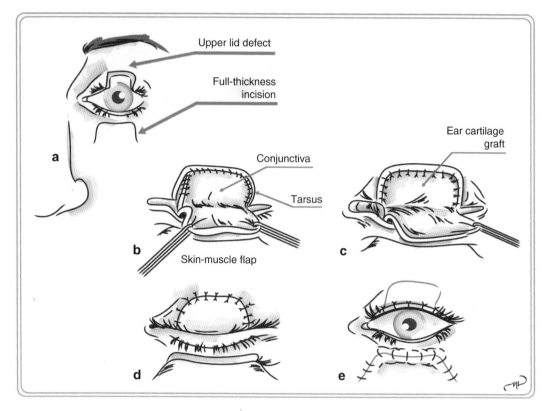

Fig. 22.21 Cutler-Beard's flap or bridged flap. (**a**) Defect area and incision lines. (**b**) Skin-muscle flap sutured in the defect area. (**c**) Ear cartilage flap in place. (**d**) Skin coverage sutured in place. (**e**) Final appearance

Medial Canthus

Loss of substance in the medial canthus area is more complex to deal with than the one in the lateral canthus area, since the presence of the lachrymal duct makes functional restoration extremely difficult.

Each flap suturing or grafting should be dealt with paying attention to the underlying tissues and preserving lachrymal and drainage pathways.

For larger loss of substance in this area, a "V-Y" shaped glabellar flap is the technique most commonly used (Fig. 22.22).

Lower Eyelid

As for the upper eyelid, full-thickness excision of tumors as large as 1/3 of the eyelid dimension can be sutured directly, with the only drawback of a reduction in length of lower orbital rim.

To gain up to 5 mm of usable tissue or to reduce the aesthetic drawbacks described above, the surgeon can perform a lateral canthoplasty, anchoring the tendon in more medial position, sutured to the periosteum with a permanent ligature.

Tenzel's semicircular rotational flap has been already described; if combination with a canthoplasty, it can be a valuable alternative technique for the reconstruction of major defects with minimal aesthetic and functional damage.

Lesions as large as 2/3 of the eyelid dimensions can be reconstructed with a tarsal-conjunctival flap, as first described by Hughes (Fig. 22.23), which involves minimal damage of the upper eyelid, skin grafting, and a persistent period of discomfort for the patient lasting through surgical events.

The abovementioned technique can also be modified according to Muller: conjunctival incision and a rotation of a flap of tarsus, conjunctiva, and muscle.

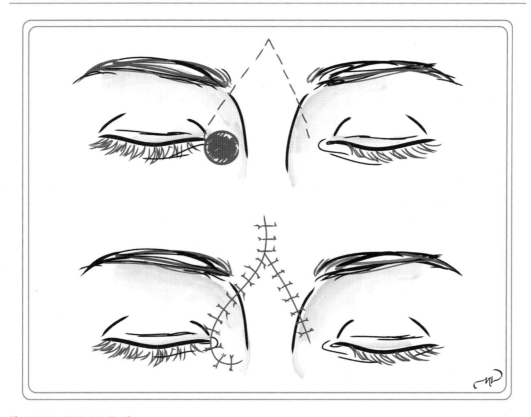

Fig. 22.22 V-Y glabellar flap

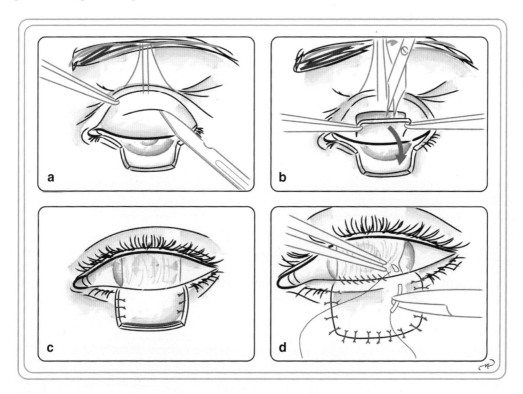

Fig. 22.23 Hughes' tarsal-conjunctival flap. (**a**) Incisions' line. (**b**) Harvesting of the tarsal-conjunctival flap. (**c**) Suture in the surgical excision site. (**d**) Final suture appearance

Fig. 22.24 Mustardé's flap

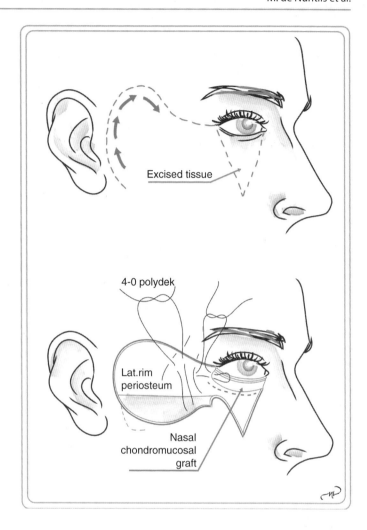

Excised tissue

4-0 polydek

Lat.rim
periosteum

Nasal
chondromucosal
graft

Full thickness or larger loss of substance of the lower eyelid can be reconstructed with a rotation flap harvested from the cheek area, as described by Mustardé (Fig. 22.24). The technique can be associated to tarsal grafting, harvested from the contralateral or homolateral upper eyelid, as described by Hughes' technique, to give proper support. Greater upward traction can be obtained anchoring the flap's apex to the periosteum and/or by tenorrhaphy that is to be removed after 1 week.

A Mustardé's flap alternative is a rotational flap of malar anterior skin (prenasal), in which a cartilage grafting has been placed. Performing this technique, surgeons must pay attention to the nasolacrimal apparatus.

Nose

Although forming a single aesthetic unit, nose reconstruction has different solutions, depending not only on the extent but also on the localization of the tumor. Following this reasoning, some authors have divided the nose into subunits [47].

Small lesions can be sutured directly or by means of tissue transplantation such as a pedicled island flap, in order to avoid excessive strain on the wound margins. Even the use of cutaneous or musculocutaneous "V-Y" shaped flaps may serve as a viable solution.

The nose root can be easily reconstructed with the help of local flaps or rotational fronto-glabellar

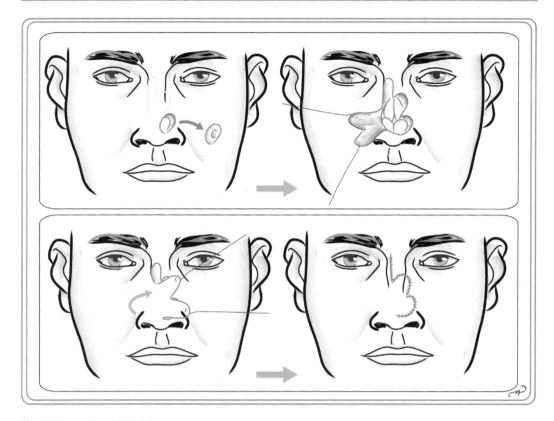

Fig. 22.25 Zitelli's bilobed flap

one, with a good cosmetic results and minimal discomfort for the patient.

The nose dorsum can be reconstructed with
Zitelli's bilobed flap (Fig. 22.25) if interested by
minor injuries or using frontal region flaps (pedicled or Indian) if interested by total or subtotal
amputation and in severe cases of loss of substance (Fig. 22.26).

A glabellar "V-Y" flap harvested on the skin
of the dorsum of the nose can be used for the
reconstructions of the lower part of the dorsum
and of the tip of the nose itself.

Nasolabial rotation flap or naso-buccal flap is
usually the surgical solution for the reconstruction of the hemidorsum of the nose (Fig. 22.27).

In reconstructing the tip of the nose, the surgeon can take advantage of all the techniques
described. Larger injuries require a frontal island
flap or a septum mucous membrane flap, although
the latter technique, being of difficult usage,

arduous, and complications arise so easily, is
rarely used.

Cheek

Generally the excision of small tumors are easily
reconstructed using local advancement, rotational,
Limberg's, Zitelli's, and island flaps. Minor injuries
can be reconstructed with a purse-string suture.

Major injuries may require rotational flaps from
the cheek area, such as Mustardé's flap or rotational
flaps (cervicofacial), even harvested on the neck
skin. Seldom pectoral or trapezium myocutaneous
flaps are used for the reconstruction of the cheek.

Grafting is to be avoided and should be used only
if complete excision is dubious while expecting for
the histological response and as a temporary closure.

Treatments of greater loss of substance do
require microsurgical reconstructive surgery.

Fig. 22.26 Frontal flaps

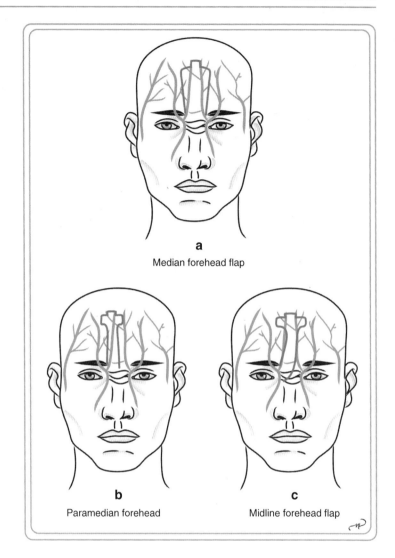

a
Median forehead flap

b
Paramedian forehead

c
Midline forehead flap

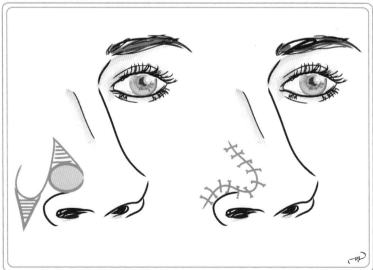

Fig. 22.27 Rotation flap

As a guideline, the reconstructive treatment of the cheek can be schematized as shown below, dividing the area into subunits:

1. Infraorbital
2. Preauricular
3. Oromandibular

Infraorbital Area

Direct closure
Local flaps
Major flaps (Mustardé or frontal)
Microsurgery

Preauricular Area

Direct or purse-string suture
Local flaps
Facelift (for preauricular localization)
For the lower part: cervicofacial flaps
Microsurgery

Oromandibular Area

Direct suture
Local flaps (for the upper area a naso-buccal flap is usually the best surgical choice)
For the lower part: cervicofacial flaps
Major flaps
Microsurgery

Upper Lip

In case of tumors not infiltrating the muscle, direct suture is always possible, trying to preserve the vermilion line, the lip folds, and in particular the filter anatomical aspect, in order for the resulting scars to lay inside or along the physiological wrinkles, so as not to alter the shape of the lip and to maximize aesthetical outcome [48].

Nasolabial flaps can be used to repair hemilabial area demolitions and are the preferred choice for major reconstructions in case of excision of noninfiltrating tumors.

More aggressive tumors or those following nerve pathways are to be treated with the amputation of part of the lip (including muscle and mucosa) and require reconstruction with direct suture if the amputation area is less than 1/3 of the lip; otherwise, the use of flaps will be necessary.

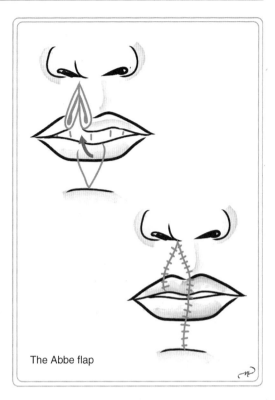

The Abbe flap

Fig. 22.28 Abbé's flap

For injuries that do not affect the angle of the mouth area, the most commonly used is the Abbé's flap, which consists in the rotation of a full-thickness triangle of lower lip (up to 1/3) to cover the breach of the superior lip, reconstructing the remaining loss of substance with local flaps. The Abbé's flap should be left in place for a period of time of 2–3 weeks, in order for its autonomization, and then severed from the donor site (Fig. 22.28). The discomfort for the patient concerns undergoing a double operation, impaired function, and deformity of the mouth between the first and second operation.

For the record, this flap invented by an Italian, Dr. Peter Sabatini in 1838, has been modified by Buck after a few years but published in 1898 by Abbé, who assumed the authorship.

If the tumor excision involves the commissure of the lip, Eastlander's flap should be used for coverage; this flap resembles the previous flap described (Fig. 22.29).

Major defects require different solutions, such as the Webster's combined flap (Fig. 22.30), which is characterized by multiple flaps, Abbé's

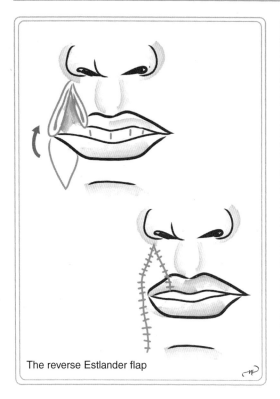

The reverse Estlander flap

Fig. 22.29 Eastlander's flap

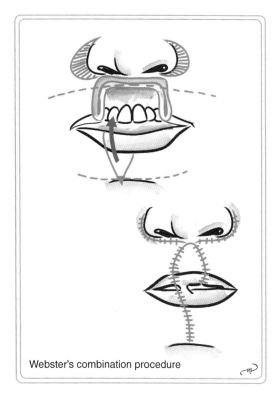

Webster's combination procedure

Fig. 22.30 Webster's flap

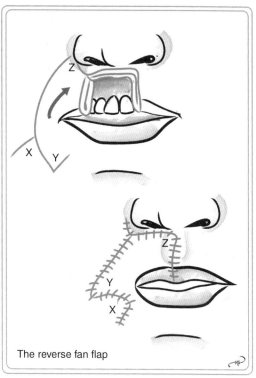

The reverse fan flap

Fig. 22.31 The reverse fan flap. (**x–z**) Advancement flap

flap to reconstruct the filter area, two advancement flaps, one for each side, following removal of perioral skin, or even the outdated inferior Z flap, used to increase the amount of tissue available (reverse fan flap, which is characterized by good motility but poor residual sensitivity – Fig. 22.31); the nasolabial flaps designed by Von Bruns in 1857 (and modified by many authors – Fig. 22.32); or the flap by Karapandzic having an upper peduncle (in the variation of rotation or movement) and later modifications (Fig. 22.33).

A solution for the reconstruction of the whole upper lip is the Kazanjian and Converse flap, which is a vascular flap with superior pedicle (Fig. 22.34).

An alternative solution to this flap is Gillies' flap, which will be described later.

Lower Lip

The principles listed for the upper lip also apply to the lower one. Differently from the above, in this area a nasolabial flap is not available. Cheeks

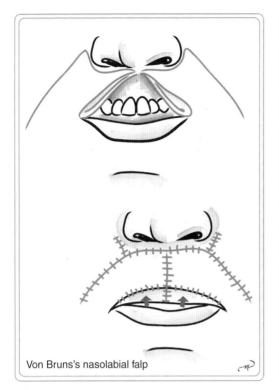

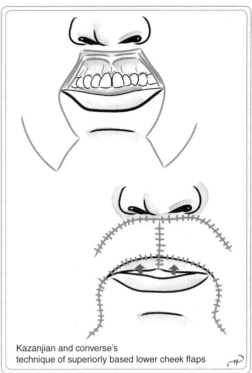

Fig. 22.32 Von Brun's flap

Fig. 22.34 Kazanjian and Converse flap

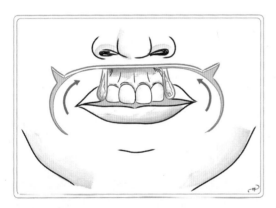

Fig. 22.33 Karapandzic's flap

and chin represent good tissue supply and in some cases reconstruction can be done harvesting flaps from the neck area (see above).

Flaps used for full-thickness reconstruction of this area are the same as of the upper lip (Abbé's, Eastlander's, etc.) for defects of various sizes.

A flap harvested on the depressor labii inferioris is the Tobin's flap, technically simple and allowing an extensive skin rotation, which leaves

a lack of sensitivity in the area, still granted by a branch of the trigeminal nerve.

A good alternative of a major defect reconstruction of the lower lip (up to 1/2 or even 2/3 of the lip) can be obtained with Bernard-Burow's flap, which utilizes cheek tissues to let the two ends of the breach approach so to close the lip tissue loss (Fig. 22.35).

Even larger excisions, up to 3/4 of the lower lip may be closed with Karapandzic's flap. Anatomically based on the Eastlander's flap, the Gillies' one allows total reconstruction of the lower lip (Fig. 22.36).

Another technique for total reconstruction of the lower lip is the one proposed by Webster, using tissue of the cheeks, which is slide into place to reconstruct the loss of substance (Fig. 22.37).

Even the chin is used as donor site for the reconstruction of defects of the lower lip, but this choice is almost never considered, being the described techniques easier to implement, more satisfactory for the patient and resulting of a more acceptable aesthetic result.

Fig. 22.35 Bernard-Burow's flap

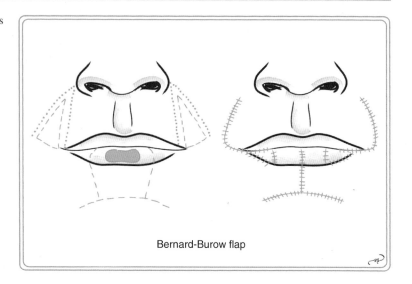

Bernard-Burow flap

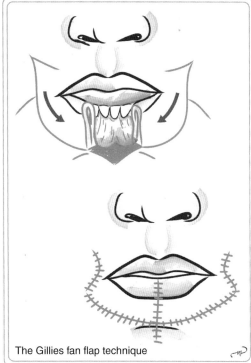

The Gillies fan flap technique

Fig. 22.36 Gillies' flap

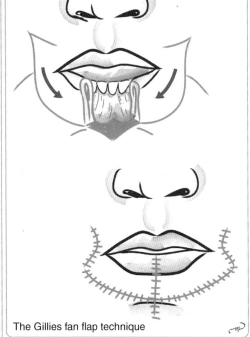

Fig. 22.37 Webster's flap

One of those surgical techniques of gradual advancement is the "step technique" proposed by Blomgren et al. [49], although it has been used only in 165 cases (Fig. 22.38), creating a visible aesthetic damage in the chin area.

Buric et al. [50] proposed in 2003 a "V-Y" island flap to reconstruct the lower lip harvested from the chin, but this technique has been used in one patient only and needs further follow-up.

Fig. 22.38 Step technique by Blomgren et al.

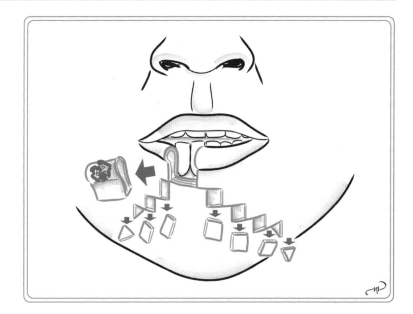

Fig. 22.39 Chondro-cutaneous helix flap

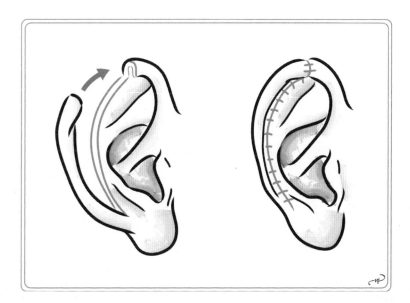

When the surgeon is planning major reconstructions, it is imperative that the margins of excision are free from cancerous infiltration and that the patient is informed of the need for different operations to improve the aesthetical and functional result.

In literature, many other flaps for lip reconstruction are described; all are very similar to each other, but the surgeon usually follows the experience.

Ear

Small and superficial cancer excisions in the ear area can be reconstructed with direct suture or removing a small wedge of underlying cartilage and simple helix flaps (Fig. 22.39).

Larger excisions require reconstructive techniques depending on the anatomical localization and on the size.

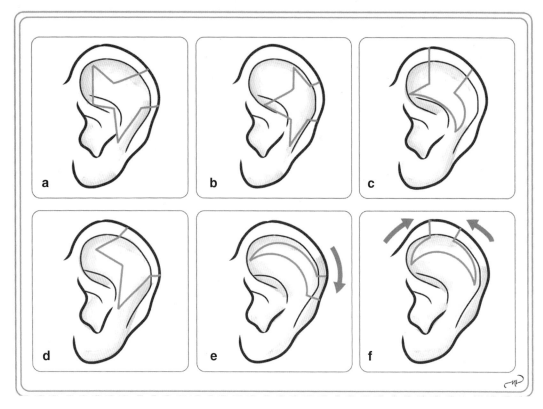

Fig. 22.40 (a–f) different incision lines with respect of the excisions areas

A tumor of few centimeters in diameter, localized on the helix, can be removed en bloc with the underlying cartilage or with a full-thickness slice of the ear, depending on the position and/or the tumor size (Fig. 22.40). This solution will leave a smaller ear but can lead to a direct closure of the excision.

A useful reconstructive technique for large helix excisions is the creation of a tubular flap (inside which cartilage from contralateral ear or taken form a different donor site can be included). The flap is sutured at the ends in the course of three operations, with a time gap of at least 3 weeks. This solution gives good reconstruction results for large portions of the ear but with a great discomfort for the patient (Fig. 22.41).

However, if the need to call for the removal of the tumor and part of the helix arises, the surgeon can reconstruct the ear by utilizing Antia-Buch's procedure, consisting of a sliding flap harvested in the helix area surrounding the loss of substance:

this solution preserves the size of the ear, the shape of which results but minimally modified. This technique is used in reconstructing excisions of localized tumors, not large in size.

A two-stage reconstruction of even larger helix defects is possible with retroauricular flaps, paying attention not to reconstruct the ear using hairy skin. This method is used to harvest cartilage grafts for a more aesthetic result. The donor site is then grafted.

Surgical ablation of the helix and surrounding tissue can be reconstructed with skin and cartilage harvested in the retroauricular or conchal area, especially if the case involves an amputation involving the upper 1/3 of the ear.

A possible reconstructive alternative for the upper 1/3 of the ear, although not often used, is grafting the skin from the concha, along with a fragment of the antihelix, then rotating it to cover the surgical excision, and then suturing on the residual loss of substance (conchal and retroauricular) skin grafts.

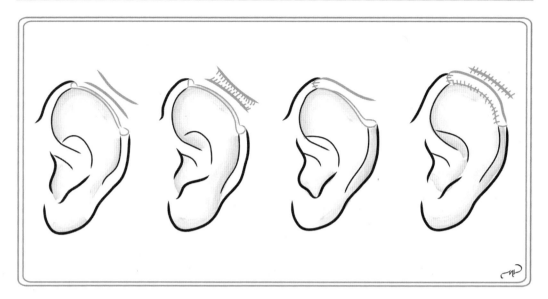

Fig. 22.41 Tubular flap for the reconstruction of the helix

The retroauricular skin is also indicated for reconstructive purposes of virtually every part of the ear, even of the concha. Minor defects can be treated in a single stage with an island flap twice the size of the defect to be reconstructed and folded on itself.

Retroauricular tissues can be used to reconstruct the earlobe or for grafting skin excisions of the ear especially if the perichondrium remains intact. This area requires close postoperative monitoring, being at high risk of keloid formation.

Keloids can be treated either early with pressure therapy or later with injection of steroids.

Hand Surgery [51]

Introduction [52]

In almost all cases, the treatment of skin cancer is through surgery. Depending on the tumor location and staging, and age and general condition of the patient, the surgeon can choose among a wide range of procedures available. Usually, these operations are performed under local anesthesia; the lesion is removed completely beyond its limits and with a macroscopic untouched margin of macroscopically healthy tissue.

The goal of the surgical therapy is the complete tumor removal and consequent disease recovery while trying to get a result as satisfactory as possible on the aesthetic and functional side.

In minor extension excisions, the resulting breach is directly sutured simply addressing the margins. In cases of a more extensive resection with larger loss of substance, the surgeon can choose to use more sophisticated surgical techniques, requiring more elaborate use of grafts, flaps, and skin plasty [53, 54].

The excision of a skin cancer can be addressed as a single-time surgery or may require two or more operations, especially if the need for widening the margin of the resection, for the removal of lymph nodes, or even for surgical procedures to achieve aesthetic purposes comes [55].

At times, in performing the histological examination of the tissues excised and the evaluation of lymph nodes draining the district affected through sentinel node biopsy, a prophylactic lymphadenectomy may become necessary.

Surgical Removal of Melanoma

A particular problem arises if the melanoma is found on the fingers of the foot or of the hand. If the tumor is located on the distal phalanx, widening of the margins of the excision could not be reconstructed using flaps or grafting, and the only possible solution remaining is the disarticulation of the finger affected.

If, on the contrary, the tumor is located on the proximal or intermediate phalanx, reconstruction is dealt with using flaps (from the palmar or plantar areas) or, in severe cases, with carpal-metacarpal or tarsometatarsal amputation.

Finally, if the melanoma is located in the interdigital area, amputation can be avoided, being the area easily reconstructed with the use of local flaps [56].

Depending on the thickness of the tumor, oncological protocols prescribe the sentinel node biopsy in the groin or armpit area. If the result of the histological examination of the lymph node is positive for metastases, inguino-iliac or axillary lymph node dissection must be carried out.

Epithelioma

The excision of these lesions is usually done under local or block anesthesia, if the tumor affects the phalangeal area.

Excision's general criteria follow the elliptical incision rule, in which margins should never be closer than 3 mm from the outer macroscopical margin of the lesion itself. Thus, if possible, with the major diameter oriented parallel to the skin, tension lines and the depth of the incisions should reach the underlying fat.

In case of a neoplasm involving the periungual area, onychectomy must be associated as surgical protocol [57].

Skin Grafts

Skin grafts are used to cover small- and medium-sized losses of substance of the fingers and hand. These flaps are predominantly used for the dorsal side of extremities, in case of a well-vascularized recipient site. In other cases, healing by secondary intention is the way to follow.

The use of skin grafting should be avoided at the commissure level. The most commonly used donor sites are the plica of the elbow, of the wrist, or of the hypothenar region of the hand.

There are two types of skin grafts: dermal-epidermal (or partial-thickness) and full-thickness grafts.

Partial-thickness grafts are rarely used to reconstruct tumors excisions when localized on the skin of the hand's fingers and of the commissure. Complications related to this kind of grafting concern mainly the mechanical and sensorial aspects, inasmuch as these grafts are thin and adherent to the underlying tissues, do not provide adequate texture, and do not adapt to sensory functions of the fingertip region. In general, they are not usually chosen to reconstruct the palmar region of the hand, due to the low sensitivity and to the excessive skin retraction.

On the contrary, full-thickness skin grafting used in the same areas rarely undergoes excessive retraction, providing good mechanical outcome and offering greater recovery sensitivity and a stable and adaptable coverage.

Flaps [58]

Skin transposition flaps [59]

They are defined as pedicled skin flaps including epidermis, dermis, and hypodermis. These flaps are harvested maintaining one of the four sides of the incision intact, so to ensure blood supply and tissues' survival.

Classifications are different but substantially distinguishing advancement, rotation, and transposition flaps.

Also the so-called geometric flaps are worth remembering: the Limberg, the Dufourmentel, and the Celsus' bipedunculate flap, used to reconstruct tumor excisions done in the back of the hand.

Island Flaps

Harvesting an island flap is done practicing an extensive incision in the medial-lateral skin of

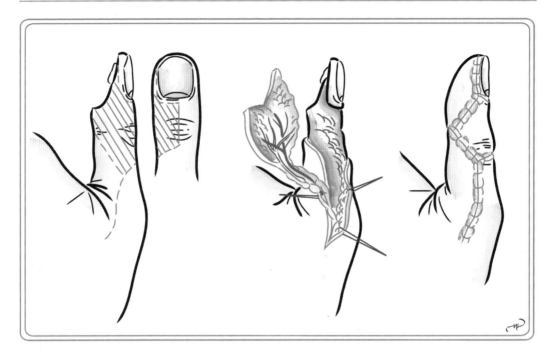

Fig. 22.42 Homodigital island flap

the hand dorsum, including adipose tissue to ensure venous drainage.

An example of homodigital island flap is the Joshi and Pho one, used to repair defects of the fingertip. The flap overlaps the dorsal surface of the finger; proximally the collateral pedicle is isolated and mobilized, thus determining a good mobilization of the flap itself, according to the rotation angle that the dissection of the vascular pedicle allows (Fig. 22.42).

The drawback for this flap is represented by the reduced thickness of the skin of the hand dorsum with respect to the fingertip skin; in addition, some authors (Wallace and Coupland) deny the existence of nerve fibers coming from collateral palmar branches reaching the dorsum of the hand [60, 61].

Further reconstructive techniques are represented by the island flap harvested from the heterodigital fingertip (Fig. 22.43), heterodigital island flap from the skin of the dorsum of the finger (kite flap) (Fig. 22.44), and free flap harvested from the skin of the fingertip, according to the principle of "skin sparing finger" [62, 63].

The problem arising if the heterodigital island flap is chosen in an anesthesiological error, being interpreted at the brain level referred to the original donor site, despite the new positioning (ulnar side of third-fourth finger); more even the residual aesthesia of the donor finger should be evaluated, along with the possible inadequate skin coverage offered for the fingertip.

Finally, the free flap harvested according to the "skin sparing finger" principle (Fig. 22.45), even remaining conceptually valid, finds its restriction of use in being unlikely for badly injured finger to provide suitable nerve-vascular pedicles for reconstructive purposes [64].

Excisions made in the middle palmar segment of the thumb can be treated with a heterodigital dorsal island flap (kite flap).

The flap is defined as being an axial neurovascular island flap, employable for the coverage in the dorsal area of the thumb, at the first commissure and the thenar region level. Is graved in the skin of the dorsal area of the second finger, its distal limit corresponding to the extensional crease of the interphalangeal joint. Once the flap is carved by means of a curved incision, on the

Fig. 22.43 Drawing of the
incisions: (**a**) Access to the
pedicle in the palm area. (*1*)
Ligation of the V finger's
radial collateral artery. (*2*)
Intraneural dissection of the
common digital nerve of the
IV space. (**b**) Tunneling (*2*)
and positioning of the flap
(*1*), grafting of the donor site
(*3*). (**c**) "Débranchement-
rebranchement" technique

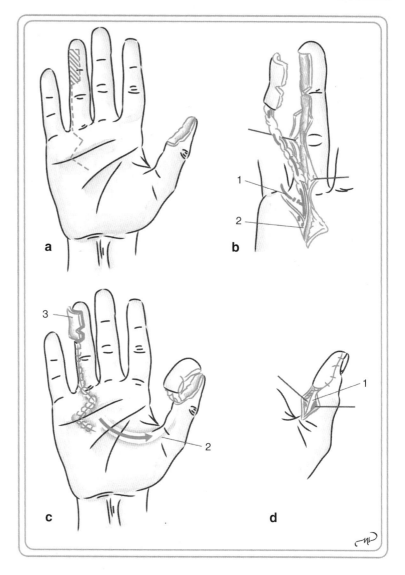

radial side of the second metacarpus and the artery, perivascular loose tissue, vein, and nerve are isolated; it is brought on the thumb through a subcutaneous tunnel.

The advantages are that no major artery is sacrificed and that, in addition, the small size of the flap can lead to direct closure of the donor site.

In this case, the sensitivity problems arising are considered of secondary importance, the issue of sensory discrimination being less important with respect to the fingertip level. It is however subordinated to anatomical and functional thumb recovery [65].

Another explanatory example of island flap is represented by Kutler's "V-Y" advancement

flap, harvested from the lateral sides of the finger whose apical side is affected by neoplasia.

Even in this case, advancement triangles of full-thickness skin flaps are obtained carving the dermis. Once elevated from the underlying bone, they are used to cover the loss of substance at the fingertip level. The two triangular flaps, directly sutured, are then anchored at the midline level of the fingertip [66, 67].

Although it is a manageable flap to harvest, it has the disadvantage of failing in ensuring an effective recovery of the sensitivity of the fingertip and often leads to hypersensitivity and paresthesia in the suture line area.

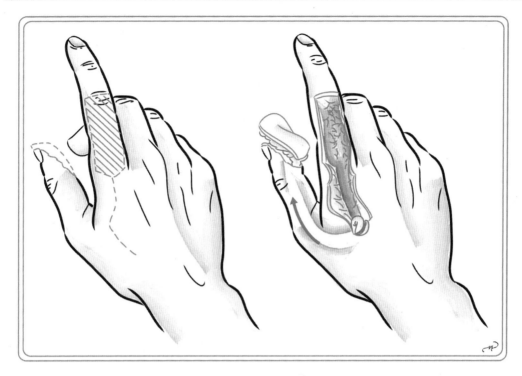

Fig. 22.44 The use of the "kite flap" to cover pulp tissue loss of the thumb. a) Planning of the flap. b) Tunneling at the level of the first commissure

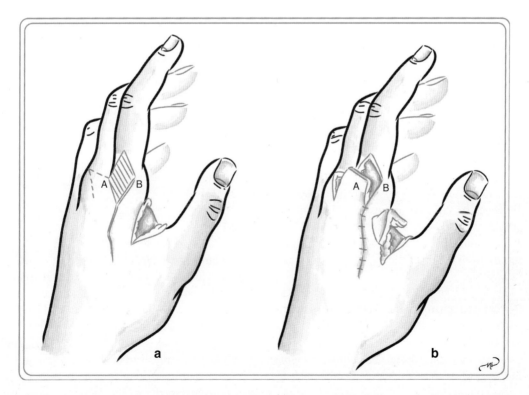

Fig. 22.45 Free flap harvested according to the "skin sparing finger" principle. (**a**) Planning of the flap. (**b**) Transferring the flap at the level of the first commissure (A: covering flap, B: transferring flap)

Sliding Flaps

Tranquilli-Leali's flap technique (known even as Atasoy's flap) design a triangular flap on the palmar surface of the hand, with downward tip, and includes the whole skin thickness above the periosteum of the distal phalanx. The flap is used for surgical reconstructions after tumors excisions interesting the apex of the tip of the long fingers, especially if the tumor is not too large.

The advancement of the flap is stabilized by a small needle transfixing the flap and attached to the distal phalanx.

The flap edges should not be sutured, being vascular damaging possible if excessive strain is exerted on the margins of the flap itself.

Vascularization of the flap is entrusted to ascending branches.

In a substantially overlapping modality, the Kutler's flap and Moberg's flap are harvested. However, O'Brien's bipedicled flap offers greater guarantees of coverage; the flap is quadrilateral in shape and includes skin and adipose tissue surrounding the palmar collateral pedicle, which is essential for venous drainage. Total advancement is attested around 10 mm.

Medication should be carried out carefully, since the pedicle should never be compressed, reducing the risk of compromising blood circulation and the vitality of the flap.

Collateral vascular pedicles are mobilized in order to cover, without tension, the loss of substance.

To cover the loss of substance of the donor area, free grafts harvested from the hypothenar eminence or the wrist are used. This technique provides satisfactory results both aesthetically and functionally, conserves bone, and maintains sensitivity at the tip of the flap.

Reconstruction of the First Commissure

The first commissure is a functional unit consisting of two subunits, dorsal and palmar, triangular in shape, whose base is identified in the free edge of the commissure.

The anatomical structures involved are the skin, the connective tissue, the adductor pollicis muscle and the first dorsal interosseous muscle, and the trapezium-metacarpal articulation [68].

Lesions and their consequences of these structures result in retraction of the commissure with considerable functional impairment of the thumb.

"Z" Plasty

The use is indicated for the reconstruction of lesions of the commissural free edge, when the retraction does not result in a significant functional limitation.

If the grade of the retraction requires a great amount of stretching or widening of the commissure, four-flap plasty finds better indications.

In this case the edges of the "Z" plasty will have a reflection angle of 120°; therefore, splitting each of them in two is necessary (Fig. 22.46).

In case of asymmetric or one side prevailing retraction of the commissural subunits, "butterfly" or "trident" plasty is more helpful for the surgeon.

Transposition Flaps

The kite flap from the hand dorsum skin and the posterior interosseous flap can be used: the advantage of the last is represented by the fact that they are not sacrificed, during harvesting, major arteries; thus, given the small dimensions of the flap, the donor site can be repaired by direct suture.

Flag Flap

It is a homodigital flap, of square shape, which is indicated in cases where tumor excision requires amputation of the proximal apical portion of the nail matrix, preserving the finger skeletal length. It is, then, rotated to cover the loss of substance from the dorsal surface of the same finger, and the donor site is reconstructed using a skin graft. Limitations of use are identifiable in the lack of sensitivity and mediocre appearance.

Fig. 22.46 "Z" plasty. (**a**) Incisions' lines. (**b**) Incision angle. (**c**) Flap transposition. (**d**) Final appearance

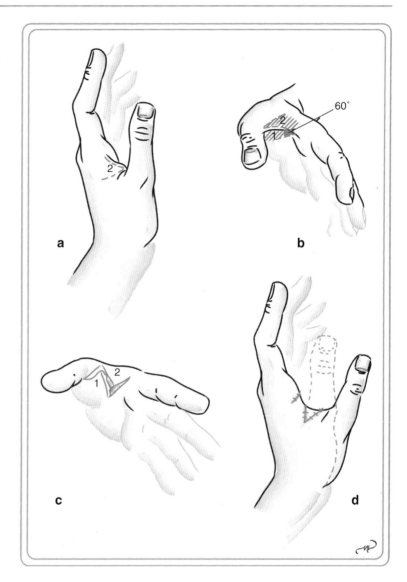

Hueston's Flaps

For this type of flap, the main indication is the apical, lateral, and oblique loss of substance of the long fingers of the hand.

It is a homodigital palmar lateral advancement-rotation axial flap, harvested carving an L-shaped incision, whose vertical arm is placed at the hand dorsal-palmar skin junction of the interested finger, while the horizontal arm is placed in level of the metacarpophalangeal palmar plica.

The donor area is reconstructed with a skin graft.

Compared to the Atasoy's flap or to Kutler's flap, this flap has the advantage of greater mobilization and distance covered.

Brunelli's Flaps

They are monopediculate island homodigital flaps, suitable for the reconstruction of the fingertip of the long fingers.

They can be direct or reverse vascularized: the first is harvested from the ulnar side of the index or middle finger, or on the radial side of the ring and little finger, as often the radial collateral artery of the second finger and collateral ulnar artery of the fifth finger are not present. Those reverse vascularized are used, for coverage of substance loss at the distal phalanx level, with a harvested flap at the proximal phalanx level. Moreover, it allows reconstructions of losses of substance at the middle phalanx level, with flaps harvested from the hand palmar area.

Reverse Flow Subcutaneous Laterodigital Flap

It is a very versatile flap used to cover losses of substance of the dorsal finger area, even in cases complicated by tendon or bone exposure.

This flap's blood supply is based on perforating vessels coming from the collateral digitalis artery or the dorsum district. The flap is harvested preserving the subcutaneous tissue.

Once elevated two dermal flaps for each side of the incision, the vasculo-nervous pedicle is identified and isolated at the base of the finger; the subcutaneous flap, which reaches the first dorsal arteria perforans level, proximally to the proximal or distal interphalangeal joint, is lifted, rotated, and placed on the loss of substance without tension.

Skin grafting is placed over the perforans arteries and the donor site is sutured; in this way the vascular pedicle is always preserved.

Glossary

Flap is a transfer of a one or more tissue from a donor site to a receiving site while maintaining integrum the vascular network.

Mohs surgery is a seriate surgical technique for progressive removal of tumor tissue using immediate microscope histological controls to determine the extent of the tumor. This procedure ensures the radical operation and at the same time allows to better preserve the surrounding healthy tissue.

Plastic surgery is a branch of surgery that aims to correct and repair morphological defects or functional losses of substance of different tissues that make up the human body either congenital or acquired as a result of trauma, cancer or degenerative diseases.

Skin expander are silicone devices used to stretch and grow the skin. They are temporarily inserted under the skin and over subsequent months, they are gradually expanded through regular saline injections. When the skin has been adequately stretched, the tissue expanders are removed.

Skin graft is a segment of one or more tissues that have lost all connection with the donor area, does not contain a network of blood vessels of its own, and that can be transferred from a donor site to an receiving area of substance loss (deficit), for reconstructive purposes, resulting from trauma or tumor excision.

References

1. Lever WF. Histopathology of the skin. 4th ed. Philadelphia: Lippincott; 1967.
2. Lever WF. Pathology of common skin tumors. J Surg Oncol. 1971;3:235.
3. Burton RC, Howe C, Adamson L, et al. General practitioner screening for melanoma: sensitivity, specificity and effect of training. J Med Screen. 1998;5:156–61.
4. Hall HI et al. Update on the incidence and mortality from melanoma in the United States. J Am Acad Dermatol. 1999;40:35–42.
5. Joshi BB. A local dorso-lateral Island flap for restoration of sensation after injury fingertip pulp. Plast Reconstr Surg. 1974;54:175–82.
6. Mathes SJ. Plastic surgery, vol. 1/8. 2nd ed. Philadelphia: Saunders/Elsevier; 2006.
7. Donati L, Farneti A, Tallacchini MC. Aspetti medico-legali e normativi dei prodotti dell'ingegneria tessutale. Milano: Giuffrè Editore; 1998.
8. Hewitt CW, Black KS, editors. Composite tissue transplantation. Austin: R.G. Landes; 1999.
9. Burg G et al. Histographic surgery: accuracy of visual assessment of the margins of basal-cell epithelioma. J Dermatol Surg. 1975;1:21.
10. Taylor GA, Barisoni D. Ten years' experience in the surgical treatment of basal cell carcinoma. A study of factors associated with recurrence. Br J Surg. 1973;60:522.
11. Griffiths RW. Audit of histologically incompletely excised basal cell carcinomas: recommendations for management by re-excision. Br J Plast Surg. 1999;52:24.
12. Renner GJ, Clark D. Facial skin malignancy. Otolaryngol Clin North Am. 1993;26.
13. Roenigk RK et al. Trends in the presentation and treatment of basal cell carcinomas. J Dermatol Surg Oncol. 1986;12:860.
14. Smith JW, Aston SJ. Grabb and Smith's plastic surgery. Boston: Little, Brown and Co.; 1991.
15. Urbach F. Geographic distribution of skin cancer. J Surg Oncol. 1971;3:219.
16. Rowe DE, Carroll RJ, Day Jr CL. Prognostic factors for local recurrence, metastasis, and survival rates in

squamous cell carcinoma of the skin, ear, and lip. Implications for treatment modality selection. J Am Acad Dermatol. 1992;26:467.

17. McCarthy JG. Plastic surgery, vol. I. Philadelphia: W.B. Saunders Co.; 1990.

18. Brodland DG, Zitelli JA. Surgical margins for excision of primary cutaneous squamous cell carcinoma. J Am Acad Dermatol. 1992;27:108.

19. Graham JH. Selected precancerous skin and mucocutaneous lesions. In: Neoplasms of skin and malignant melanoma. Chicago: Year Book; 1976. p. 69–121.

20. Kricker A, Armstrong BK, English DR, et al. Does intermittent sun exposure cause basal cell carcinoma? Int J Cancer. 1995;60:489.

21. Marks R, Rennie G, Selwood TS. Malignant transformation of solar keratoses to squamous cell carcinoma. Lancet. 1988;1:795.

22. Ron E et al. Radiation-induced skin carcinomas of the head and neck. Radiat Res. 1991;125:318.

23. Strom SS, Yamamura Y. Epidemiology of nonmelanoma skin cancer. Clin Plast Surg. 1997;24(4):627.

24. Wolfe JT. The role of screening in the management of skin cancer. Curr Opin Oncol. 1999;11:123–8.

25. Veronesi U, Cascinelli N. Narrow excision (1-cm margin). A safe procedure for thin cutaneous melanoma. Arch Surg. 1991;126:438–41.

26. Strauch N, Vasconez LO. Grabb's encyclopedia of flaps, vol. I/III. Boston: Little, Brown and Co.; 1990.

27. Mathes SJ, Nahai F. Clinical atlas of muscles and musculocutaneous flaps. St. Louis: C.V. Mosby Co.; 1979.

28. Strauch B, Yu HL. Atlas of microvascular surgery. New York: Thieme; 1993.

29. Cormack GC, Lamberty GH. The arterial anatomy of skin flaps. London: Churchill Livingstone; 1986.

30. Buncke H, Furnas D, editors. Clinical frontiers in reconstructive microsurgery. St. Louis: C.V. Mosby Co.; 1984.

31. Tranquilli-Leali E. Ricostruzione dell'apice delle falangi ungueali mediante autoplastica volare peduncolata per scorrimento. Infort Traum Lavoro. 1935; 1:148–54.

32. Song YG, Chen ZG, Song YL. The free thigh flap: a new free flap concept based on septocutaneous artery. Br J Plast Surg. 1984;37:149–59.

33. Bernstein PE. Mohs '98: single procedure Mohs' surgery with immediate reconstruction. Otolaryngol Head Neck Surg. 1999;120:184.

34. Cottel WI, Proper S. Mohs' surgery, fresh-tissue technique. Our technique with a review. J Dermatol Surg Oncol. 1982;8:576.

35. Mohs FE. Chemosurgery. Clin Plast Surg. 1980;7:349.

36. Rowe DE, Carroll RJ, Day CL. Mohs' surgery is the treatment of choice for recurrent (previously treated) basal cell carcinoma. J Dermatol Surg Oncol. 1989;15:424.

37. Gonzales-Ulloa M, Mayer R, Smith JM, Zaoli G. In: Piccin, editor. Chirurgia Plastica Estetica, vol. 1/7. 2006.

38. Cohen PR et al. The cuticular purse string suture: a modified purse string suture for the partial closure of round postoperative wounds. Int J Dermatol. 2007; 46:746–53.

39. Peled IJ et al. Purse-string suture for reduction and closure of skin defects. Ann Plast Surg. 1985;14(5): 465–9.

40. Bozikov K, Arnez ZM. Factors predicting free flap complications in head and neck reconstruction. J Plast Reconstr Aesthet Surg. 2006;59:737–42.

41. Gonzalez-Ulloa M. Restoration of the face covering by means of selected skin in regional aesthetic units. Br J Plast Surg. 1956;9(3):212–21.

42. Demirkan F, Chen HC, Wei FC, et al. The versatile anterolateral thigh flap: a musculocutaneous flap in disguise in head and neck reconstruction. Br J Plast Surg. 2000;53:30–6.

43. Genden EM, Rinaldo A, Suàrez C, et al. Complications of free flap transfer for head and neck reconstruction following cancer resection. Oral Oncol. 2004;40:979–84.

44. Khouri RK, Cooley BC, Kunselman Allen R, et al. A prospective study of microvascular free-flap surgery and outcome. Plast Reconstr Surg. 1998;102(3):711–21.

45. Koshima I, Fukuda H, Yamamoto H, Moriguchi T, Soeda S, Otha S. Free anterolateral thighs flaps for reconstruction of head and neck defects. Plast Reconstr Surg. 1993;92:412.

46. Myers EN, Suen JY, Myers JN, Hanna EY, editors. Cancer of the head and neck. Philadelphia: Saunders; 2003.

47. Fata MD et al. Nasal reconstruction, principles and techniques. 2011. Published on: http://emedicine. medscape.com/article/1820512-overview.

48. Rowe DE, Carroll RJ, Day CL. Prognostic factors for local recurrence, metastasis, and survival rates in squamous cell carcinoma of the skin, ear, and lip: implications for treatment modality selection. J Am Acad Dermatol. 1992;26:976.

49. Blomgren I et al. The step technique for reconstruction of lower lips defects after cancer resection. A follow-up of 165 cases. Scand J Plast Reconstr Surg. 1988;22:103.

50. Buric N et al. Reconstruction of the lower lip by mental V-Y island neurovascular advancement flap. Acta Stomatol Naissi. 2003;19(41).

51. Wang HT, Fletcher JW, Erdmann D, Levin LS. Use of the anterolateral thigh free flap for upper-extremity reconstruction. J Hand Surg Am. 2005;30:859–64.

52. Koshima I, Kawada S, Etoh H, et al. Flow-through anterior thigh flaps for one-stage reconstruction of soft tissue defects and revascularization of ischemic extremities. Plast Reconstr Surg. 1995;95:252.

53. Foucher G, Thomas M, Braun FM, et al. Le traitement des pertes de substance en sifilet des doigts. Ann Chir Plast Esthet. 1984;29:64–8.

54. Patel KK et al. A "round block" purse-string suture in facial reconstruction after operations for skin cancer surgery. Br J Oral Maxillofac Surg. 2003;41:151–6.

55. Chung-Scheng L, Sin-Daw L, Chin-Chiang Y. The reverse digital artery flap for fingertip reconstruction. Ann Plast Surg. 1989;22:495–500.

56. Litter JW. Principles of reconstructive surgery of the hand. In: Converse JM, editor. Reconstructive plastic surgery VI: the hand and upper extremity. Philadelphia: WB Saunders; 1977. p. 3138–42.

57. Regnard PJ, Renard JF, Barry P, et al. Le lambeau en llot d'avancement hèmi-pulpaire: une technique séduisante pour le traitement des amputations digitales distales. Ann Chir Plast Esthet. 1985;30:287–90.

58. Adani R, Tarallo L, Marcoccio I, Cipriani R, Gelati C, Innocenti M. Hand reconstruction using the thin anterolateral thigh flap. Plast Reconstr Surg. 2005;1116: 467–73.

59. Masquelet AC, Gilbert A. Atlante dei lembi cutanei nella ricostruzione degli arti. Roma: Antonio Delfino Editore; 2000.

60. Backhouse KM. Innervation du bras et de la main. In: Tubiana R, editor. Chirurgie de la main. Paris: Masson; 1980. p. 309–24.

61. Schernberg F, Amiel M. Etude anatomo-clinique d'un lambeau unguéal complet. Ann Chir Plast Esthet. 1985;30:127–31.

62. Atsoy E. Reversed cross finger subcutaneous flap. J Hand Surg. 1982;7:481.

63. Atsoy E, Igakidimis E, Kaspaki ML, Kutz JE, Kleinert HC. Reconstruction in amputated fingertip with a triangular volar flap: a new surgical procedure. J Bone Joint Surg. 1970;52A:921–6.

64. Dautel G, Merle M. Vascularization of palmar digital nerves. J Hand Surg Br. 1992.

65. Foucher G. Complications and bad results of toe partial transfers in thumb reconstructions. Ann Chir Main. 1991;10:529.

66. Foucher G, Merle M, Michon J. Le traitement des mutilations traumatiques du pouce: aspects nouveaux at apport microchirurgical. Chirurgie. 1984;110:56–62.

67. Merle M, Dautel L, Valenti L. La mano traumatica. L'urgenza. Paris: Masson; 1993.

68. Netter FH. Atlante di Anatomia Umana. 1998.

Cryosurgery

23

Paola Pasquali

Key Points

- Relatively simple, inexpensive, and fast surgical technique
- Long healing process since it requires second-intention wound healing
- Useful in the most common types of skin cancers and in palliative treatment

Introduction

Cryosurgery is the surgical technique where sub-zero temperatures are used to induce destruction of undesirable tissues. It was first used for destruction of tissues by James Arnott of England (1883) for palliation of breast, cervical, and skin cancers.

Destruction of skin tissues by cold follows certain basic principles that should be known by those who use cryosurgery. In dermatology, liquid nitrogen (LN) has proven to be the ideal cryogen, thanks to its safety and, most importantly, because it has a freezing point at −193 °C. It is easily available and inexpensive, making cryosurgery cost effective and convenient to patients and institutions. In the 1960s, LN was formally introduced in dermatologist offices, thanks to the work started by a neurosurgeon, Irving Cooper, later followed and improved by Douglas Torry and Setrag Zacarian (both dermatologists) and an engineer Michael Bryne (founder of Brymill Corporation), the latter responsible for developing the first commercially available handheld device.

The term cryosurgery refers to the surgical technique. Cryotherapy is a term that should be reserved to exposure of a tissue to cold temperature, usually not below freezing point and not necessarily aiming tissue destruction; it includes the uses of cold as a therapeutic agent to reduce physiological reactions like pain or swell (local inflammation or heat, pain reduction, or vasoconstriction). In cryotherapy, living tissues are exposed to temperatures well above freezing point. In cryopreservation, instead [1], cold is used to preserve tissues for future uses. No destruction is aimed.

Living cells have a certain temperature. Cryosurgery generates a flow of heat out of the cell that can eventually destroy it, depending on the speed of freezing and the temperature drop obtained. Fast freezing followed by low thawing cycles at temperatures below −50 °C kills cancerous cells.

The flow of the heat will be dependent on the material present between the lesion to be treated and the cryogen. Air is a poor conducting medium. Therefore, the further away we are from the lesion, the less flow of heat (FH) will occur. If the intervening material is water (as it occurs when a lesion is wet with water-soaked gauze),

P. Pasquali
Department of Dermatology,
Pius Hospital De Valls, Carrer Paul Cezanne 36C,
Cambrils, Tarragona 43850, Spain
e-mail: pasqualipaola@gmail.com

A. Baldi et al. (eds.), *Skin Cancer*, Current Clinical Pathology,
DOI 10.1007/978-1-4614-7357-2_23, © Springer Science+Business Media New York 2014

Fig. 23.1 *Arrows* show the flow of heat (FH) differences between different materials

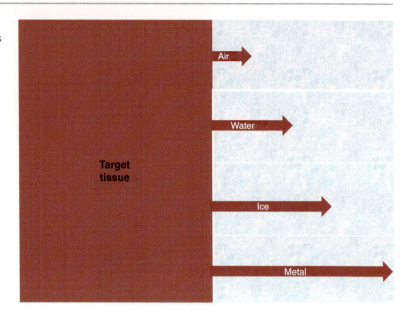

then the FH will be higher. An ice medium (like the one occurring in a second freezing of a cancerous cell) and finally a metal one (occurring when a metal probe is used) will have increasingly larger FH (Fig. 23.1).

In a fast frozen tissue, temperature drops can be visualized as isotherms being at the center of the lesion, the area with the lowest temperature. The cryosurgeon will need to guarantee that the required −50 °C needed to destroy cancer cells is at the bottom of the tumor. The easiest way is to measure it at the periphery of the tumor (Fig. 23.2). The knowledge of the shape of the tumor will be important in determining the required margins. As a general rule, the margins to be frozen are the same than when removing a tumor by surgery.

Basic Principles

The molecular basis for destruction with sub-zero temperature can be summarized as follows [2–4] (Table 23.1):

1. *Direct injury*. With initial freezing, water crystals form outside the cells. This generates a hyperosmotic environment and subsequent water movement out of the cell. Internal dehydration initiates membrane and organelle damage. As freezing is maintained, there is water crystal formation inside the cell which results in cell bursting. As the tissue thaws, crystals reorganize forming newer and larger crystals that cause further destruction.

In addition, the mechanical damage generated at the membrane level adds to the metabolic failure caused by ionic changes, pH decrease, and lipid alteration, all leading to further permeability alterations.

Most of the direct damage occurs during the freezing period, causing cell death by necrosis mainly at the center of the lesion.

2. *Vascular injury*. Cold generated severe vasoconstriction with subsequent decrease in the blood flow. With thawing, the tissue becomes congested due to vasodilation and vascular damage. Eventually, there is platelet aggregation and microthrombi formation which leads to vascular stasis. Thawing brings about hyperperfusion, free radical formation, and further membrane damage. Blood supply due to microcirculation failure occurs in about 1 h from freezing and causes death by ischemia, evident at the periphery of the cryoinjury.

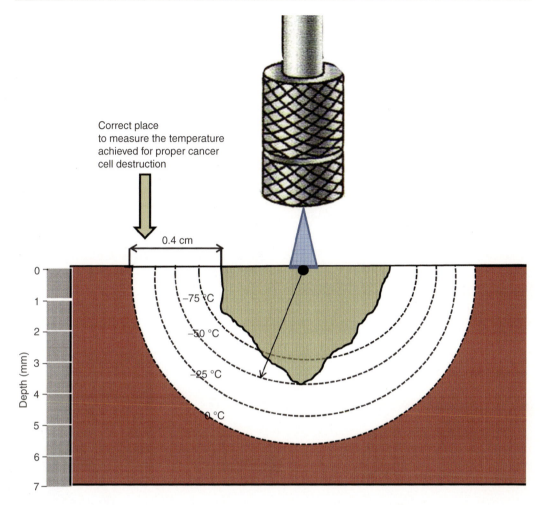

Correct place
to measure the temperature
achieved for proper cancer
cell destruction

0.4 cm

Fig. 23.2 Schematic view of the isotherms. As we move further down from the freezing source, temperatures are higher in depth and laterally

Table 23.1 Molecular basis of cryosurgical injury		Mechanism	Time of cycle	Location
	Direct injury	Intracellular ice crystal formation; followed after days by coagulation necrosis	Freezing phase	Center
	Vascular injury	Microcirculatory failure	Thawing phase	Periphery
	By apoptosis	Cell death by apoptosis	Up to 8 h after rewarming	Periphery
	Immunological[a]	Dendritic cell mediated	Late event	Periphery

[a]Animal studies

3. *Apoptosis.* Cell death by apoptosis is a phenomenon seen at the periphery of the cryoinjury that occurs as a late event (2–8 h after freezing) [5].

4. *Immunological effect.* Sub-zero temperature also produces death at distant sites from the cryoinjury, and it is a late event

probably induced by cytokines [6, 7] (see Immunocryosurgery Chap. 24).

Equipments

The equipment required for office cryosurgery is commercially available through different manufacturers. It consists of a unit to deliver the LN, diverse attachments, tank to store LN, and other accessories (Fig. 23.3).

Handheld Unit

These units are used to deliver the cryogen. They have to hold enough LN to allow the cryosurgeon to perform several procedures without filling the tank every time. Large units hold more LN but weigh more and are cumbersome to handle. Excess in weight or in diameter of the units can result in loss of accuracy. This is the reason why the ideal unit size ranges from 300 to 500 cc. The most popular commercially

available units are made by Brymill Corporation. Further developments in the unit have produced the Cry-Ac® Tracker (Brymill) which is the only unit that measures the temperature on the skin as LN is delivered to the target lesion and the newest Cry-Ac® TrackerCam™ which measures temperatures, monitors freezing, and records the procedure.

Other manufactures are Erbokryo derm, Wallach (UltraFreeze tm; units available in 300 and 500 cc), or Cortex (Cryopro, in 500 and 350 cc units).

Attachments and Other Delivery Gadgets (Fig. 23.4)

Tips or apertures are devices that can be screwed at the open end of the unit and allow the output of LN through openings of predetermined size. They are named with letters: A, 0.04 in.; B, 0.03 in.; C, 0.022 in.; and D, 0.016 in. The larger the openings, the larger the release of LN. They are used for cryospray technique.

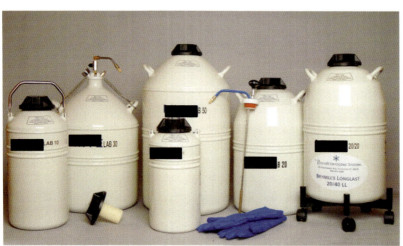
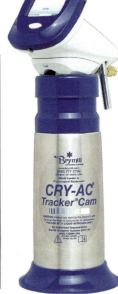

Fig. 23.3 Dewars, gloves, withdraw device, and Cry-Ac® TrackerCam™

Probes are metal extensions usually covered by Teflon (to avoid sticking to the surface). They come in different sizes (cylindrical, conical, ball shaped, half-moon, sharp-pointed conical, concave, flat elongated). They have an internal conduit line that freezes the metal from the inside maintaining a continuous low temperature. They are used for close cryosurgery.

Chambers are metal cylinders with one of the endings screwed onto the opening of the unit while the free open end has a rubber ring to

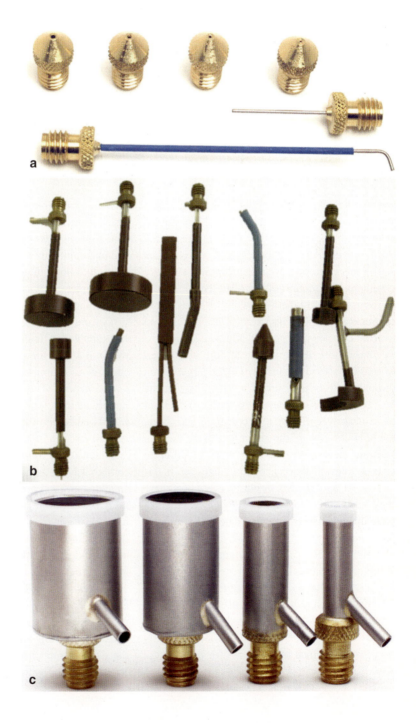

Fig. 23.4 (**a**) Spray tips. (**b**) Probes. (**c**) Chambers. (**d**) Cones. (**e**) Tweezers

Fig. 23.4 (continued)

d

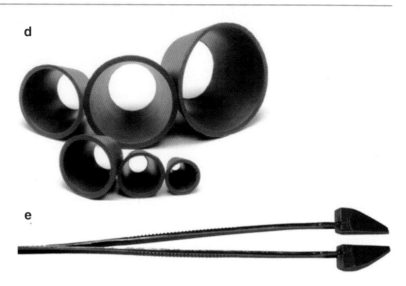

e

protect the skin. Once applied over the target lesion, LN is released and maintained inside the chamber (by applying a discrete pressure on the skin). LN turbulence generates inside the chamber and allows extremely powerful freezing. They are considered a variation of the open technique and its use is limited to the treatment of lesions where destruction in depth is important. They are reserved to advance malignancies like skin metastasis.

Cones are cylinders, open at both ends, used to confine LN as it is delivered to the target lesion through a tip or aperture. They help protect the healthy skin that surrounds the target (not meant to be destroyed). They also constrain and direct the flow of LN to the delimited area, making freezing more effective. They come in different sizes and are made of neoprene (sizes are 6, 11, 16, 25, 30, and 38 mm) or plastic (very useful are the ones used in otoscope). A device called cryoplate that consists of a Lexan plate with four conical openings (4, 7, 9, and 12 mm) is another alternative. These are all variants of the open technique. It is usually used in benign lesions.

Tweezers have been designed for benign lesions. However, they can be used to grasp exophytic tumors. A modified tweezer (with one ending attached at the unit for continuous LN flow) was designed by our team for use in large vascular tumors (Fig. 23.5).

Extensions (bend or straight) are meant to attach applicators or probes. They are used to treat hard-to-reach lesions, keeping the unit straight and maintaining precision. Luer lock adapters can be used to hook in needles or other probes. Back vent adapter eliminates intermittent spray (useful for continuous flow over a large tumor).

Dewars. LN needs to be stored in special dewars capable of maintaining the gas restrained within it and at the same time, allow some small amounts to evaporate to avoid pressure build up on the insides. The quality of the cover is very important in determining the duration of stored LN. They come in different sizes: 5, 10, 20, 30, and 50 L capacity. The intermediate sizes (20–30 L) tend to be more practical because they hold enough LN to last for 1–2 months unlike the smaller ones and are more manageable than the 50 L. A 5 L dewar can be used to place the residual LN of a larger dewar while waiting to get it filled again. There is a LN generator (MMR technology® ideal for offices located away from distribution networks.

Gloves, Roller Base for Dewars, Withdrawal Device. These are optional gadgets that can be useful for manipulating LN. Gloves protect from accidental spilling and the roller base helps move the dewar from one side to another (meant for large ones); the withdrawal device comes in two

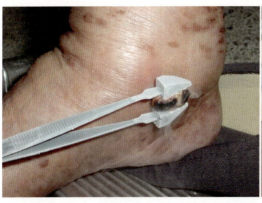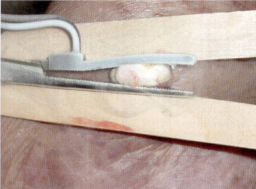

Fig. 23.5 Tweezers used in SK tumors of the leg

models: one that affixes to dewars and stays there until new refill. LN is released by opening a faucet; the other is meant to be fit every time the unit has to be refilled and offers instant pressurization, and once the unit is filled, it is removed, and the dewar cap is placed back.

Techniques

These are basically:
1. Spray or open technique
2. Cone or semi-open technique
3. Probe or close technique
4. Chamber or semi-closed technique
5. Tweezer
6. Intralesional

In skin cancer, the most commonly used are spray, probe, and chamber.

Spray or Open Technique

The open technique is probably the most common one. It is the technique of choice for benign lesions and in numerous skin cancers. LN is released through tips with apertures of known diameter. The most commonly used is the C tip (0.022 in./0.56 mm). Other apertures are A, 0.04 in./1.02 mm; B, 0.031 in./0.079 mm; D, 0.016 in./0.41 mm; and E, 0.013 in./0.33 mm. Luer lock adapters will be useful to use in differ-

ent gauge needles, whenever in need of a more delimited freezing.

Extensions can be located between the unit and the tip to allow the operator to reach areas not readily exposed, such as mouth, earlobe, or canal. There are 1″ × 20 g Straight Spray and 3″ × 20 g Bent Spray.

The larger tips will release largest amounts of LN and therefore, freezing will be faster and deeper. Distance from the target tissue and direction of the spray are also elements to take into consideration (Fig. 23.6).

In skin cancer, it is the ideal technique for:
(a) Flat, superficial lesions, like actinic keratosis or superficial basal cell carcinomas.
(b) Whenever contact cryosurgery cannot be applied either because (1) the surface of the tumor is too irregular and cannot be flattened down by curettage or (2) tumors whose size exceed that of the probes available.
(c) For difficult-access regions. In the latter case, bend or straight adapter can help. Thick tumors are rich in keratin, a bad cold conductant. Therefore, the surgeon has to guarantee to reach the bottom of the lesion. Spraying applied in a brushing manner can give false freezing fronts because the surface will freeze while the deeper areas still maintain temperatures above −50 °C. Temperature control (with the tracker) lets the surgeon know that the temperature reached is the desired one.

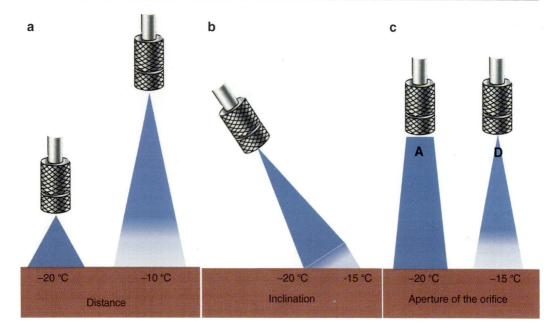

Fig. 23.6 Effects of (**a**) distance (the closer to the skin, the lower the final temperature in the skin) (**b**) inclination: the area closer to the freezing tip will have a lower final temperature (**c**) aperture of the orifice the larger the orifice, more LN will get to skin resulting in a lower final temperature. Aperture (*A*) is 0.04 in and aperture (*D*) is 0.016 in

Spraying has to be done from the center and allow the freezing front to extend radially until the desired frozen margin is reached. The freezing front has to advance just to the area outside the lesion that would be removed if conventional surgery was performed.

For premalignant lesions, a 2 mm margin is sufficient. For basal cell carcinomas, leave a 4 mm margin. For squamous cell carcinomas, leave a 5–6 mm margin.

For large tumors (over 3 CMS), there are two alternatives: (1) segmental and (2) fractional cryosurgery.

Segmental cryosurgery was first described by Zacarian. It consists in dividing a large tumor with imaginary lines and treats each segment separately. Each freezing front is allowed to overlap, in order to guarantee a complete freezing of the tumor (Fig. 23.7).

Fractional cryosurgery is a staged freezing method described by Gonçalves [8]. It consists of freezing the center of a large tumor, leaving the periphery untreated. Once the center has healed, the remaining tumor will be smaller due to the shrinkage generated by the central scar. A sec-

ond freezing, again at the center, can then cover the whole remaining tumor or be part of a series of freezes aimed at creating a small final tumor. Usually, one step is sufficient for most common tumors. Fractional cryosurgery is not limited to spraying technique. Probes can also be used for this sequential freezing process.

Cone or Semi-open Technique

It is a spray technique that limits the LN to an area bounded by a cone (plastic or rubber), reducing damage to areas peripheral to the tumor. Used primarily for well-circumscribed lesions.

Probe or Close Technique

This is the ideal technique for skin cancer. LN is released inside a close system that maintains the sub-zero temperature, freezes the metal probe, and is then released through a rubber hose. The metal which they are made is usually copper, which is an excellent conductant.

Fig. 23.7 Zacarian's segmental (*upper part*) versus Goncalves fractional (*lower part*) cryosurgery. In segmental cryosurgery, the tumor is divided in equal parts using imaginary lines. Each segment is frozen separately. It can be done part by part or all at once. In fractional cryosurgery, tumor is frozen in the center (**a**), let neal (**b**), leaving a final smaller tumor with a central scar (**c**)

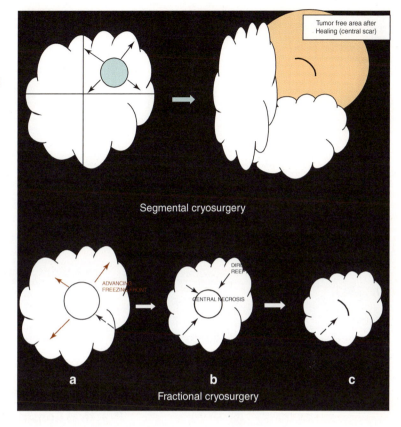

The sub-zero temperature is maintained as they go through metal, much more than when passing though air (as it occurs in the open technique). It is a way to guarantee that the sub-zero temperature reaches the tumor and the desired lethal temperature is achieved.

It is the ideal technique for (a) skin cancer in general and (b) in the treatment of tumors provided that the appropriate probe is available particularly in tumors with a regular surface or as flat as possible, in order to reduce the interphase (area of air spaces left between the probe and tumor surfaces due to inadequate contact) (Fig. 23.8). (c) Vascular/Cyst tumours the probe has to firmly attach to the skin.

Chamber or Semi-closed Technique

It is a variation to the spray technique. LN is released through a tip inside a chamber that has been firmly applied over the tumor. Correct placement is important in order to avoid spilling LN from the sides. Once the cryogen starts being released inside the chamber, a turbulent movement of the LN generates a fast and deep freezing of the tumor, which tends to be faster than with probe.

It is a very powerful tool that should be reserved for nodular malignancies, especially metastatic lesions.

Tweezer Technique

A technique reserved to pendular lesions. It can also be useful in large vascular tumors (like Kaposi sarcomas) for palliative treatments (Fig. 23.5). It can be useful to grasp and freeze a lesion for biopsy (cryobiospy).

Intralesional Technique

Originally developed for keloids, it could be an option for ultrasound directed freezing of

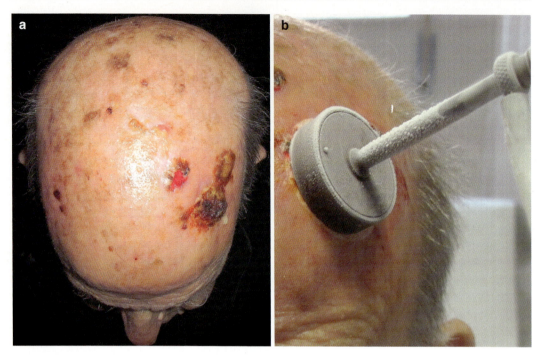

Fig. 23.8 Probe or close cryosurgery on a squamous cell carcinoma of the scalp previous curettage of the lesion, in a 92-year-old patient with severe skin cancerization of the scalp

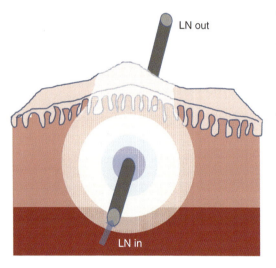

Fig. 23.9 Intralesional cryosurgery. A needle (attached through a luer lock to the unit) is passed through the tumor allowing the open end to come out of the other side of the skin to allow LN release

metastatic lesions. A needle, connected to the unit, is passed through the tumor, leaving the outlet end of the needle outside the skin. The freezing front will advance from the inside of the tumor towards the periphery (Fig. 23.9).

Practical Considerations and Applications

Indications and Contraindications [9]

Actinic keratosis (AK) and actinic cheilitis are probably the most popular indications for cryosurgery. It is important to keep in mind that some AK might have lots of keratin (hypertrophic AK). It is therefore important to either remove the keratotic part or wet it first (to improve cold conductivity through the tissue). Freezing has to include a 2 mm margin at the periphery of the lesion. AK is mostly present in skin cancerized areas. It is then important to treat the area as a whole with topical treatments (i.e., 5 % 5-fluorouracil, imiquimod, or topical diclofenac) before and then treat the remaining lesions (Fig. 23.10). One cryospray cycle is usually sufficient, making sure to include an appropriate margin (2 mm).

Superficial tumors (superficial BCC, in situ squamous cell carcinomas). Superficial BCC are, as the word says, very superficial lesions, with small islands of clustered cells scattered over areas that can range from few millimeters to

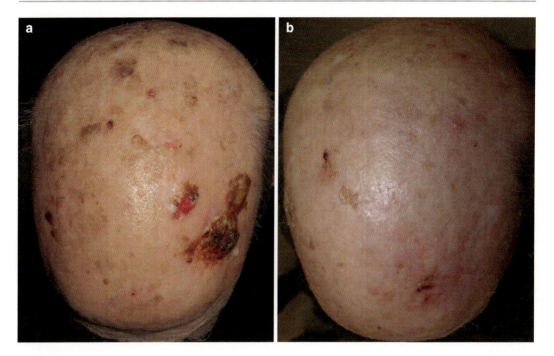

Fig. 23.10 Severe skin cancerization of the scalp (**a**) in the same patient as Fig 23.8. (**b**) after 3 months of topical 3 % diclofenac (Solaraze®), close cryosurgery of the large tumors and spraying of the residual AK

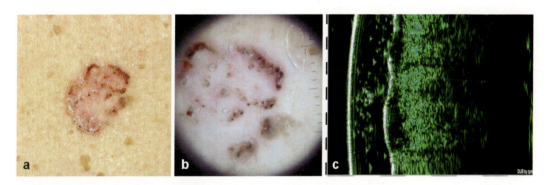

Fig. 23.11 Previous view of a superficial BCC prior to freezing, in order to determine the depth of freeze. Clinical (**a**), dermoscopic (**b**) and ultrasound (22 MHz, TPM®) (**c**) (US) view of a superficial BCC treated with a double cycle probe technique. The US shows that the tumor depth is below 1 mm

several centimeters. The treatments should therefore focus on the depth as much as on the horizontal spread (Fig. 23.11). This is the main reason why cryosurgery, PDT, laser, or topical treatments are ideal for their treatment. Same goes for *Bowen's disease* (in situ squamous cell carcinomas) and *erythroplasia of Queyrat*. Two freezing cycles should be performed, either with the spray or probe technique, making sure that the temperature reached at the bottom (and hence perilesional)

is around −50 °C. For large lesions, it is convenient to do segmental or fractional cryosurgery to avoid unnecessary depth destruction.

Nodular lesions (nodular BCC, well-differentiated and moderately differentiated squamous cell carcinomas/keratoacanthomas). Nodular lesions with a surface that can be flattened (i.e., previous curettage) are better treated with probes. If the nodule is small enough, the pressure applied with the probe will be sufficient to adhere

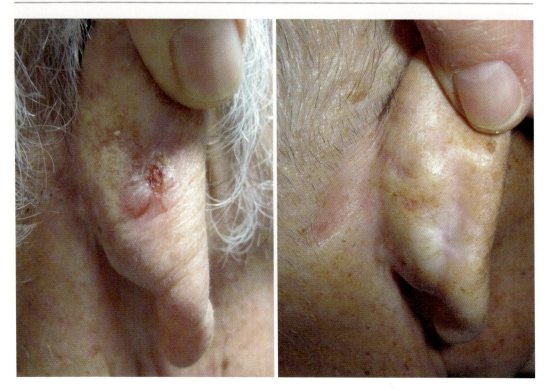

Fig. 23.12 Ulcerated BCC (*left*) treated with closed double freeze-thaw cycle. On the *right*, 1 1/2 years later

to the metal surface into the tumor. With probes, freezing is faster and deeper. If the appropriate size of probe is not available, it is possible to do segmental or fractional cryosurgery. Whenever we feel that the surface is too irregular to guarantee the proper application of the probe, we should use the open technique. Chambers should be reserved for metastatic lesions or deeply seated tumors.

In BCC, two freeze-thaw cycles are the rule (Fig. 23.12) and for squamous cell, 2–3 freeze-thaw cycles.

The knowledge of the surface temperature thanks to the new equipments available (Cry-Ac® TrackerCam™) has been a breakthrough in the management of skin cancer with cryosurgery. The excellent results reported in the past on experienced hands [10–13] can now be further documented.

Another fundamental aim is the use of high-frequency ultrasound (22 MHz HFUS) to determine the size and shape of the tumor [14] (Fig. 23.11). A clinical picture, a dermoscopic

diagnosis, and an HFUS determination of dimensions will be of outmost importance in deciding the technique and the number of cycles. Furthermore, HFUS can be used to visualize the freezing from. By applying the HFUS probe immediately after freezing, the surgeon will be able to visualize the depth of the freezing from and the advancement of the thawing as it advances from the surface towards the depth. Additionally, one can see the changes in the tissue caused by the freezing procedure at the first cycle and the further damage at the second cycle.

Cryobiopsy; for diagnostic purposes a shaving of a previously spray-frozen lesion allows to obtain non altered tissue for biopsy. No local anesthesia is required.

Pigmentary lesions. Any correct skin cancer treatment requires a previous correct diagnosis of the lesion. If for any tumor this is the case, for pigmentary lesions, it is of primary importance to know the correct diagnoses. Freezing a melanoma thinking that it is a hyperpigmented seborrheic keratosis can result in a fatal error.

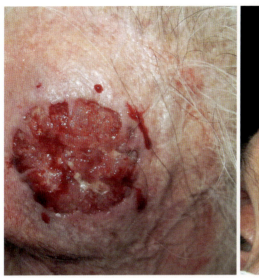
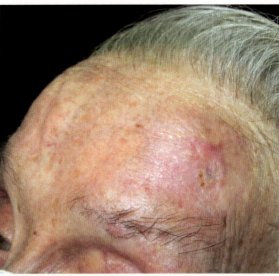

Fig. 23.13 Palliative treatment of a BCC of over 8 cm in the front of a 99-year-old woman. One treatment, double cycle, cryospray, −55 °C. No recurrence after 1 year of treatment

Melanocytes are extremely sensitive to cold. They are rapidly destroyed. Cryosurgery has been reserved to palliative treatments in inoperable melanomas (Fig. 23.13) and in some large lentigo maligna, using inmunocryosurgery [15].

Postoperative Care

Postoperative care is simple but long in comparison to conventional surgery where the procedures are more laborious and post-ops relatively fast. During the first hour, the patient might feel discomfort and occasionally pain, depending on the treated area and the sensitivity to cold.

For superficial treatments, like the ones applied in premalignant lesions, there is no need to cover. The area can be washed daily, with water and soap. Depending on the anatomical area, total healing will occur between 3 and 7 days (face) up to 2–3 weeks (other anatomical areas). For deep freezes, as in cancerous lesions, healing takes longer: for a lesion in the face, 7–12 days, 2–4 weeks in the trunk, and over a month for leg lesions. After 24–48 h, a blister will form which can have clear or bloody (in previously curettage lesions) content. From the moment the blister breaks, there will be

oozing which can last for several days (depending on the depth of freeze). Deeper freezes will require covering the lesion after the daily cleanup.

It is convenient to use antibiotic ointments over the healing lesion. Crust formation should be avoided to speed up healing and reduce the possibility of infection.

Expected Side Effects

There are expected occurrences after a cryosurgical procedure.

One of the most characteristic is edema. Several conditions will determine the edema: (1) the freezing depth, (2) the total volume of tissue that is frozen, (3) the skin type, (4) individual susceptibility to cold, (5) anatomical site of the tumor, and (6) age.

In general, deep freezing of large tumors in white skins will present a larger edema. As an expected effect, patients have to be properly informed, both orally and in a written manner. Cryosurgeons must be prepared to reassure the patient about it.

Edema and swelling are not painful. The presence of pain, which could occur after a week of the cryosurgical procedure, tends to be a sign of infection. Freezing around eyelids or in the frontal area tends to result in larger swellings; older people treated of tumors in the face can have edemas that last several days. Edema caused by treating lesions in the front tends to localize in the superior part of the face in the morning and tends to relocate in the neck in the evening, due to gravity.

It does not tend to respond to anti-inflammatory treatment neither oral nor topical.

Bullae or vesicles can also occur. They tend to appear 24–48 h after the procedure and break spontaneously where skin is thinner. They can be filled with clear liquid or, if previous curettage was performed, with bloody secretion.

Some cryosurgeons leave the bullae or vesicle. Others prefer to remove it to fasten healing time.

Exudation of liquid material occurs when the bullae/vesicle breaks. The amount of liquid will depend on the freezing depth. Inform your patients in order to avoid unnecessary calls and worries.

Complications

As with every method, pitfalls can occur. In cryosurgery, postoperative sequelae may be temporary or occasionally permanent. Most pitfalls attributed to cryosurgery are the result of inappropriate technique. Therefore, correct training will reduce many unwanted secondary effects. The equipment is readily available and the apparent simplicity of the method has facilitated indiscriminate use without following proper patient selection.

Temporary complications include:

- Bleeding: possible in deep freezing once the necrosis of the tissue sets in and small vessels become exposed. It can be controlled by hemostatic solution but occasionally requires electrocoagulation or even ligation of the vessel with a suture.
- Headache: if the treated area was in the scalp or face.
- Infection: can be recognized by the presence of pus, excessive redness, and pain that appear days after the treatment.

- Nitrogen gas insufflation: can occur if the open technique is used on a previously drained cyst.
- Hypertrophic scarring, cold urticaria, or paresthesia: these have also been described.
- Hyperpigmentation.
- Milia formation at the site of bulla formation. Occasional permanent complications include:
- Retraction of tissue, when cryosurgery has been performed near the lips, ala nasi, or eyebrows
- Alopecia
- Ectropion
- Permanent hypopigmentation
- Others: tendon rupture, ulceration, and tissue defect

Future Considerations

The combination of a cytology diagnosis (which requires a minimum tissue removal), refined dermoscopic diagnosis, and tumor US size and shape and the capability to measure and record the temperature at the site of freezing have been essential in bringing cryosurgery into a more reproducible method.

The use of noninvasive diagnosis techniques like confocal microscopy [16] (CM) or optical coherence tomography [17] (OTC) will further facilitate the cryosurgeons' work.

With time, equipments will include more than one of the following options. Further developments in the area of immunocryosurgery (see next chapter) will be crucial in the development of a technique that is showing to have an effect beyond the simple in situ destruction of cancerous cells.

Glossary

Close technique is the technique where LN is contained within a close conduits system called probe.

Cryobiopsy is a cryosurgical technique by which a biopsy is taken by previously freezing the site to be biopsied without the need to apply local anesthesia.

HFUS High Frequency Ultrasound

Open technique is the cryosurgical techniques that utilized open tips for spraying.

Semi-open technique refers to the cryosurgical technique that bounds the sprayed LN by means of a cone.

Semi-closed technique limits the LN inside a chamber in contact with the skin.

References

1. Stańczyk M, Telega JJ. Thermal problems in biomechanics- a review. Part III. Cryosurgery, cryopreservation and cryotherapy. Acta Bioeng Biomech. 2003;5(2):3–22.
2. Baust JG, Gage AA. The molecular basis of cryosurgery. BJU Int. 2005;95(9):1187–91.
3. Gage AA, Baust JG. Mechanisms of tissue injury in cryosurgery. Cryobiology. 1998;37:171–86.
4. Gage AA, Baust JM, Baust JG. Experimental cryosurgery investigations in vivo. Cryobiology. 2009. doi:10.1016/j.cryobiol.2009.10.001.
5. Forest V, Peoc'h M, Campos L, Guyotat D, Vergnon JM. Effects of cryotherapy or chemotherapy on apoptosis in a non-small- cell lung cancer xenografted into SCID mice. Cryobiology. 2005;50:29–37.
6. den Brok MH, Sutmuller RP, Nierkens S, Bennink EJ, Frielink C, Toonen LW, et al. Efficient loading of dendritic cells following cryo and radiofrequency ablation in combination with immune modulation induces antitumour immunity. Br J Cancer. 2006;95(7):896–905.
7. Redondo P, del Olmo J, López-Díaz A, Inoges S, Marquina M, Melero I, et al. Imiquimod enhances the systemic immunity attained by local cryosurgery destruction of melanoma lesions. J Invest Dermatol. 2007;127(7):1673–80.
8. Gonçalves JC. Fractional cryosurgery for skin cancer. Dermatol Surg. 2009;35(11):1788–96.
9. Pasquali P. Cryosurgery. In: Rigel D, Robinson J, Ross MI, Friedman R, Cockerell CJ, Lim H, Stockfleth E, editors. Edited by John M Kirkwood. Cancer of the skin, expert consult. 2nd ed. New Year: Elsevier; 2011. p. 450–461.
10. Lindemalm-Lundstam B, Dalenbäck J. Prospective follow-up after curettage-cryosurgery for scalp and face skin cancers. Br J Dermatol. 2009;161(3):568–76.
11. Nordin P, Stenquist B. Five-year results of curettage-cryosurgery for 100 consecutive auricular non-melanoma skin cancers. J Laryngol Otol. 2002; 116(11):893–8.
12. Suhonen RE, Kuflik EG. Cryosurgical methods for eyelid lesions. J Dermatolog Treat. 2001;12(3):135–9.
13. Pasquali P, Trujillo B. Manejo crioquirúrgico del cáncer de piel: curativo y paliativo. Gac Med Caracas. 2007;115(2):138–43.
14. Wortsman X. Common applications of dermatologic sonography. J Ultrasound Med. 2012;31(1): 97–111.
15. Bassukas ID, Gamvroulia C, Zioga A, Nomikos K, Fotika C. Cryosurgery during topical imiquimod: a successful combination modality for lentigo maligna. Int J Dermatol. 2008;47(5):519–21.
16. Ahlgrimm-Siess V, Horn M, Koller S, Ludwig R, Gerger A, Hofmann-Wellenhof R. Monitoring efficacy of cryotherapy for superficial basal cell carcinomas with in vivo reflectance confocal microscopy: a preliminary study. J Dermatol Sci. 2009;53(1):60–4.
17. Mogensen M, Thrane L, Jørgensen TM, Andersen PE, Jemec GB. OCT imaging of skin cancer and other dermatological diseases. J Biophotonics. 2009; 2(6–7):442–51.

Immunological Aspects of Cryosurgery

24

Eduardo K. Moioli and Aleksandar L. Krunic

Key Points

- Cryosurgery is minimally invasive, minimally damaging to surrounding structures, generally well tolerated, has relatively low cost, and often results in good cosmetic results.
- Cryosurgery has been demonstrated for the treatment of both primary tumors and metastases.
- The mechanism of cell death and tissue injury during cryosurgery is complex and results from both direct and indirect mechanisms of injury involving apoptosis and necrosis.
- Cryoimmunology describes a process that involves a specific immune response that is formed against antigens and debris derived from cells and tissues destroyed by cryosurgery.

- Initial local inflammation and systemic immune system activation after cryosurgery play key roles during the primary destruction of cryoablated tissue as well as the continued immune surveillance via memory immune cells.
- Future directions include elucidating specific cytokines and cellular pathways associated with cryoinjury as well as standardization of techniques for its various applications.

Introduction

Therapeutic approaches to treat tumors have included surgical resection, chemotherapy, radiation, thermal ablation, and cryodestruction. In comparison to other modalities, cryosurgery is minimally invasive, is less damaging to surrounding structures, and has better patient comfort (anesthetic effect), lower cost, and often better cosmetic results. Furthermore, frozen tumor remains "in situ" for the body to absorb, producing stimulation of immunologic response to tumor-specific antigens derived from the frozen tissue [1]. Many earlier reports of regressing metastatic foci after cryoablation of primary tumors (prostate cancer, breast cancer, lung metastases) have raised some interest in the likely immunological effects of cryosurgery; however, it had not been clear whether the immune response was indeed responsible or not.

E.K. Moioli
Section of Dermatology,
University of Chicago,
5841 S.Maryland Ave, Chicago, IL, USA

A.L. Krunic, MD, PhD, FAAD, FACMS (✉)
Department of Dermatology,
University of Illinois College of Medicine,
Chicago, IL, USA

Department of Dermatology,
Northwestern University Feinberg School of Medicine,
Chicago, IL, USA
e-mail: krunic@uic.edu

A. Baldi et al. (eds.), *Skin Cancer*, Current Clinical Pathology,
DOI 10.1007/978-1-4614-7357-2_24, © Springer Science+Business Media New York 2014

At the time, immunological assays were limited, and as such, conclusions regarding the "immunoprotective" or "immunodepressive" aspects of cryoablation were not possible, rendering the true role of the immune system difficult to verify.

Cryoimmunology describes a process that involves a specific immune response that is formed against antigens and debris derived from the cells and tissues after cryodestruction. Comparable to the immune response that modulates anticancer activity with recent monoclonal antibodies, the innate, humoral, and cytotoxic arms of immunity may become activated after cryosurgery and participate in further tumor destruction [2]. The initial inflammatory process secondary to the ablation of tissue plays a critical role in the initiation and mediation of the immune response against tumors [3]. For instance, inflammatory cytokines such as IFN-γ, which are upregulated by cryotherapy, may induce maturation of immune cells such as antigen-presenting cells (APCs), which in turn guide immune activation against the cells/tissues destroyed by freezing [4]. Some of the key players during the immunological response that follows cryoablation and cryosurgery include macrophages, dendritic cells, neutrophils, and CD4+ and CD8+ cells [5].

The benefits of cryoablation in treating both primary tumors and metastases have been described historically, especially in prostate cancer [6, 7]. Other types of tumors have also been demonstrated to regress after cryosurgery including breast, myosarcoma, hepatic, and rectal, among others [8–12]. More recently, some of the mechanisms in which cryoablation results in immune-mediated destruction of tumors and metastases have been elucidated. Interestingly, conflicting results from animal experiments evaluating tumor response to cryoablation have ranged from the desired destruction of the primary tumor and shrinking of distant metastases to the unwarranted growth of tumors and hastened experimental animal death. More recent studies have shed light and suggested theories for the mechanisms for such varied results. The current chapter will discuss the mechanisms behind cryoimmunology, including how the immune system becomes activated after cryoablation, as well as some of the evidence both for and against the use of this approach to treating tumors.

Mechanisms of Cell Death and Tissue Injury During Cryosurgery

The mechanism of cell death and tissue injury during cryosurgery is complex. There are multiple processes that occur related to the rates of temperature change, target temperature, distance from freezing center, and extracellular/cellular solute concentrations after freezing, among others. Depending on some of these processes, either necrosis or apoptosis occurs secondary to direct or indirect cellular injury. The direct process occurs due to the sequelae of direct freezing of water. First, ice crystals form in the extracellular space, increasing the osmolar concentration of that environment. Consequently, water leaves the cell to dilute the extracellular matrix in order to reach intra- and extracellular space osmolar balance, which results in cell dehydration. The resulting high solute concentration and lower temperatures intracellularly cause reversible conformational change of cytoplasmic enzymes that may lead to direct cell death [13]. However, if freezing rates are rapid, not enough time is allowed for this process of cellular dehydration to unfold because ice crystals form quickly within the cell as well as extracellularly, leading to direct mechanical damage to organelles and cell membranes which cause immediate cell death [14]. This is more commonly observed near the cooling probe (center of cryolesion), where freezing rates are rapid and the temperatures are lowest (Fig. 24.1). Moreover, upon slow thawing of the tissue after freezing, free water rushes into the cells, increasing intracellular ice crystal formation or resulting in cell bursting [15].

The direct cell damage described above results in necrosis and release of intracellular contents, as well as extracellular matrix damage, all leading to activation of the short-lived, nonspecific innate immune response and inflammation. The direct mechanical injury resulting in cell necrosis is typical at short distances from the center of the cryogenic lesion given the lower temperatures achieved. Temperatures

Fig. 24.1 Necrosis and apoptosis zones after cryoablation. Areas closest to the center of the cryolesion reach lower temperatures with higher freezing rates resulting in rapid intracellular ice crystal formation, cell bursting, and necrosis (direct injury). At longer distances from the cryoprobe, only milder freezing temperatures are reached, resulting in a transition from necrosis to apoptosis. The lower freezing rate at distant sites results in intracellular osmolar dehydration, necrosis secondary to extracellular ice crystal formation, or enzymatic changes that result in apoptosis

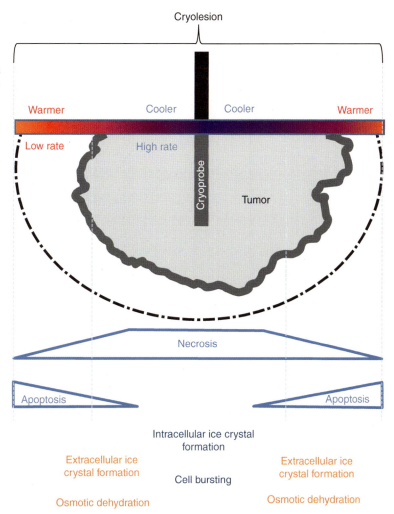

of approximately −20 °C have been suggested for adequate tissue destruction; however, it is worthwhile to note that malignant cells may be more resistant to cryoinjury and require lower temperatures [16]. Human primary prostatic adenocarcinoma cell lines cryoablated at two different cooling rates of 5 or 25 °C/s required temperatures lower than −40 and −19 °C, respectively, for complete destruction of cells [17]. Other groups have also suggested that tissue temperatures should at least approach −40 °C in tumors for effective ablation of malignant tissue [15, 16]. When human colon carcinoma cells were exposed to a temperature range of −6 to −36 °C, approximately 98.5 % of cells that reached −36 °C were dead by direct

cryolysis after 4 h, while only approximately 50 % underwent cryolysis if they only reached −10 °C. Current standards for cryoablation of malignant tumors recommend −50 to −60 °C degrees.

Within higher, sublethal temperature ranges, cryoablated cells in malignant tissues such as in human colon carcinomas have been shown to undergo apoptosis instead of necrosis [18]. Markers for apoptosis can be observed in cells 4 h after freezing. The percent of apoptotic colon carcinoma cells is maximized at −25 °C with approximately 28 % of cells demonstrating elevated apoptosis markers. Colder temperatures result in lower apoptotic rates likely secondary to a shift toward the mechanism of cell injury described

Table 24.1 Mechanisms of cell death and tissue injury after cryosurgery

Direct injury	Indirect injury
Extracellular matrix ice crystal formation	Thrombus formation
Intracellular osmotic dehydration	Vascular stasis and ischemia
Enzymatic conformational changes	Innate and adaptive immune system-driven injury
Intracellular ice crystal formation and cell bursting	

above, namely, a predominantly cryolytic type of cell death and tissue necrosis (Fig. 24.1). It is important to note that cell death by apoptosis is the primary mechanism of cryoablation in the peripheral zone of the cryogenic lesion (away from the center of cryolesion), given the inherent higher temperatures found away from the source of freezing. Also notable is that apoptotic cell death does not induce an inflammatory response as seen during necrosis. The balance between apoptosis and necrosis may play an important role in whether a tumor undergoing cryoablation is destroyed or not.

Indirect cell damage also occurs after cryoablation. Ice crystals form in blood vessels damaging the lining endothelium. After thawing and reperfusion of affected vessels, platelets become activated causing thrombus formation and subsequent local tissue ischemia [19]. The vascular stasis results in further tissue damage post-cryoablation. Furthermore, indirect damage occurs due to immunological injury that follows an initial inflammatory response (Table 24.1). This process of immune system activation is described by cryoimmunology and is discussed in the following sections.

Inflammation and Immune System Activation After Cryosurgery: The Cornerstone of Cryoimmunology

Cryoimmunology can be described as a process involving inflammation and immune attack against damaged target tissue that follows local cryoablation. As described above, antigens are released after cryosurgery secondary to membrane disruption and cell death. In addition, preformed inflammatory cytokines are also released from the surrounding extracellular matrix, initiating an immediate inflammatory response. For instance, studies have demonstrated that levels of IL-1β, IL-6, and TNF-α are elevated after cryoablation of large hepatic metastases [20, 21]. IL-12 and IFN-γ have also been detected shortly after freezing [1]. Prostate tumor cell gene expression of several cytokines implicated in stimulating immunity, such as IL-2, IL-15, IL-12p40, IL-18, and TNF-α, was demonstrated to increase after cryoablation. Cells including neutrophils, macrophages, and lymphocytes are recruited by the ongoing inflammatory process and add to the cytokine milieu by secreting other inflammatory mediators marking the activation of the innate immune response [22–24]. Cell infiltration including APCs and T cells may be mediated by the expression of proteins such as heat-shock protein 70 (HSP 70) from tumors undergoing cell death [25]. As quickly as within a few hours after cryosurgery, polymorphonuclear (PMN) leukocytes are also recruited to the lesion site and infiltrate the area. Their migration peaks after 3 days and occurs along with an increasing macrophage infiltration that peaks at 7 days [26]. NK cell activity was also shown to increase in a mammary adenocarcinoma mouse model after cryoablation [1].

Following innate immunity activation, the acquired immune response begins with the actions of antigen-presenting cells (APCs). APCs, namely, macrophages and dendritic cells (DCs), engulf the antigens released by cryoablation and present them to T cells via major histocompatibility complex (MHC) classes I and II. A cytotoxic and humoral response develops with APC presentation of antigen to lymphocytic cells. Once antigens are endocytosed by DCs, these cells migrate to lymph nodes where they undergo maturation, becoming efficient APCs able to prime naïve antigen specific T cells. In response to inflammatory and antigenic signals, DCs that have been loaded with endocytosed cryotreated tumor cell fragments upregulate their maturation gene expression including IL-1, Fas, CDKN1A, osteoprotegerin, and CXCR4, as

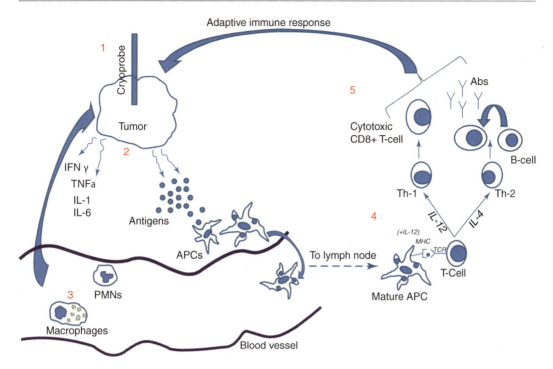

Fig. 24.2 Inflammation and immune system activation after cryoablation. (*1*) Cryoprobe freezes tumor and associated stroma resulting in (*2*) the release of antigens and inflammatory cytokines (i.e., IFN-gamma, TNF-alpha, IL-1, IL-6) from tumor and extracellular matrix. (*3*) Innate immune cells such as macrophages and polymorphonuclear cells (PMNs) migrate to cryolesion in response to chemotaxis caused by inflammatory cytokines and contribute to the inflammatory milieu. (*4*) Antigen-presenting cells (APCs) including dendritic cells and macrophages endocytose antigens, migrate to lymph nodes where they mature, and present antigens to naïve T cells in the presence of cytokines such as IL-12. (*5*) T cells differentiate into Th1 or Th2 cells in the presence of IL-12 or IL-4, respectively. Th1 cells undergo differentiation into cytotoxic T cells, whereas Th2 cells contribute to the differentiation of B cells into antibody producing cells marking the initiation of the adaptive immune response

well as their expression of immunostimulatory cytokines including IL-1β, IL-12p40, IL-15, TNF-α, and IFN-γ. DC maturation estimated by flow cytometric measurement of the surface marker CD86, a ligand that participates in T-cell priming, was shown to increase 8-fold after freezing prostate cancer cells [27]. Moreover, the expression of class-II MHC, which is a required component of antigen presentation and activation of T cells, was doubled.

As APCs present antigens to naïve helper T cells (Th) in the presence of IL-12, T-cell differentiation into Th1 cells occurs. Th1 cells release IL-2, IL-12, IFN-γ, TNF-α, and GM-CSF, which in turn participate in activating cytotoxic (CD8) T cells. B-cell proliferation and differentiation into antibody-producing cells also occur upon expression of IL-4 by naïve helper T cells, resulting in T-cell differentiation into Th2 cells. Th2 cells express IL-4 and IL-5 cytokines, promoting B-cell differentiation into antibody-producing cells. The above-described cascade of events marks the initiation of the adaptive arm of the immune response triggered by cryoablation. This response is specific against the antigens derived from cryoablated cells, possibly priming systemic antitumor activity (Fig. 24.2).

Immunity vs. Tumor Microenvironment

Tumor survival and progression are partly due to their ability to evade the host immune system. Tumor microenvironments appear to modulate immune response by regulating immune cell phenotype and function both locally and systemically. For instance, patients with progressing hepatocellular carcinoma (HCC) have been demonstrated to have increasing levels of peripheral CD4+CD25+ cells, detected by flow cytometry [28]. CD4+CD25+ cells are some of the best-described regulatory T cells (Treg) that down-regulate the immune system. Increases in Treg cell levels have also been shown in other cancers including gastric, lung, pancreatic, and breast cancers [29]. It has been speculated that the response to cryoablation may vary depending on tumor type and the level of Treg cells present. For instance, patients' HCC response after cryoablation with argon-helium cryoprobes to freezing temperatures of −135 °C appeared to be dependent on to the quantities of circulating CD4+Cd25+ Treg cells prior to treatment. Patients with HCC regression after cryoablation showed significantly decreased Treg frequency by flow cytometry. In contrast, patients with HCC progression and recurrence showed increased Treg cells. Treg frequencies were approximately 6.9 % in early stage HCC, 8.8 % in intermediate stage, 10.3 % in advanced stage, and 13.4 % in terminal stage HCC. These results indicate the role of immune downregulation in tumor survival, even after therapy. These data may also help explain why cryoablation is at times ineffective in treating certain tumors. It is likely that adjunctive therapy may be necessary to obtain the full potential antitumor effects of cryotherapy.

Other studies have suggested that cryotherapy may counteract the tumor microenvironment anti-immune activity. The immunological response to cryoablation in a renal cell cancer animal model demonstrated higher IFN-γ to IL-4 levels, suggesting an increase in Th1:Th2 ratio and demonstrating the interplay between inflammatory cytokines and activation of the immune system after cryosurgery. The increase in Th1 to Th2 ratio opposes the anti-immune response effects of renal cell carcinoma (RCC) previously shown [30].

Sabel and colleagues have elegantly demonstrated how rate of freeze could affect the resulting immune response after cryoablation of 4T1 breast carcinoma in BALB/c mice [31]. Two weeks after inoculation of mice with the tumor cells, the animals were divided in four groups (control, surgical resection group, and low- and high-freeze group). High-freeze technique used argon cryoprobe for 30s and duty cycle of 100 %, while low-freeze used the same probe, but with duty cycle of 10 % for several minutes. One week later, high-freeze group demonstrated significant reduction in CD4+CD25+ T-regulatory cells in examined tumor lymph nodes, while the number of cytotoxic CD8+ cells was not significantly affected. Both, low-freeze group and surgery group had dramatically higher Treg levels, producing more immunosuppression and increased levels of lung metastases in the latter. Furthermore, the cytotoxic CD8 T-cell responses to exposure to tumor cells in vitro were almost tripled in the high-freeze group in comparison to low-freeze, surgery, and control. Specific evidence of antitumor activity following cryoablation is discussed in more detail in the following section.

Primary and Metastatic Antitumor Activity

The formation of autoantibodies against cryoablated tissues was demonstrated many decades ago. Early experiments with cryoablation of the rabbit benign prostate, seminal vesicle, and bulbourethral glands showed that autoantibodies specific to these tissues could be isolated from the serum of respective animals. These antibodies did not react with other autologous tissues such as the kidney, liver, or thyroid and did not recognize human-derived tissues, demonstrating the specificity of the antibodies for the cryoablated tissue [32]. Autoantibody formation was detected as early as within 7–10 days of cryoablation. These data led to subsequent studies exploring the generation of immune system-targeted therapy against malignant tissues with cryosurgery. Treatment of prostate cancer with cryoablative techniques has been described more extensively and has shed light into the widespread potential applications of cryoimmunology as primary or adjuvant therapy for cancer. Similar to the above-mentioned investigations with benign prostates, studies performing cryoablation of malignancy-laden prostates demonstrated that serum antibodies specific to prostate cancer antigens were found in the serum after cryosurgery [33]. Interestingly, despite increased antibody levels, actual secondary tumor growth and tumor histology were unchanged. Several other reports have suggested similar contradictory data in regard to the actual efficacy of tumor regression after cryotherapy and are discussed in more detail in a separate section below.

Despite some of the skepticism and contradiction in the data, other investigators have demonstrated impressive benefits of cryotherapy for cancer treatment in human patients. A retrospective study comparing the effects of targeted cryoablation of prostate cancer and control therapies including brachytherapy, external beam radiation, or 3-dimensional conformal radiation demonstrated that cryotherapy resulted in equal or superior disease-free rates [34]. The mean follow-up time was 5.3 years and the outcome measures were prostate-specific antigen (PSA)-based cutoffs. No serious complications were reported and only minimal morbidity was observed.

Patients with nonmetastatic prostate cancer have also been treated using a percutaneous approach to cryoablation [35]. Biopsy of treated tissue after percutaneous cryotherapy showed elevated levels of TNF-α and IFN-γ as well as increased Th1:Th2 ratio. A significant increase in peripheral blood mononuclear cells was also shown along with increased cytolytic activity of cytotoxic T lymphocytes against autologous prostate cancer cells. This activity was specific to prostate tissue. It is prudent to note, however, that despite evidence of immune system activation, this approach was not sufficient to prevent cancer relapse. Moreover, the level of differentiation of the prostate tumor cells also plays a role in the effectiveness of cryosurgery. More differentiated tissue proved to be associated with advantageous survival in patients [36], since the capacity for proliferation decreases in cells as they mature and differentiate.

Some of the rationale for the limited effectiveness of cryotherapy in eradicating tumors may be explained by the expression of inhibitory T-cell coreceptor CTLA-4. CTLA-4 binds B-7 at the surface of APCs. Their interaction inhibits T-cell activation by reducing the expression of IL-2. CTLA-4 is the target of a recently FDA-approved antibody drug, ipilimumab, which can diminish this immune inhibitory process and allow a more robust response. Given the potential to enhance the antitumor effects of thermal ablation, the adjuvant use of ipilimumab along with cryotherapy was demonstrated in a recent study [37]. A mouse model of primary prostate cancer treated with combination of cryoablation and ipilimumab was utilized, showing that the growth of secondary tumors seeded at distant sites after initial thermal ablation of the primary tumor (also known as tumor rechallenge) was slowed and tumor rejection was triggered. The secondary tumors were found to be highly infiltrated by CD4+ T cells, as well as CD8+ T cells, and relatively less T-regulatory cells. This cessation in growth was not observed after cryoablation alone. These results are promising and suggest augmentation of antitumor immunity with combination therapy.

Many other types of cancers have been targeted using cryoimmunology. For instance, tumors created by human melanoma cell lines that were xenografted in mice and treated with cryoablation were evaluated for necrosis-induced recruitment of inflammatory cells and induction of immune-mediated activity [26]. After freezing, congestion, edema, and endothelial cell activation were detected, as well as a polymorphonuclear leukocytes infiltration into the tumor. Antibodies against the tumor cells were also detected.

In mammary adenocarcinoma, a striking reduction in the development of tumors was demonstrated in mice after treatment with cryoablation [1]. Mice were first treated with either surgical resection or cryoablation of the primary mammary adenocarcinomas. Later, the same two groups of mice were subjected to rechallenge with the same tumor type, and while the group that had been treated with surgical resection alone developed new tumors 86 % of the time, only 16 % of the group previously treated by cryoablation had recurrence. These data exemplify that cryoablation of the primary tumors likely resulted in an adaptive immune response with memory specific to the tumor type, reducing the development of new tumors/recurrences. The investigators also noted that natural killer (NK) cell activity was increased.

In human studies involving patients with rectal carcinoma, 13 patients with inoperable cases were subjected to cryosurgery [38]. The investigators reported raised concentrations of IgG and IgA in biopsies of the tumors, detected by direct immunofluorescence. Although no prognostic factors were evaluated, the authors proposed that the immunoglobulin increase would likely result in antitumor properties, similar to previous studies in other organ systems. Patients with colon cancers were also treated with cryoablation of their metastatic liver masses [39]. The levels of serum total gangliosides (STGs) and antibody titers against these STGs were measured as an indicator of cryoablative-related necrosis and induction of humoral immunity against colon cancer-specific gangliosides. IgM titers were increased significantly after cryoablation, correlating to the increase in serum ganglioside levels. No increase in IgM was observed against normal tissue gangliosides, again, illustrating the tissue specific immunity.

Given that the immune response against malignant cells is specific and systemic, activity against metastatic cancers have also been shown. It has been proposed that cryoablation of breast cancer prior to surgical resection can be an effective adjuvant therapy in preventing recurrence and reducing metastases in mice [40]. These investigations led to the illustration of increased fraction of tumor-specific T cells as shown by IFN-γ release assay. Strikingly, the number of pulmonary metastases was reduced after cryoablation when compared to surgery alone or controls. The progression of metastasizing comedo-type breast adenocarcinoma in rats were also evaluated after cryotherapy in comparison to surgical resection alone [41]. Ten weeks after local cryotherapy of tumors, rats were rechallenged with breast adenocarcinoma cells. The investigators reported an increased rejection rate of secondary tumors in the cryoablation group compared to surgery alone. Moreover, the number of lymph node metastases and tumor weight was also lower.

Splenic and lymph node reaction to cryotherapy of metastasizing mammary tumor cells were studied in a rat model [2]. It was shown that the spleen increased in weight by 1 week post-treatment and regressed to preoperative values

by 6 weeks. Lymph nodes draining the site of tumor implantation and treatment showed paracortical hyperplasia, histiocytosis, and germinal center hyperplasia, indicating T-cell activation and increased B-cell and macrophage activity. Furthermore, tumor rechallenge after cryosurgery resulted in increased resistance rate that peaked at 10 weeks post-cryoablation.

Conflicting Data

The size and amount of tissue that is cryoablated may play a significant role in whether the immune response is stimulated or actually suppressed. For instance, when myosarcoma and carcinosarcoma tumors were treated with cryosurgery, regression of secondary tumors was observed if a large portion of the cryoablated tumor was also concomitantly removed surgically during therapy. Interestingly, the antitumor immune response was suppressed if most of the cryoablated tissue was not removed [42]. Perhaps the anti-immunity properties of the tumor microenvironment involving CD25+ Treg cells, even after cryoablation as discussed previously, may overcome immune activation and protect against immune attack locally. Surviving malignant cells may then repopulate the area and reform tumors resulting in cancer recurrence.

Similarly, liver metastases appear to respond in the same fashion [43]. When only a single colon cancer-derived metastatic liver nodule was treated with cryoablation in a mouse model, the overall number of metastatic liver nodules and size of primary tumor was reduced. However, if multiple nodules were treated, an actual increase in the number of lesions was found, although this difference was not statistically significant.

It is important to mention that many of the studies reporting conflicting results (including actual tumor progression upon cryodestruction) did not standardize their methodology entirely, which has varied significantly from the type of the tumor studied, the presence or absence of pre-existing immune recognition of the tumor by the host, the method and volume of tissue frozen, as well as the timing of the monitoring and detection of immune response.

Fig. 24.3 Immunology
of cryoinjury – a summary

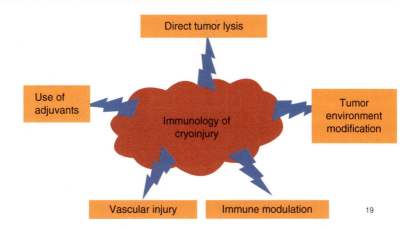

Cryosurgery Adjuvants

Molecular adjuvants can be used to enhance cryodestruction within frozen tumors. The use of adjuvants is bifactorial; first, it could increase control of local disease in the area of cryoinjury, reducing risk for local recurrence; second, it could decrease complications due of overfreezing into adjacent healthy tissues near the treatment site, enhancing the wound healing and postsurgical recovery. The adjuvants can be broadly categorized into three groups: (a) thermophysical adjuvants, which enhance the injury caused by ice formation; (b) chemotherapeutic approaches that act at a molecular level to induce apoptosis; and (c) cytokines or vascular-based agents that modulate the inflammatory response or stimulate immune cells to enhance tissue destruction. The most common thermophysical adjuvants are glycine and eutectic salts, studied in human breast and rat prostate tumors, respectively. Chemotherapy agents, like 5-FU and doxorubicin, have been used systemically 1–4 days before cryoablation of prostate or hepatoma, respectively. The potential for tumor necrosis factor-alpha (TNF-α) and imiquimod in enhancing vasodilatation, apoptosis, and immune response upon cryoablation has been analyzed in prostate and breast cancers as well.

Some common factors to be considered once cryosurgery adjuvants are selected include (a) the sensitivity of the tumor to the adjuvant, (b) the selectivity of the adjuvant toward the tissue, (c) the dose of the adjuvant needed to enhance injury in the temperature range (up to −0.5 °C), (d) side effects associated with the adjuvant, (e) the mode of delivery of the adjuvant, and (f) the time of application of the adjuvant relative to cryosurgery procedure [44]. A summary of some of the mechanisms involved in the immunology of cryoinjury is shown in Fig. 24.3.

Conclusion

It is not surprising that there is tremendous interest in immunological aspects of cryosurgery, since cryoablation has the potential for both local and systemic therapy, i.e., direct ablation of the tumor and eradication of micrometastases through the immune system with minimal systemic toxicity. However, the generation of antitumor immune response is complex, and several factors may contribute not only to a positive response but also tilt it to the opposite direction, including immune suppression. Further directions would possibly include clarification of (1) cytokine profile triggered by cryoablation, (2) the availability of the antigens and the forms of their presentation to be processed by antigen-presenting cells, (3) the timing of the immune response post cryoinjury, (4) ideal ratio of apoptosis vs. necrosis for induction of immunoprotective and not immunosuppressive response, (5) the type and subsets of phagocytic cells responsible for clearing of tumor debris (dendritic cells vs. macrophages), and (6) the effects of freezing on tumor microenvironment, vascularity, and suppressive T-regulatory cells.

As the field of cryosurgery continues to expand, extensive research in the mechanism of the immunomodulatory effects of cryo-injury is mandatory as any potential for further decrease of immune response could be detrimental for the patient. On the contrary, induction or augmentation of positive immune response, if triggered by use of proper and controlled cryotechnique, especially with the use of adjuvants, could make this modality a very attractive approach to cancer treatment. The use of single modality for the destruction of tumor and control of its micrometastases with little toxicity has always been the ultimate, although not yet achieved, goal of modern cancer therapy.

Glossary

APCs Antigen-presenting cells
Cryoimmunology process that involves a specific immune response formed against antigens and debris derived from cells and tissues destroyed by cryosurgery.
DCs Dendritic cells
MHC Major histocompatibility complex
RCC Renal cell carcinoma

References

1. Sabel MS, Nehs MA, Su G, Lowler KP, Ferrara JL, Chang AE. Immunologic response to cryoablation of breast cancer. Breast Cancer Res Treat. 2005; 90:97–104.
2. Miya K, Saji S, Morita T, Niwa H, Takao H, Kida H, et al. Immunological response of regional lymph nodes after tumor cryosurgery: experimental study in rats. Cryobiology. 1986;23:290–5.
3. Osada S, Imai H, Tomita H, Tokuyama Y, Okumura N, Matsuhashi N, et al. Serum cytokine levels in response to hepatic cryoablation. J Surg Oncol. 2007; 95:491–8.
4. He T, Tang C, Xu S, Moyana T, Xiang J. Nterferon gamma stimulates cellular maturation of dendritic cell line DC2.4 leading to induction of efficient cytotoxic T cell responses and antitumor immunity. Cell Mol Immunol. 2007;4:105–11.
5. Matin SF, Sharma P, Gill IS, Tannenbaum C, Hobart MG, Novick AC, et al. Immunological response to renal cryoablation in an in vivo orthotopic renal cell carcinoma murine model. J Urol. 2010;183:333–8.
6. Gursel E, Roberts M, Veenema RJ. Regression of prostatic cancer following sequential cryotherapy to the prostate. J Urol. 1972;108:928–32.
7. Ablin RJ, Soanes WA, Gonder MJ. Immuno-cryourogenital treatment of benign and malignant diseases of the prostate. Gerontol Clin. 1970;12:302–13.
8. Staren ED, Sabel MS, Gianakakis LM, Wiener GA, Hart VM, Gorski M, et al. Cryosurgery of breast cancer. Arch Surg. 1997;132:28–33; discussion 4.
9. Wong LL, Limm WM, Cheung AH, Fan FL, Wong LM. Hepatic cryosurgery: early experience in Hawaii. Hawaii Med J. 1995;54:811–3.
10. Crews KA, Kuhn JA, McCarty TM, Fisher TL, Goldstein RM, Preskitt JT. Cryosurgical ablation of hepatic tumors. Am J Surg. 1997;174:614–7; discussion 7–8.
11. Wang ZS. Cryosurgery in rectal carcinoma–report of 41 cases. Zhonghua Zhong Liu Za Zhi. 1989; 11:226–7.
12. Blackwood CE, Cooper IS. Response of experimental tumor systems to cryosurgery. Cryobiology. 1972;9: 508–15.
13. Privalov PL. Cold denaturation of proteins. Crit Rev Biochem Mol Biol. 1990;25:281–305.
14. Mazur P, Rall WF, Leibo SP. Kinetics of water loss and the likelihood of intracellular freezing in mouse ova. Influence of the method of calculating the temperature dependence of water permeability. Cell Biophys. 1984;6:197–213.
15. Baust JG, Gage AA. The molecular basis of cryosurgery. BJU Int. 2005;95:1187–91.
16. Yang G, Zhang A, Xu LX. Intracellular ice formation and growth in MCF-7 cancer cells. Cryobiology. 2011;63:38–45.
17. Tatsutani K, Rubinsky B, Onik G, Dahiya R. Effect of thermal variables on frozen human primary prostatic adenocarcinoma cells. Urology. 1996;48:441–7.
18. Hanai A, Yang WL, Ravikumar TS. Induction of apoptosis in human colon carcinoma cells HT29 by sublethal cryo-injury: mediation by cytochrome c release. Int J Cancer. 2001;93:526–33.
19. Weber SM, Lee Jr FT, Chinn DO, Warner T, Chosy SG, Mahvi DM. Perivascular and intralesional tissue necrosis after hepatic cryoablation: results in a porcine model. Surgery. 1997;122:742–7.
20. Glasgow SC, Ramachandran S, Csontos KA, Jia J, Mohanakumar T, Chapman WC. Interleukin-1beta is prominent in the early pulmonary inflammatory response after hepatic injury. Surgery. 2005;138:64–70.
21. Seifert JK, Junginger T. Cryotherapy for liver tumors: current status, perspectives, clinical results, and review of literature. Technol Cancer Res Treat. 2004;3:151–63.
22. Bishoff JT, Chen RB, Lee BR, Chan DY, Huso D, Rodriguez R, et al. Laparoscopic renal cryoablation: acute and long-term clinical, radiographic, and pathologic effects in an animal model and application in a clinical trial. J Endourol. 1999;13:233–9.
23. Chosy SG, Nakada SY, Lee Jr FT, Warner TF. Monitoring renal cryosurgery: predictors of tissue necrosis in swine. J Urol. 1998;159:1370–4.

24. Campbell SC, Krishnamurthi V, Chow G, Hale J, Myles J, Novick AC. Renal cryosurgery: experimental evaluation of treatment parameters. Urology. 1998;52:29–33; discussion 33–4.

25. Todryk S, Melcher AA, Hardwick N, Linardakis E, Bateman A, Colombo MP, et al. Heat shock protein 70 induced during tumor cell killing induces Th1 cytokines and targets immature dendritic cell precursors to enhance antigen uptake. J Immunol. 1999;163:1398–408.

26. Gazzaniga S, Bravo A, Goldszmid SR, Maschi F, Martinelli J, Mordoh J, et al. Inflammatory changes after cryosurgery-induced necrosis in human melanoma xenografted in nude mice. J Invest Dermatol. 2001;116:664–71.

27. Ismail M, Morgan R, Harrington K, Davies J, Pandha H. Immunoregulatory effects of freeze injured whole tumour cells on human dendritic cells using an in vitro cryotherapy model. Cryobiology. 2010;61: 268–74.

28. Zhou L, Fu JL, Lu YY, Fu BY, Wang CP, An LJ, et al. Regulatory T cells are associated with post-cryoablation prognosis in patients with hepatitis B virus-related hepatocellular carcinoma. J Gastroenterol. 2010;45:968–78.

29. Baecher-Allan C, Anderson DE. Regulatory cells and human cancer. Semin Cancer Biol. 2006;16: 98–105.

30. Rayman P, Wesa AK, Richmond AL, Das T, Biswas K, Raval G, et al. Effect of renal cell carcinomas on the development of type 1 T-cell responses. Clin Cancer Res. 2004;10:6360S–6.

31. Sabel MS, Su G, Griffith KA, Chang AE. Rate of freeze alters the immunologic response after cryoablation of breast cancer. Ann Surg Oncol. 2010;17:1187–93.

32. Shulman S, Brandt EJ, Yantorno C. Studies in cryo-immunology. II. Tissue and species specificity of the autoantibody response and comparison with iso-immunization. Immunology. 1968;14: 149–58.

33. Hoffmann NE, Coad JE, Huot CS, Swanlund DJ, Bischof JC. Investigation of the mechanism and the effect of cryoimmunology in the Copenhagen rat. Cryobiology. 2001;42:59–68.

34. Bahn DK, Lee F, Badalament R, Kumar A, Greski J, Chernick M. Targeted cryoablation of the prostate: 7-year outcomes in the primary treatment of prostate cancer. Urology. 2002;60:3–11.

35. Si TG, Guo Z, Wang HT, Han YP, Hao XS. Cryoablation for prostate cancer induces tumor-specific immune response. Zhonghua Nan Ke Xue. 2009; 15:350–3.

36. Petersen DS, Milleman LA, Rose EF, Bonney WW, Schmidt JD, Hawtrey CE, et al. Biopsy and clinical course after cryosurgery for prostatic cancer. J Urol. 1978;120:308–11.

37. Waitz R, Solomon SB, Petre EN, Trumble AE, Fasso M, Norton L, et al. Potent induction of tumor immunity by combining tumor cryoablation with anti-CTLA-4 therapy. Cancer Res. 2012;72:430–9.

38. Kogel HGR, Fohlmeister I, Pichlmaier H. Cryotherapy of rectal cancer. Immunologic results. Zentralbl Chir. 1985;110:147–54.

39. Ravindranath MH, Wood TF, Soh D, Gonzales A, Muthugounder S, Perez C, et al. Cryosurgical ablation of liver tumors in colon cancer patients increases the serum total ganglioside level and then selectively augments antiganglioside IgM. Cryobiology. 2002;45:10–21.

40. Sabel MS, Arora A, Su G, Chang AE. Adoptive immunotherapy of breast cancer with lymph node cells primed by cryoablation of the primary tumor. Cryobiology. 2006;53:360–6.

41. Misao A, Sakata K, Saji S, Kunieda T. Late appearance of resistance to tumor rechallenge following cryosurgery. A study in an experimental mammary tumor of the rat. Cryobiology. 1981;18:386–9.

42. Sabel MS. Cryo-immunology: a review of the literature and proposed mechanisms for stimulatory versus suppressive immune responses. Cryobiology. 2009;58:1–11.

43. Urano M, Tanaka C, Sugiyama Y, Miya K, Saji S. Antitumor effects of residual tumor after cryoablation: the combined effect of residual tumor and a protein-bound polysaccharide on multiple liver metastases in a murine model. Cryobiology. 2003; 46:238–45.

44. Goel R, Anderson K, Slaton J, Schmidlin F, Vercellotti G, Belcher J, et al. Adjuvant approaches to enhance cryosurgery. J Biomech Eng. 2009;131:074003.

Photodynamic Therapy

25

Raffaella Sala, Maria Teresa Rossi, and Piergiacomo
Calzavara-Pinton

Key Points

- In the treatment of AK and superficial BCC, MAL-PDT is at least as effective as other types of treatment such as cryosurgery and surgery.
- MAL-PDT shows some important advantages: excellent cosmetic results, a non-invasive technique without bleeding and local anaesthesia.
- MAL-PDT seems useful in the treatment of patients with multiple lesions or wide lesions and patients with lesions in surgically difficult areas.

Introduction

Photodynamic therapy (PDT) is a therapeutic technique involving the delivery of a photosensitiser followed by irradiation with visible light at doses that are not harmful in themselves. The photoactivated drug sensitises intracellular molecular oxygen to generate reactive oxygen species (ROS), such as singlet oxygen, hydroxylic radical, superoxide anion and hydrogen peroxide, that

damage cells by inducing necrosis, apoptosis and the production of inflammatory mediators [1].

In the past decade, PDT with topical application of protoporphyrin IX (PpIX)-inducing precursors like 5-aminolevulinic acid (ALA) and its methyl ester (methyl aminolevulinate, MAL) (Metvix®, Galderma, F) showed promising results in the treatment of actinic keratosis (AK), Bowen's disease (BD) and basal cell carcinoma (BCC).

Basic Principles

ALA is not a photosensitiser by itself but it is metabolised to photosensitive PpIX via the intrinsic cellular haem biosynthetic pathway. The only regulatory inhibitor of PpIX production is the intracellular availability of ALA or MAL [1].

MAL is a lipophilic molecule that penetrates cell membranes at a larger extent than hydrophilic ALA. Soon after penetration, MAL is quickly demethylated to ALA, and therefore, the following metabolic steps are the same [2].

ALA through a series of enzymatic conversions is converted into PpIX that diffuses from the mitochondrion into the endoplasmic reticulum as well as the plasma membrane which are the other known sites of cellular damage through PDT [3].

The accumulation of PpIX and other porphyrin intermediates is critically dependent on the activity of ferrochelatase and the availability of iron.

R. Sala • M.T. Rossi
P. Calzavara-Pinton, MD (✉)
Department of Dermatology, University of Brescia,
Piazzale Spedali Civili 1, Brescia 25123, Italy
e-mail: calzavar@mail.unibs.it

A. Baldi et al. (eds.), *Skin Cancer*, Current Clinical Pathology,
DOI 10.1007/978-1-4614-7357-2_25, © Springer Science+Business Media New York 2014

The rate of ALA-induced porphyrin synthesis and accumulation has been shown to be higher in malignant and premalignant cells than in their normal counterparts [4], and a 10:1 ratio of PpIX accumulation in tumours of the keratinocyte lineage in comparison to surrounding healthy skin has been found [5].

In addition, selectivity is strongly favoured by the greater permeability of the abnormal stratum corneum overlying tumoural and inflammatory skin diseases.

PpIX, through its extensive network of alternating double bonds, is essential for transfer of singlet oxygen species and the generation of ROS. These species are relatively short lived, with a radius of only 0.01 μm, and thus have low mutagenic potential for nonlocalised DNA damage [6].

Light Sources

PDT of dermatological conditions is made easy by the accessibility of the skin to light application. The most suitable light source has the emission spectrum (i.e. the plot of the power output at any single wavelength) matching the absorption spectrum (i.e. the plot of the absorption coefficient at any single wavelength) of the photosensitiser. PpIX has a high absorption peak corresponding to the Soret band at about 405 nm and other lower absorption maxima, the Q bands, at approximately 510, 545, 580 and 630 nm. However, 625–633 nm red light is generally used in clinical practice because it allows for a deeper penetration into the skin.

Light sources available for PDT belong to three broad groups: broadband lamps, diode lamps and lasers.

Broadband metal-halogen, e.g. slide projector lamps, or fluorescent lamps are cheap and have a high power density that keeps light exposure times within practical limits. The emission of metal-halogen lamps is white spanning over the whole visible range or can be equipped with optical filters that allow a waveband of 100–200 nm to pass. The only fluorescent lamp useful for PDT is the Blu-U® light system with an emission peak in the Soret band.

Light-emitting diodes (LEDs) are small solid-state semiconductors with a high and reliable emission in a narrow bandwidth of 20–50 nm. They are cheap, simple to use and can be arranged in grids or panels in order to give a broad field of illumination.

Lasers provide a high fluence of monochromatic light and a highly homogeneous light beam, but they are expensive, have low reliability and portability and can illuminate only small areas of the skin surface.

Light doses are principally related to the emission spectrum of the light dose and the peak of absorption of the drug. For example, after MAL sensitisation, 37 J/cm² of light from a LED lamp peaking at 630 nm or 75–100 J/cm² of a filtered incoherent lamp centred in the red waveband gives similar biological effects [7].

Practical Considerations and Applications

The only topical photosensitising product that is licensed in Europe is Metvix® cream (Galderma, F) containing 160 mg/g of the methyl-derivative ester. It is approved for the treatment of actinic keratosis (AK), Bowen's disease (BD) and basal cell carcinoma (BCC) (see Figs. 25.1, 25.2 and 25.3). The optimal treatment protocol has been standardised: Metvix® is applied on the lesion and 3–5 mm of the surrounding healthy skin under an occlusive and light-protecting dressing before being irradiated with 75 J/cm² of red light from a high-pressure filtered lamp or 37 J/cm² of light from a diode lamp with an emission peak at 632 nm. The irradiation should be carried out at the time of maximum concentration in the target tissue. With ALA this is variable and not easily predictable (4–6 h), whereas with MAL it is after about 3 h.

Crusts and scales, if any, should be removed with keratolytic agents or a superficial curettage before applying the cream [8].

During light exposure, patients may experience a burning sensation or stinging pain. Cooling of the lesions with a fan or spraying iced water during and soon after the treatment is widely used for reducing pain, but, if an extended irradiation

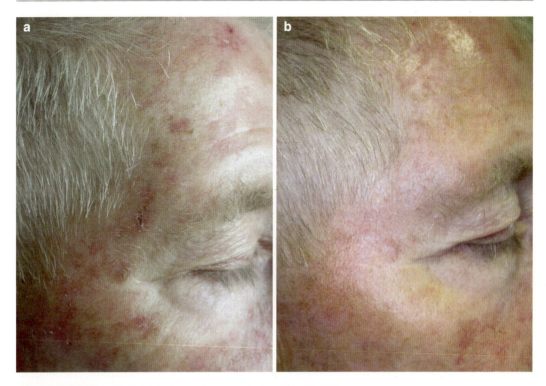

Fig. 25.1 Actinic keratosis of the face before (**a**) and after (**b**) MAL-PDT

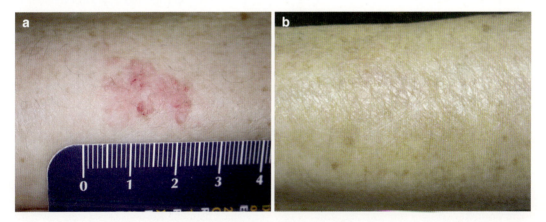

Fig. 25.2 Bowen's disease of the forearm before (**a**) and after (**b**) MAL-PDT

field or severely photodamaged skin has to be treated, the administration of oral analgesics is also necessary [9]. The application of local analgesics like eutectic mixtures of lidocaine/prilocaine prior to irradiation overlapping the incubation period of MAL is not recommended as their high pH might chemically inactivate the photosensitiser [10].

In addition, various inexpensive ALA preparations are on the market and commonly used. However, ALA is included in the European list of orphan drugs to be used only in the photodiagnosis of bladder cancer. Therefore, their use must be authorised by the local Ethical Committee. Other main limitations are that the treatment protocol is not standardised and treatment results are not

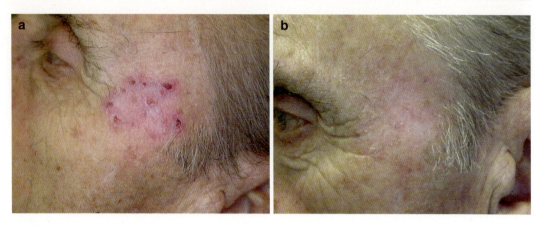

Fig. 25.3 Basal cell carcinoma of the zygomatic area before (**a**) and after (**b**) MAL-PDT

comparable. A 20 % ALA emulsion (Levulan® Kerastick, Dusa Pharmaceuticals, INC., Wilmington, MA) is registered for the treatment of AKs in the USA but is not yet available in the EU countries.

Therapeutic Applications

Actinic Keratosis (AKs)

A European multicentre randomised prospective study compared MAL-PDT and cryosurgery for AK. A total of 193 patients with 699 lesions received either a single treatment with MAL-PDT (repeated after 1 week in 8 % of cases) or a double freeze-thaw course of liquid nitrogen cryosurgery. The overall complete response (CR) rates after 3 months were not significantly different: 69 % with MAL-PDT and 75 % with cryosurgery. However, the cosmetic outcomes were deemed excellent (no scarring or hypopigmentation) in 96 % of patients treated with MAL-PDT and in 81 % of those treated with cryosurgery, and the difference was statistically significant [7].

A higher overall complete response rate after 3 months was observed with MAL-PDT (91 %) in 204 Australian patients who received another treatment session after 1 week (Table 25.1). CRs with a single treatment session of cryosurgery (68 %) and placebo (30 %) were significantly lower. Cosmetic outcome was rated excellent in 81 % of MAL-PDT patients versus 51 % of patients treated with cryosurgery [11].

Similar results (89 % CR) were found in 80 American AK patients treated with two sessions of MAL-PDT in a multicentre, randomised, double-blind, placebo-controlled study. The cosmetic outcome was scored good to excellent in more than 90 % of patients [12].

In an open prospective study, 211 patients with 413 thin to moderately thick AKs were randomised to undergo either a single treatment with MAL-PDT (regimen I; $n=105$) or 2 treatments at weekly intervals (regimen II; $n=106$). Thirty-seven lesions (19 %) showing an incomplete response 3 months after a single treatment were retreated. All patients were followed up 3 months after the last treatment. The complete response rate for thin lesions after a single treatment was 93 %, which was similar to 89 % after repeated treatment. Response rates were lower for thicker lesions: 70 % versus 84 %, respectively. However, the overall response rate in patients randomised for the single treatment improved after the second treatment: 88 %. The conclusion of this study was that a single MAL-PDT session is effective for thin AK and repeated treatments are recommended for thicker or non-responding lesions [13].

In a randomised multicentre trial using a side-by-side design, 119 patients with 1,501 lesions

Table 25.1 Clinical trials using topical MAL-PDT for treatment of actinic keratoses

Study	Design	Study size	Dosage regimen	Results
Szeimies et al. [7]	Multicentre randomised prospective study	193 pts with 699 lesions	MAL-PDT with MAL applied 3 h before broad-spectrum red light ($75\ J/cm^2$) vs. single treatment with cryotherapy	CR after 3 months: MAL-PDT, 69 %; cryotherapy, 75 % CO: MAL, 96 %; cryotherapy, 81 %
Freeman et al. [11]	Randomised prospective study	204 pts	MAL-PDT with MAL applied 3 h before broad-spectrum red light ($75\ J/cm^2$) two treatment sessions at weekly intervals vs. single treatment with cryotherapy	CR after 3 months: MAL-PDT, 91 %; cryotherapy, 68 %; placebo, 30 % CO: excellent in MAL-PDT, 81 %; cryotherapy, 51 %
Pariser et al. [12]	Multicentre, randomised, double-blind study	80 pts	MAL-PDT with MAL applied 3 h before broad-spectrum red light ($75\ J/cm^2$) two treatment sessions at weekly intervals vs. placebo	CR at 3 months: MAL, 89 %; placebo,38 % Excellent or good CO >90 %
Tarstedt et al. [13]	Randomised multicentre trial	211 pts with 413 thin to moderately thick AKs	MAL-PDT with MAL applied 3 h before light-emitting diode system (634 nm), $37\ J/cm^2$; one or two treatment sessions at weekly intervals	CR: 89–93 % thin AK, 70–88 % thicker AK
Morton et al. [14]	Randomised multicentre, intraindividual (right-left) study	119 patients with 1,501 lesions	MAL-PDT with MAL applied 3 h before light-emitting diode system (634 nm), $37\ J/cm^2$; one treatment session vs. cryotherapy	CR after 6 months: MAL-PDT, 89.1 %; cryotherapy, 86.1 %. CO better with MAL-PDT
Dragieva et al. [15]	Randomised double-blind trail (transplant recipients)	17 pts with a total number of 129 mild to moderate AKs	MAL-PDT with MAL applied 3 h before broad-spectrum red light ($75\ J/cm^2$) vs. placebo	CR: 90 % MAL-PDT vs. 0 % placebo

CR complete response, *MAL* methyl aminolevulinate, *PDT* photodynamic therapy, *pts* patients, *CO* cosmetic outcome

were treated with MAL-PDT or cryotherapy [14]. Twenty-four weeks after treatment, no significant difference of complete remission rates (MAL-PDT, 89.1 %; cryotherapy, 86.1 %) was seen but patients had a significant better cosmetic result with PDT.

Transplant patients have an increased propensity to develop multiple AKs and an increased transformation rate into invasive squamous cell carcinoma (SCC). Seventeen transplant recipients with a total number of 129 mild to moderate AKs were enrolled in a prospective, randomised, double-blind, placebo-controlled study. Two lesional areas of a patient were randomised for MAL-PDT or placebo cream plus light exposure. MAL-PDT cleared lesional areas in 13 of 17 patients, whereas placebo did not improve treated areas [15]. In an open trial from the same group, 20 transplant recipients and 20 controls with AK or BD underwent either a single or two consecutive treatments of 20 % ALA-PDT [16] and showed similar cure rates after 4 weeks. However, the rates were significantly lower in immunosuppressed patients after 12 and 48 weeks [15, 16]. Table 25.1 summarises the results obtained in the aforementioned studies.

Basal Cell Carcinoma (BCC)

A few multicentre, randomised, prospective and controlled studies of MAL-PDT of both superficial and nodular BCC have been done in the USA, Australia and Europe (Table 25.2). In 59 patients with 350 superficial (thickness <2 mm) BCCs, the complete-clearance response

Table 25.2 Clinical trials using topical MAL-PDT for treatment of basal cell carcinoma

Study	Design	Study size	Dosage regimen	Results
Soler et al. [17]	Retrospective study	350 superficial (thickness <2 mm) BCC	MAL-PDT with MAL applied 3 h before incoherent halogen lamp (50–200 J/cm²)	CR: 89 % after 3 months 79 % after 24–48 months CO excellent or good in 98 % after 24–48 months
Basset-Séguin et al. [18]	Randomised study	60 pts with 114 lesions were treated with MAL and 58 with 105 lesions received cryotherapy (2 freeze-thaw cycles)	MAL-PDT with MAL applied 3 h before broad-spectrum red light (75 J/cm²) two treatment sessions at weekly intervals vs. single treatment with cryotherapy	CR at 5 years: MAL-PDT, 78 %; cryotherapy, 80 % CO excellent in MAL-PDT, 60 %; cryotherapy, 16 %
Foley [19]	Double-blind controlled study	66 pts with nodular BCC	MAL-PDT with MAL applied 3 h before broad-spectrum red light (75 J/cm²) 2–4 treatment sessions depending on response vs. placebo	CR: 73 % MAL-PDT vs. 21 % placebo CO excellent or good in 98 %
Rhodes et al. [20]	Prospective, randomised, multicentre study	97 patients, 50 with 53 lesions treated with MAL-PDT and 47 with 52 lesions treated by excision surgery	MAL-PDT with MAL applied 3 h before broad-spectrum red light (75 J/cm²) 2–4 treatment sessions depending on response	CR at 5 years: MAL-PDT, 76 %; surgery, 96 % CO good to excellent in: MAL-PDT, 87 %; surgery, 54 %
Szeimies et al. [21]	Multicentre, randomised, controlled, open study	196 pts with s-BCC	MAL-PDT with MAL applied 3 h before light-emitting diode system (634 nm), 37 J/cm²; two sessions, 1 week apart, vs. surgery	CR at 3 months: MAL-PDT, 92.2 %; surgery, 99.2 % CR at 12 months: MAL-PDT, 90 %; surgery, 99.2 % CO good to excellent in: PDT, 94 %; surgery, 60 %
Vinciullo et al. [22]	Prospective, multicentre, noncomparative study	102 pts with "difficult-to-treat" lesions	MAL-PDT with MAL applied 3 h before broad-spectrum red light (75 J/cm²), 1–3-cycle treatment	CR: 90 % after 3 months, 84 % after 12 months and 78 % after 24 months CO excellent or good in 79 % after 12 months and 84 % after 24 months

CR complete response, *MAL* methyl aminolevulinate, *PDT* photodynamic therapy, *pts* patients, *CO* cosmetic outcome, *s-BCC* superficial basal cell carcinoma

rate was 89 % after 3 months and 79 % after a follow-up of 24–48 months (median, 35 months). Cosmetic outcome was reported as excellent or good in 98 % of cases [17].

A randomised study compared MAL-PDT (60 patients with 114 superficial BCC) with cryotherapy (58 patients with 105 lesions) (2 freeze-thaw cycles). Patients with an incomplete response at 3 months received 2 further MAL-PDT sessions ($n=20$) or repeated cryotherapy ($n=16$). Hundred lesions treated with MAL-PDT and 93 lesions treated with cryotherapy

were in complete response at 3 months' follow-up. There was no difference in 5-year recurrence rates with either treatment (20 % with cryotherapy vs. 22 % with MAL-PDT, $p=0.86$). However, more patients had an excellent cosmetic outcome with MAL-PDT (60 % vs. 16 % with cryotherapy, $p=0.00078$) [18].

Sixty-six patients with nodular BCC received two sessions of either MAL-PDT or placebo cream plus light exposure in a randomised, double-blind controlled study from Australia. Before MAL application, lesions were surgically debulked. The overall complete response rates were 73 % for MAL-PDT and 21 % for placebo after 6 months [19].

In 97 patients affected by nodular BCC, 50 with 53 lesions were treated with two treatment sessions with MAL-PDT a week apart, and 47 with 52 lesions were treated by excision surgery. After 3 months, the overall cure rates were similar (91 % vs. 98 %). After 24 months, the recurrence rates were higher (10 %) for MAL-PDT than for surgery (2 %). At 5 years, recurrence was documented in 14 % of lesions treated with MAL-PDT versus 4 % of excised lesions ($p = .09$). The cosmetic outcome was good to excellent in 87 % of the patients receiving MAL-PDT versus 54 % with surgery [20].

In a recent multicentre, randomised, controlled, open study of 196 patients with superficial BCC, two sessions of MAL-PDT, 1 week apart (repeated 3 months later if incomplete clinical response), were less effective than excision surgery, 92.2 % versus 99.2 % and, after 12 months, 9.3 % lesions with MAL-PDT recurred and none with surgery. However, cosmetic outcome was statistically superior for MAL-PDT at all time points [21].

Because of the excellent cosmetic results and the lack of surgical invasiveness, MAL-PDT seems particularly well suited for lesions that would otherwise require extensive surgical procedures and/or for patients with contraindications to surgery. In an open, prospective, multicentre, noncomparative study, 102 patients with "difficult-to-treat" superficial and/or nodular BCC, i.e. large lesions, lesions located in the H-zone of the face or in cases where there was a high risk of surgical complications, were treated with MAL-PDT. The estimated complete response rate (assessed using a time-to-event approach) was 90 % after 3 months, 84 % after 12 months and 78 % after 24 months. Overall cosmetic outcome was judged as excellent or good in 79 % of the patients after 12 months and 84 % after 24 months [22]. Similar results were obtained in 94 patients with 123 BCC, who were at risk of complications or who had had poor results using conventional therapies [23].

Bowen's Disease (BD)

BD is approved for MAL-PDT since 2006. BD is an excellent target for PDT given a very low propensity to progress to invasive SCC, estimated at approximately 3 % [24]. The first trials of PDT for BD have used ALA. In general, they enrolled small case series with a total of approximately 200 lesions when results are pooled and cure rates ranged from 82 to 100 % CR of lesions after 6–12 months of follow-up [25–29]. However, widely different application time of ALA (range 4–20 h) and different light sources (red light, green light, blue light, 630-nm laser, 585-nm laser) make it difficult to decipher the optimal treatment parameters using ALA for these lesions.

The efficacy of MAL-PDT in comparison to cryotherapy or 5-FU for BD was investigated in a randomised multicentre trial with 24-month follow-up [30]. Of the 124 lesions treated with MAL-PDT, 93 % had a CR at 3 months versus 86 % with cryotherapy and 83 % with 5-FU. At 12 months, MAL-PDT had statistically greater CR rates compared with cryotherapy (80 % vs. 67 %, $p = 0.047$). At 24 months, relapse rates were 18 % for MAL-PDT, 23 % for cryotherapy and 21 % for 5-FU. Cosmetic outcome was significantly better with MAL-PDT than with the other treatments at 3- and 12-month follow-ups.

With MAL-PDT [31], the 24-months' CR rate for BD was 71 %, whereas microinvasive and invasive SCCs had CR rates of 58 and 26 %, respectively. Clinical thickness, histological depth of invasion and degree of cell atypia were found to negatively impact long-term CR on univariate analysis.

Contraindications

Use of MAL-PDT is contraindicated in patients with a history of porphyria, allergies to porphyrins, sensitivity to any excipients contained in MAL cream or those with sensitivity to any wavelengths of light used for photoactivation. It is not registered for use during pregnancy and in children.

PDT is not recommended for the treatment of pigmented BCCs because of pigment obscuring penetration of light and sclerosing/morpheaform BCCs given their unpredictable borders and dense composition.

Adverse Effects

Local transitory erythema and oedema develop on the sensitised skin during light exposures, and the patients may experience a burning sensation, stinging pain or itching restricted to the irradiated area. These symptoms are usually restricted to the period of irradiation but may last a couple of hours thereafter. With ALA, patients with AK seem to experience more pain than patients with BCC or BD, and the degree of pain correlates with gender (men more than women), size of the lesion (large more than small lesions) and body site (head more than trunk and extremities), but does not depend on treatment dose, age, fluorescence intensity or Fitzpatrick skin type [32].

Postinflammatory hypo- or hyper-pigmentation may occur after irradiation but scarring is rarely seen.

Topical MAL or ALA preparations have no systemic toxicity. MAL, ALA and PpIX have no genotoxic and mutagenic potential because they are excluded from the nucleus [33].

The case of an 82-year-old patient who developed a malignant melanoma on the site of repeated PDT for AKs has been reported. However, the causative connection remains unclear because the patient was previously treated with ultraviolet B phototherapy, a well-known carcinogenic agent [34].

Future Considerations

MAL- or ALA-PDT has proved to eradicate the malignant lesions while causing minimal damage to the normal surrounding tissue.

In the treatment of AK and superficial BCC, MAL-PDT is at least as effective as other types of treatment such as cryosurgery and surgery. However, MAL-PDT shows some important advantages: excellent cosmetic results, a non-invasive

technique without bleeding and local anaesthesia. It seems particularly useful in the treatment of patients with multiple lesions or wide lesions and patients with lesions in surgically difficult areas, e.g. near orifices or on the central part of the face. If results are partial or in case of relapse, MAL-PDT can be repeated several times until clinical remission occurs because it does not create a cumulative toxicity, nor does it preclude the use of other methods of treatment in the future.

Glossary

ALA   Aminolevulinic acid
CO   Cosmetic outcome
CR   Complete response
LEDs   Light-emitting diodes
MAL   Methyl aminolevulinate
PDT   Photodynamic therapy
PpIX   Protoporphyrin IX

References

1. Henderson BW, Dougherty TJ. How does photodynamic therapy work? Photochem Photobiol. 1992;55:145–57.
2. Gaullier JM, Berg K, Peng Q, et al. Use of 5-aminolevulinic acid esters to improve photodynamic therapy on cells in culture. Cancer Res. 1997;57:1481–6.
3. Barr H, Kendall C, Reyes Goddard J, et al. Clinical aspects of photodynamic therapy. Sci Prog. 2002;85:131–50.
4. Datta SN, Loh CS, MacRobert AJ, et al. Quantitative studies of the kinetics of 5-aminolaevulinic acid induced fluorescence in bladder transitional cell carcinoma. Br J Cancer. 1998;78:1113–8.
5. Fritsch C, Homey B, Stahl W, et al. Preferential relative porphyrin enrichment in solar keratoses upon topical application of 5-aminolevulinic acid methyl ester. Photochem Photobiol. 2000;71:640–7.
6. Kennedy JC, Pottier RH, Pross DC. Photodynamic therapy with endogenous protoporphyrin IX: basic principles and present clinical experience. J Photochem Photobiol B. 1990;6:143–8.
7. Szeimies RM, Karrer S, Radakovic-Fijan S, et al. Photodynamic therapy using topical methyl 5-aminolevulinate compared with cryotherapy for actinic keratosis: a prospective, randomized study. J Am Acad Dermatol. 2002;47:258–62.
8. Morton CA. Methyl aminolevulinate (Metvix) photodynamic therapy – practical pearls. J Dermatolog Treat. 2003;14 Suppl 3:23–6.

9. Touma D, Yaar M, Whitehead S, et al. A trial of short incubation, broad-area photodynamic therapy for facial actinic keratoses and diffuse photodamage. Arch Dermatol. 2004;140:33–40.

10. Peng Q, Soler AM, Warloe T, et al. Selective distribution of porphyrins in skin thick basal cell carcinoma after topical application of methyl 5-aminolevulinate. J Photochem Photobiol B. 2001;62:140–5.

11. Freeman M, Vinciullo C, Francis D, et al. A comparison of photodynamic therapy using topical methyl aminolevulinate (Metvix) with single cycle cryotherapy in patients with actinic keratosis: a prospective, randomised study. J Dermatolog Treat. 2003;14: 99–106.

12. Pariser DM, Lowe NJ, Stewart DM, et al. Photodynamic therapy with topical methyl aminolevulinate for actinic keratosis: results of a prospective randomised multicenter trial. J Am Acad Dermatol. 2003;48:227–32.

13. Tarstedt M, Rosdahl I, Berne B, et al. A randomized multicenter study to compare two treatment regimens of topical methyl aminolevulinate (Metvix)-PDT in actinic keratosis of the face and scalp. Acta Derm Venereol. 2005;85:424–8.

14. Morton C, Campbell S, Gupta G, et al. Intraindividual, right-left comparison of topical methyl aminolevulinate-photodynamic therapy and cryotherapy in subjects with actinic keratosis: a multicentre, randomized controlled study. Br J Dermatol. 2006;155:1029–36.

15. Dragieva G, Prinz BM, Hafner J, et al. A randomized controlled clinical trial of topical photodynamic therapy with methyl aminolaevulinate in the treatment of actinic keratoses in transplant patients. Br J Dermatol. 2004;151:196–200.

16. Dragieva G, Hafner J, Dummer R, et al. Topical photodynamic therapy in the treatment of actinic keratoses and Bowen's disease in transplant recipients. Transplantation. 2004;77:115–21.

17. Soler AM, Warloe T, Berner A, et al. A follow-up study of recurrence and cosmesis in completely responding superficial and nodular basal cell carcinomas treated with methyl 5-aminolevulinate-based photodynamic therapy alone and with prior curettage. Br J Dermatol. 2001;145:467–71.

18. Basset-Seguin N, Ibbotson SH, Emtestam L, et al. Topical methyl aminolaevulinate photodynamic therapy versus cryotherapy for superficial basal cell carcinoma: a 5 year randomized trial. Eur J Dermatol. 2008;18(5):547–53.

19. Foley P. Clinical efficacy of methyl aminolevulinate (Metvix) photodynamic therapy. J Dermatolog Treat. 2003;14 Suppl 3:15–22.

20. Rhodes LE, de Rie MA, Leifsdottir R, et al. Five-year follow-up of a randomized, prospective trial of topical methyl aminolevulinate photodynamic therapy vs surgery for nodular basal cell carcinoma. Arch Dermatol. 2007;143(9):1131–6.

21. Szeimies RM, Ibbotson S, Murrell DF, et al. A clinical study comparing methyl aminolevulinate photodynamic therapy and surgery in small superficial basal cell carcinoma (8–20 mm), with a 12-month follow-up. J Eur Acad Dermatol Venereol. 2008;22(11):1302–11.

22. Vinciullo C, Elliott T, Francis D, et al. Photodynamic therapy with topical methyl aminolaevulinate for 'difficult-to-treat' basal cell carcinoma. Br J Dermatol. 2005;152:765–72.

23. Horn M, Wolf P, Wulf HC, et al. Topical methyl aminolevulinate photodynamic therapy in patients with basal cell carcinoma prone to complications and poor cosmetic outcome with conventional treatment. Br J Dermatol. 2003;149:1242–9.

24. Kao GF. Carcinoma arising in Bowen's disease. Arch Dermatol. 1986;122:1124–6.

25. Stables GI, Stringer MR, Robinson DJ, et al. Large patches of Bowen's disease treated by topical aminolaevulinic acid photodynamic therapy. Br J Dermatol. 1997;136:957–60.

26. Morton CA, Whitehurst C, Moore JV, et al. Comparison of red and green light in the treatment of Bowen's disease by photodynamic therapy. Br J Dermatol. 2000;143:767–72.

27. Britton JE, Goulden V, Stables G, et al. Investigation of the use of the pulsed dye laser in the treatment of Bowen's disease using 5-aminolaevulinic acid photo-therapy. Br J Dermatol. 2005;153:780–4.

28. Svanberg K, Andersson T, Killander D, et al. Photodynamic therapy of non-melanoma malignant tumours of the skin using topical delta-amino levulinic acid sensitization and laser irradiation. Br J Dermatol. 1994;130:743–51.

29. Fijan S, Honigsmann H, Ortel B. Photodynamic therapy of epithelial skin tumours using delta-aminolaevulinic acid and desferrioxamine. Br J Dermatol. 1995;133:282–8.

30. Morton C, Horn M, Leman J, et al. Comparison of topical methyl aminolevulinate photodynamic therapy with cryotherapy or fluorouracil for treatment of squamous cell carcinoma in situ: results of a multicenter randomized trial. Arch Dermatol. 2006;142: 729–35.

31. Calzavara-Pinton PG, Venturini M, Sala R, et al. Methylaminolaevulinate-based photodynamic therapy of Bowen's disease and squamous cell carcinoma. Br J Dermatol. 2008;159:137–44.

32. Grapengiesser S, Ercson M, Gudmundsson F, et al. Pain caused by photodynamic therapy of skin cancer. Clin Exp Dermatol. 2002;27:493–7.

33. Fuchs J, Weber S, Kaufmann R. Genotoxic potential of porphyrin type photosensitizers with particular emphasis on 5-aminolevulinic acid: implications for clinical photodynamic therapy. Free Radic Biol Med. 2000;28:537–48.

34. Wolf P, Fink-Puches R, Reimann-Weber A, et al. Development of malignant melanoma after repeated topical photodynamic therapy with 5-aminolevulinic acid at the exposed site. Dermatology. 1997;194: 53–4.

Lasers for Skin Cancer

26

Michael P. McLeod, Katherine M. Ferris,
Sonal Choudhary, Yasser A. Alqubaisy,
and Keyvan Nouri

Key Points

- The optimal skin cancer laser therapy should directly target the neoplastic cells, destroy them in a reproducible manner, and only require one treatment.
- Experience on lasers explored for treating skin cancers be be presented including the argon, carbon dioxide (CO_2), erbium-doped yttrium aluminum garnet (Er:YAG), and, most recently, pulse dye lasers will be presented.

- A laser such as CO_2 or Er:YAG may be useful as an adjunctive treatment with secondary use of photodynamic therapy.
- Future considerations include combination of various mapping techniques such as reflectance confocal microscopy or a variant may be able to specifically locate the tumor cells so that a laser may directly target them.

M.P. McLeod, MS • S. Choudhary, MD
Y.A. Alqubaisy, MD
Department of Dermatology and Cutaneous Surgery,
University of Miami Leonard M. Miller School
of Medicine, 1475 N.W. 12 Ave #2175,
Miami, FL 33136, USA

K.M. Ferris, BA
Department of Dermatology and Cutaneous Surgery,
University of Miami Hospital,
Miami, FL, USA

K. Nouri, MD (✉)
Department of Dermatology and Cutaneous Surgery,
University of Miami Leonard M. Miller School
of Medicine, 1475 N.W. 12 Ave #2175,
Miami, FL 33136, USA

Department of Dermatology, Sylvester Comprehensive
Cancer Center/University of Miami Hospital and Clinics,
1475 N.W. 12 Ave #2175, Miami, FL 33136, USA
e-mail: knouri@med.miami.edu

Introduction

Lasers are currently not an effective treatment for skin cancer. However, considerable research has been carried out which has led to a greater understanding of how to develop a laser that is effective for treating skin cancer. The optimal laser therapy should directly target the neoplastic cells, destroy them in a reproducible manner, and only require one treatment.

Lasers offer a number of advantages over the current standards of care, which include Mohs micrographic surgery (MMS), surgical excision, curettage and electrodessication, cryosurgery, and radiation. Available dermatologic lasers are less invasive than standard surgical approaches and are likely to conserve more tissue than MMS. Lasers generally do not produce as large of a scar and are also less likely to lead to a loss of anatomical integrity in delicate areas such as the eye, ear, or genitalia when compared to standard surgical methods.

A. Baldi et al. (eds.), *Skin Cancer*, Current Clinical Pathology,
DOI 10.1007/978-1-4614-7357-2_26, © Springer Science+Business Media New York 2014

Basic Principles

Mohs micrographic surgery uses mapped staged surgical excision along with histological analysis of frozen sections to determine where the surgical margins of the tumor exist in relation to normal tissue. The horizontal histological sections allow nearly 100 % of the surgical margins to be observed under the microscope. Unfortunately, MMS is time-consuming and is limited to fellowship-trained dermatologists.

Surgical excision uses a predetermined surgical margin in relationship to the clinically observed tumor. The surgical margins are determined by the tumor type; for example, basal cell carcinoma requires 4 mm margins, squamous cell carcinoma needs 5 mm margins, and melanoma is dependent upon the Breslow depth with surgical margins varying from 5 mm to 2+ cm. Surgical excisions can be associated with large scars and the large margins can compromise functionality as well as anatomical integrity. Neither surgical excision nor MMS is an optimal treatment for patients with multiple and diffusely located skin cancers such as patients affected by nevoid BCC syndrome, xeroderma pigmentosa, Rothmund-Thomson syndrome, or Gorlin-Goltz syndrome.

Curettage and electrodessication is primarily used for more superficial tumors. It applies an electric current to desiccate the tumor and allows for secondary curetting of the more friable tumor remnants. Unfortunately, this method does not allow for histological analysis and does not successfully treat deeper tumors.

Cryosurgery uses liquid nitrogen to lower the tumor temperature to approximately −50 to −60 °C. It is associated with pain, hypopigmentation, higher recurrence rates for certain tumor types, and also a lack of histological analysis.

Radiation uses X-rays or electron beam therapy to destroy neoplastic tissue. Tissue exposed to radiation therapy tends to atrophy, which worsens with time. This is in contradistinction to scars associated with surgical methods that generally improve with time. This technique can also be time-consuming and, in addition to atrophy, may induce alopecia and even radionecrosis, especially over bony surfaces, since bone is an avid absorber of radiation.

Laser therapy aims to confer sufficient energy to neoplastic tissue in order to cause destruction. The therapeutic approach has evolved from causing diffuse destruction, of both diseased and normal tissue, to more selective targeted therapy. One such target that has shown promise is the vasculature within a tumor, such as that found in basal cell carcinomas. Many newer lasers exploit this target to cause localized tumor destruction. In addition, recent approaches have attempted to apply two different laser wavelengths sequentially or have used lasers as an adjunct to other modalities in order to achieve greater efficacy.

Lasers as a Single Treatment

A number of lasers have been explored for treating skin cancers including the argon, carbon dioxide (CO_2), erbium-doped yttrium aluminum garnet (Er:YAG), and, most recently, the 585 and 595 nm pulse dye lasers. The first lasers used to treat skin cancers and premalignant conditions were the continuous wave (CW), CO_2, and argon lasers. The continuous wave lasers are associated with a significant risk of nonspecific thermal heating and secondarily can result in hypertrophic and atrophic scarring [1, 2]. The pulsed lasers were developed in an effort to minimize these side effects [3–5].

Argon Lasers

The argon laser emits a continuous wavelength of 457–514.5 nm but can also be used in gated and shuttered manners. Originally developed to treat pigmented lesions and port-wine stains, this laser remains limited in application due to its superficial depth of penetration of approximately 1 mm. Based on histological studies, the mechanism of the argon laser involves nonspecific thermal damage owing to exposure intervals beyond the thermal relaxation time of superficial vessels [6]. It has been effectively used to treat Kaposi's sarcoma, a tumor with a well-known vascular component [7]. Similarly, it has been used to effectively treat bowenoid papulosis and Bowen's disease located on the genitalia, both of which are superficial cutaneous tumors [8]. In cases where surgical excision is contraindicated, the argon laser has been used to treat lentigo maligna, albeit not successfully likely due to the atypical melanocytes extending down the adnexal structures deeper than the penetration depth of this laser [9, 10]. This laser has also been used to treat leukoplakia, malignant melanoma, and even metastatic melanoma; however, such reports included insufficient patient numbers to effectively evaluate this treatment [11, 12].

Nd:YAG Lasers

The Nd:YAG lasers penetrate much deeper (4–6 mm) than the argon lasers due to their longer wavelength of 1,064 nm [13]. This particular wavelength targets both normal and neoplastic tissue and destroys them by coagulation necrosis [13]. It has been successful in treating perianal condyloma acuminata as well as hemangiomas [14, 15]. The Nd:YAG has been explored for a diverse number of tumors including Bowen's disease, basal cell carcinoma, actinic keratosis, leukoplakia, Kaposi's sarcoma, and bowenoid papulosis [16–18]. The most successful reports have come from the Russian literature where the pulsed Nd:YAG laser has been used to successfully treat squamous cell carcinoma, basal cell carcinoma, malignant melanoma, and cutaneous metastases of melanoma [7, 19, 20]. One large-scale study involving BCC and SCC by Moskalik et al. [21] demonstrated recurrence rates of 1.8 % for BCCs treated with a pulsed Nd laser, 2.5 % for BCCs treated with the pulsed Nd:YAG laser, while 4.4 % of SCCs treated with pulsed Nd recurred (no SCCs were treated with the Nd:YAG). The follow-up intervals ranged from 3 months to 5 years. These results indicate that the Nd and Nd:YAG lasers may be an effective treatment for BCC and SCC; however, further study is warranted.

Ruby Lasers

The 694 nm ruby laser has been used for treating basal cell carcinoma, squamous cell carcinoma, melanoma, mycosis fungoides, and Kaposi's sarcoma with limited success [12, 22]. Tumors with pigmentation such as pigmented BCC, Kaposi's sarcoma, and melanoma avidly absorb the 694 nm wavelength in comparison to non-pigmented tumors [13]. Despite this feature, the ruby laser has not outperformed other treatment options and further study is not warranted at this time.

CO$_2$ Lasers

The 10,600 nm infrared CO$_2$ laser was the predominant laser previously (prior to the PDL) studied in the treatment of cutaneous skin tumors [1, 8, 14, 22–27]. The 10,600 nm wavelength targets water and can be used for vaporization, coagulation, and cutting. In fact, blood and lymphatic vessels smaller than 0.5 mm in diameter can be sealed by the laser [13]. The CO$_2$ laser can be used to excise the tumor; however, since it causes coagulation to the edges where it cuts, histological analysis is not as accurate as that which occurs with scalpel excisions [13]. The CO$_2$ laser has demonstrated poor results when treating basal cell carcinoma in vaporization mode [23]. It has been used more successfully to treat SCC in situ, including genital lesions which can be associated with significant morbidity following surgical excision [28]. Additionally, the laser has demonstrated clinical efficacy in treating bowenoid papulosis, leukoplakia, actinic cheilitis, and solar keratosis [27, 29–32]. In fact, the CO$_2$ laser in vaporization mode can be considered a treatment of choice for actinic cheilitis, erythroplasia of Queyrat, and bowenoid papulosis due to its success at removing the neoplastic lesion and excellent cosmesis [27, 29, 31].

Erbium-Doped Yttrium Aluminum Garnet Lasers (Er:YAG)

The Er:YAG laser emits light at the 2,940 nm wavelength and has been used for treating actinic keratosis, but has not been extensively explored for treating skin cancers [33, 34]. One retrospective study demonstrated that all actinic keratoses were cleared in 24 patients and 14 (58.3 %) of these patients remained clear at 2-year follow-up [35]. Thus, the Er:YAG may have a role in prophylaxis, but has not been pursued as a therapeutic option for cancerous lesions. Clearly, more study is warranted for actinic keratoses.

Pulse Dye Lasers

The pulse dye lasers may be uniquely suited for treating basal cell carcinoma due to the fact that a unique microvasculature supplies the tumor [36]. The 585 and 595 nm pulse dye lasers (PDL) have been investigated for treating basal cell carcinoma. The pulse dye laser is known to target primarily vascular structures. Oxyhemoglobin has a light absorption peak at 577 nm, while deoxyhemoglobin has a broader peak which overlaps both the 542 and 577 nm peaks of oxyhemoglobin [37]. These wavelengths are close to the yellow light emitted by both the 585 and 595 nm wavelengths of pulse dye lasers. Basal cell carcinoma is known to exhibit a small microvasculature system (telangiectasias) of approximately 20 μm in diameter [36]. The pulse dye laser can be used to specifically target basal cell carcinoma's vascular system, rather than the actual tumor cells itself. Shah et al. used the 595 nm PDL along with a fluence of 15 J/cm^2, a 7 mm spot size, 10 % overlap, and 4 mm of normal surrounding skin irradiated in a series of four treatments with a follow-up time of 2–4 weeks to destroy 91.7 % of the BCCs under 1.5 cm. However, larger BCCs (those greater than 1.5 cm in diameter) only cleared 25 % of the time [38]. In a study with a longer follow-up time of 1 year and a higher number of basal cell carcinomas, Konnikov et al. reported that 19 of 20 or 95 % of BCCs, irrespective of size, were cleared with four treatments with the 595 nm PDL at similar settings as the previous study but with 20/30 ms of dynamic cooling device (DC), irradiating the tumor with one pass and also 4 mm of normal surrounding skin [39]. Unfortunately, 7 out of the 20 patients refused to allow any form of histological analysis after 21 months. This makes it difficult to conclude that 19/20 tumors did not recur in the following 21 months but also

highlights a strength or advantage to laser therapy and, notably, that the cosmetic results were so good that the patients did not want to mar their lasered site with a surgical scar [39]. Campolmi et al. used only clinical observation as a measure of efficacy and reported that 16/20 BCCs were cleared with the pulse dye laser. Unfortunately, and similar to the Konnikov et al. study, it is very difficult to ascertain whether residual BCC exists when no histological measurements are taken. It should also be noted that even if residual BCC exists, the ensuing inflammatory response triggered by the laser (tissue damage) may actually assist in removing the remainder of the tumor, as biopsy alone cures 23.5 % of BCCs.

Laser Combined with Photodynamic Therapy

A laser such as the CO_2 or Er:YAG ablative laser may be useful as an adjunctive treatment with secondary use of photodynamic therapy. It is thought that the initial laser can reduce the tumor size so that PDT can readily clear the remaining tumor cells. PDT is already used to treat actinic keratoses, but is limited by its depth of penetration of only 2 mm [40]. In 2007, a combined approach using the CO_2 ablative laser along with photodynamic therapy using methyl aminolevulinate as a photosensitizer demonstrated that all 13 BCCs responded to treatment with no recurrences noted during a mean follow-up period of 18.1 months [41]. In 2008, another combined laser and PDT approach was explored using the Er:YAG laser and topical aminolevulinic acid as the photosensitizer [40]. This study compared three different treatment regimens: the Er:YAG laser alone, PDT alone, and the Er:YAG laser to the basal cell carcinoma first for debulking, followed by PDT [40]. The combined approach with the Er:YAG laser followed by PDT demonstrated the most clinical efficacy with an overall clearance rate of 98.97 % compared to 91.75 % for the Er:YAG laser alone and 94.85 % for PDT alone. It should also be noted that the combined Er:YAG laser with PDT had the best cosmetic outcome in comparison to the other two approaches [40].

Future Considerations

Current laser technology does not specifically target the neoplastic cells. Future techniques are likely to directly target the tumor cells and destroy them with one treatment. Additionally, various mapping techniques such as reflectance confocal microscopy or a variant may be able to specifically locate the tumor cells so that a laser may directly target those cells. This technology utilizes a focused near-infrared light to illuminate a small tissue site which is imaged onto a detector through a small aperture. The result is visualization of thin tissue planes in vivo, with resolution comparable to traditional histology [6]. This and/or its variant will likely facilitate localization of the tumor cells within the cutaneous tissue, so that the laser could be aimed in the appropriate direction to eradicate the tumors, without the need for biopsy or other invasive approaches.

Glossary

CW Continuous wave
Er:YAG Erbium-doped yttrium aluminum garnet
Nd-YAG Neodymium-doped yttrium aluminum garnet

References

1. Wheeland RG, Bailin PL, Ratz JL, et al. Carbon dioxide laser vaporization and curettage in the treatment of large or multiple superficial basal cell carcinomas. J Dermatol Surg Oncol. 1987;13:119–25.
2. Olbricht SM, Stern RS, Tang SV, et al. Complications of cutaneous laser surgery. A survey. Arch Dermatol. 1987;123:345–9.
3. Kauvar AN, Waldorf HA, Geronemus RG. A histopathological comparison of "char-free" carbon dioxide lasers. Dermatol Surg. 1996;22:343–8.
4. Trelles MA, David LM, Rigau J. Penetration depth of ultrapulse carbon dioxide laser in human skin. Dermatol Surg. 1996;22:863–5.
5. Cotton J, Hood AF, Gonin R, et al. Histologic evaluation of preauricular and postauricular human skin after high-energy, short-pulse carbon dioxide laser. Arch Dermatol. 1996;132:425–8.
6. Tanzi EL, Lupton JR, Alster TS. Lasers in dermatology: four decades of progress. J Am Acad Dermatol. 2003;49:1–31; quiz 31–4.
7. Wheeland RG, Bailin PL, Norris MJ. Argon laser photocoagulative therapy of Kaposi's sarcoma: a clinical and histologic evaluation. J Dermatol Surg Oncol. 1985;11:1180–5.
8. Landthaler M, Haina D, Brunner R, et al. Laser therapy of bowenoid papulosis and Bowen's disease. J Dermatol Surg Oncol. 1986;12:1253–7.
9. Arndt KA. New pigmented macule appearing 4 years after argon laser treatment of lentigo maligna. J Am Acad Dermatol. 1986;14:1092.
10. Arndt KA. Argon laser treatment of lentigo maligna. J Am Acad Dermatol. 1984;10:953–7.
11. Goldman L. Surgery by laser for malignant melanoma. J Dermatol Surg Oncol. 1979;5:141–4.
12. Goldman L, Schwartz RA. Current development for laser surgery for skin cancer. In: Schwartz RA, editor. Skin cancer- recognition and management. New York: Spring; 1988. p. 346.
13. Geronemus R, Ashinoff R. Lasers in the treatment of skin cancer. Dermatol Clin. 1991;9:765–76.
14. Stein BS. Laser treatment of condylomata acuminata. J Urol. 1986;136:593–4.
15. Achauer BM, Vander Kam VM. Capillary hemangioma (strawberry mark) of infancy: comparison of argon and Nd:YAG laser treatment. Plast Reconstr Surg. 1989;84:60–9; discussion 70.
16. Brunner R, Landthaler M, Haina D, et al. Treatment of benign, semimalignant, and malignant skin tumors with the Nd:YAG laser. Lasers Surg Med. 1985;5:105–10.
17. Landthaler M, Haina D, Brunner R, et al. Neodymium-YAG laser therapy for vascular lesions. J Am Acad Dermatol. 1986;14:107–17.
18. Wishnow KI, Johnson DE. Effective outpatient treatment of Kaposi's sarcoma of the urethral meatus using the neodymium:YAG laser. Lasers Surg Med. 1988;8:428–32.
19. Keller GS, Doiron DR, Fisher GU. Photodynamic therapy in otolaryngology – head and neck surgery. Arch Otolaryngol. 1985;111:758–61.
20. Wagner RI, Kozlov AP, Moskalik KG. Laser radiation therapy of skin melanoma. Strahlentherapie. 1981;157:670–2.
21. Moskalik K, Kozlov A, Demin E, et al. The efficacy of facial skin cancer treatment with high-energy pulsed neodymium and Nd:YAG lasers. Photomed Laser Surg. 2009;27:345–9.
22. Goldman L, Wilson RG. Treatment of basal cell epithelioma by laser radiation. JAMA. 1964;189:773–5.
23. Adams EL, Price NM. Treatment of basal-cell carcinomas with a carbon-dioxide laser. J Dermatol Surg Oncol. 1979;5:803–6.
24. Bailin PL. Use of the CO_2 laser for non-port-wine-stain cutaneous lesions. In: Arndt K, Noe JM, Rosen S, editors. Cutaneous laser therapy: principles and methods. New York: Wiley; 1983. p. 187–99.

25. Bilik R, Kahanovich S, Rubin M, et al. Morbidity and recurrence rates after surgical treatment of malignant melanoma by scalpel versus CO2 laser beam. Surg Gynecol Obstet. 1987;165:333–8.
26. Lejeune FJ, Van Hoof G, Gerard A. Impairment of skin graft take after CO2 laser surgery in melanoma patients. Br J Surg. 1980;67:318–20.
27. Stanley RJ, Roenigk RK. Actinic cheilitis: treatment with the carbon dioxide laser. Mayo Clin Proc. 1988;63:230–5.
28. Shimizu I, Cruz A, Chang KH, et al. Treatment of squamous cell carcinoma in situ: a review. Dermatol Surg. 2011;37:1394–411.
29. Bain L, Geronemus R. The association of lichen planus of the penis with squamous cell carcinoma in situ and with verrucous squamous carcinoma. J Dermatol Surg Oncol. 1989;15:413–7.
30. Eliezri YD. The toluidine blue test: an aid in the diagnosis and treatment of early squamous cell carcinomas of mucous membranes. J Am Acad Dermatol. 1988;18:1339–49.
31. Greenbaum SS, Glogau R, Stegman SJ, et al. Carbon dioxide laser treatment of erythroplasia of Queyrat. J Dermatol Surg Oncol. 1989;15:747–50.
32. King CM, Yates VM, Dave VK. Multicentric pigmented Bowen's disease of the genitalia associated with carcinoma in situ of the cervix. Br J Vener Dis. 1984;60:406–8.
33. Wollina U, Konrad H, Karamfilov T. Treatment of common warts and actinic keratoses by Er:YAG laser. J Cutan Laser Ther. 2001;3:63–6.
34. Jiang SB, Levine VJ, Nehal KS, et al. Er:YAG laser for the treatment of actinic keratoses. Dermatol Surg. 2000;26:437–40.
35. Iyer S, Friedli A, Bowes L, et al. Full face laser resurfacing: therapy and prophylaxis for actinic keratoses and non-melanoma skin cancer. Lasers Surg Med. 2004;34:114–9.
36. Grunt TW, Lametschwandtner A, Staindl O. The vascular pattern of basal cell tumors: light microscopy and scanning electron microscopic study on vascular corrosion casts. Microvasc Res. 1985;29:371–86.
37. DeFatta RJ, Krishna S, Williams 3rd EF. Pulsed-dye laser for treating ecchymoses after facial cosmetic procedures. Arch Facial Plast Surg. 2009; 11:99–103.
38. Shah SM, Konnikov N, Duncan LM, et al. The effect of 595 nm pulsed dye laser on superficial and nodular basal cell carcinomas. Lasers Surg Med. 2009;41:417–22.
39. Konnikov N, Avram M, Jarell A, et al. Pulsed dye laser as a novel non-surgical treatment for basal cell carcinomas: response and follow up 12–21 months after treatment. Lasers Surg Med. 2011;43:72–8.
40. Smucler R, Vlk M. Combination of Er:YAG laser and photodynamic therapy in the treatment of nodular basal cell carcinoma. Lasers Surg Med. 2008; 40:153–8.
41. Whitaker IS, Shokrollahi K, James W, et al. Combined CO(2) laser with photodynamic therapy for the treatment of nodular basal cell carcinomas. Ann Plast Surg. 2007;59:484–8.

Radiation Therapy in Dermatology

27

Stephan Lautenschlager

Key Points

- Highly relevant as a therapeutic alternative or under certain conditions even as the treatment of choice to treat basal cell carcinomas, squamous cell carcinomas, extensive precancerous lesions, lentigo maligna and lentigo maligna melanoma.
- Excellent alternative when surgery is not feasible in patients over 60 and in those with underlying medical conditions.
- Palliative radiotherapy may be indicated for Kaposi's sarcoma, T- and B-cell lymphoma and even curative for primary cutaneous B-cell lymphoma.
- Fractional low-dose treatments are better tolerated and give better cosmetic results.

Introduction

In spite of advances in the local treatment of malignant skin tumours and other skin diseases, radiotherapy remains highly relevant as a therapeutic alternative or under certain conditions even as the treatment of choice. Hardly any other procedure is capable of treating superficial as well as deep skin tumours with such precision according to their depth and without causing serious damage to healthy tissue. In particular, curative radiotherapy is used to treat basal cell carcinomas, squamous cell carcinomas, extensive precancerous lesions, lentigo maligna, lentigo maligna melanoma and Merkel cell carcinoma [1]. Ideally, moderately to larger-sized non-melanoma skin cancers in the facial region in patients over the age of 60 are treated with radiotherapy when surgery is not feasible.

Palliative treatment is administered for malignant skin lymphomas of the B- or T-cell type, Kaposi's sarcoma and also skin metastasis. The possibilities of radiation therapy for benign relapsing skin changes should also not be forgotten, but some basic rules must be adhered to in these cases, e.g. failure of other therapeutic methods and exact diagnosis with histological confirmation, as is also the case for tumours. The advantages and disadvantages of the treatment with X-rays must be weighed up precisely (Table 27.1).

Improved X-ray technology with new devices, maintenance of safety rules and accurate

S. Lautenschlager, PhD
Dermatologisches Ambulatorium Stadtspital Triemli,
Herman Greulich-Strasse 70, Zurich CH-8004,
Switzerland

Outpatient Clinic of Dermatology,
Triemli Hospital, Zurich, Switzerland
e-mail: stephan.lautenschlager@triemli.stzh.ch

A. Baldi et al. (eds.), *Skin Cancer*, Current Clinical Pathology,
DOI 10.1007/978-1-4614-7357-2_27, © Springer Science+Business Media New York 2014

Table 27.1 Advantages and disadvantages of radiotherapy

Advantages
Outpatient treatment, even for tumours covering large areas
Healthy tissue can be preserved
Large safety margins possible (a decisive advantage over surgical excision margins that tend to be marginal in size, in particular in the facial region)
High effectiveness
Cosmesis usually good or very good (face > trunk and extremities)
Most functional results are excellent
Anaesthesia not required
Also possible for anticoagulation
Disadvantages
Only for selected patients
Several appointments required
No subsequent radiation treatment possible in the same location after treatment of tumours
Permanent loss of hair
Cosmetic results are inferior on the trunk and the extremities compared to the facial area
Chronic radiodermatitis tends to become more extensive over time when compared with surgical scarring

dosimetry have reduced the side effects to a minimum. To achieve optimal results, knowledge of some technical issues are essential [2]. There are three main forms of radiation therapy: teletherapy (external beam radiation therapy including X-rays and electrons, brachytherapy and systemic radioisotope therapy). In dermatology teletherapy is by far most often used.

Physical Background

In addition to fast electrons used during the therapeutic application of ionising radiation in dermatology, very soft, i.e. low-energy, Grenz and soft X-rays are preferred, as these are mainly absorbed by the outermost layers of tissue. Voltages in the range of 10–50 kV are usually used to generate these X-rays, rarely up to 100 kV. The treatment of skin diseases with soft X-rays requires an understanding of some important parameters like radiation quality and homogeneity and symmetry of the radiation fields. An understanding of two basic physical laws is of great importance here: (1) inverse square law (the intensity of the dose (dose rate) of X-rays emitted from a point source is inversely proportional to the square of the distance from that source) and (2) absorption law (the absorption of x-rays is proportional to the thickness, density and atomic number of the material and inversely proportional to the energy of the x-ray quanta).

Radiation Quality

Radiation quality determines the depth of penetration of radiation into the tissue. This is set by selection of the voltage (kV) on the X-ray equipment and the associated filtering. The voltage range for soft X-ray equipment lies between 10 and 100 kV. The limit is 50 kV for most equipment used in dermatology.

Selection of additional filtering is dependent on the tube potential. Plastic foil (Cellon) is generally used in the 12 kV range of Grenz rays. Aluminium filters of different thicknesses are used for higher voltages of up to 100 kV.

In order to avoid faulty irradiation, the equipment must be fitted with a filter-safety device or with fixed voltage-filter combinations appropriate to the type of equipment. The combinations are pre-installed in the newest equipment (Fig. 27.1). In addition to information on the

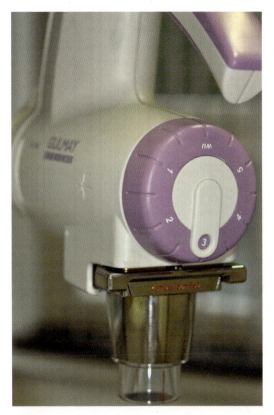

Fig. 27.1 Pre-installed voltage-filter combinations in newest equipment

voltage and the selected filters, a full description of radiation quality must also include the half-value layer thickness (HVL). HVL refers to the layer thickness that reduces the intensity of the radiation to half its initial strength. It increases with hardening of the beam.

Half-Value Depth in Tissue

The depth of penetration into the tissue determined by the radiation quality is usually described by the half-value depth in tissue (HVD). This is the depth in the tissue at which the intensity of the radiation or the dose rate has been reduced to half of the surface dose rate. HVD also increases with hardening of the beam. However, due to the inverse square law, it is also dependent on the focus-skin distance (FSD), i.e. on the length of the tube.

Half-value layer thicknesses can now be measured simply using foils and plates made of materials with equivalent water contents. Tables on HVL can be found in the literature. Particular care is required if cartilage or bone is located immediately under the skin in the radiation field. Low-energy X-ray quanta are mainly absorbed due to the photo effect, and this results in three to four times more energy being deposited in bone than in water or tissue located at the same depth. This can cause dangerous overdoses in the bone.

Radiation Quantity

Radiation quantity is described by the dose rate at the surface of the skin. Dosing in radiotherapy is measured using the energy dose unit Gray ($1\ Gy = 1\ J/kg$). The surface dose is dependent on several parameters. The most important parameters are tube current, voltage and filtration, as well as field size. Radiation quantity or the dose rate basically increases linearly with tube current (in mA).

A high percentage of X-ray quanta in the voltage range of up to 100 kV are backscattered due to their interactions with molecules in the tissue. This results in an increase in the surface dose for the tissue. This backscatter contribution increases with field size and voltage. It can be neglected for small fields and low voltages, whereas it can be up to 30 % at 50 kV and more for larger radiation fields.

The therapeutic approach for different skin diseases is shown in Table 27.2.

Radiation Therapy for Malignant Skin Tumours

Indications

Curative Treatment

In general, patients over the age of 60 with moderately to larger-sized tumours in the facial region can be treated with radiotherapy (RT) when the expected outcome is better than with alternative methods [4]. Locations like the eyelids (Fig. 27.2),

Table 27.2 Recommended doses for different skin diseases

Diagnosis	Voltage (kV)	Field (cm)	Fractionation (Gy)	Total dose (Gy)	Interval (days)
BCC and SCC	20–50	<2	5–6 × 8	40–48	4–7
		2–5	10–12 × 4		3–4
		>5	26–28 × 2	52–56	Daily
Merkel cell tumour/SCC metastasis	20–50	>5	26–28 × 2	52–56	Daily
Mycosis fungoides/other lymphomas	20–50		3–7 × 2	6–14	3–4
Kaposi's sarcoma	20–50	<2	3–5 × 8	24–40	4–7
		>2	5–10 × 4	20–40	3–4
Lentigo maligna/melanoma metastasis	20–50		7–10 × 6	42–60	2–7
Lentigo maligna	12	<2	5–6 × 20	100–120	4–7
		>2	10–12 × 10	100–120	3–4
Bowen's disease/Queyrat erythroplasia	20	<2	3–4 × 8	24–32	4–7
		>2	8–10 × 4	32–40	3–4
Actinic keratosis	12	<2	2–3 × 8	16–24	4–7
	20	>2	5–7 × 4	20–28	3–4
Chronic eczema	12		6–12 × 1	6–12	4–7
	20		6–12 × 0.5	3–6	4–7
Psoriasis	12		4–12 × 2	8–24	4–7
	20		4–12 × 1	4–12	4–7
Lichen planus	20–50		6–12 × 0.5	3–6	4–7
Painful venous ulcer	20–50		5–10 × 0.2	1–2	Daily
Pruritus ani/vulvae	12		4–8 × 1	4–8	4–7

Adapted from Panizzon and Cooper [1] and Panizzon [2, 3]

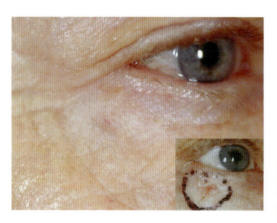

Fig. 27.2 Nodular BCC in a 67-year-old patient 4 years after 12 × 4 Gy, 30 kV

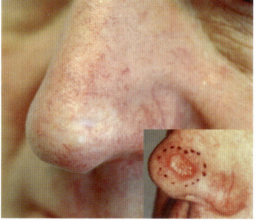

Fig. 27.3 SCC in a 64-year-old patient 5 years after 12 × 4 Gy, 40 kV

nose (Fig. 27.3), lips and ears produce particularly satisfactory results, both cosmetically and functionally. It is likewise an excellent option for patients receiving anticoagulants [4].

The half-value depth in tissue (HVD) must always correspond to the approximate thickness

of the tumour. This usually results in optimum protection of the skin lying underneath, while simultaneously destroying the tumour. When suspecting the presence of possible invasive tumours, a magnetic resonance imaging (MRI) is required prior to therapy as tumours that have infiltrated cartilage or bone are not an indication including soft X-ray and surface therapy.

Radiation treatment is only carried out after a histopathological examination. The histology provides information not only on the type and extent of the tumour but also on potential special histological subtypes, such as sclerodermiform growth patterns in basal cell carcinomas [5]. The latter are less sensitive to radiation – probably due to the concomitant fibrosis – and often exhibit a tendency to relapses, partly due to the difficulties in clinical delimitation. However, this does not necessarily mean that radiation therapy must be excluded as an option for inoperable patients. The radiation parameters should, however, be adapted, for example, through higher individual doses or higher total doses or through treatment with faster electrons. As a rule, basal cell carcinomas (BCCs) and squamous cell carcinomas (SCCs) can be treated in the same way. There is a general tendency towards using higher total doses for SCCs. Local control rates in BCCs range from 90 to 95 % [4], and careful patient selection can result in even higher cure rates [6–8]. In a prospective trial, where 93 patients with BCC were randomised to receive either cryosurgery or radiation therapy, the 2-year cure rate for the RT group was 96 % [9]. Cosmesis is rated in over 90 % as excellent or good [6]. Most important long-term side effects (after 4 years) are hypopigmentation and telangiectases in 92 and 82 %, respectively [10] (Fig. 27.4). Factors influencing

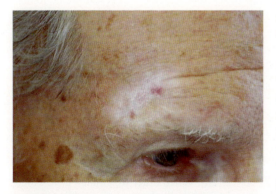

Fig. 27.4 Marked hypopigmentation and telangiectases 9 years after RT (especially in sun-exposed areas)

cosmetic results are in order of importance: time after treatment, site, tumour thickness, field size and treatment parameters [10, 11].

The risk of radiation-induced malignancy is probably lower than 1:1,000 after 10–15 years [12]. Radiotherapy can be used to treat many types of BCC, even those overlying bone and cartilage, although it is probably less suitable for the treatment of large tumours in critical sites, as very large BCC masses are often both resistant and require radiation doses that closely approach tissue tolerance.

Local control rate is lower for SCC by 10–15 % than an equivalent-sized BCC [13]. Poorly differentiated SCCs recur in up to 50 % and therefore should not be treated with X-rays [1]. For high-risk SCCs, Mohs surgery should be preferred [14].

In special circumstances – especially in larger SCCs on the lower lip – brachytherapy may be used alternatively. In these cases a radiation source is placed inside or next the tumor area. For example Cobalt-60 can be used to generate gamma rays, produced by spontaneous decay of the nucleus.

Electron beam therapy – where electrons are directed to a tumor site – is produced by a linear accelerator. An electron beam will penetrate to a certain depth and spare any underlying tissue from radiation damage. Therefore this form of radiation is best used to irradiate large skin cancers in sites overlying cartilage or bone.

Safety margins in any kind of teletherapies should be chosen from 0.5 to 1 cm. Treatment of Merkel cell carcinoma is primarily surgery, with adjuvant radiotherapy becoming standard since recent data have shown that radiotherapy improves both locoregional control and survival.

Precancerous Lesions

The recommendation of modern RT for precancerous skin lesions is usually limited to patients where the cosmetic and/or functional outcome is likely to be better with radiotherapy compared with surgery or other various treatment modalities. RT is especially suited for elderly patients with various comorbidities suffering from extensive and widespread actinic keratoses of the scalp, Bowen's disease and lentigo maligna.

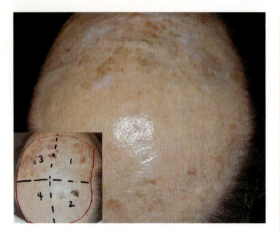

Fig. 27.5 Disseminated actinic keratosis in a 66-year-old patient 7 years after 6 × 4 Gy, 12 kV

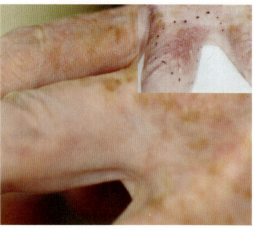

Fig. 27.6 Bowen's disease 6 years after RT (8 × 4 Gy, 20 kV)

Actinic Keratoses

Actinic keratoses (AK) are seen in up to 25 % of adults in the northern hemisphere, mostly in the older fair-skinned population with a worldwide increase [15–17]. Mostly, AK therapy is simple, but widespread actinic keratoses of the scalp, especially in the elderly population, can be a therapeutic challenge. For giant or widespread lesions, fractionated Grenz or superficial soft X-ray radiation is very efficient [2, 18, 19]. As radiation may induce dose-dependent alopecia and even more important secondary tumours, younger patients have to be excluded [20], although the risk of developing radiogenic ulcers and tumours after soft X-ray therapy is not very high [20]. Usually the required total dose varies from 20 to 28 Gy with single dose 4–8 Gy once or twice per week with 12–20 kV [2]. If the entire scalp is affected, the radiation field has to be subdivided in different sections (Fig. 27.5). The prolonged treatment time (usually 6–8 sessions), and higher costs compared to cryotherapy, electrodesiccation or topical agents are offset by the longer remission time with less future treatments after radiotherapy [2]. Patients have to be advised that transient inflammatory reactions occur during treatment. Sun protection counselling is mandatory. This treatment is preferably carried out during the winter months.

Bowen's Disease

These intra-epidermal neoplasias can be very extensive, occasionally exophytic, occurring in locations exposed to the sun but also in the anogenital region [21–23]. Often the pilosebaceous apparatus is involved [24]. Various RT techniques (soft X-rays, orthovoltage or electron therapy) and regimens have been used to treat BD, but there are no studies directly comparing other treatments with RT, and data are sparse regarding dosing and toxicity. RT is advantageous in patients who refuse surgery, for lesions in cosmetically sensitive areas (Fig. 27.6), for large and multiple lesions and for patients with keloid formation [22]. Several retrospective studies indicate local control rates from 89 to 100 % although the doses reported were very different. Recent review articles on managing patients with BD emphasise the multitude of treatments for these patients [25, 26]. Despite this, RT remains an excellent and well-tolerated therapeutic option in selected patients with BD (in particular on digital, penile or perianal sites), but risk factors for poor healing on the lower leg, such as poor vascularity, size of the lesion (>4 cm) and large fraction size (>4 Gy), should be taken into account, especially when orthovoltage X-rays are used [21, 22, 25]. When other treatments have failed, RT can be effective [27].

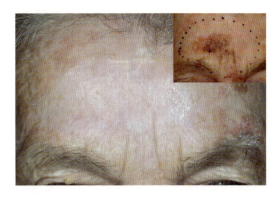

Fig. 27.7 Lentigo maligna in an 82-year-old patient 5 years after 12 × 10 Gy, 12 kV

Lentigo Maligna

Lentigo maligna (LM) is a macular pigmented skin lesion usually found in patients in their seventh–eighth age decade, with actinic skin damage, and located in the head and neck region in 90 % of the cases. LM is regarded as a form of melanoma in situ with slow horizontal growth and, if untreated, may progress to lentigo maligna melanoma [28]. For this reason, early treatment is mandatory, but the diffuse nature of melanocytic overgrowth makes LM difficult to treat, with recurrence rates ranging up to 50 % [28]. Surgical excision with clear margins was previously considered as the first-line treatment [29]. Since patients seem to be unsuitable for excision, especially because of advanced age, large size of the lesion and proximity of the eye, ear or nose, RT has been used in Europe for decades as the primary treatment with control rates of 95 % [30]. Using the Miescher technique, high doses of Grenz or soft X-rays are applied, affecting only the epidermis and the upper dermis [31]. This technique often induces a severe acute radiodermatitis with only limited long-term side effects with excellent cosmetic results when used on the face. Farshad et al. [30] reported a recurrence rate of 7 % after a mean time of 45.6 months in 101 treated patients with LM and LMM. They emphasised a safety margin of at least 10 mm. Schmid-Wendtner et al. [32] reported in 42 patients a success rate of even 100 % (10 × 10 Gy, 14.5 kV, 50 % depth dose

1.1 mm, mean follow-up 23 months). Based on the excellent cosmetic result, the low recurrence rate and the lack of systemic side effects, RT can be seen as the first-line treatment for elderly patients with facial LM (Fig. 27.7).

Palliative RT

Kaposi's Sarcoma

Kaposi's sarcoma is a multifocal neoplasm of the skin and internal organs that originates in the lymph or blood vessels and is associated with human herpes virus 8.

All forms of Kaposi's sarcoma (classic, endemic African, transplant-related and AIDS-related epidemic) are highly radiosensitive and can be treated palliatively using radiotherapy in a few appointments and lead to optimum cosmetic results.

Cutaneous Lymphomas

RT is a suitable method for the treatment of uni-locular mycosis fungoides and in tumour stage IIb and further stages of development. In general, T-cell and B-cell lymphomas are highly radiosensitive, but with the exception of certain B-cell lymphomas [33] and CD-30 positive lymphomas, radiotherapy is mostly not curative but palliative [34]. Pseudolymphomas are also highly sensitive to radiation.

Radiation Therapy for Benign Skin Diseases

The basic rules governing this application must be taken into consideration prior to radiation therapy for benign skin changes.

The dermatologist should have some knowledge on the depth of the different skin lesions, similar to what is required for RT of malignant skin changes. The rule of thumb is (analogous to tumours) that the HVD should be equivalent to the depth of the inflammatory lesion (50 % isodose). It must be pointed out that the total dose for soft X-rays for benign diseases should, as a rule, be 12 Gy per field and life and the total dose for Grenz rays is 50 Gy.

Indications

Eczema

RT is hardly the therapy of first choice for eczemas, but can by all means be indicated in cases of persistent, tylotic, rhagadiform and chronic cumulative contact eczemas. Among other things, this causes a reduction in the Langerhans cells. Grenz rays with a half-value depth in tissue of 1 mm are the first option, for economic reasons with reference to radiation exposure. In hyperkeratotic skin conditions, it may also be meaningful to initially conduct a keratolysis with 10 % salicylic Vaseline and to use Grenz rays only afterwards. RT offers high rates of improvement or complete remission even with low-dose irradiation, e.g. 2×0.5 Gy weekly for 4–5 weeks [35].

Psoriasis

Even today, treatment of psoriasis remains difficult for some locations, especially on the scalp and fingernails. In addition, psoriasis of the scalp can cause itching and be difficult to approach therapeutically. The hair does not necessarily need to be cut short in the case of psoriasis of the scalp. It can also be parted and then treated with radiation. It is important to also point out that Grenz rays do not cause alopecia as the matrix of the hair lies deeper than 1 mm, while the HVD for Grenz rays is 1 mm. The approach is similar for psoriasis of the fingernails [2]. Attention must be paid to the fact that the nails are often thickened. In this case, a similar approach to that for tylotic, hyperkeratotic eczema is recommended, i.e. also pretreating with keratolytic agents (up to 40 % salicylic acid).

Keloids

It is important to point out in this case that the prophylactic use of X-rays must take place as early as possible, i.e. on the same day as the operation or no later than the day after surgery. This requires good coordination between the surgeon and the radiotherapist. The sole treatment with X-rays of keloids is not indicated.

Other Indications

Other indications are painful paronychia, hidradenitis, therapy-resistant verruca vulgaris and painful ulcers on the lower leg, in particular when local treatment and analgesics are unsuccessful. Another example is pemphigus chronicus familiaris benignus (Hailey-Hailey disease). This disease causes painful and erosive changes in the anogenital region, is highly resistant to therapy and responds very well to Grenz rays. A few appointments produce rapid positive results. In this case, low-dose radiation therapy is a highly effective form of therapy and economic with reference to radiation exposure.

In conclusion, fractionated radiotherapy is an effective and well-tolerated outpatient treatment modality which should be considered according to the exact diagnosis, age of the patient, comorbidities, goals of treatment, lesion characteristics including location and not least patient preference.

Glossary

Absorption law the absorption of X-rays is proportional to the thickness, density and atomic number of the material and inversely proportional to the energy of the X-ray quanta.

Electron beam radiation therapy is a radiation therapy that uses a linear accelerator where electrons are directed to the tumour site. It has low penetration and spares deeper tissues.

Gray it is the international energy dose unit of absorbed radiation dose of ionising radiation (IR). It is measured as the absorption of 1 J of IR by 1 kg of matter (1 Gy = 1 J/kg).

Grenz or soft-energy (low-energy) therapy involves exposing the skin to low-energy, non-penetrating radiation. It is mostly used in inflammatory skin conditions.

Half-value depth in tissue (HVD) is the depth in the tissue at which the intensity of the radiation or the dose rate has been reduced to half of the surface dose rate focus-skin distance (FSD), i.e. on the length of the tube.

Half-value layer thickness (HVL) refers to the layer thickness that reduces the intensity of the radiation to half its initial strength. It increases with hardening of the beam. It is measured in aluminium.

Inverse square law the intensity of the dose (dose rate) of X-rays emitted from a point source is inversely proportional to the square of the distance from that source.

Ionising radiation (IR) is the radiation that removes an electron from an atom. In medicine, it is used in radiography (diagnostic X-rays, 20–150 kV, used to obtain images from inside the body), in nuclear medicine as tracer method and in radiation therapy for its damage on DNA cells (superficial X-rays, 50–200 kV; orthovoltage X-rays, 200–500 kV; and megavoltage X-rays, 1–25 MV).

Miescher technique it is a type of external beam radiotherapy. It involves the use of an X-ray tube with a beryllium window set at a determined energy, with the target lesion positioned at 20 cm, a 50 % depth dose at 1–1.3 of skin, a dose of 20 Gy per treatment with 5 treatments given 3–4 days apart and a 5-mm margin of normal skin included, with an accumulated dose of 10,000 rads.

Orthovoltage therapy or, "deep" X-rays, are produced by X-ray generators, in the range of 22–500 kV and penetration of about 4–6 mm.

Palliative treatment is the treatment to alleviate symptoms without curing the disease.

Radiation field homogeneity refers to the homogenous dose distribution in the area of radiation

Radiation field symmetry maximum ratio of doses at 2 symmetric points relative to the central axis of the field.

Radiation quality is the spectrum of radiant energy produced by a given radiation source with respect to its penetration or its suitability for a specific application. It determines the depth of penetration of radiation into the tissue.

Radiation quantity is the dose rate at the surface of the skin. It is expressed in Grays.

Radiotherapy it is the treatment of a disease using radiation, especially by selective irradiation with X-rays or other ionising radiation and by ingestion of radioisotopes.

X-ray quanta Individual units of X-ray energy.

References

1. Panizzon RG, Cooper JS. Radiation Treatment and Radiation Reactions in Dermatology. 1st ed. Berlin/Heidelberg/New York: Springer; 2004.
2. Panizzon RG. Dermatologische radiotherapie. Hautarzt. 2007;58:701–10, quiz.
3. Panizzon R. Radiotherapy. In: Wolff K, Goldsmith LA, Katz SI, Gilchrest BA, Paller AS, Leffell DJ, editors. Fitzpatrick's dermatology in general medicine. 7th ed. New York: McGraw Hill; 2008. p. 2279–84.
4. Veness MJ. The important role of radiotherapy in patients with non-melanoma skin cancer and other cutaneous entities. J Med Imaging Radiat Oncol. 2008;52:278–86.
5. Zagrodnik B, Kempf W, Seifert B, et al. Superficial radiotherapy for patients with basal cell carcinoma: recurrence rates, histologic subtypes, and expression of p53 and Bcl-2. Cancer. 2003;98:2708–14.
6. Schulte KW, Lippold A, Auras C, et al. Soft X-ray therapy for cutaneous basal cell and squamous cell carcinomas. J Am Acad Dermatol. 2005;53:993–1001.
7. Locke J, Karimpour S, Young G, Lockett MA, Perez CA. Radiotherapy for epithelial skin cancer. Int J Radiat Oncol Biol Phys. 2001;51:748–55.
8. Hernandez-Machin B, Borrego L, Gil-Garcia M, Hernandez BH. Office-based radiation therapy for cutaneous carcinoma: evaluation of 710 treatments. Int J Dermatol. 2007;46:453–9.
9. Hall VL, Leppard BJ, McGill J, Kesseler ME, White JE, Goodwin P. Treatment of basal-cell carcinoma: comparison of radiotherapy and cryotherapy. Clin Radiol. 1986;37:33–4.
10. Rupprecht R, Lippold A, Auras C, et al. Late side-effects with cosmetic relevance following soft X-ray therapy of cutaneous neoplasias. J Eur Acad Dermatol Venereol. 2007;21:178–85.
11. Veness M, Richards S. Role of modern radiotherapy in treating skin cancer. Australas J Dermatol. 2003;44:159–66.
12. Feigen M. Should cancer survivors fear radiation-induced sarcomas? Sarcoma. 1997;1:5–15.
13. Silva JJ, Tsang RW, Panzarella T, Levin W, Wells W. Results of radiotherapy for epithelial skin cancer of the pinna: the Princess Margaret Hospital experience, 1982–1993. Int J Radiat Oncol Biol Phys. 2000;47:451–9.
14. Motley R, Kersey P, Lawrence C. Multiprofessional guidelines for the management of the patient with primary cutaneous squamous cell carcinoma. Br J Dermatol. 2002;146:18–25.
15. Hemminki K, Zhang H, Czene K. Time trends and familial risks in squamous cell carcinoma of the skin. Arch Dermatol. 2003;139:885–9.
16. Diepgen TL, Mahler V. The epidemiology of skin cancer. Br J Dermatol. 2002;146 Suppl 61:1–6.
17. Christenson LJ, Borrowman TA, Vachon CM, et al. Incidence of basal cell and squamous cell carcinomas in a population younger than 40 years. JAMA. 2005;294:681–90.
18. Barta U, Grafe T, Wollina U. Radiation therapy for extensive actinic keratosis. J Eur Acad Dermatol Venereol. 2000;14:293–5.
19. Pipitone MA, Gloster HM. Superficial squamous cell carcinomas and extensive actinic keratoses of the scalp treated with radiation therapy. Dermatol Surg. 2006;32:756–9.

20. Landthaler M, Hagspiel HJ, Braun-Falco O. Late irradiation damage to the skin caused by soft X-ray radiation therapy of cutaneous tumors. Arch Dermatol. 1995;131:182–6.

21. Dupree MT, Kiteley RA, Weismantle K, Panos R, Johnstone PA. Radiation therapy for Bowen's disease: lessons for lesions of the lower extremity. J Am Acad Dermatol. 2001;45:401–4.

22. Lukas VanderSpek LA, Pond GR, Wells W, Tsang RW. Radiation therapy for Bowen's disease of the skin. Int J Radiat Oncol Biol Phys. 2005;63:505–10.

23. Cox NH. Body site distribution of Bowen's disease. Br J Dermatol. 1994;130:714–6.

24. Kossard S, Rosen R. Cutaneous Bowen's disease. An analysis of 1001 cases according to age, sex, and site. J Am Acad Dermatol. 1992;27:406–10.

25. Cox NH, Eedy DJ, Morton CA. Guidelines for management of Bowen's disease: 2006 update. Br J Dermatol. 2007;156:11–21.

26. Moreno G, Chia AL, Lim A, Shumack S. Therapeutic options for Bowen's disease. Australas J Dermatol. 2007;48:1–8.

27. McKenna DJ, Morris S, Kurwa H. Treatment-resistant giant unilateral Bowen's disease of the scalp responding to radiotherapy. Clin Exp Dermatol. 2009;34:85–6.

28. Bosbous MW, Dzwierzynski WW, Neuburg M. Lentigo maligna: diagnosis and treatment. Clin Plast Surg. 2010;37:35–46.

29. Coleman III WP, Davis RS, Reed RJ, Krementz ET. Treatment of lentigo maligna and lentigo maligna melanoma. J Dermatol Surg Oncol. 1980;6:476–9.

30. Farshad A, Burg G, Panizzon R, Dummer R. A retrospective study of 150 patients with lentigo maligna and lentigo maligna melanoma and the efficacy of radiotherapy using Grenz or soft X-rays. Br J Dermatol. 2002;146:1042–6.

31. Miescher G. Die Behandlung der Malignen Melanome der Haut mit Einschluss der Melanotischen Praecancerose. Strahlentherapie. 1960;46:25–35.

32. Schmid-Wendtner MH, Brunner B, Konz B, et al. Fractionated radiotherapy of lentigo maligna and lentigo maligna melanoma in 64 patients. J Am Acad Dermatol. 2000;43:477–82.

33. Senff NJ, Hoefnagel JJ, Neelis KJ, Vermeer MH, Noordijk EM, Willemze R. Results of radiotherapy in 153 primary cutaneous B-cell lymphomas classified according to the WHO-EORTC classification. Arch Dermatol. 2007;143:1520–6.

34. Holloway KB, Flowers FP, Ramos-Caro FA. Therapeutic alternatives in cutaneous T-cell lymphoma. J Am Acad Dermatol. 1992;27:367–78.

35. Sumila M, Notter M, Itin P, Bodis S, Gruber G. Long-term results of radiotherapy in patients with chronic palmo-plantar eczema or psoriasis. Strahlenther Onkol. 2008;184:218–23.

Electrochemotherapy in Dermatological Oncology

28

Enrico P. Spugnini

Key Points

- It is a safe and effective therapy in the treatment of a wide variety of cutaneous and subcutaneous lesions that can be used alone or in adjuvance to surgery.
- It is useful for treatment of multiple and metastatic lesions and those that have undergone multimodal therapies.
- The procedure can be performed under local or systemic anesthesia, mostly depending on the number of lesions and their location.
- Might result to be an excellent alternative for the treatment of bulky tumors.

Introduction

Electroporation is associated with the creation of aqueous pathways (electropores) in the cell membrane as a result of applied short intensive electric field. This phenomenon allows molecules, ions, and water to pass from one side of the membrane to the other. The electroporation is reversible if the membrane returns into the normal state after the end of the field exposure, which is possible

when its parameters have been appropriately selected. Otherwise, the pores cannot be resealed. The process that becomes irreversible leads to cell death.

Theoretical Background

For over 30 years, the use of electroporation has been reported in bacterial, plant, and mammal cells, as well as in fungi and protozoans. Importantly, in the early 1990s, the first studies on the in vivo electropermeabilization in laboratory animals were reported [1–5]. The first clinical study on the use of electropermeabilization to increase the uptake of a chemotherapeutic agent in human tumors was reported by Belehradek et al. [6]. Since then, several investigations have been published in humans [7–11] and in companion animals with spontaneous neoplasms [12–14]. Nowadays, electropermeabilization has been proven effective for the targeted delivery to living cells of ions, dyes, radiotracers, drugs, antibodies, oligonucleotides, DNA, and RNA and is under consideration for virtually any molecule [15]. Below some basic data referred to typical mammalian cells exposed to direct current are reported. It is known that their resting transmembrane potential differences are comprised between 50 and 70 mV and are due to the difference in ionic strengths inside and outside the cell. The transmembrane potential needed to induce their electropermeabilization is similar in different cell types and ranges, on average, from 250 to 350 mV.

E.P. Spugnini, DVM, PhD
S.A.F.U. Department, Regina Elena Cancer Institute,
Viale C.T. Odescalchi 10, Rome 00147, Italy
e-mail: info@enricospugnini.net, spugnini.vet@tiscali.it

A. Baldi et al. (eds.), *Skin Cancer*, Current Clinical Pathology,
DOI 10.1007/978-1-4614-7357-2_28, © Springer Science+Business Media New York 2014

Cell electropermeabilization from the clinical standpoint can be either transient or irreversible, depending on the magnitude and the time length of the imposed transmembrane potential, which in turn is related to the external applied field. Characteristic DC field strengths required for electropermeabilization are in the range of $1 \ kV \cdot cm^{-1}$ for most of these cell types, whose size is typically comprised between 10 and 40 μm.

The commonly accepted interpretation of the membrane permeabilization includes the following states: (i) *initial hydrophobic*, characterized by the original orientation of the lipids; (ii) *creation of initial hydrophilic pores* under strong electric field; and (iii) *reorientation of the lipids* adjacent to the aqueous inside a pore in a manner that their hydrophilic heads are facing the pore, while the hydrophobic tails are hidden inside the membrane.

For practical (i.e., experimental and clinical) purposes, the process of electroporation has been divided into five steps defined as induction, expansion, stabilization, resealing, and memory effect. They happen within microseconds, milliseconds, seconds, and hours, respectively. In a simplified description, the cell is surrounded by a conductive matrix and has an inner conducting cytoplasm, and the two compartments are separated by a lipid bilayer formed by the cytoplasmic membrane. Calling the external conductivity λ_{ext}, the cytoplasmic conductivity λ_{int}, the membrane conductivity λ_{memb}, and E the electric field intensity, the induced potential difference ($\Delta\Psi_E$) as a function of the time t can be expressed [16] as:

$$\Delta\Psi_E(t) = g(\lambda_{ext}, \lambda_{memb}, \lambda int)$$
$$E \ k \ r \cos\theta \ (1 - \exp(-t/\tau))ss$$

where k is a form factor accounting for the impact of the cell on the extracellular field distribution, r is the radius of the cell (assumed to be spherical), θ is the angle between the cell membrane and the field direction, τ is a membrane charging time constant, and g is a function of the three involved conductivities [16].

The permeabilization occurs when and where the potential difference crosses a critical poration value ($\Delta\Psi_p$), which has been estimated as being not less than 200 mV [17]. Clearly, E controls the poration, and a critical threshold has been defined also for this variable (E_p), so that when $E > E_p$, the permeabilization becomes possible [17]. According to the above equation, E_p is cell size-dependent, and indeed it roughly ranges from $0.1 \ kV \ cm^{-1}$ for large cells (e.g., muscle cells) to $1–2 \ kV \ cm^{-1}$ for small cells (e.g., bacteria) [17]. While the expansion is progressing, the membrane goes through a transition characterized by abnormally high conductance and permeability. During this phase, the electric field intensity controls the geometry of the part of the cell affected, while the pulse duration controls the density of the perturbation of the cell membrane. Interrupting the administration of the electric field induces the stabilization process; when the electric field becomes subcritical ($E < E_p$), there is a decrease of the conductance in the permeabilized part of the cell membrane, and the plasmalemma shifts from highly permeable to variously leaky [16].

During the resealing, the membrane leaks are annihilated. As stated before, sealing kinetics require seconds and are therefore generally much slower than the electric field relaxation, because pushing water out of the formed hydrophilic pore and the rearrangement of the lipid bilayer into the normal state require the overcoming of relatively high free energy barriers [18]. The picture emerging from this research is that of a pore that is initiated close to a head group defect (fluctuation) in which a cluster of polar heads points inwardly, with respect to the zero field average conformation. At the location of these defects, induced on the outer side of the membrane by the external electric field, water molecules start to penetrate the lipid bilayer, eventually forming hydrogen-bonded chains of molecules. The phenomenon is dynamically driven by the electric field, which tends to orient the dipoles of both water and head groups. The time scale on which the pore is formed is around 200 ps. At later times the pore becomes stabilized and presents an inner hydrophilic interface. If the field is removed, the pore gradually collapses and resealing is eventually observed (Fig. 28.1).

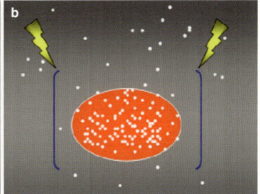

Fig. 28.1 Schematic representation of the enhanced uptake of lipophobic drug (*white dots*) by a tumor cell (approximated to a sphere) following the creation of an electric field (*blue bars*) and the administration of permeabilizing pulses (*yellow sparks*). (**a**) Drug uptake by the tumor cell before the administration of permeabilizing pulses. (**b**) Drug uptake by the tumor cell after administration of permeabilizing pulses (Modified from Spugnini et al. [19])

Electrochemotherapy

Electroporation is defined as permeability change in the cell membrane following exposure to short pulse of high electric field. Due to the low conductivity of the lipid bilayer, application of high external electric field generates a potential difference across the membrane. As the cross-membrane potential difference reaches a threshold value of about 200 mV, a sudden increase in membrane permeability is observed. Processes leading to this electroporation phenomenon are not fully understood on the molecular level. However, there is a general agreement that cross-membrane potential difference contributes to stabilization of transient membrane defects and to their expansion to large metastable hydrophilic pores. Both transient and stable pores can be the sites of extrinsic material entry into the cell [16, 17]. Electropermeabilization typically uses high-voltage pulses of μs to ms duration to generate the necessary electric field for opening pores in the cell membrane [20]. Optimum electroporation parameters vary depending upon the cell type and purpose. Electric field strengths of 1,200 V/cm and 100 μs pulses are applied for drug delivery. Experimental studies supported that (i) the percentage of porated cells is related to the increase of the pulse amplitude and duration and (ii) poration occurs when the pulse amplitude exceeds a threshold value. Electropermeabilization is very often performed using bursts of rectangular pulses. Their typical durations are in the range from hundreds of μs to tens of ms, while the intervals between the pulses vary from several ms to several s. The most common types of waves have been, since the pioneering years, the square, which has a defined intensity and duration [2–11] and maintains the voltage throughout the life of the pulse [2–11], and the exponentially decaying one [1]. More recently, other waves have been proposed for electroporation, in the attempt to achieve higher efficiency and greater adaptability to the in vivo setting in particular the bipolar oscillating pulses [21], such as the bipolar square pulse, which gives higher membrane permeabilization levels than unipolar pulses [21] administered in bursts (i.e., pulse trains with short interpulse intervals [21–23] for reducing the electroporation morbidity).

Many cancers are resistant to multimodal treatments, and there is a need for therapeutic innovations and discovery. The ideal treatment of cancer should effectively control local and systemically recurrent disease, be applicable to a diversity of tumor types and anatomical locations, facilitate multimodal and systemic therapies, be minimally intrusive, and improve patient well-being and life expectancy by tumor control and cure. Electrochemotherapy (ECT) has been defined as the enhanced uptake of chemotherapy agents by solid tumors, following the application of permeabilizing pulses [2]. The first and most actively studied ECT agent has been bleomycin. This drug can penetrate the cell membrane only through protein receptors due to its lipophobic nature, thus resulting in slow and quantitatively limited uptake under normal conditions [24]. The complex formed by bleomycin and its carrier is transported in the cytosol by means of endocytotic vesicles, but the mechanism of its release is still unknown. Following internalization by the cell, this drug induces single and double deoxyribonucleic acid (DNA) breaks [25] which are seen as chromosomal gaps, deletions, and DNA fragmentation that can ultimately lead to cell death [26]. Bleomycin requires oxygen and metals as cofactors to cause DNA damage [27]. It forms a complex with Cu^{2+}, and the complex is internalized into the cell [26]. There is some evidence that the bleomycin-Cu^{2+} complex is a prodrug, which once inside the cell is converted to the biologically potent Fe^{2+}-bleomycin [26]. The Fe^{2+}-bleomycin complex binds to O_2 and then to DNA, and this quaternary complex (Fe^{2+}-bleomycin-O_2-DNA) results in DNA cleavage. The binding of Fe^{2+}-bleomycin complex to O_2 happens very rapidly and is stabilized by the presence of DNA [26]. The interaction with the DNA takes place at the minor groove with clear nucleotide selectivity, e.g., preferentially at the level of the GC base pairs [26–28].

Bleomycin cuts the chromatin at the level of the linker DNA between nucleosomes [28, 29] inducing single- and double-strand DNA breaks with a ratio of six to ten single-strand to one double-strand break [26, 28, 29]. The attack to the opposite strand is not as sequence specific as the first cleavage but is cut within one nucleotide of the first attack site [28]. It has been calculated that one molecule of bleomycin can make eight to ten DNA breaks [28, 29] and that 3×10^6 bleomycin molecules can create about 5×10^6 double-strand breaks in one cell [18, 29]. Bleomycin-induced DNA fragmentation is a very rapid phenomenon: it happens within 30 s. of drug entry within the cell [28, 29]. Bleomycin may induce cell damage through other mechanisms such as release of free nucleic bases without strand cleavage, oxidative degradation of RNA, an attack on small organic molecules, and lipid peroxidation [26, 27, 29]. The high toxicity of bleomycin when it reaches the intracellular environment is impaired by its inability to freely diffuse through the cytoplasmic membrane [28, 29]. In vitro studies evidenced that less than 0.1 % of bleomycin added to culture medium becomes associated to the cell [24]. It is on this background that the cytotoxicity of bleomycin can be enhanced by 300–700-folds by electroporation [30].

In particular, one study [29] using electroporation as a mechanism to enhance the cellular internalization of bleomycin suggested two possible mechanisms of cell killing that were dependent on the number of internalized molecules of bleomycin:

1. When only a few thousands molecules were internalized, the cells arrested in the G_2–M phase and became enlarged and polynucleated before dying, thus mimicking the behavior of lethally radiated cells.
2. When several million molecules where internalized following electroporation, the cells died showing swelling and nucleus dissolution, changes suggestive of apoptotic death.

The first use of electrochemotherapy with bleomycin in humans was published in 1991 on head and neck tumor nodules [1]. Since that time, the therapy has undergone significant advances in terms of the systems used and the cancers demonstrated to be suitable for treatment [2–5]. A number of companies, including IGEA (IGEA, Carpi, Italy) and Inovio (Inovio Biomedical Corporation, CA, USA), have developed pulse generators with approval for use in humans. In the past decade since their development, electrochemotherapy has become established as a safe and effective therapy in the treatment of a wide variety of cutaneous and subcutaneous lesions. Electrochemotherapy may be given with conventional anticancer treatments, and experiences to date suggest it may also be a significant adjunct in combination with surgery. While several cancer types appeared to be responsive to

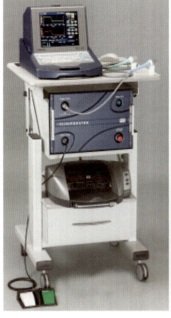
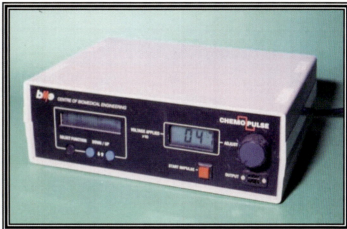

Fig. 28.2 (**a**) Cliniporator IGEA. (**b**) Chemopulse

electrochemotherapy, its clinical application to date has been confined to cutaneous malignancies, often recurrent, multiple, and metastatic after multimodal therapies [6–11, 21, 22].

The treatment is associated with minimal side effects for patients, is easy to perform in a day-hospital setting, and is inexpensive. Most of the treated neoplasms have been Kaposi sarcoma, squamous and basal cell carcinoma, fibrosarcoma, and mammary carcinoma [6–11, 21, 22, 31]. Moreover cutaneous metastases of hypernephroma, ovarian cancer, mammary carcinoma, and Merkel's tumor have been reported [32–35]. Pooling together partial and complete responses observed in the first studies, the overall response rate of the first trials with bleomycin or cisplatin was around 86 % (with a range from 62 to 100 %) [36, 37]. Figure 28.2 shows two electrochemotherapy equipments currently used in clinical oncology, and Figs. 28.3 and 28.4 show different electrodes.

After the first successful trials on electrochemotherapy, using bleomycin or cisplatin, a broader multicentric European trial named ESOPE (European Standard Operating Procedure on Electrochemotherapy) has been conducted, and its results have been published in 2006 [39]. The aim of the study was the standardization of the different electrochemotherapy protocols adopted by the various groups investigating the technique. It has been a 2-year multi-institutional prospective nonrandomized study evaluating response to the different drugs bleomycin and cisplatin (administered intralesionally or systemically) and treatment-associated toxicity. The study obtained an overall 84.8 % response for the treatment of cutaneous nodules (11.1 % partial responses and 73.7 % complete responses, respectively) [39]. The study failed to show a difference in response for the groups receiving bleomycin systemically or locally or cisplatin intralesionally [39].

Standard Operating Procedure

Drugs

Bleomycin
The currently adopted dose of intravenous bleomycin is similar to those used in conventional chemotherapeutic regimens (15,000 IU/m^2) [39].

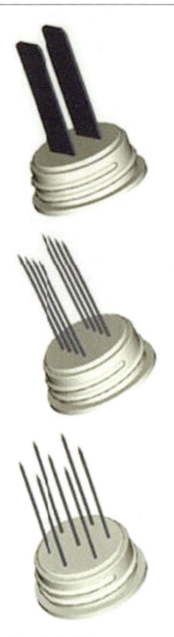

Fig. 28.3 Electrodes for Cliniporator

Cisplatin

As with bleomycin, the dosage for intratumoral cisplatin therapy (1 mg/cm^3) is tumor volume dependent [39]. This results in much lower therapeutic dose and prevents the neurotoxicity, nephrotoxicity, and hematological toxicity associated with its systemic administration.

Anesthesia

The procedure can be performed under local or systemic anesthesia, mostly depending on the number of lesions and their location. In the case of head and neck tumors, for example, treatment is often carried out under general anesthesia to minimize patients' discomfort secondary to electrically induced muscular contractions. When smaller, discrete tumors are involved, treatment may be carried out under local anesthesia using, for example, lidocaine, often in combination with adrenaline to promote vasoconstriction that will lead to increased drug permanence.

Choice of the Electrodes and Pulse Protocol

Needle array or plate electrodes are chosen accordingly to the tumor characteristics. The repetition frequency is decided on the basis of number and size of the nodules and the expected morbidity for the patient. The electrodes are sequentially applied until complete coverage of the whole tumor volume has been achieved.

Patient Follow-Up

In general, most patients are treated with electrochemotherapy on a day-hospital regimen. Relative indications for hospitalization include patients with history of adverse reactions to anesthesia or patients with other pathologies that might result in a high anesthetic risk. Patients are rechecked after 6–8 weeks post-treatment. The number of treatments required

Noteworthy, being electrochemotherapy effective after a single treatment, the cumulative dose of bleomycin is much lower than that of conventional chemotherapy protocols. Intralesional bleomycin doses are based on tumor volume (500 IU/cm^3) [39]. The route of drug administration is decided on the number of lesions to be treated.

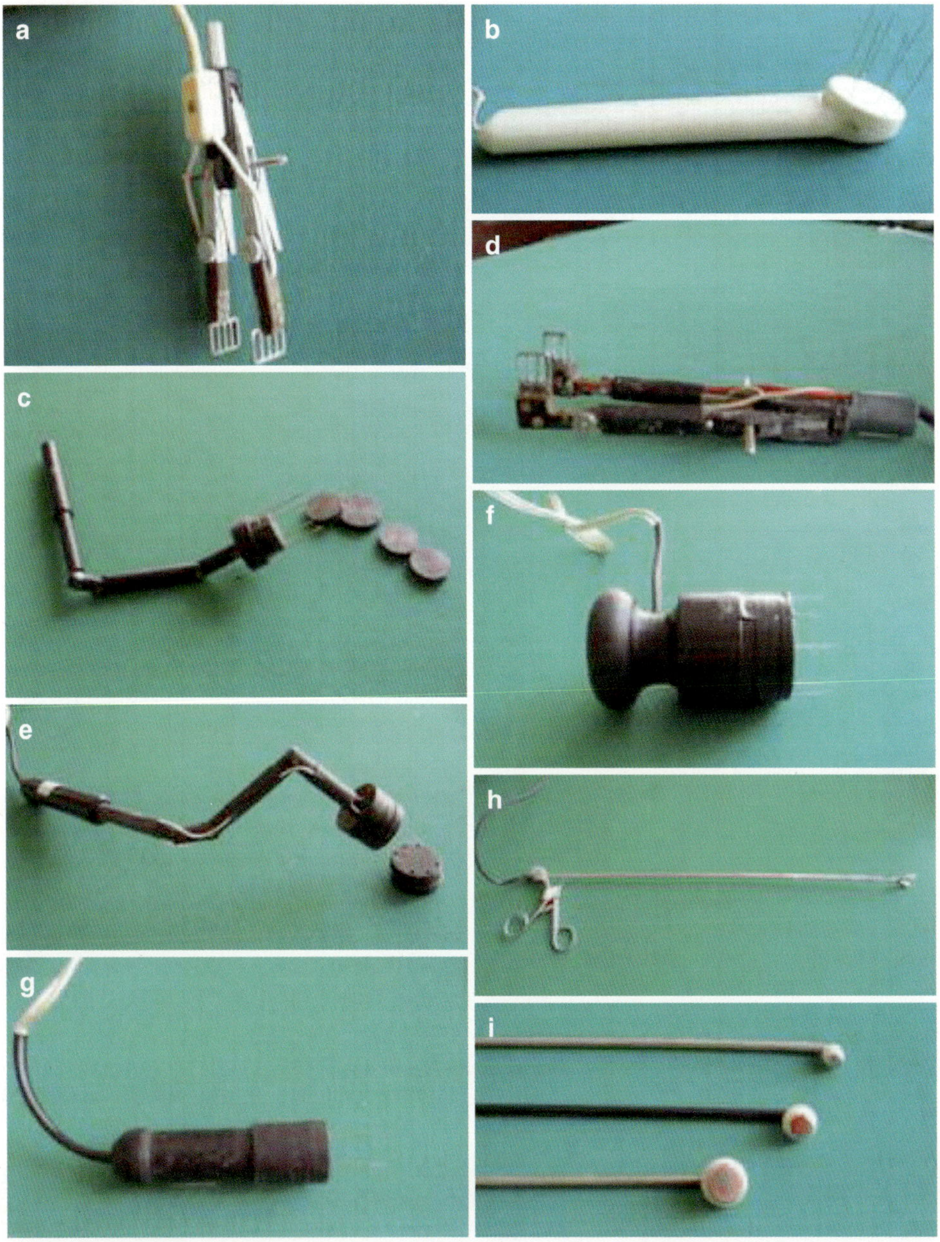

Fig. 28.4 Electrodes adopted with chemopulse (**a**) Steel and bakelite symmetrical compass electrode with perforated metal plates. Plate dimensions (length × height × width): 17 × 12 × 1 mm (Fig. 28.1a). (**b**) Six-needle array with long plastic handle and steel needles. Needle length: 45 mm; array diameter: 50 mm. (**c**) Six-needle array electrode with flexible plastic handle and steel needles. Needle length: 28 mm; array diameter: 25 mm. The electrode has six movable disks (whose thickness is 4 mm) that allow the modulation of needle insertion. (**d**) Modified monolateral compass electrode in steel, bakelite, and plastic with perforated metal plates. Plate dimensions: 22 × 10 × 1 mm. (**e**) Sharp and thin six-needle array electrode with flexible plastic handle and steel needles. Needle length: 28 mm; array diameter: 25 mm. This electrode has six movable disks of 4 mm thickness. (**f**) Sharp and thin six-needle array electrode with short handle and steel needles. Needle length: 40 mm; array diameter: 45 mm. This electrode comes with four movable disks a having thickness of 4 mm. (**g**) Vaccine type twin needle array electrode with plastic handle and steel needles. Needle length: 20 mm; array diameter: 20 mm. (**h**) Laparoscopic pinch steel electrode. This device has a metal clam shell pinch whose length is 20 mm long. Active part dimensions: 11 × 7 × 1 mm. (**i**) Unipolar plate steel electrodes whose active part is a little segment of sphere having an approximate diameter size of 10, 15, and 20 mm, respectively. (Modified from Spugnini et al. [38])

will be dependent upon the size, number, and responsiveness of the tumor nodules.

Response Criteria

Tumor response is determined by tumor volume. Tumor volume (V) is calculated from measured dimensions using the formula

$$V = \frac{\pi \times A \times B^2}{6}$$

where (A) is the longest diameter of the lesion (in mm) and (B) is the longest diameter (in mm) perpendicular to A.

Conclusion

Electrochemotherapy has proven to be an easy and effective treatment for the palliation of skin metastases, whose side effects are limited to muscular contractions and, seldom, skin burns at the site of electrodes' application. The major result has been so far obtained in the palliation of hemorrhaging melanomas [9] with a significant benefit for the patients. There are some strategies currently explored to enhance its efficacy and broaden its field of application. One of the most intriguing is its coupling with surgery in an adjuvant fashion (like a substitute of radiation therapy) for the treatment of bulky tumors, like reported in veterinary oncology [12–14]. Otherwise, its use in combination with direct tumor electrical destruction (irreversible electroporation) could be extremely proficient for the therapy of large soft tissue and deep cancers [40, 41].

Glossary

Bleomycin A G2-acting chemotherapy drug, whose efficacy is greatly amplified by electrochemotherapy. It is the first choice drug in electrochemotherapy practice.

Cisplatin A G1-acting chemotherapy drug, used as a second choice agent in electrochemotherapy.

Electrochemotherapy A therapy combining the administration of chemotherapy agents with permeabilizing electric pulses to improve drug efficacy.

Membrane pores Membrane perturbations caused by electric pulses that increase drug uptake.

References

1. Okino M, Mohri H. Effects of a high-voltage electrical impulse and an anticancer drug on in vivo growing tumors. Jpn J Cancer Res. 1987;78:1319–21.
2. Belehradek Jr J, Orlowski S, Poddevin B, Paoletti C, Mir LM. Electrochemotherapy of spontaneous mammary tumours in mice. Eur J Cancer. 1991;27:73–6.
3. Mir LM, Orlowski S, Belehradek Jr J, Paoletti C. Electrochemotherapy potentiation of antitumour effect of bleomycin by local electric pulses. Eur J Cancer. 1991;27:68–72.
4. Salford LG, Persson BR, Brun A, Ceberg CP, Kongstad PC, Mir LM. A new brain tumour therapy combining bleomycin with in vivo electropermeabilization. Biochem Biophys Res Commun. 1993;194:938–43.
5. Sersa G, Cemazar M, Miklavcic D. Antitumor effectiveness of electrochemotherapy with cis-diamminedichloroplatinum (II) in mice. Cancer Res. 1995;55:3450–5.
6. Belehradek M, Domenge C, Luboinski B, Orlowski S, Belehradek Jr J, Mir LM. Electrochemotherapy, a new antitumor treatment. First clinical phase I-II trial. Cancer. 1993;72:3694–700.
7. Mir LM, Glass LF, Sersa G, Teissié J, Domenge C, Miklavcic D, et al. Effective treatment of cutaneous and subcutaneous malignant tumours by electrochemotherapy. Br J Cancer. 1998;77:2336–42.
8. Panje WR, Hier MP, Garman GR, Harrell E, Goldman A, Bloch I. Electroporation therapy of head and neck cancer. Ann Otol Rhinol Laryngol. 1998;107:779–85.
9. Gehl J, Geertsen PF. Efficient palliation of haemorrhaging malignant melanoma skin metastases by electrochemotherapy. Melanoma Res. 2000;10:585–9.
10. Sersa G, Stabuc B, Cemazar M, Miklavcic D, Rudolf Z. Electrochemotherapy with cisplatin: clinical experience in malignant melanoma patients. Clin Cancer Res. 2000;6:863–7.
11. Sersa G, Stabuc B, Cemazar M, Miklavcic D, Rudolf Z. Electrochemotherapy with cisplatin: the systemic antitumour effectiveness of cisplatin can be potentiated locally by the application of electric pulses in the treatment of malignant melanoma skin metastases. Melanoma Res. 2000;10:381–5.
12. Spugnini EP, Baldi A, Vincenzi B, Bongiorni F, Bellelli C, Citro G, et al. Intraoperative versus postoperative electrochemotherapy in high grade soft tissue sarcomas: a preliminary study in a spontaneous feline model. Cancer Chemother Pharmacol. 2007;59:375–81.
13. Spugnini EP, Vincenzi B, Citro G, Santini D, Dotsinsky I, Mudrov N, et al. Adjuvant electrochemotherapy for

the treatment of incompletely excised spontaneous canine sarcomas. In Vivo. 2007;21:819–22.

14. Spugnini EP, Vincenzi B, Citro G, Dotsinsky I, Mudrov T, Baldi A. Evaluation of Cisplatin as an electrochemotherapy agent for the treatment of incompletely excised mast cell tumors in dogs. J Vet Intern Med. 2011;25:407–11.

15. Spugnini EP, Biroccio A, De Mori R, Scarsella M, D'Angelo C, Baldi A, et al. Electroporation increases antitumoral efficacy of the bcl-2 antisense G3139 and chemotherapy in a human melanoma xenograft. J Transl Med. 2011;9:125.

16. Teissie J, Golzio M, Rols MP. Mechanisms of cell membrane electropermeabilization: a minireview of our present (lack of?) knowledge. Biochim Biophys Acta. 2005;1724:270–80.

17. Rols MP. Electropermeabilization, a physical method for the delivery of therapeutic molecules into cells. Biochim Biophys Acta. 2006;1758:423–8.

18. Tounekti O, Kenani A, Foray N. The ratio of single to double-strand DNA breaks and their absolute values determine cell death pathway. Br J Cancer. 2001;84:1272–9.

19. Spugnini EP et al. Potential role of electrochemotherapy for the treatment of soft tissue sarcoma: first insights from preclinical studies in animals. Int J Biochem Cell Biol. 2008;40:159–63.

20. Rodamporn S, Beeby SP, Harris NR, Brown AD, Chad JE. Design and construction of a programmable electroporation system for biological applications. Proc ThaiBME. 2007; 234–8.

21. Daskalov I, Mudrov N, Peycheva E. Exploring new instrumentation parameters for electrochemotherapy. Attacking tumors with bursts of biphasic pulses instead of single pulses. IEEE Eng Med Biol Mag. 1999;18:62–6.

22. Peycheva E, Daskalov I. Electrochemotherapy of skin tumours: comparison of two electroporation protocols. J BUON. 2004;9:47–50.

23. Peycheva E, Daskalov I, Tsoneva I. Electrochemotherapy of Mycosis fungoides by interferon-alpha. Bioelectrochemistry. 2007;70:283–6.

24. Pron G, Belehradec Jr J, Mir LM. Identification of a plasma membrane protein that specifically binds bleomycin. Biochem Biophys Res Commun. 1993;194:333–7.

25. Byrnes RW, Templin J, Sem D, Lyman S, Petering D. Intracellular DNA strand scission and growth inhibition of Ehrlich ascites tumor cells by bleomycin. Cancer Res. 1990;50:5275–86.

26. Lazo JS. Bleomycin. In: Chabner BA, editor. Cancer chemotherapy and biotherapy. Philadelphia: Lippincott-Raven Publishers; 1996. p. 379–93.

27. Burger RM. Cleavage of nucleic acids by bleomycin. Chem Rev. 1998;98:1153–69.

28. Mir LM, Tounekti O, Orlowski S. Bleomycin: revival of an old drug. Gen Pharmacol. 1999;27:745–8.

29. Tounekti O, Pron G, Belehradek Jr J, Mir LM. Bleomycin, an apoptosis-mimetic drug that induces two types of cell death depending on the number of molecules internalized. Cancer Res. 1993;53: 5462–9.

30. Mir LM, Banoun H, Paoletti C. Introduction of definite amounts of nonpermanent molecules into living cells after electropermeabilization: direct access to cytosol. Exp Cell Res. 1988;175:15–25.

31. Trifonov D, Katev N, Daskalov I. Intra-arterial chemotherapy of breast cancer combined with electroporation. J BUON. 2001;6:331.

32. Sersa G, Cufer T, Cemazar M, Rebersek M, Zvonimir R. Electrochemotherapy with bleomycin in the treatment of hypernephroma metastases: case report and literature review. Tumori. 2000;86:163–5.

33. Kubota Y, Mir LM, Nakada T, Sasagawa I, Suzuki H, Aoyama N. Successful treatment of metastatic skin lesions with electrochemotherapy. J Urol. 1998;160:1426.

34. Rodríguez-Cuevas S, Barroso-Bravo S, Almanza-Estrada J, Cristóbal-Martínez L, González-Rodríguez E. Electrochemotherapy in primary and metastatic skin tumors: phase II trial using intralesional bleomycin. Arch Med Res. 2001;32:273–6.

35. Curatolo P, Mancini M, Clerico R, Ruggiero A, Frascione P, Di Marco P, et al. Remission of extensive merkel cell carcinoma after electrochemotherapy. Arch Dermatol. 2009;145:494–5.

36. Sersa G, Stabuc B, Cemazar M, Jancar B, Miklavcic D, Rudolf Z. Electrochemotherapy with cisplatin: potentiation of local cisplatin antitumour effectiveness by application of electric pulses in cancer patients. Eur J Cancer. 1998;34:1213–8.

37. Sersa G. The state of the art of electrochemotherapy before the ESOPE study; advantages and clinical uses. Eur J Cancer. 2006;4:52–9.

38. Spugnini EP et al. Rational design of new electrodes for electrochemotherapy. J Exp Clin Cancer Res. 2005;24:245–54.

39. Mir LM, Gehl J, Sersa G, Collins CG, Garbaya JR, Billard V, et al. Standard operating procedures of the electrochemotherapy: instructions for the use of bleomycin or cisplatin administered either systemically or locally and electric pulses delivered by the CliniporatorTM by means of invasive or non-invasive electrodes. Eur J Cancer (Suppl). 2006;4:14–25.

40. Neal 2nd RE, Rossmeisl Jr JH, Garcia PA, Lanz OI, Henao-Guerrero N, Davalos RV. Successful treatment of a large soft tissue sarcoma with irreversible electroporation. J Clin Oncol. 2011;29:e372–7.

41. Thompson K, Kee ST. Clinical research on irreversible electroporation of the liver. In: Kee ST, Gehl J, Lee EW, editors. Clinical aspects of electroporation. New York: Saunders Publisher; 2011. p. 237–46.

Systemic Treatment of Primary Cutaneous Lymphomas

29

Pablo Luis Ortiz-Romero and Evangelia Papadavid

Key Points

- Primary cutaneous lymphomas (PCL) are a group of non-Hodgkin's lymphomas originating in the skin in the absence of extracutaneous involvement.
- Emphasis will be made on skin-directed therapies. Different treatment modalities will be presented for both T-cell and B-cell lymphomas.

Introduction

Primary cutaneous lymphomas (PCL) are a heterogeneous group of non-Hodgkin's lymphomas that characteristically present on the skin. By definition, extracutaneous involvement at the moment of diagnosis must be absent.

P.L. Ortiz-Romero, MD, PhD (✉)
Department of Dermatology,
Instituto de investigación i + 12, hospital 12 de Octubre, Facultad de Medicina,
Universidad Complutense,
Avenida de Córdoba s/n, Madrid 28041, Spain
e-mail: portiz.hdoc@salud.madrid.org

E. Papadavid
Department of Dermatology,
Athens University Medical School, Attikon University Hospital and Andreas Syggros Cutaneous Lymphoma Clinic,
Athens, Greece

PCL are rare diseases. Annual incidence is around 0.4–1/100.000. About two-thirds have T-cell origin and, the rest, B-cell origin.

It is very important to consider that PCL have frequently a behaviour and prognosis totally different than their systemic counterparts that can involve secondarily the skin. Until the publication of the EORTC-WHO classification [1], it was not rare that PCL were treated with the same therapeutic approach of systemic lymphomas. Frequently, patients received treatments more aggressive than necessary for lymphomas with an indolent behaviour. More recently, WHO Blue Book classification of lymphomas has included almost all primary cutaneous lymphomas as separate entities (Table 29.1) [2].

Several guidelines to help clinicians to treat PCL have been published [3–7]. However, due to the rarity and heterogeneity of PCL, randomised clinical trials are usually lacking (with few exceptions) and levels of evidence are usually low.

Given that PCL can be easily reached, skin-directed treatments (alone or in combination with systemic agents) are frequently used (phototherapy, photochemotherapy, radiotherapy, topical treatments or intralesional infusion of several drugs). Skin-directed therapies are out of the scope of this chapter and will be treated elsewhere.

The choice of treatment will depend on the type of PCL and the stage of the disease. Some of our cases will need systemic approach from the beginning, and others will not be treated systemically, almost never.

A. Baldi et al. (eds.), *Skin Cancer*, Current Clinical Pathology,
DOI 10.1007/978-1-4614-7357-2_29, © Springer Science+Business Media New York 2014

Table 29.1 WHO-EORTC classification of primary cutaneous lymphomas

Cutaneous T-cell and NK-cell lymphomas

  Mycosis fungoides

  MF variants and subtypes

    Folliculotropic MF

    Pagetoid reticulosis

    Granulomatous slack skin

  Sézary syndrome

  Adult T-cell leukaemia/lymphoma

  Primary cutaneous CD30+ lymphoproliferative disorders

    Primary cutaneous anaplastic large cell lymphoma

    Lymphomatoid papulosis

  Subcutaneous panniculitis-like T-cell lymphoma

  Extranodal NK/T-cell lymphoma, nasal type

  Primary cutaneous peripheral T-cell lymphoma, unspecified

  Primary cutaneous aggressive epidermotropic CD8+ T-cell lymphoma (provisional)

  Cutaneous γ/δ T-cell lymphoma (provisional)

  Primary cutaneous CD4+ small/medium-sized pleomorphic T-cell lymphoma (provisional)

Cutaneous B-cell lymphomas

  Primary cutaneous marginal zone B-cell lymphoma

  Primary cutaneous follicle centre lymphoma

  Primary cutaneous diffuse large B-cell lymphoma, leg type

  Primary cutaneous diffuse large B-cell lymphoma, other

    Intravascular large B-cell lymphoma

Precursor hematologic neoplasm

  CD4+/CD56+ hematodermic neoplasm (blastic NK-cell lymphoma)

Table 29.2 Staging of mycosis fungoides

Ia: Patches/plaques covering <10 % body surface area
Ib: Patches/plaques covering ≥10 % body surface area
IIa: Patches or plaques, any surface + palpable, nonspecific lymph nodes
IIb: Tumoural stage
IIIa: Erythrodermic without peripheral blood involvement
IIIb: Erythrodermic with light peripheral blood involvement
IVa1: Any skin involvement with severe peripheral blood involvement
IVa2: Any skin involvement with lymph nodes infiltration
IVb: Any skin involvement with visceral involvement

than 20 years. If we consider MF stages, in early MF (stages Ia–IIa), stage Ia MF does not have impact in survival; in stages Ib and IIa, 10-years survival is >90 % and around 80 %, respectively. In advanced MF, stages IIb–IVb, median disease-specific survival is reached in around 7 years for stage IIb, around 4 years for stages III and IVa1, around 3 years for stage IVa2 and around 2 years for stage IVb [8, 9] (Table 29.2).

On the other hand, to date, no treatment has demonstrated to be able to modify natural history of the disease, and no treatment has been able to cure MF (except probably radiotherapy in unilesional MF).

So, our main interest should not be to cure MF but to increase quality of life (QoL), to achieve and maintain complete response, if possible, and to produce minimal toxicities during and after treatment.

Three MF variants are considered, based on their outcome, different from classical MF. Pagetoid reticulosis is characterised by the presence of localised patches or plaques with an intraepidermal proliferation of neoplastic T cells. The neoplastic T cells are CD3+ and may have either a CD4+ or CD8+. Prognosis is excellent and almost never need systemic therapies [1].

Follicular MF is characterised by the presence of folliculotropic or syringotropic infiltrates, often sparing the epidermis. Most cases show follicular mucinous degeneration. Lesions are frequently located on the head and neck area. Prognosis of follicular MF is worst than classical MF.

Primary Cutaneous T-Cell Lymphomas

Mycosis Fungoides and Variants

Mycosis fungoides (MF) is the most common primary cutaneous T-cell lymphoma, encompassing around 50 % of all PCLs. It characteristically evolves in patch, plaque and tumour stages and eventually can affect lymph nodes, peripheral blood and viscera. It is produced by proliferation of epidermotropic small to medium-sized T cells with cerebriform nuclei. Most of them are CD4+.

Before treating MF, doctors should have in mind that most cases have an indolent behaviour. Median survival of MF (in global) is not reached after more

Perifollicular location of the infiltrates renders them frequently less responsive to skin-directed therapies. So, systemic treatments will be used earlier in follicular MF than in classical MF.

Granulomatous slack skin (GSS) is characterised by the development of folds of lax skin, mostly on the axillae or inguinal groins. Histology shows a granulomatous infiltrate with elastophagocytosis and clonal T cells. Usually GSS has a very indolent behaviour.

Immunomodulators

Cytokines

IFNα

Interferons (IFNs) are cytokines that exhibit pleiotropic cellular effects, including antiviral, immunomodulatory, antiproliferative and proapoptotic effects [10, 11].

IFNα is indicated (alone or in combination) in early MF as a second-line treatment and in advanced MF as first-line treatment.

IFNα has been used subcutaneously in monotherapy at doses between 3 and 36 MU, 3 times a week. As high doses have much more adverse events and do not provide clearly better responses, usually low to intermediate doses (3–9 MU) are preferred.

In monotherapy, overall response rate (ORR) is around 88 % for early MF and 66 % for advanced MF. Between 10 and 35 % of patients achieve complete response. Intralesional IFNα is used in tumoural lesions, combining systemic effect with very high local doses.

Time to response is 8–12 weeks (some patients need >6 months to respond) and mean duration of response is between 30 and 40 months [12, 13].

Most common adverse events are fatigue, anorexia and a flu-like syndrome, more intense at the beginning of treatment. Usually it is well controlled with acetaminophen but occasionally is dose limiting. Leukopenia, thrombopenia and hypertransaminasemia are common too. Thyroid function should be monitored. Long-term users can develop depression [12–14].

IFNα is frequently used in combination with PUVA, retinoids, rexinoids or extracorporeal photopheresis.

Combination with PUVA seems to increase RR of PUVA with a 90–100 % ORR and 62–84 % CRs [15–18]. Stadler et al. [19] conducted a randomised clinical trial comparing PUVA alone vs. PUVA + IFNα. They reported that the combination was able to save UVA irradiation and to increase duration or response vs. PUVA alone.

Combination of IFNα with etretinate or acitretin should not be recommended because it produces similar response rates to IFN alone [20] and worst results than combination IFN + PUVA [21].

Other cytokines have been used to treat MF, trying to reverse the TH1/TH2 imbalance typical of the disease. Experience with IFNγ is much more limited and efficacy seems to be lower than IFNα. Response rates of 30 % without CRs have been reported in a phase II study with 16 patients. Duration of response was 10 months [22].

A phase II clinical trial with interleukin 12 (IL12) in early MF with 23 cases reported 43 % of RR (lasting 3 to >45 weeks) without CRs. Main toxicity was asthenia, headache, fatigue, chills, arthralgia, myalgia and increasing of GOT and GPT [23].

Results with IL2 have been poor, with 18 % of RR without CRs in a phase II clinical trial including 22 heavily pretreated MFs [24].

Retinoids/Rexinoids

Retinoids are derivatives of vitamin A that inhibit proliferation and induce differentiation in different tumours. In MF, etretinate, its metabolite acitretin and mostly bexarotene have been used.

Combined treatment of acitretin + PUVA achieves the same response of PUVA alone (73 % vs. 72 % CRs, respectively), but the cumulative dose of PUVA to achieve CR was lower in the combined treatment group [25]. Combination is recommended as second-line therapy in MF stages Ia to IIa and as first line for MF IIb or III [4].

Bexarotene (Bxt) is a rexinoid (specific agonist of RXR receptors). Bxt has multiple activities (blocks tumour growth, induces apoptosis, blocks NFKB, modifies microenvironment, etc.). Oral Bxt has been approved by FDA for resistant, recurrent MF (EMEA label includes "advanced").

It is recommended to start with 150 mg/m² and increase to 300 mg/m², if possible.

In monotherapy, response rates in refractory early MF are 54 %, with 7 % of CRs. Median time to response is about 8 weeks. Response rates in refractory advanced MF are 45 % with 2 % of CRs. Median time to response is >20 weeks [26, 27].

Most common adverse event is hypertriglyceridemia appearing between 80 and 100 % of cases. It is the most dose-limiting toxicity of Bxt. It usually starts 1–2 days after beginning and disappears 2–4 days after withdrawal of bexarotene. Second most common AE is central hypothyroidism, appearing between 70 and 80 % of cases. It starts and disappears 2–4 days after beginning and withdrawal of Bxt, respectively.

Other adverse events appearing in >20 % of cases are neutropenia (usually late), skin peeling, leukopenia, elevated LDH, headache and hypercholesterolemia. Very importantly, it does not produce photosensitivity, allowing combination with PUVA.

It is recommended to normalise serum lipids and thyroid function before starting Bxt. One or two hypolipidemic agents should be introduced one week before Bxt (fenofibrate ± statin are the most usual). Gemfibrozil is contraindicated because it produces paradoxical hypertriglyceridemia when combined with Bxt.

Most authors recommend to associate thyroid hormone replacement from the beginning (50μg/day) but is not always needed.

Blood tests should include lipid profile, free T4 (not TSH), muscle enzymes (to detect early myopathy induced by hypolipidemics) and pancreatic enzymes (to detect pancreatitis) and should be performed periodically, starting 1 week before and at 7, 14 and 28 days time points; after that, monthly [28, 29].

Bxt can be combined with different therapies as PUVA, IFN, extracorporeal photopheresis or denileukin diftitox.

Different series reporting combination of PUVA + Bxt have been published. In global, response rates vary from 60 to 78 % depending on the dosage of Bxt [30, 31]. A randomised clinical trial with PUVA + two different doses of Bxt (150 vs. 300 mg/day) (MILL-61896) did not find differences in response

rate. Interestingly, patients included in the trial seemed to need less UVA irradiation than historical doses needed in the centre that performed the study [32]. The EORTC CLTF has finished a randomised clinical trial (EORTC 21011) comparing Bxt+PUVA vs. Bxt alone. The study was underpowered but no significant differences in response rate or response duration was observed. There was a trend towards fewer PUVA sessions and lower UVA dose required to achieve CCR in the combination arm (PUVA + bexarotene) [3, 19, 30, 80].

A phase II clinical trial [33] reported that responses of the combination of IFN+Bxt were similar to Bxt alone. However, clinical practice shows that frequently patients achieving a tableau with Bxt or IFN alone respond with the combination [34].

Extracorporeal Photopheresis (ECP)

ECP is an immunomodulatory therapy involving leukapheresis. Lymphocytes are treated ex vivo with 8-methoxypsoralen + UVA irradiation and reinfused to the patient. First reported in 1987 [35], it was approved by FDA 1 year later for treatment of CTCL. More than 1,000 patients have been published with CTCL treated with ECP. RRs of 43–100 % and CRs from 0 to 62 % have been reported. Recently, UK consensus on the use of ECP has been published [36].

Mechanism of action is not well understood, but clinical and laboratory findings support the hypothesis of a vaccination-like effect. It seems that malignant T lymphocytes suffer cell cycle stop and apoptosis. After that, phagocytosis, antigen presentation and elicitation of specific immune responses mediated through cytotoxic T lymphocytes with antitumour specificity would occur.

ECP should be restricted to erythrodermic CTCL, either stage III or IVa demonstrating a peripheral blood involvement with T-cell clone and/or circulating Sézary cells >10 % and/or CD4/CD8 ratio >10. Patch/plaque or tumoural stages are not suitable for ECP. Treatment of stage IVb or erythrodermic patients without peripheral blood involvement is not recommended following UK consensus, but there are some publications reporting response in some of these patients. Patients with very high tumour burden in peripheral blood respond poorly and should be considered for combination (e.g. alemtuzumab) or alternative treatments.

Schedule includes 1–2 cycles per month (two procedures performed on two consecutive days per cycle).

Adverse events are rare. Venous access can originate infections.

UK consensus recommends maintaining treatment for at least 6 months. If no response is achieved, combination with other drugs (Bxt, IFN or multiple combinations are frequently used) [37–39] is done for three additional months. If no response, treatment should be stopped. International guidelines are under preparation (several workshops held to date in Minden and Lisbon) that probably could modify these recommendations. ECP treatment is recommended early as patients become more immunosuppressed with time.

Median time to maximum response is 10 months. Patients achieving response should be maintained with the same schedule and eventually reduce frequency (every 6–12 weeks) before stopping. Median time to treatment failure is 18 months.

Transimmunisation is a modification of ECP consisting in incubating overnight at body temperature the buffy coat after photoactivation. This allows co-incubation of the apoptotic malignant T cells with the newly formed antigen-presenting cells prior to reinfusion [40].

Monoclonal Antibodies

Denileukin diftitox (Ontak™, Onzar™), DAB389–IL-2, is a recombinant fusion protein that selectively binds high-affinity IL-2 receptor (CD25). The molecule consists of sequences for the enzymatically active domain of diphtheria toxin and the IL2. After joining receptor, DAB389-IL2 is internalised in the cell, diphtheria toxin is released and protein synthesis is blocked, resulting in cell death.

Denileukin diftitox was approved by FDA in 1999 (not by EMEA) for resistant, recurrent MF expressing IL2. Dose schedule is 18 mcg/kg/day by IV infusion once daily for 5 days every 3 weeks for up to 8 cycles.

Phase III clinical trials [41, 42] including patients with stages Ib-IVa and at least 20 % of cells expressing IL2 have reported RRs between 30 and 49 % with 10 % of CRs. Median time to response is 3–4 months and median duration of response is 6.9 months.

Most common adverse events are fever, myalgia, chills, nausea and vomiting and a mild increase in transaminase levels. Acute hypersensitivity occurs in 60 %, always in the first 24 h and during the initial infusion. Vascular leak syndrome (hypotension, hypoalbuminaemia and oedema) occurs in 25 % of cases within the first 14 days of a given dose. Myelosuppression is very rare. Adverse events drop and response rates increase to 60 % if patients are pretreated with corticosteroids [43].

Response rate is higher in CD25+ MF cases. Different papers have reported 30–78 % of response in cases with >20 % of cells expressing CD25 and 20–30 % in cases with low CD25 expression. However, a recent review considering only patients achieving CR with denileukin diftitox did not find differences between CD25 +ve and −ve cases. More than 36 % of patients relapsing after a first course of denileukin diftitox treatment respond again to this drug [44–46].

Combination of denileukin diftitox with bexarotene is based on the rationale that Bxt can induce expression of IL2 on malignant T cells. A phase I clinical trial combining Ontak + Bxt reported 67 % of RR [47].

Alemtuzumab (Campath™) is a humanised monoclonal antibody that targets CD52. CD52 is found in normal and malignant B and T cells. Granulocytes, macrophages or thrombocytes do not express CD52. Alemtuzumab is usually administered at a dose of 30 mg intravenously three times per week, for up to 12 weeks.

A phase II clinical trial [48] with 22 patients with heavily pretreated MF or SS patients reported an ORR of 55 % with 32 % of CRs. Sézary cells were cleared from the blood in 6 of 7 (86 %) patients, and CR in lymph nodes was observed in 6 of 11 (55 %) patients. The effect was better on erythroderma (OR, 69 %) than on plaque or skin tumours (OR, 40 %) and in patients who had received 1 to 2 previous regimens (OR, 80 %) than in those who had received 3 or more prior regimens (OR, 33 %). Time to treatment failure was 12 months.

The main problem with alemtuzumab is the severe immunosuppression produced, with high-risk viral, bacterial and fungal infectious complications that may be life-threatening [49].

Patients should be monitored for CMV reactivation using periodically PCR studies every 2–3 weeks. If viremia is increasing, ganciclovir should be recommended. On the other hand, acyclovir and sulfamethoxazole trimethoprim to prevent herpes virus and Pneumocystis carinii pneumonia should be given to patients. Mantoux test with booster and chest X-ray to detect latent infection by Mycobacterium tuberculosis should be performed. Active or latent hepatitis B or C infections should be treated before using alemtuzumab. Serology for Strongyloides is recommended for patients living in endemic areas.

Recently, a new approach with low subcutaneous dose (10 mg s.c. eod) has been reported with very good results (14 patients, 3 CRs and 9 PRs) and very importantly, without infectious complications [50].

Finally, patients should have cardiac monitorisation. In a series of patients treated with standard IV dose, 4 of 8 patients with no prior history of cardiac problems developed significant cardiac toxicity (congestive heart failure or arrhythmia) that mostly improved after alemtuzumab discontinuation [51].

Other monoclonal antibodies are under investigation.

Zanolimumab is a fully human anti-CD4 antibody directed against CD4 molecules on surface of T cells. There are 2 phase II clinical trials finished, including 47 patients [52]. Patients were initially treated with intravenous zanolimumab at a dose of 280 mg/week, which was increased to 560 mg/week in early-stage patients and 980 mg/week in patients with advanced disease. In MF, RRs were low in the low dose (15 %) vs. high dose (56 % of RR with 2 CRs and 10 PRs). In SS, RR was only 22 % with high dose, showing a greater efficacy of zanolimumab in MF compared to SS.

In the high-dose arm, median time to response was less than 8 weeks and median response duration, 81 weeks. Most frequent adverse events are eczematous dermatitis, low-grade infections, flu-like symptoms and asthenia. Zanolimumab produces a very prolonged CD4 reduction, lasting even >24 months. There is an ongoing pivotal

phase III clinical trial comparing 3 dose levels (4 vs. 8 vs. 14 mg/kg). The first two doses were stopped because of low RRs. Trial was stopped in Europe but is ongoing in the USA.

Recombinant *CD3 immunotoxin* (A-dmDT (390)-bisFv(UCHT1)) is composed of the catalytic and translocation domains of diphtheria toxin fused to two single-chain Fv fragments of an anti-CD3 epsilon monoclonal antibody. The drug was administered to 5 MF patients. Two of them had PR lasting 1 and >6 months [53].

SGN30 and a more active drug (SGN35, brentuximab vedotin (BV)) are anti CD30 monoclonal antibodies. Brentuximab vedotin is a chimeric protein targeting CD30 on cell surface. The molecule is conjugated with monomethyl auristatin E (MMAE), a microtubule disruptor. After joining receptor, MMAE is internalized and blocks mitosis. In two different trials recently reported, ORR is between 40 and 68 % depending on the level of CD30 expression. Time to response was 6-10.5 weeks. Most frequent adverse events are peripheral neuropathy, rash, fatigue and diarrhea. Neutropenia can be severe [54, 96, 97].

Mogamulizumab (KW-061), a humanized, defucosilated monoclonal antibody targeting CCR4 produces antibody dependent cellular cytotoxicity. ORR in a recent phase II clinical trial was 37 % (29 % in mycosis fungoides, 47 % in Sézary syndrome).

Inhibitors of Histone Deacetylases (HDACi)

HDACi are a new group of compounds involved in the balance of acetylation/deacetylation of proteins within the cell. Histones are the main proteic component of the chromatin. Its main function is to allow DNA strand to roll around and form nucleosomes. Protein queues of histones can suffer different chemical modifications (phosphorylation, methylation, acetylation, etc.). Depending on the level of histone acetylation, chromatin has a more or less relaxed or packed disposition. Relaxed chromatin allows gene expression, while packed chromatin does not. HDACi produce histone hyperacetylation, chromatin has a more relaxed disposition, and cells modify their behaviour.

Very importantly many other proteins in the cell can suffer acetylation/deacetylation (p53, bcl6, cMyc, NFKB, HSP90, etc.). In global all these proteins are called acetiloma. The final result of HDACi is a group of transcriptional and non-transcriptional effects with cell cycle stop, induction of apoptosis, increase of immunogenicity, antiangiogenic activity, chaperone inhibition, mitotic catastrophe, autophagy and senescence [55–57].

Vorinostat

Vorinostat (Zolinza™) is the first HDACi approved by FDA in 2006 (not approved by EMEA) for the treatment of CTCL progressive, persistent or recurrent after two systemic therapies. Recommended dose is 400 mg daily, oral [58, 59].

Phase IIb clinical trial with 74 patients (most of them stage at least IIb) showed a RR of 29.7 % without CRs (including 30 % of showed a RR in advanced disease, a 33 % of RR in Sézary syndrome and a 22 % of RR in tumoural stage). Median time to response was around 2 months and time to progression, 4.9 months (in cases with stage at least IIb median time to progression was 9.8 months).

The most common adverse events (AE) were diarrhoea (49 %), fatigue (46 %), nausea (43 %) and anorexia (26 %); most were grade 2 or lower but those grade 3 or higher included fatigue (5 %), pulmonary embolism (5 %), thrombocytopenia (5 %) and nausea (4 %).

Post hoc analysis has demonstrated safety of vorinostat after at least 2 years of long-term maintenance [60].

Immunohistochemical analysis of STAT1 and phosphorylated STAT3 (pSTAT3) in skin biopsies obtained from CTCL patients enrolled in the vorinostat phase IIb trial showed that nuclear accumulation of STAT1 and high levels of nuclear pSTAT3 in malignant T cells correlate with a lack of clinical response [61]. On the other hand, HR23B expression pretreatment is considered a biomarker for response to vorinostat [62].

Romidepsin

Romidepsin (Istodax ®) is the second HDACi approved by FDA (2009) for the treatment of adult patients with cutaneous T-cell lymphoma (CTCL) or peripheral T-cell lymphoma (PTCL) who have received at least one prior systemic therapy. Romidepsin is given IV at a dose of 14 mg/m^2 on days 1, 8 and 15 every 28 days [63, 64].

Pooled analysis of 2 clinical trials included 167 (71 + 96) patients, 76 % of them at least stage IIb. RR was 41 % with 6 % of CRs. RR in Sézary syndrome was 58 %.

A clinically meaningful improvement in pruritus was observed in 43 % of patients, including patients who did not achieve an objective response.

Time to response was 2 months and median duration of response was 15 months.

Very interestingly, it has been shown that romidepsin increases CD25 expression, giving a rational basis to possible future treatments combined with denileukin diftitox.

Most common drug-related adverse events (AE), all grades, included nausea (67 %), fatigue (49 %), anorexia (37 %), ECG T-wave changes (29 %), anaemia (26 %), dysgeusia (23 %), neutropenia (22 %) and leukopenia (20 %).

Other HDACi are under investigation. *Panobinostat* (20 mg, oral, days 1, 3 and 5 of every week). A phase II clinical trial reported with Seventy-nine bexarotene-exposed and 60 bexarotene-naïve patients. The ORR was 17.3 % (15.2 % and 20.0 % in the bexarotene-exposed and -naïve groups, respectively). The most common adverse events were thrombocytopenia, diarrhoea, fatigue and nausea [65].

Proteasome Inhibitors: Bortezomib (Velcade™)

Bortezomib is a reversible inhibitor of the 26S proteasome in mammalian cells that degrades ubiquitinated proteins, thereby maintaining homeostasis within cells. Inhibition of the 26S proteasome can affect multiple signalling cascades within the cell, produces stress of the endoplasmic reticulum and can lead to cell death [66].

Bortezomib is FDA approved for the treatment of multiple myeloma patients and mantle cell lymphoma patients who have received at least 1 prior therapy.

In MF, a phase II study [67] with 12 previously treated CTCL (stage III or IVb) patients who received bortezomib as monotherapy for a total of six cycles (1.3 mg/m^2 iv, days 1, 4, 8 and 11 out of 21). The overall response rate was 67 %, with two (17 %) CRs and six (50 %) PRs. All responses were durable, lasting from 7 to 14 or more months. The most common grade 3 toxicities were neutropenia ($n=2$), thrombocytopenia ($n=2$) and sensory neuropathy ($n=1$).

Chemotherapeutic Agents

MF is relatively chemoresistant due to the low proliferative rate that frequently have the tumour cells. Both single and multiagent chemotherapy have been used in MF. Chemotherapy should be restricted for advanced MF (stages IIb–IV). There is evidence against its use in early MF. Kaye et al. reported a randomised clinical trial comparing chemotherapy: cyclophosphamide, adriamycin, vincristine and etoposide (CAVE)+total skin electron beam irradiation (TSEB) vs. conservative palliative therapy, consisting of topical mechlorethamine, superficial radiotherapy and phototherapy. RR was better in the chemotherapy group (38 % vs. 18 %), but very importantly, there were no significant differences in disease-free survival or overall survival between the two groups. Toxicity was much higher in the aggressive arm [68].

Single-Agent Chemotherapy

A systematic review including 526 MF patients treated with different single-agent chemotherapeutic agents reported a response rate of 66 % (median duration 3–22 months) with 33 % or CRs [69].

Gemcitabine is a pyrimidine nucleoside analogue that, after phosphorylation, inhibits ribonucleotide reductase and DNA synthesis. It is used IV 1,000–1,200 mg/m^2 on days 1, 8 and 15 out of 28. RRs between 50 and 70 % with CRs between 8 and 16 % have been reported. Adverse events include myelosuppression that can oblige to dose reduction, haemolytic uremic syndrome, pulmonary embolism, congestive heart failure, acute myocardial infarction, angina, increased hepatic transaminases, mucositis, lethargy, fever, cutaneous hyperpigmentation, infusion-related maculopapular rash and radiation recall [70, 71].

Chlorambucil is a nitrogen mustard derivative that works as a bifunctional alkylating agent. It is recommended for erythrodermic MF or SS. Usual dose is 2–6 mg/day, combined with prednisone (20–40 mg/day). Other authors recommend pulses every 2 weeks consisting of chlorambucil 10–12 mg/day for 3 consecutive days+flucortolone 75 mg first day, 50 mg second day and 25 mg third day [72, 73].

Methotrexate (MTX) is an antineoplastic antimetabolite with immunosuppressant properties. It is an inhibitor of tetrahydrofolate dehydrogenase and prevents the formation of tetrahydrofolate, necessary for synthesis of thymidylate, an essential component of DNA. Oral weekly doses between 5 and 125 mg have been used.

In patch/plaque stage (Ib), Zackheim and colleagues reported 12 % patients with CR and 22 % of PR. Median time to treatment failure was 15 months [74].

However, MTX has been used mostly for erythrodermic MF or SS. PRs of 17–35 % with 40 % of CRs have been reported [75, 76].

Most common side effects of MTX include ulcerative stomatitis, leukopenia, abdominal distress, fatigue and decreased resistance to infection. Long-term use can produce hepatic fibrosis or even cirrhosis.

Pentostatin (2′-deoxycoformycin) is a purine analogue and a potent inhibitor of adenosine deaminase, producing apoptosis of lymphocytes. Dose is 5 mg/m^2 intravenous (IV) bolus for three consecutive days of every 3-week cycle. Most patients do not have toxicity but cardiac or pulmonary events can be life-threatening. Open studies in MF and SS have reported RRs of 35–71 % with 10–33 % of CRs [77, 78].

Pegilated liposomal doxorubicin (Caelyx™) is an anthracycline glycoside antineoplastic antibiotic. The drug's precise mechanism of action is not fully understood, but it appears to be a DNA-damaging agent. Dose recommended is 20 mg/m^2, days 1 and 14 out of 28 days. Several papers have been published in MF. The EORTC conducted a phase II clinical trial (21012) inclinding 49 patients and reported 40.8 % of response rate (6.1 % had complete responses and 34.7 % experienced PRs). Median time to progression and median duration of response were 7.4 and 6 months, respectively. Most frequent toxicity is palmoplantar erythrodysesthesia. Cardiomyopathy should be monitored, but cardiac toxicity of liposomal doxorubicin is low [79, 80].

Pralatrexate (Folotyn ™) is a novel antifolate designed for preferential tumour uptake and accumulation. It inhibits dihydrofolate reductase (DHFR). Pralatrexate is given intravenously. Optimal dose is 15 mg/m^2/week/6 weeks + vitamin B12 (1 mg i.m. every 8–10 weeks) + folic acid (1 mg/day orally). The subgroup of 12 MF patients included in the PROPEL study, central analysis showed 25 % of response rate with 1.7 months of disease free survival. Investigator analysis of the same group of patients reported a 58 % of response rate with 5.3 months of progression free survival [81, 82].

Most frequent toxicity was mucositis. Pralatrexate was approved by FDA in 2009 but asked post-marketing requirements (a clinical trial comparing pralatrexate + bexarotene vs. bexarotene alone).

Forodesine is a purine nucleoside phosphorylase inhibitor that selectively induces T-cell apoptosis. It is under investigation in CTCL. Recommended dose is 10 mg oral/12 h. There are reports about a phase I/II clinical trial with 64 cases (80 % were at least stage IIb). Overall RR was 39 % (with 3 CRs). Importantly, erythrodermic MF had higher RR (65 %). Median time to response was 42 days and median duration or response was 127 days+. Main toxicities were nausea, headache, diarrhoea, fatigue, pruritus and peripheral oedema. Grade 3 adverse events were pneumonia, cellulites and diarrhoea [83].

Polychemotherapy

Multiagent chemotherapy should be restricted to advanced MF after failure of several other systemic treatments, including monochemotherapy. The exception is maybe stage IVb in which multiple-agent chemotherapy should be offered early to patients. As commented before, polychemotherapy in early MF achieves higher RR than conservative, skin-directed treatment but gives much higher toxicity without impact in overall survival [68]. Moreover, it is frequent that relapses after polychemotherapy are relatively rapid and frequently aggressive.

A systematic review including 331 patients treated with different combinations [69] reported 31 % of CRs. Median duration of responses was between 5 and 41 months.

Most popular multiple-agent chemotherapy is CHOP (cyclophosphamide, doxorubicin, vincristine and prednisone).

BMTransplantation

Autologous stem cell transplantation (*SCT*) is not recommended for MF because, although patients achieve response, usually it is very transient, with disease progression occurring within months after the procedure [84]. Even after careful manipulation of the stem cell harvest, most cases present the T-cell clone in the reinfusion sample. Interestingly, the presence or not of the clone does not predict duration of response [85]. A meta-analysis performed to compare the outcome of allogeneic vs. autologous SCT in patients with MF/Sézary syndrome showed a more favourable outcome of patients who received allogeneic SCT [86].

Recently a paper by the European Group for Blood and Marrow Transplantation has been published reporting MF/SS cases after allo-SCT [87]. They reported an OS of 66 % at 1 year and 54 % at 3 years in the whole group. Overall survival is better in cases with family-related donor, with less advanced disease (less systemic therapies used) and with reduced intensity conditioning (to reduce the toxicity related to induction therapy and to increase graft-vs.-lymphoma effect). Their suggestion is to perform the allo-SCT as soon as possible, using relative donors and reduced intensity conditioning. The problem is that mortality without relapse in the first year (probably in most cases is mortality caused by procedure) is around 20 %. In other words, around 20 % of patients die in the first year probably caused by the SCT.

Overall survival (including relapse and non-relapse mortality) is around 60 % in the first year. After that curves reach a plateau meaning that some patients could be cured or at least are manageable with other non-chemotherapeutic therapies. Very interestingly, some patients who experience relapse can successfully undergo rescue treatment with donor lymphocyte infusions (looking for graft vs. lymphoma effect), and relapses seem to be more indolent and frequently respond to nonaggressive therapies.

Allo-SCT should be considered in young patients with advanced MF resistant to several previous systemic therapies. The best moment to perform the procedure is not well defined yet. The risk of mortality within the first 1 or 2 years and the quality of life related to lymphoma and to graft vs. host should be bear in mind.

Spectrum of CD30+ Lymphoproliferative Disorders

This group of diseases encompasses a clinico-pathologic spectrum that goes from primary cutaneous anaplastic large cell lymphoma (PC-ALCL) on one side to lymphomatoid papulosis (LyP) on the other with borderline cases in the middle. They are the second most common group of primary cutaneous lymphomas, accounting around 30 % of all PCL.

PC-ALCLs are characterised by the presence of different kinds of cells in the infiltrate (not only anaplastic), but, as a diagnostic criteria, more than 75 % of them must express CD30 antigen. Previous mycosis fungoides, LyP or systemic ALCL should be discarded. Clinically, most patients present solitary or grouped cutaneous tumours, frequently ulcerated. Partial or total spontaneous remission appears in about one-third of lesions. Around 10 % can spread to regional lymph nodes [1]. Prognosis is very good with 90 % 10-year survival. Lymph node involvement does not seem to worsen prognosis of PC-ALCL [88]. Recently consensus recommendations of the EORTC, ISCL and USCCL for treatment of this lymphoma have been published [6]. Solitary or grouped lesions should not be treated with systemic therapies. Treatment of choice is surgical excision or radiotherapy.

For PC-ALCL with multifocal lesions, poly-chemotherapy (frequently CHOP) has been used, achieving around 90 % of CRs but with 70 % of relapses [6]. Experience with MTX (5–25 mg/sem) for multilesional PCALCL is limited, but there is a generalised expert consensus that its use is reasonable.

Alternatives to MTX are interferon alpha, bexarotene or thalidomide, but reported cases are scarce. Polychemotherapy is discouraged except for cases with extracutaneous spread beyond locoregional lymph nodes.

A phase II clinical trial with a monoclonal antibody anti-CD30 (SGN30) included 11 patients with PC-ALCL. Six of them (55 %) achieved CR and 3 of them (27 %), PR [54]. Three of the six cases with more than one problem (different combinations of MF, LyP and pcALCL) achieved CR too. Most frequent AEs were fatigue, pruritus and diarrhoea. A clinical trial with SGN35 including both CD30+ MF and PC-ALCL is ongoing. SGN35 is a chimeric protein composed of the same monoclonal antibody of SGN30 linked to auristatin E, an antitubulin agent that produces mitotic catastrophe [54, 89].

LyP is characterised by the presence of multiple papulonodular generalised, recurrent, self-curative lesions, appearing chronically over years. Histologically, four variants have been described, but a particular patient can have several of them at the same moment or in different time points. In type B LyP, CD30+ cells are frequently absent. Prognosis is excellent with almost a 100 % of 10-year survival. Between 10 and 20 % of LyP are associated (pre or post LyP) with other lymphomas, mostly MF, Hodgkin's disease and ALCL. To date, no treatment has demonstrated to modify natural course of LyP, and no treatment has demonstrated a risk reduction to transformation into more aggressive lymphomas.

In patients with limited number of lesions and not leaving disfiguring scars, "wait and see" is acceptable. High-power topical corticosteroids accelerate regression of lesions but do not prevent appearance of new lesions, and relapses are rapid. Oral corticosteroids are not effective.

For cases with important number of lesions or leaving scars, phototherapy or low-dose weekly MTX (5–25 mg) are the best choices (reviewed in [6]).

Different phototherapy approaches have been tried in LyP: PUVA, UVA1, UVB, nbUVB, and heliotherapy. No comparative study has been performed. With any of them, most patients have reduction in number of lesions and faster regression of the lesions. RRs are around 95 %. Relapses appear shortly after cessation of therapy in around

80 % of patients. Maintenance therapy could increase the risk of skin cancer.

Low-dose methotrexate is also very effective for LyP, with RRs around 100 % but rapid relapses after discontinuation oblige to maintenance therapy, increasing the risk of toxicity for long-term therapy.

Experience with other systemic treatments (IFN, retinoids, rexinoids) is more limited.

Polychemotherapy should not be used in LyP. Clearance of lesions is the usual, but relapses appear immediately after the end of the cycles (or even during cycles) [6].

In the same phase II clinical trial with SGN30 commented before, 3 LyP cases were included. One patient each achieved CR or PR. With SGN35, a previously cited phase II clinical trial included 6 LyP patients. All of them achieved response (5 of them CR) after a median of 3 weeks. Duration of response was 22 weeks [54].

Subcutaneous Panniculitis-Like T-Cell Lymphoma (SP-TCL)

SP-TCL is characterised clinically for the presence of subcutaneous nodules or deep plaques, usually multiple or generalised, located more frequently on the legs but any body area can be involved. Ulceration is rare.

Nineteen percent of the patients present associated autoimmune diseases (mostly lupus erythematosus). Differentiation from LE panniculitis can be difficult.

Infiltrate is generally confined to the subcutis. Cells are pleomorphic with predominance of small- to medium-sized cells. Rimming around individual adipocytes, fat necrosis and karyorrhexis are typical. Immunophenotype is usually CD4−, CD8+ CD56−, and betaF1+; strongly expresses cytotoxic proteins; and frequently loses panT markers. Haemophagocytic syndrome (HPS) appears in 17 % of cases. Five years OS in cases without HPS is >90 % vs. 46 % in cases with HPS [1, 90]. Given the excellent prognosis of SP-TCL without HPS, polychemotherapy is not recommended. In the paper by the EORTC CLTF, 55 % of the cases reached sustained complete remission after prednisone or other immunosuppressive agents (even in relapsed cases). CHOP(−like) courses resulted in a sustained complete remission of 64 % of the patients, with much higher toxicity. Patients with solitary lesions respond to surgery or radiotherapy without additional systemic treatments.

Patients with SP-TCL with HPS have a very poor outcome even despite treatment with CHOP or CHOP-like combinations. Auto-SCT or allo-SCT have been proposed as options for these patients, but experience is limited [90–92].

Other Primary Cutaneous T-Cell Lymphomas

Except primary cutaneous CD4+ small/medium-sized pleomorphic T-cell lymphoma, the rest of PCLs (*NK/T cell, nasal type*; *cutaneous gamma-delta TCL and aggressive epidermotropic CD8+*) are aggressive diseases with median survivals around 12–36 months. Treatment with polychemotherapy should be given as first option, but results are disappointing. Auto or allo-SCT should be considered.

Primary cutaneous CD4+ small/medium-sized pleomorphic T-cell lymphoma has a very good prognosis with a 5-year survival between 60 and 80 %, especially in cases with solitary or localised lesions. In these cases, surgery and radiotherapy are the treatments of choice. Interferon, cyclophosphamide or bexarotene has been used [1].

Cutaneous B-Cell Lymphomas

Primary cutaneous B-cell lymphomas (CBCL) represent 20–25 % of all PCL. This group includes 3 main diseases: primary cutaneous marginal zone lymphoma (PCMZL), primary cutaneous follicular centre lymphoma (PCFCL) and primary cutaneous diffuse large B-cell lymphoma, leg type (PCLBCL,LT) [1]. In the WHO classification, PCFCL and PCLBCL,LT are considered separate entities, whereas PCMZL has been included among the rest of extranodal marginal zone B-cell lymphomas [2].

Primary Cutaneous Marginal Zone B-Cell Lymphoma

PCMZL is an indolent disease. It is clinically characterised for the presence of solitary or multiple nodules, mostly on extremities. In endemic areas, it can be associated to *B. Burgdorferi* infection. Infiltrate is composed of small B cells, including marginal zone cells (centrocyte-like), lymphoplasmacytoid cells and plasma cells. Immunophenotype shows monotypic cIg, CD20+, Bcl2+, Bcl6−, and MUM1−(+ on plasma cells). Extracutaneous progression is exceptional and 5-year survival is 95–100 % [1, 2]. Recently, the EORTC CLTF and the ISCL have published a paper with consensus recommendations for treatment of CBCL [7].

Given that PCMZL is an indolent disease, observation (with close follow-up of patients) is an acceptable possibility. Those cases positive for Borrelia should be treated with antibiotics first. Forty-three percent of them achieve CR after different antibiotic regimens. No comparative studies have been performed but cephalosporins seem to be superior to tetracyclines (reviewed in [7]).

In cases with solitary or scarce number of lesions, surgery or radiotherapy are the therapies of choice. More than 40 % of cases relapse, but relapse does not mean worsening of prognosis.

Intralesional corticosteroids depot has been rarely reported but with good results. In a series with 9 patients, 4 CR and 5 PRs were reported. Median duration of response was 47 months [93].

Intralesional IFN has been reported [94] in a series of 8 cases, using 3 MU, 3 times a week. All patients responded; 25 % relapsed but responded again with IFN.

Rituximab (MabThera™, antiCD20 monoclonal antibody) has been used both intravenously (375 mg/m^2/week, 4 weeks) and intralesionally in very limited number of cases. CRs between 67 and 89 %, respectively, have been reported [7]. Spanish Cooperative Group on Cutaneous Lymphomas [98] has recently published a paper including 17 cases of PCMZL (10 mg per lesion, 3 injections per week, only 1 week a month). Sixty-seven percent of them achieved CR with very low cumulative doses of Rituximab (median 150 mg). Interestingly, non-injected lesions responded frequently, showing systemic effect of intralesional rituximab.

Chlorambucil has been used as single-agent chemotherapy in several papers. All patients responded with 64 % of CRs.

Multiagent chemotherapy has been used, mostly in multilesional cases, achieving 85 % of CRs. However, adverse events caused by polychemotherapy do not support its use in this indolent lymphoma. In a paper by Bekkenk et al., they reported that in patients with primary cutaneous immunocytoma (probably most of them would be now classified as PCMZL) or PCFLC (see below), outcome is similar with radiotherapy or with multiagent chemotherapy [95].

Primary Cutaneous Follicle Centre Lymphoma

PCFCL is a tumour of neoplastic follicle centre cells. It usually presents as solitary or multiple nodules or tumours located mainly on the trunk or head. Infiltrate can be follicular, follicular and diffuse or diffuse, composed of a mixture of neoplastic centrocytes and centroblasts. Immunophenotype shows monotypic or absent cIg, CD20+, Bcl2−, Bcl6+ and MUM1−, FoxP1− [1, 2]. Outcome is good, with 5-year survival of 95 %. Between 5 and 10 % of cases present extracutaneous dissemination.

Similar as recommended for PCMZL, a wait-and-see policy is acceptable for PCFLC asymptomatic with low number of lesions.

Most frequently reported treatment for PCFCL is radiotherapy, with almost 100 % CRs and 47 % or relapses. The EORTC/ISCL paper recommends doses of at least 30 Gy (but probably much lower doses are enough) and a margin of clinically uninvolved skin of at least 1 to 1.5 cm.

Similar to PCMZL, patients with unilesional or low number of lesions, surgical excision is also an excellent choice, with 98 % of CRs.

Responses with IFN or intralesional rituximab are quite similar to those reached with PCMZL. In the paper by the Spanish Cooperative Croup on Cutaneous Lymphomas, they included 18 cases of PCFCL treated with intralesional rituximab. Almost 80 % achieved CR with very low cumulative doses (median, similar to PCMZL).

Intravenous rituximab with the standard dose (375 mg/m^2) has been reported in several papers (reviewed in [7]) with 75 % of CRs. Duration of treatment was 1–8 weeks in different reports. Some patients relapse after CR, but all relapses were confined to the skin. The EORTC/ISCL consensus paper considers rituximab as the first choice of treatment in cases with very extensive skin lesions. According to this paper, combination chemotherapy (R-COP; R-CHOP) or chemoradiotherapy should be considered only in exceptional cases, such as patients with progressive disease not responding to rituximab or patients developing extracutaneous disease.

In a similar way as PCMZL, relapses are usually confined to the skin and should not be interpreted as an upgrade in the aggressiveness of the disease. Cutaneous relapses usually respond to the same treatments previously used.

Primary Cutaneous Diffuse Large B-Cell Lymphoma, Leg Type

This is a lymphoma characterised for a monomorphic proliferation of large transformed B cells, arising most commonly on the legs [1, 2]. Malignant cells express monotypic sIg and/or cIg, CD20+, CD79a+, Bcl2+, bcl6+(−), MUM1+ and FoxP1+. PCLBCL,LT is an aggressive disease with frequent relapses and extracutaneous dissemination. Five-year survival is 55 %. Outcome seems to be better in cases with solitary lesions.

Radiotherapy for PCLBCL,LT achieves 88 % or CRs, but extracutaneous relapses around 30 % have been reported. Treatment of choice is R-CHOP [7].

Glossary

Bxt Bexarotene It is a rexinoid specific agonist of RXR receptors
CAVE Cyclophosphamide-adriamycin-vincristine-etoposide
CBCL Cutaneous B-cell lymphomas
CHOP Cyclophosphamide, doxorubicin, vincristine and prednisone
CR Complete response
CTCL Cutaneous T-cell lymphoma
DHFR Dihydrofolate reductase
ECP Extracorporeal photopheresis
EMA European Medicines Agency
EORTC European Organization for Research and Treatment of Cancer
GSS Granulomatous slack skin
HDACi Inhibitors of histone deacetylases
IFNs Interferons
MF Mycosis fungoides
MU Million units
NFKB Nuclear factor kappa-light-chain-enhancer of activated B cells
ORR Overall response rate
PCFCL Primary cutaneous follicle centre lymphoma
PCL Primary cutaneous lymphomas
PCMZL Primary cutaneous marginal zone B-cell lymphoma
QoL Quality of life
RR Response rate
SCT Stem cell transplantation
SP-TCL Subcutaneous panniculitis-like T-cell lymphoma
TSEB irradiation Total skin electron beam irradiation
WHO World Health Organization Classification

References

1. Willemze R et al. WHO-EORTC classification for cutaneous lymphomas. Blood. 2005;105(10):3768–85.
2. Swerdlow SH, Campo E, Harris NL, Pileri SA, Stein H, Thiele J, et al., editors. WHO classification of tumours and haematopoietic and lymphoid tissues. Lyon: IARC; 2008.
3. Whittaker SJ et al. Joint British Association of Dermatologists and U.K. Cutaneous Lymphoma Group guidelines for the management of primary cutaneous T-cell lymphomas. Br J Dermatol. 2003;149(6):1095–107.
4. Trautinger F et al. EORTC consensus recommendations for the treatment of mycosis fungoides/Sezary syndrome. Eur J Cancer. 2006;42(8):1014–30.
5. Zelenetz AD et al. NCCN Clinical Practice Guidelines in Oncology. Non-Hodgkin's lymphomas. Version 1.2013. NCCN.org.
6. Kempf W et al. EORTC, ISCL, and USCLC consensus recommendations for the treatment of primary cutaneous CD30-positive lymphoproliferative disorders: lymphomatoid papulosis and primary cutaneous anaplastic large-cell lymphoma. Blood. 2011;118(15): 4024–35.

7. Senff NJ et al. European Organization for Research and Treatment of Cancer and International Society for Cutaneous Lymphoma consensus recommendations for the management of cutaneous B-cell lymphomas. Blood. 2008;112(5):1600–9.

8. Agar NS et al. Survival outcomes and prognostic factors in mycosis fungoides/Sezary syndrome: validation of the revised International Society for Cutaneous Lymphomas/European Organisation for Research and Treatment of Cancer staging proposal. J Clin Oncol. 2010;28(31):4730–9.

9. Olsen E et al. Revisions to the staging and classification of mycosis fungoides and Sezary syndrome: a proposal of the International Society for Cutaneous Lymphomas (ISCL) and the cutaneous lymphoma task force of the European Organization of Research and Treatment of Cancer (EORTC). Blood. 2007; 110(6):1713–22.

10. Tracey L et al. Identification of genes involved in resistance to interferon-alpha in cutaneous T-cell lymphoma. Am J Pathol. 2002;161(5):1825–37.

11. Tracey L et al. Transcriptional response of T cells to IFN-alpha: changes induced in IFN-alpha-sensitive and resistant cutaneous T cell lymphoma. J Interferon Cytokine Res. 2004;24(3):185–95.

12. Bunn Jr PA, Ihde DC, Foon KA. The role of recombinant interferon alfa-2a in the therapy of cutaneous T-cell lymphomas. Cancer. 1986;57(8 Suppl): 1689–95.

13. Olsen EA et al. Interferon alfa-2a in the treatment of cutaneous T cell lymphoma. J Am Acad Dermatol. 1989;20(3):395–407.

14. Papa G et al. Is interferon alpha in cutaneous T-cell lymphoma a treatment of choice? Br J Haematol. 1991;79 Suppl 1:48–51.

15. Roenigk Jr HH et al. Photochemotherapy alone or combined with interferon alpha-2a in the treatment of cutaneous T-cell lymphoma. J Invest Dermatol. 1990; 95(6 Suppl):198S–205.

16. Kuzel TM et al. Effectiveness of interferon alfa-2a combined with phototherapy for mycosis fungoides and the Sezary syndrome. J Clin Oncol. 1995;13(1): 257–63.

17. Chiarion-Sileni V et al. Phase II trial of interferon-alpha-2a plus psoralen with ultraviolet light A in patients with cutaneous T-cell lymphoma. Cancer. 2002;95(3):569–75.

18. Rupoli S et al. Long-term experience with low-dose interferon-alpha and PUVA in the management of early mycosis fungoides. Eur J Haematol. 2005;75(2): 136–45.

19. Stadler RKA, Luger T, Sterry W. Prospective, randomized, multicentre clinical trial on the use of interferon a-2a plus PUVA versus PUVA monotherapy in patients with cutaneous T-cell lymphoma, stages I and II. J Clin Oncol. 2006;24(Suppl):18s (abstr 7541).

20. Dreno B et al. The treatment of 45 patients with cutaneous T-cell lymphoma with low doses of interferon-alpha 2a and etretinate. Br J Dermatol. 1991;125(5): 456–9.

21. Stadler R et al. Prospective randomized multicenter clinical trial on the use of interferon -2a plus acitretin versus interferon -2a plus PUVA in patients with cutaneous T-cell lymphoma stages I and II. Blood. 1998;92(10):3578–81.

22. Kaplan EH et al. Phase II study of recombinant human interferon gamma for treatment of cutaneous T-cell lymphoma. J Natl Cancer Inst. 1990;82(3):208–12.

23. Rook AH et al. The role for interleukin-12 therapy of cutaneous T cell lymphoma. Ann N Y Acad Sci. 2001;941:177–84.

24. Querfeld C et al. Phase II trial of subcutaneous injections of human recombinant interleukin-2 for the treatment of mycosis fungoides and Sezary syndrome. J Am Acad Dermatol. 2007;56(4):580–3.

25. Thomsen K et al. Retinoids plus PUVA (RePUVA) and PUVA in mycosis fungoides, plaque stage. A report from the Scandinavian Mycosis Fungoides Group. Acta Derm Venereol. 1989;69(6):536–8.

26. Duvic M et al. Bexarotene is effective and safe for treatment of refractory advanced-stage cutaneous T-cell lymphoma: multinational phase II-III trial results. J Clin Oncol. 2001;19(9):2456–71.

27. Duvic M et al. Phase 2 and 3 clinical trial of oral bexarotene (Targretin capsules) for the treatment of refractory or persistent early-stage cutaneous T-cell lymphoma. Arch Dermatol. 2001;137(5):581–93.

28. Assaf C et al. Minimizing adverse side-effects of oral bexarotene in cutaneous T-cell lymphoma: an expert opinion. Br J Dermatol. 2006;155(2):261–6.

29. Gniadecki R et al. The optimal use of bexarotene in cutaneous T-cell lymphoma. Br J Dermatol. 2007; 157(3):433–40.

30. Ortiz-Romero PL et al. Treatment of mycosis fungoides with PUVA and bexarotene. Actas Dermosifiliogr. 2006;97(5):311–8.

31. Papadavid E et al. Safety and efficacy of low-dose bexarotene and PUVA in the treatment of patients with mycosis fungoides. Am J Clin Dermatol. 2008; 9(3):169–73.

32. Guitart J. Combination treatment modalities in cutaneous T-cell lymphoma (CTCL). Semin Oncol. 2006;33(1 Suppl 3):S17–20.

33. Straus DJ et al. Results of a phase II trial of oral bexarotene (Targretin) combined with interferon alfa-2b (Intron-A) for patients with cutaneous T-cell lymphoma. Cancer. 2007;109(9):1799–803.

34. McGinnis KS et al. Low-dose oral bexarotene in combination with low-dose interferon alfa in the treatment of cutaneous T-cell lymphoma: clinical synergism and possible immunologic mechanisms. J Am Acad Dermatol. 2004;50(3):375–9.

35. Edelson R et al. Treatment of cutaneous T-cell lymphoma by extracorporeal photochemotherapy. Preliminary results. N Engl J Med. 1987;316(6): 297–303.

36. Scarisbrick JJ et al. U.K. consensus statement on the use of extracorporeal photopheresis for treatment of cutaneous T-cell lymphoma and chronic graft-versus-host disease. Br J Dermatol. 2008;158(4): 659–78.

37. McGinnis KS et al. The addition of interferon gamma to oral bexarotene therapy with photopheresis for Sezary syndrome. Arch Dermatol. 2005;141(9):1176–8.

38. Dippel E et al. Extracorporeal photopheresis and interferon-alpha in advanced cutaneous T-cell lymphoma. Lancet. 1997;350(9070):32–3.

39. Tsirigotis P et al. Extracorporeal photopheresis in combination with bexarotene in the treatment of mycosis fungoides and Sezary syndrome. Br J Dermatol. 2007;156(6):1379–81.

40. Berger CL et al. Transimmunization, a novel approach for tumor immunotherapy. Transfus Apher Sci. 2002; 26(3):205–16.

41. Olsen E et al. Pivotal phase III trial of two dose levels of denileukin diftitox for the treatment of cutaneous T-cell lymphoma. J Clin Oncol. 2001;19(2):376–88.

42. Prince HM et al. Phase III placebo-controlled trial of denileukin diftitox for patients with cutaneous T-cell lymphoma. J Clin Oncol. 2010;28(11):1870–7.

43. Foss FM et al. Biological correlates of acute hypersensitivity events with DAB(389)IL-2 (denileukin diftitox, ONTAK) in cutaneous T-cell lymphoma: decreased frequency and severity with steroid premedication. Clin Lymphoma. 2001;1(4):298–302.

44. Talpur R et al. CD25 expression is correlated with histological grade and response to denileukin diftitox in cutaneous T-cell lymphoma. J Invest Dermatol. 2006; 126(3):575–83.

45. Negro-Vilar A, Dziewanowska Z, Groves E, et al. Phase III Study of Denileukin Diftitox (ONTAK®) to evaluate efficacy safety in CD25+ and CD25– cutaneous T-cell lymphoma (CTCL) patients. Blood (ASH Annual Meeting Abstracts). 2006;108: Abstract 696.

46. Foss F, Duvic M, Olsen EA. Predictors of complete responses with denileukin diftitox in cutaneous T-cell lymphoma. Am J Hematol. 2011;86(7):627–30.

47. Foss F, Demierre MF, DiVenuti G. A phase-1 trial of bexarotene and denileukin diftitox in patients with relapsed or refractory cutaneous T-cell lymphoma. Blood. 2005;106(2):454–7.

48. Lundin J et al. Phase 2 study of alemtuzumab (anti-CD52 monoclonal antibody) in patients with advanced mycosis fungoides/Sezary syndrome. Blood. 2003; 101(11):4267–72.

49. Bernengo MG et al. Low dose intermittent alemtuzumab in the treatment of Sezary syndrome: clinical and immunologic findings in 14 patients. Haematologica. 2007;92(6):784–94.

50. Thursky KA et al. Spectrum of infection, risk and recommendations for prophylaxis and screening among patients with lymphoproliferative disorders treated with alemtuzumab*. Br J Haematol. 2006;132(1):3–12.

51. Lenihan DJ et al. Cardiac toxicity of alemtuzumab in patients with mycosis fungoides/Sezary syndrome. Blood. 2004;104(3):655–8.

52. Kim YH et al. Clinical efficacy of zanolimumab (HuMax-CD4): two phase 2 studies in refractory cutaneous T-cell lymphoma. Blood. 2007;109(11):4655–62.

53. Frankel AE et al. Anti-CD3 recombinant diphtheria immunotoxin therapy of cutaneous T cell lymphoma. Curr Drug Targets. 2009;10(2):104–9.

54. Duvic M, Tetzlaff M, Clos AL, Gangar P, Talpur R. Results of a Phase II Trial of Brentuximab Vedotin (SGN-35) for CD30+ Cutaneous TCell Lymphomas and Lymphoproliferative Disorders. Blood (ASH Annual Meeting Abstracts) 2012;120: Abstract 3688.

55. Marks PA. The mechanism of the anti-tumor activity of the histone deacetylase inhibitor, suberoylanilide hydroxamic acid (SAHA). Cell Cycle. 2004;3(5):534–5.

56. Marks PA, Jiang X. Histone deacetylase inhibitors in programmed cell death and cancer therapy. Cell Cycle. 2005;4(4):549–51.

57. Wozniak MB et al. Vorinostat interferes with the signaling transduction pathway of T-cell receptor and synergizes with phosphoinositide-3 kinase inhibitors in cutaneous T-cell lymphoma. Haematologica. 2010;95(4):613–21.

58. Duvic M et al. Phase 2 trial of oral vorinostat (suberoylanilide hydroxamic acid, SAHA) for refractory cutaneous T-cell lymphoma (CTCL). Blood. 2007;109(1):31–9.

59. Olsen EA et al. Phase IIb multicenter trial of vorinostat in patients with persistent, progressive, or treatment refractory cutaneous T-cell lymphoma. J Clin Oncol. 2007;25(21):3109–15.

60. Duvic M et al. Evaluation of the long-term tolerability and clinical benefit of vorinostat in patients with advanced cutaneous T-cell lymphoma. Clin Lymphoma Myeloma. 2009;9(6):412–6.

61. Fantin VR et al. Constitutive activation of signal transducers and activators of transcription predicts vorinostat resistance in cutaneous T-cell lymphoma. Cancer Res. 2008;68(10):3785–94.

62. Khan O et al. HR23B is a biomarker for tumor sensitivity to HDAC inhibitor-based therapy. Proc Natl Acad Sci U S A. 2010;107(14):6532–7.

63. Piekarz RL et al. Phase 2 trial of romidepsin in patients with peripheral T-cell lymphoma. Blood. 2011; 117(22):5827–34.

64. Whittaker SJ et al. Final results from a multicenter, international, pivotal study of romidepsin in refractory cutaneous T-cell lymphoma. J Clin Oncol. 2010;28(29):4485–91.

65. Duvic M et al. Panobinostat activity in both bexarotene-exposed and – naïve patients with refractory cutaneous T-cell lymphoma: Results of a phase II trial. European Journal of Cancer 49. 2013;386–394.

66. Adams J et al. Proteasome inhibitors: a novel class of potent and effective antitumor agents. Cancer Res. 1999;59(11):2615–22.

67. Zinzani PL et al. Phase II trial of proteasome inhibitor bortezomib in patients with relapsed or refractory cutaneous T-cell lymphoma. J Clin Oncol. 2007;25(27): 4293–7.

68. Kaye FJ et al. A randomized trial comparing combination electron-beam radiation and chemotherapy with topical therapy in the initial treatment of mycosis fungoides. N Engl J Med. 1989;321(26):1784–90.

69. Bunn Jr PA et al. Systemic therapy of cutaneous T-cell lymphomas (mycosis fungoides and the Sezary syndrome). Ann Intern Med. 1994;121(8):592–602.

70. Duvic M et al. Phase II evaluation of gemcitabine monotherapy for cutaneous T-cell lymphoma. Clin Lymphoma Myeloma. 2006;7(1):51–8.

71. Zinzani PL et al. Gemcitabine treatment in pretreated cutaneous T-cell lymphoma: experience in 44 patients. J Clin Oncol. 2000;18(13):2603–6.

72. Coors EA, von den Driesch P. Treatment of erythrodermic cutaneous T-cell lymphoma with intermittent chlorambucil and fluocortolone therapy. Br J Dermatol. 2000;143(1):127–31.

73. Winkelmann RK, Diaz-Perez JL, Buechner SA. The treatment of Sezary syndrome. J Am Acad Dermatol. 1984;10(6):1000–4.

74. Zackheim HS, Kashani-Sabet M, McMillan A. Low-dose methotrexate to treat mycosis fungoides: a retrospective study in 69 patients. J Am Acad Dermatol. 2003;49(5):873–8.

75. Zackheim HS, Kashani-Sabet M, Hwang ST. Low-dose methotrexate to treat erythrodermic cutaneous T-cell lymphoma: results in twenty-nine patients. J Am Acad Dermatol. 1996;34(4):626–31.

76. Zackheim HS, Epstein Jr EH. Low-dose methotrexate for the Sezary syndrome. J Am Acad Dermatol. 1989;21(4 Pt 1):757–62.

77. Kurzrock R, Pilat S, Duvic M. Pentostatin therapy of T-cell lymphomas with cutaneous manifestations. J Clin Oncol. 1999;17(10):3117–21.

78. Dearden C, Matutes E, Catovsky D. Pentostatin treatment of cutaneous T-cell lymphoma. Oncology (Williston Park). 2000;14(6 Suppl 2):37–40.

79. Wollina U, Graefe T, Kaatz M. Pegylated doxorubicin for primary cutaneous T-cell lymphoma: a report on ten patients with follow-up. J Cancer Res Clin Oncol. 2001;127(2):128–34.

80. Dummer R, Quaglino P, Becker JC et al. Prospective international multicenter phase II trial of intravenous pegylated liposomal doxorubicin monochemotherapy in patients with stage IIB, IVA, or IVB advanced mycosis fungoides: final results from EORTC 21012. J Clin Oncol. 2012:20;30(33):4091–7.

81. Horwitz SM, Kim YH, Foss FM, et al. Identification of an active, well-tolerated dose of pralatrexate in patients with relapsed or refractory cutaneous T-cell lymphoma (CTCL): final results of a Multicenter Dose-Finding Study. Blood (ASH Annual Meeting Abstracts). 2010;116: Abstract 2800.

82. Foss F, Horwitz SM, Coiffier B et al. Pralatrexate is an effective treatment for relapsed or refractory transformed mycosis fungoides: a subgroup efficacy analysis from the PROPEL study Clin Lymphoma Myeloma Leuk. 2012;12(4):238–43.

83. Duvic M, Forero-Torres A, Foss F, Olsen E, Kim Y. Response to oral forodesine in refractory cutaneous T-cell lymphoma: interim results of a phase I/II study. ASH Annual Meeting Abstracts. 2007;110(11):122.

84. Olavarria E et al. T-cell depletion and autologous stem cell transplantation in the management of tumour stage mycosis fungoides with peripheral blood involvement. Br J Haematol. 2001;114(3):624–31.

85. Russell-Jones R et al. Autologous peripheral blood stem cell transplantation in tumor-stage mycosis fungoides: predictors of disease-free survival. Ann N Y Acad Sci. 2001;941:147–54.

86. Wu PA et al. A meta-analysis of patients receiving allogeneic or autologous hematopoietic stem cell transplant in mycosis fungoides and Sezary syndrome. Biol Blood Marrow Transplant. 2009;15(8):982–90.

87. Duarte RF et al. Allogeneic hematopoietic cell transplantation for patients with mycosis fungoides and Sezary syndrome: a retrospective analysis of the Lymphoma Working Party of the European Group for Blood and Marrow Transplantation. J Clin Oncol. 2010;28(29):4492–9.

88. Bekkenk MW et al. Primary and secondary cutaneous CD30(+) lymphoproliferative disorders: a report from the Dutch Cutaneous Lymphoma Group on the long-term follow-up data of 219 patients and guidelines for diagnosis and treatment. Blood. 2000;95(12):3653–61.

89. Katz J, Janik JE, Younes A. Brentuximab vedotin (SGN-35). Clin Cancer Res. 2011;17(20):6428–36.

90. Willemze R et al. Subcutaneous panniculitis-like T-cell lymphoma: definition, classification, and prognostic factors: an EORTC Cutaneous Lymphoma Group Study of 83 cases. Blood. 2008;111(2):838–45.

91. Hashimoto H et al. Effective CD34+ selected autologous peripheral blood stem cell transplantation in a patient with subcutaneous panniculitic T cell lymphoma (SPTCL) transformed into leukemia. Bone Marrow Transplant. 1999;24(12):1369–71.

92. Ichii M et al. Successful treatment of refractory subcutaneous panniculitis-like T-cell lymphoma with allogeneic peripheral blood stem cell transplantation from HLA-mismatched sibling donor. Leuk Lymphoma. 2006;47(10):2250–2.

93. Perry A, Vincent BJ, Parker SR. Intralesional corticosteroid therapy for primary cutaneous B-cell lymphoma. Br J Dermatol. 2010;163(1):223–5.

94. Cozzio A et al. Intra-lesional low-dose interferon alpha2a therapy for primary cutaneous marginal zone B-cell lymphoma. Leuk Lymphoma. 2006;47(5):865–9.

95. Bekkenk MW et al. Treatment of multifocal primary cutaneous B-cell lymphoma: a clinical follow-up study of 29 patients. J Clin Oncol. 1999;17(8):2471–8.

96. Krathen M, Sundram U, Bashey S, Sutherland K, Salva K, Wood GS et al. Brentuximab Vedotin Demonstrates Significant Clinical Activity in Relapsed or Refractory Mycosis Fungoides with Variable CD30 Expression Blood (ASH Annual Meeting Abstracts) 2012;120: Abstract 797.

97. Duvic M, Pinter-Brown L, Foss F, Sokol L, Jorgensen J, Ni X et al. Correlation of Target Molecule Expression and Overall Response in Refractory Cutaneous T-Cell Lymphoma Patients Dosed with Mogamulizumab (KW-0761), a Monoclonal Antibody Directed Against CC Chemokine Receptor Type 4 (CCR4). Blood (ASH Annual Meeting Abstracts) 2012;120: Abstract 3697.

98. Peñate Y, Hernández-Machín B, Pérez-Méndez LI et al. Intralesional Rituximab in the Treatment of Indolent Primary Cutaneous B-Cell Lymphomas. An Epidemiologic Observational Multicentre Study: the Spanish Working Group on Cutaneous Lymphoma. Br J Dermatol. 2012;167(1):174–9.

Systemic Therapy in Melanoma

30

Carmen Nuzzo, Maria Simona Pino,
and Francesco Cognetti

Key Point

The incidence of malignant melanoma (MM) is continuously rising representing today the second most common cancer in women and the third in men younger than 40 years. Recognized risk factors for MM are exposure to sunlight (ultraviolet radiation [UV]), a susceptible host phenotype, namely people with fair complexion, blond or red hair, blue eyes, freckles, with a tendency to burn rather than tan when exposed to sunlight. The prognosis of metastatic melanoma remains poor. Different chemotherapeutic agents such as dacarbazine, temozolamide, and fotemustine, have shown clinical activity when used as single agent. No combination regimens have shown, in controlled, randomized studies, to held a significant benefit in survival compared with single agents. A number of new approaches for the treatment of patients with metastatic melanoma are undergoing evaluation in clinical trials. These new biological drugs have shown for first time in 30 years of clinical trials to increase survival.

C. Nuzzo • M.S. Pino • F. Cognetti, MD (✉)
Division of Medical Oncology "A", Medical Oncology
Department, National Cancer Institute Regina Elena,
Via Elio Chianesi, 53, Rome 00144, Italy
e-mail: fcognetti@alice.it

Introduction

Current estimates are that 70,230 new cases of invasive melanoma will be diagnosed in 2011 and 8,790 patients will die from malignant melanoma (MM) in the USA. The incidence continues to rise, making MM the leading cause of death from cutaneous malignancies. Comparing rates in the current year with those in the 1990, cancer death rates for MM increased by 4.74 % [1]. Recognized risk factors for MM are exposure to sunlight (ultraviolet radiation [UV]) and a susceptible host phenotype, namely, people with fair complexion, blond or red hair, blue eyes, and freckles and with a tendency to burn rather than tan when exposed to sunlight. An increased number of benign moles (melanocytic nevi) are a factor linked to melanoma risk. From 18 to 85 % of MM arise from melanocytic nevi. The presence of atypical moles or dysplastic nevi also increases the risk. The risk of MM is as high as 80 % for patients with dysplastic nevi and a family history positive for MM. A personal history of skin cancers, immunosuppression, and xeroderma pigmentosum are other risk factors for MM.

MM prognosis is strictly associated with clinical and histopathological factors. The depth of invasion (Breslow thickness) of the original lesion, the level of invasion (Clark level), ulceration, mitotic rate, presence of tumor-infiltrating lymphocytes, and the presence of microscopic satellites all affect prognosis [2]. Primary tumor location, patient age, and gender are clinical variables associated with prognosis. In general, patients with MM of the extremities have a better prognosis than those with lesions of the trunk and head. Increased patient age and male sex are associated with a worse outcome. The involvement of regional lymph nodes is a poor prognostic factor, regardless of Breslow thickness or Clark levels. The staging system for melanoma, developed by the American Joint Committee on Cancer and updated in 2002, classifies patients into stages I and II for clinically localized primary melanoma to the skin, stage III in the presence of lymph nodes or in-transit metastases, and stage IV if metastatic disease is beyond regional lymph nodes. It is estimated that 82–85 % of melanoma patients present with localized disease, 10–13 % with regional disease, and 2–5 % with distant metastases. For patients with localized melanomas, more than 1.0 mm in thickness, survival rates range from 50 to 90 %. When regional nodes are involved, survival rates are roughly halved. However, within stage III, 5-year survival rates range from 20 to 70 %, depending primarily on the nodal tumor burden. Patients with stage IV disease generally have median survival of only 6–8 months. Long-term survival in patients with distant metastatic melanoma, taken as a whole, is less than 10 %.

Adjuvant Therapy of Melanoma

The primary treatment for most patients with stage I and II melanoma is surgical resection. Postoperative adjuvant therapy must be considered in patients with high-risk MM, that is, patients with melanoma that is more than 4 mm thick (stage IIB) or with node positive (stage III). Adjuvant treatment may be considered for patients with resected in-transit melanoma or for those patients with stage IV free of disease following surgical resection of metastases. Multiple strategies such as chemotherapy, biological therapy, and radiation therapy have been used as adjuvant therapy for melanoma [3].

INF-alpha

So far, interferon alfa-2b (IFNα-2b) is the only drug to demonstrate a significant overall survival (OS) benefit in patients with high-risk melanoma

in randomized controlled trial [4]. In the Eastern Cooperative Oncology Group (ECOG) trial 1684, a total of 287 patients with stage IIB or III were enrolled [5]. All patients were treated with wide local excision and complete regional lymph node dissection and then randomized to either high-dose INFα-2b (HDI 20 MU/m^2 intravenously [IV] 5 days per week for 4 weeks, followed by 10 MU/m^2 3 days per week subcutaneously [SC] for 48 weeks) or observation. After a median follow-up of 6.9 years for survivors, both median disease-free survival (DFS) and median overall survival (OS) were significantly better for the HDI group when compared to the observation group (DFS 1.72 vs 0.98 years and OS 3.82 vs 2.78 years, respectively). At 5 years, the HDI arm was found to have a DFS rate of 37 % and OS of 46 %, while the observation arm patients had a DFS rate of 26 % and an OS of 37 %. Since an attempt was made to administer maximally tolerated doses of INF, it is not surprising that toxicity was significant among those treated with HDI. Grade 3 toxicities occurred in 67 % of patients, grade 4 in 9 %, and two patients died due to hepatotoxicity. The most prevalent toxicities were constitutional symptoms, myelosuppression, and hepatotoxicity. Nonetheless, HDI appeared to alter the natural history of melanoma in high-risk patients and extend median DFS and OS by approximately 1 year. This landmark study resulted in the approval of HDI by the US Food and Drug Administration (FDA) in 1995 for use in high-risk melanoma patients. In the intergroup trial E1690/S9111/C9190, 642 patients with high-risk melanoma, with similar inclusion criteria as the E1684 study, were treated with wide local excision, followed by randomization to HDI, low-dose INF (LDI 3 MU/m^2 three times per week SC for 2 years), or observation [6]. It is important to note that unlike in the E1684, regional lymph node dissection was not mandatory. The results of this trial confirmed the DFS advantage of HDI seen in the E1684, but not the OS advantage. LDI did not significantly affect DFS when compared to observation. Intriguingly a statistically significant difference in 5-year OS was observed for patients in the observation arms between the E1690 and E1684 (55 % in E1690 and 37 % in E1684, $P = .001$). A post hoc analysis of the E1690 revealed that 31 % of patients in the observation arm who relapsed received interferon salvage therapy, including all but one of the patients with resectable regional recurrences. These patients had a prolonged OS when compared to those not receiving salvage interferon therapy (mean 2.2 vs 0.8 year, $P=.0024$), so selection bias may have played a role in this difference. It is important to note that approximately one third of the observation patients who experienced a relapse had disease confined to a regional lymph node basin that had not been previously evaluated pathologically. These patients then had a second opportunity for surgical cure in the form of lymphadenectomy and a second opportunity to receive adjuvant systemic therapy with HDI as "salvage therapy." However, it does not appear that this HDI salvage therapy alone sufficiently explains the prolonged post-relapse survival of patients on the observation arm when compared with patients on the observation arm of E1684. Significant toxicities were again observed with interferon therapy, but there were no deaths due to complications among those treated with HDI. In the intergroup trial E1694/ S9512/C509801, 880 patients with resected high-risk melanoma were randomized to 1-year course of HDI compared with a 2-year course of treatment with the GM2 ganglioside vaccine (GMK) [7]. The trial was prematurely closed in April 2000 by the external safety monitoring committee after an interim analysis indicating that GMK was significantly inferior to HDI in relation to both relapse and mortality end points. Indeed, after a median follow-up of 16 months, there was a significant increase in 2-year DFS for the HDI group versus the GMK vaccine group (62 % vs 49 %) as well as in 2-year OS (78 % vs 73 %). Analysis of the hazard of relapse and death in each stratification group demonstrated the superiority of HDI over GMK in all subsets. Again, significant toxicities were associated with HDI. A delay or dose reduction was required in 33 % of patients during the induction phase and in 38 % during the maintenance phase, but only 10 % of patients required discontinuation of therapy.

Thus, the results from a series of well-designed, randomized clinical trials indicate a significant improvement in DFS and possibly OS with the use of HDI. However, these results come with substantial cost regarding toxicities, which has limited the acceptance of HDI therapy by patients and physicians. Many clinical trials were then performed, reducing the dose of HDI and extending the treatment time. In the EORTC 18952 trial, 1,388 patients (stage IIB or III) were randomized to observation or to 13 or 25 months of treatment with subcutaneous INFα-2b. Treatment comprised 4 weeks of 10 MU of INFα-2b (5 days per week), followed by either 10 MU three times a week for 1 year or 5 MU three times a week for 2 years, to a total dose of 1,760 MU. The primary end points were distant metastasis-free interval (DMFI) and OS. At 4.5 years, the 25-month interferon group showed a 7.2 % increase in rate of DMFI and a 5.4 % improvement in OS, while the 13-month interferon group showed a 3.2 % increase in rate of DMFI and no extension of OS. Toxicity was acceptable, with 18 % of patients going off study because of toxicity or as a result of refusal of treatment because of side effects [8]. Since the duration of treatment seemed more important than dose, further attempts were made with IFN-α at low doses for an extended period of time. However, all studies have failed to demonstrate an improvement in DMFI or OS [9–11]. In the same way, the combination of interferon with chemotherapy has led to unsatisfying results. In a prospective randomized phase III trial conducted by the German Dermatologic Cooperative Oncology Group (DeCOG), a total of 444 patients with regional node involvement were randomized to receive either 3 MU SC of IFNα-2a three times a week for 2 years or combined treatment with same doses of IFNα-2a plus dacarbazine (DTIC) 850 mg/m^2 every 4–8 weeks for 2 years or to observation alone [12]. Treatment with IFNα-2a significantly improved OS and DFS in patients with melanoma as compared with patients treated with surgery alone (4-year OS rate 59 % vs 42 %, $P=.0045$), whereas no improvement of survival was found for the combined treatment with 45 % survival rate. Similarly, DFS rates showed significant benefit for IFNα-2a treatment.

In March 2011, the FDA has approved the pegylated IFNα-2b for the adjuvant treatment of melanoma patients with lymph node involvement, within

84 days from surgical resection. The approval of pegylated IFNα-2b was based on the results of an EORTC (European Organisation for Research and Treatment of Cancer) study [13]. In the EORTC 18991, 1,256 patients with stage III melanoma were randomized between observation and weekly pegylated interferon 6 μg/kg/week for 8 weeks (induction) and then 3 μg/kg/week (maintenance) for an intended duration of 5 years. Pegylated IFNα-2b significantly improved recurrence-free survival (RFS) (34.8 vs 25.5 months, $P=.011$), prespecified regulatory primary end point, but not DMFS, primary end-point, or OS, secondary end point, compared with observation. Safety analysis conducted on 608 patients treated with pegylated IFNα-2b showed that the benefit of the treatment was confined to patients with microscopic nodal metastases (stage III N1) compared to macro-metastases. The most serious adverse events due to the drug were fatigue, increased levels of liver enzymes, and pyrexia. Recently, at the ASCO 2011 annual meeting, 7.6-year outcomes of EORTC 18991 were presented [14]. Significant RFS benefit was sustained at 7.6 years follow-up, with no change in DMFS or OS observed from 2007 to 2011. Moreover, the significant benefit in RFS and DMFS, observed in 2007, from adjuvant pegylated interferon maintenance in patients with stage III N1 disease was still seen in 2011, but was no longer statistically significant. Patients with stage III N2 disease showed no benefit from adjuvant pegylated interferon maintenance in any end point. These data suggest that patients with palpable nodal involvement appeared to have more biologically aggressive disease and relapsed rapidly despite interferon.

Collectively, systematic reviews, meta-analysis, and an analysis of pooled data evaluating the benefit of interferon, published between 2002 and 2004, have demonstrated a significant advantage in DFS, with inconsistent results on OS [15–17]. More recent meta-analyses, published from 2006 to 2010, suggest that treatment with interferon produces an advantage in terms of DFS and OS for patients at high risk of recurrence. In a meta-analysis by Verna et al., high doses of interferon for patients with high risk appear to offer a statistically significant advantage in RFS and OS at 2 years [18]. No improvement in OS was observed when low-dose interferon was compared with observation only after surgery [18]. A meta-analysis conducted by Eggermont et al. recently demonstrated a prolongation of DFS in 7 % and OS benefit in 3 % of IFN-treated patients when compared with observation-only patients. No differences were observed for the dose and duration of treatment [19]. Finally, the meta-analysis conducted by Mocellin et al., which included 14 randomized controlled trials published between 1990 and 2008 evaluating different treatment schedules, showed that adjuvant IFN-α treatment was associated with a statistically significant improvement in DFS (risk reduction 18 %) and OS (risk reduction 11 %) in patients with high-risk melanoma. No optimal IFN-α dose and/or treatment duration or a subset of patients more responsive to adjuvant therapy was identified using subgroup analysis and meta-regression [20].

Immunotherapies and Cancer Vaccines

The results using granulocyte-macrophage colony-stimulating factor (GM-CSF) have also shown promise, reducing the risk of melanoma recurrence in patients with resected disease, with less toxicity than INFα-2b. GM-CSF is a hematopoietic growth factor that also modulates immune system activity by mediating the proliferation and maturation of antigen-presenting dendritic cells and moreover activating monocytes and macrophages. Spitler and colleagues tested a 3-year course of adjuvant GM-CSF in 98 patients with resected stage II (T4), III, or IV melanoma [21]. The median melanoma-specific survival rate at 5 years in this cohort was 60 % overall and 67 and 40 % for patients with resected stage III and resected stage IV disease, respectively. Based on these and other experimental data, an ongoing phase III study (ECOG 4697) is comparing a 1-year course of GM-CSF, with or without melanoma-antigen peptide vaccination, to placebo in patients with completely resected advanced melanoma [22]. The preliminary data from 735 patients demonstrated an improvement in DFS (11.8 vs 8.8 months, $P = .034$) for adjuvant GM-CSF. OS was also improved but without achieving a statistical significance (median OS 72.1 vs 59.8 months, $P = .551$).

The recent progress in tumor immunology and biotechnology has led to many attractive and potentially effective anticancer strategies. In this context, the development of therapeutic vaccines for melanoma treatment has always been pursued by many researchers. Melanoma has for a long time been considered the best candidate solid tumor because of its immunogenic characteristics such as spontaneous remissions, the prognostic importance of lymphocytic infiltration in primary melanomas, and the expression of a wide variety of antigens. However, a lack of successful translation into the clinical setting has been observed. Indeed, the development of T-cell tolerance directed toward tumor-associated antigens (TAAs) can limit the repertoire of functional tumor-reactive T cells, thus impairing the ability of vaccines to elicit effective antitumor immunity. The past decades in tumor immunology have witnessed a considerable effort in the discovery and molecular characterization of TAAs. These antigens included cancer/testis antigens (i.e., antigens expressed by tumor cells of different histology and by testicular and placental cells), differentiation antigens (i.e., proteins expressed by normal cells during their differentiation process), unique antigens (i.e., antigens expressed by a specific tumor, typically consisting in normal proteins which undergo mutations in their amino acid sequence during tumor development), and finally universal antigens (i.e., antigens expressed by most human tumors). The molecular and immunological characterization of several TAAs has allowed synthesizing TAA-derived peptides to be used in clinical trials for assessing their therapeutic potential as vaccines in cancer patients. So far, numerous TAA peptides, mostly recognized by CD8+ T cells, have been tested in clinical trials in melanoma patients. They include peptides from differentiation antigens such as Melan-A/MART-1 and gp100, cancer/testis antigens such as NY-ESO-1 and MAGE, as well as universal antigens such as survivin. Among them, only a limited number have been shown to be able to induce significant immune and clinical responses. MAGE, which stands for melanoma-associated antigen, is a protein expressed by about half of melanoma tumors. In patients with MM, this peptide vaccine in combination with certain adjuvants could induce specific T-cell response as well as durable objective response. MAGE-A3 vaccination has already shown promising results in phase II studies. A recombinant MAGE-A3 fusion protein combined with different immunological adjuvants, AS02B or AS15, has been assessed in the EORTC 16032–18031 randomized phase II trial in 68 patients with unresectable stage III or stage IV melanoma [23]. The MAGE-A3 vaccine was safe and provoked a robust immunological response, with disease regression or stabilization in approximately 15 % of treated patients. A double-blind, randomized, placebo-controlled phase III trial (DERMA) is currently evaluating the efficacy of vaccination with MAGE-A3 in combination with a CpG-based immune stimulator as adjuvant therapy in patients with MAGE-A3-positive resected stage III melanoma. Vaccinations will be administered five times at 3-week intervals during the induction phase and eight times at 3-month intervals during the maintenance phase, for a total of 30 months of treatment.

New agents, antiangiogenic drugs, such as bevacizumab, and immunomodulators, such as the anti-CTLA-4 monoclonal antibody ipilimumab, are currently been evaluated in the adjuvant setting. The encouraging results achieved with high-dose ipilimumab in advanced melanoma patients have suggested to use it alone or in combination with HDI in further clinical trials. EORTC 18071 trial is testing ipilimumab compared to placebo, while the ECOG 1609 is comparing ipilimumab and HDI.

Metastatic Melanoma Treatment

The treatment of patients with metastatic MM depends on the overall condition and age of the patient, as well as on the site and number of metastases. Excluding the rare cases of oligometastatic disease amenable by surgery, metastatic MM is almost invariably incurable with a median survival of 9 months and an estimated 5-year survival rate of 5–15 %.

Chemotherapy

Numerous chemotherapy agents have demonstrated activity in the treatment of metastatic melanoma. Dacarbazine (DTIC), an alkylating agent, is the only chemotherapy agent approved by the FDA for the treatment of metastatic melanoma. An overall response rate (ORR) of 10–20 % has been reported in initial phase II trials. Unfortunately, more recent trials have shown a lower response rates ranging from 5 to 12 % [24–26]. The duration of response is usually short, lasting a median of 3–6 months, though long-term remissions can occur in 1–2 % of patients who obtain a complete response. The most commonly used regimen is 800–1,000 mg/m^2 IV every 3–4 weeks or 200–250 mg/m^2 IV for 5 days every 3–4 weeks. The most frequently reported toxicities are hematological and gastrointestinal, with at times severe nausea and vomiting.

Temozolomide (TMZ) is a second-generation alkylating agent, analog of dacarbazine, which has demonstrated 100 % oral bioavailability, and extensive tissue distribution, including penetration of the blood–brain barrier. In a randomized phase III study of TMZ versus DTIC, similar median OS (7.7 vs 6.4 months) and RR (13.5 % vs 12.1 %) were observed, although patients treated with TMZ experienced a longer median PFS (1.9 vs 1.5 months, $P = .012$). In this study, the standard 5-day regimen of TMZ with a daily dose of 200 mg/m^2 on days 1–5 every 28 days was used [27]. Recently, a randomized phase III trial (EORTC 18032), which examined the efficacy of an extended schedule of TMZ (150 mg/m^2/day for 7 days repeated every 14 days) compared with standard dose single-agent DTIC, showed no difference in OS and PFS, with an improved RR (14.5 % vs 10 %) for TMZ treatment [28]. Thus, the antitumor activity of single-agent TMZ appears to be similar to single-agent DTIC, regardless of the dosing schedule. TMZ has the advantage of an oral administration with a better distribution in the central nervous system

and therefore is the preferred choice in patients with brain metastases. A large number of phase II studies have also investigated the combination of TMZ with interferon-α or thalidomide in patients with advanced melanoma and have reported promising activity, particularly when dose-dense regimens were used. The combination of TMZ and whole brain irradiation has been evaluated in a phase II trial in 31 patients with melanoma metastatic to the brain [29]. The median PFS and OS were 2 and 6 months, respectively, showing a limited antitumor activity of this combination. The major side effects of TMZ are mild-to-moderate myelosuppression and mild nausea and vomiting.

Fotemustine is a nitrosourea alkylating agent, which crosses the blood–brain barrier. In a European phase III trial, 229 patients were randomly assigned to receive either intravenous fotemustine (100 mg/m^2 weekly for 3 weeks) or DTIC (250 mg/m^2 for 5 consecutive days every 4 weeks). Fotemustine was associated with a better ORR (15.2 % vs 6.8 %, $P = .043$), twofold higher compared to DTIC. Similar median durations of responses (5.8 vs 6.9 months) and TTP (1.8 vs 1.9 months) were observed. Interestingly, the median time to brain metastasis was 22.7 months with fotemustine versus 7.2 months with DTIC [24]. The recommended dose of fotemustine is 100 mg/m^2 weekly for 3 consecutive weeks (days 1, 8, and 15), followed by a 5-week rest period (induction treatment), followed by a maintenance therapy in nonprogressive patients consisting of fotemustine 100 mg/m^2 every 3 weeks. The main toxicities are hematological with neutropenia and thrombocytopenia.

Several combination chemotherapy regimens have been studied. The most commonly used is the association of cisplatin, vinblastine, and dacarbazine known as CVD. As compared with DTIC or fotemustine treatment, CVD shows a higher RR of 30–45 %, with a median duration of response significantly better. However, no regimens have shown, in controlled, randomized studies, to hold a significant benefit in survival compared with single-agent DTIC. Other chemotherapeutic agents with single-agent activity include carmustine, lomustine and semustine, with

RR of 13–18 %; vinblastine and vindesine, with RR of 14 %; taxanes, with RR of 16–17 %; and carboplatin and cisplatin, with RR of 15–20 %.

IL-2 and Other Immunotherapies

Immunological therapies have been extensively studied for the treatment of advanced melanoma. Multiple clinical trials of immune modulation strategies, including cytokines, tumor vaccines, adoptive immunotherapy, and their combinations, have been tested over the years. Until recently, the only FDA-approved immunotherapy for the treatment of metastatic melanoma was high-dose interleukin 2 (HDIL2). The approval was based on phase II studies in 277 patients, showing durable complete response in 7 % of patients [30]. However, HDIL2 can cause life-threatening capillary leak syndrome, arrhythmias, renal toxicity, and hypotension. Death is a rare but well-documented adverse event during treatment. Although most of the side effects are self-limiting and resolve at discontinuation, only patients with high performance status may be considered for this regimen [31, 32]. Nevertheless, HDIL2 received US FDA approval for patient with metastatic melanoma in 1998, although it has not been approved in Europe.

Cytotoxic T-lymphocyte antigen-4, or CTLA-4, is the main negative regulator of T-cell-mediated antitumor immune responses and therefore represents a critical immunity checkpoint, controlling both the duration and the intensity of an immune response. Full T-cell activation requires two signals. The first is provided by T-cell receptor (TCR) binding to TAAs presented by antigen-presenting cells (APCs) via major histocompatibility complexes. The second signal is generated when CD28, the principal costimulatory receptor on the T cell, binds to members of the B7 family, such as CD80 and CD86, presented on the APC. The resulting dual signaling induces changes including T-cell proliferation and cytokine release, which trigger and then amplify the immune response. In response to T-cell activation, CTLA-4 is upregulated and competes with CD28 for CD80 and CD86 binding on APCs but with significantly higher affinity, therefore downregulating or deactivating the T cell. On the other hand, CTLA-4 signaling contributes to the immunosuppressive function of regulatory T cells (Tregs). Binding of Tregs-associated CTLA-4 to APCs decreases APC function and T-cell proliferation deregulating a natural homeostatic mechanism designed to prevent unwanted autoimmunity against self-antigens by inducing peripheral immune tolerance. Anti-CTLA-4 monoclonal antibody binding to CTLA-4 on T cell prolongs T-cell activation, restores T-cell proliferation, and thus amplifies T-cell-mediated immunity, which enhances the patient's capacity to mount an antitumor immune response (see Fig. 30.1) [33–36]. Ipilimumab (MDX-010) is a first-in-class fully human monoclonal antibody against CTLA-4, with a plasma half-life of 12–14 days. This drug has now been studied in more than 2,900 patients enrolled in 25 clinical trials and has shown high RR and long survival time in patients with advanced melanoma [37–39]. In a phase II multicentric trial (MDX010-08), 72 chemotherapy naïve patients with advanced melanoma were randomized to receive ipilimumab 3 mg/kg every 4 weeks for four doses either alone or in combination with up to six 5-day courses of DTIC 250 mg/m^2/die. Surprisingly, a durable objective clinical response and an encouraging OS were observed with ipilimumab treatment, both alone and in combination with chemotherapy [40]. Ipilimumab has been studied in three more randomized phase II trials at the dosage of 10 mg/kg [38, 39, 41]. In these trials, patients were treated with ipilimumab every 3 weeks for four cycles (induction therapy), followed by ipilimumab every 12 weeks beginning at week 24 (maintenance therapy). Analysis of the long-term survival of patients treated with 10 mg/kg showed an OS ranging from 10.2 months in pretreated patients to 22.5 months in untreated patients after a median follow-up, respectively, of 10.1 and 16.3 months [42]. Notably, long-term survivors included patients evaluated with a progressive disease (PD) by the World Health Organization (WHO) criteria of responses. Indeed, it is well known that response to ipilimumab is typically heterogeneous and has been seen during, at the end of, and beyond the 12-week induction period. Four distinct response patterns to

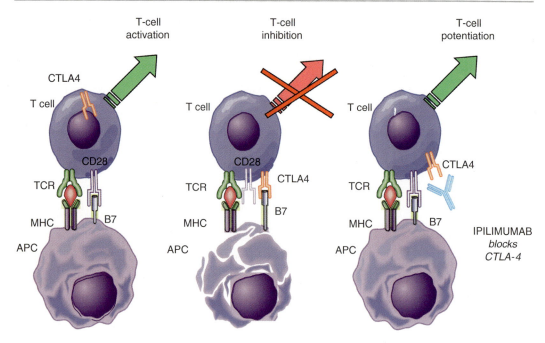

Fig. 30.1 T-cell activation and mechanism of action of ipilimumab. *APC* antigen-presenting cell, *CTLA-4* cytotoxic T-lymphocyte antigen-4, *TCR* T-cell receptor, *MHC* major histocompatibility complex

Table 30.1 Evolution of mWHO to irResponse criteria

	CR	PR	SD	PD
WHO criteria	All lesions gone	SPD of index lesions decreases 50 % from baseline new lesions *not* allowed	SPD of index lesions neither CR, PR, nor new lesions *not* allowed	SPD of index lesions increases 25 % from nadir and/or unequivocal progression of non-index and/or new lesions
	irRC	irPR	irSD	irPD
irResponse criteria	All lesions gone	SPD of index + any new lesions decreases 50 % from baseline new lesions allowed	SPD of index + any new lesions neither irRC, irPR, nor irPD new lesions allowed	SPD of index + any new lesions increases 25 % from nadir irPD is based on SPD only

Confirmation of progression whenever clinically acceptable
SPD sum of the product of the perpendicular diameters

ipilimumab have been described: (1) shrinkage of baseline index lesions without new lesions appearing; (2) durable SD followed (in some cases) by slow, steady decline in tumor burden; (3) response after an increase in tumor burden; and (4) response in the presence of new lesions [43]. To systematically characterize additional patterns of response in patients with advanced melanoma, the immune-related response criteria (irRC) were established as a necessary evolution of the WHO criteria (Table 30.1). Based on these criteria, an irRC is defined as a complete disappearance of all lesions; an irPR is defined as a decrease in tumor burden ≥50 % relative to baseline; an irSD is defined as a

disease not meeting the criteria for irRC or irPR, in absence of irPD; and, finally, an irPD is defined as an increase in tumor burden ≥25 % relative to the nadir (minimum recorded tumor burden). All the responses must be confirmed by a repeat, consecutive assessment no less than 4 weeks from the date first documented [43]. Although these proposed definitions have not been tested prospectively in a randomized clinical trial, they are helpful in patient management, as RECIST and WHO criteria can underestimate the antitumor activity of ipilimumab.

Based on preclinical data suggesting synergy between ipilimumab and vaccines in melanoma,

Fig. 30.2 Kaplan-Meier curve for overall survival

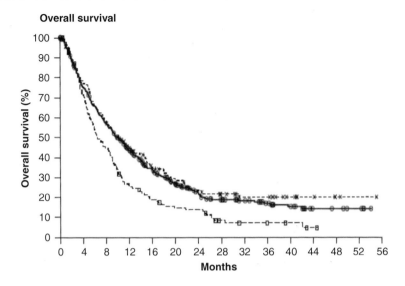

a randomized double-blind phase III trial of ipilimumab 3 mg/kg with or without a peptide vaccine, gp100, was undertaken [44]. A total of 676 HLA-A-0201-restricted melanoma patients, with unresectable stage III or IV disease, were randomized. Ipilimumab induction therapy was administered every 3 weeks for four consecutive doses without maintenance, with responding patients eligible for re-induction at relapse. The median OS in the ipilimumab alone group was 10.1 months, as compared with 10.0 months in the ipilimumab plus gp100 group, and 6.4 months in the gp100 alone group (P = .003) (Fig. 30.2). A phase III trial of ipilimumab at the dose of 10 mg/kg with DTIC versus DTIC plus placebo in untreated patients with advanced melanoma completed accrual in 2008 and survival data were published on 2011 [45]. Overall survival was significantly better in the combination arm (11.2 vs 9.1 months) with higher survival rates at 1, 2, and 3 years. A relevant result was that after 2 years, there was a stable 10 % increase in the population of patients who appeared to have longer term response and the potential of cure from this therapy: estimated 2-year overall survival was 28.5 % with ipilimumab and DTIC, compared with 17.9 % with DTIC alone. The types of adverse events were consistent with those seen in prior studies of ipilimumab. On March 2011, ipilimumab became the first drug in more than a decade to be approved by FDA for the treatment of

unresectable or metastatic melanoma. On July 2011 EMA approved Ipilimumab after first line treatment.

It is noteworthy to highlight that ipilimumab produces an uncommon, mechanism-related spectrum of autoimmune or immune-related adverse events (irAEs), creating unique challenges in diagnosis and clinical management. These irAEs are dose dependent and can occur quite rapidly. They include severe rash (50 % of cases); diarrhea and enterocolitis (10–35 % of cases); hypophysitis (5 % of cases); hepatitis (2–20 % of cases); and, more rarely, uveitis, pancreatitis, neuropathy, severe leucopenia, and red cell aplasia. Diarrhea and colitis, histologically resembling ulcerative colitis, often have a rapid onset and can, if untreated, lead to a fatal bowel perforation and septicemia. Mortality as high as 5 % has been reported. Safety guidelines recommend bowel rest and supportive care, as well as systemic steroids as first-line intervention with most patients responding to this treatment. Patients should be started on 1 mg/kg of methylprednisolone or prednisone twice daily, and the corticosteroids should be gradually tapered over 30 days or longer. When necessary, in patients with symptoms despite initiation of corticosteroids, relapse of symptoms after initial response, or partial response to corticosteroids, should be treated with the antitumor necrosis factor antibody infliximab at a dose of 5 mg/kg. Hepatitis with elevation of transaminase to over 500 U/L has also been reported. Liver function test results should be monitored before each dose of ipilimumab. Grade 3 or 4 hepatitis should be treated with steroids initially, followed sequentially by mycophenolate mofetil, tacrolimus, and, eventually, infliximab. Hypophysitis is the most commonly reported endocrine adverse reaction associated with ipilimumab. Symptoms of hormone deficiency include fatigue, insomnia, loss of libido, anorexia, weight loss, severe hyponatremia, hypothyroidism, and/or symptoms mimicking Addison disease. Unlike most other irAEs, endocrine dysfunction has a protracted course and is irreversible in many cases. It is noteworthy that patients experiencing an irAE have a higher chance of having an antitumor response to ipilimumab. In this context, the studies are in progress to identify host- or tumor-related factors that can be used as predictive biomarker. In a pooled analysis of studies CA184-007, CA184-008, and CA184-022 (and confirmed prospectively in study CA184-004), higher peripheral blood absolute lymphocyte counts (ALC) were significantly associated with clinical activity. Data have emerged recently showing that hair depigmentation develops alongside durable responses to ipilimumab in patients with advanced melanoma. Hair depigmentation suggests an association between induced autoimmunity and clinical benefit and could be a potential surrogate for response in some patients. Ipilimumab is the first-in class of a series of immunomodulating antibodies that are in clinical development such as antiPD1, antiPDL1, antiCD137. Some of these agent are being investigated in clinical trials.

Emerging Therapies for Patients with Metastatic Melanoma

Among the pathways deregulated in melanoma, the RAS/RAF/MEK/ERK pathway is an attractive target based on its role in promoting cell proliferation, invasion, and resistance to apoptosis. Beyond the presence of *NRAS* mutations in approximately 20 % of all melanomas, the basis for this constitutive activation was not well understood. In 2002, the *BRAF* mutation was discovered in a screen for mutations in the *RAF* genes. Subsequent biochemical investigations confirmed the role of mutated *BRAF* in constitutive ERK signaling and in stimulating proliferation and survival. *BRAF* mutations have been found in approximately 60 % patients, primarily in young individuals with melanoma originating on non-chronically sun-damaged skin [46, 47]. One of the earlier *BRAF* inhibitors investigated was the multikinase inhibitor sorafenib, which targets BRAF, CRAF, and the VEGF and PDGF receptor tyrosine kinases. As sorafenib was a relatively nonselective *BRAF* inhibitor, not significant clinical activity was demonstrated in patients with advanced melanoma [48]. However, when combined with chemotherapeutic agents, including carboplatin and paclitaxel, or temozolomide, it showed greater activity leading to phase III trials, which eventually failed both in first line and second line [49, 50]. The failure of sorafenib suggested the need for a more potent and targeted approach. The most common *BRAF* mutation (in approximately 90 % of clinical pathology samples) is the T1799A point mutation, in which a T$\rightarrow$A transversion results in an amino acid substitution at position 600 in BRAF, from a valine (V) to a glutamic acid (E). This mutation occurs within the activation segment of the kinase domain, resulting in the protein taking on a constitutive active configuration [51]. Given the prevalence of this mutation in melanoma, there has been an intense interest in selective *BRAF* inhibitors. In a recent phase I trial, vemurafenib (PLX4032), an oral selective inhibitor of oncogenic BRAF V600E kinase, induced an objective clinical response in 81 % of patients with *BRAF V600E* mutation-positive melanoma [52]. The most frequent adverse events were arthralgia, rash, nausea, photosensitivity, fatigue, pruritus, and palmar-plantar dysesthesia. Interestingly, squamous cell carcinomas, keratoacanthoma subtype, developed in 31 % of the patients. The majority were resected and none led to discontinuation of treatment. A phase II trial (BRIM 2) involving patients who had received previous treatment for melanoma, positive for the *BRAF V600E* mutation, showed a best ORR greater than 52 %, with a median duration of response of nearly 7 months, and a median PFS greater than 6 months [53]. A phase III (BRIM 3)

Fig. 30.3 Overall survival. Kaplan-Meier estimates of survival in patients in the intention-to-treat population

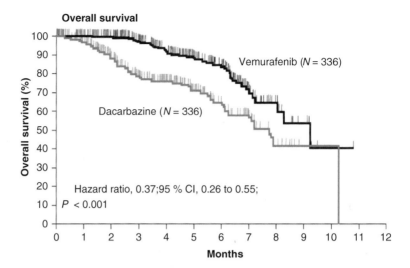

trial comparing the efficacy of PLX4032 with that of DTIC in 675 patients with previously untreated, metastatic melanoma positive for the *BRAF V600E* mutation was published recently [54]. In the interim analysis for OS (see Fig. 30.3) and final analysis for PFS, vemurafenib was associated with a relative reduction of 63 % in the risk of death and of 74 % in the risk of either death or disease progression, as compared with DTIC (*P*<.001 for both comparisons). Response rates were 48 % for vemurafenib and 5 % for DTIC. On August 2011, FDA approved Vemurafenib tablets (Zelboraf, made by Hoffmann –La Roche Inc.) for the treatment of patients with unresectable or metastatic melanoma with the BRAF V600E mutation as detected by an FDA approved test. On February 2012 EMA approved Vemurafenib in monotherapy for the treatment of adult patients with BRAF V600 mutation positive unresectable or metastatic melanoma. The second selective BRAF inhibitor to enter clinical development was GSK2118436. In a phase I/II clinical trial, patients with metastatic melanoma harboring *BRAF* mutations were accrued [55]. At the two highest doses evaluated, 150 and 250 mg twice daily, objective responses were observed in 10 of 16 patients with *BRAF V600E*. Of note, five patients with the *BRAF V600K* mutations were enrolled at the highest doses evaluated, and all had evidence of tumor regression. In addition to seeing responses at various sites of visceral metastatic disease, evidence of regression was observed early

in the course of therapy in several patients with small previously untreated brain metastases [56]. The most common toxicities observed were mild-to-moderate fever, fatigue, headache, nausea, and vomiting. A first-line trial comparing GSK2118436 to DTIC in treatment naive metastatic melanoma patients documented that Dabrafenib significantly improved progression free survival compared with Dacarbazine [57].

Although dramatic clinical activity has been shown with single-agent BRAF-targeted therapy, the antitumor effect is of limited duration. Resistance to BRAF-inhibitor therapy is common and rapidly acquired in the majority of patients [58, 59]. No Mek inhibitor has demonstrated significant clinical activity in BRAF – mutated melanoma in the phase II setting; Selumetinib had a RR of only 10 % in BRAF- mutant melanoma [60] and PD 0325901 was poorly tolerated [61, 62]. In the first published phase III trial Trametinib (GSK 1120212), as compare with chemotherapy improved rates of progression free and overall survival among patients who had metastatic melanoma with a BRAF V600E e V600K mutation [63]. The combination of Dabrafenib and Trametinib increase the rate of pirexia instead PFS significantly improve [64]. Phase III combination of BRAF and Mek inhibitors studies are currently being tested.

KIT is a receptor tyrosine kinase that plays an important role in proliferation, development, and survival of melanocytes, hematopoietic cells, and germ cells and is ubiquitously expressed in mature melanocytes. Activating mutations and gene amplification of KIT have been found in 39 % of mucosal, 36 % of acral, and 28 % of melanomas that arise in chronically sun-damaged skin [65]. Recent reports, although limited in number, describe dramatic and durable responses to treatment with imatinib mesylate and other KIT inhibitors. Several multicenter phase II trials are currently under way to evaluate KIT-targeted agents, including imatinib, sunitinib, nilotinib, and dasatinib, in melanoma patients whose tumors harbor KIT aberrations. A randomized phase III trial will evaluate nilotinib, a multitarget kinase inhibitor, compared with DTIC as first-line therapy in patients with advanced melanoma harboring *KIT* mutations. Finally, as with BRAF-targeted therapies, understanding the potential mechanisms of resistance to KIT-targeted therapy is an active area of investigation.

Glossary

Adjuvant therapy is a treatment that is given in addition to the primary, main or initial treatment.

BRAF is a human gene that makes a protein called B-Raf. The gene is also referred to as proto-oncogene B-Raf and v-Raf murine sarcoma viral oncogene homolog B1, while the protein is more formally known as serine/threonine-protein kinase B-Raf.

Interferon-alpha is a pleiotropic cytokine belonging to type I IFN, currently used in cancer patients.

References

1. Siegel R, Ward E, Brawley O, Jemal A. Cancer statistics, 2011: the impact of eliminating socioeconomic and racial disparities on premature cancer deaths. CA Cancer J Clin. 2011;61(4):212–36.
2. Corona R, Mele A, Amini M, et al. Interobserver variability on the histopathologic diagnosis of cutaneous melanoma and other pigmented skin lesions. J Clin Oncol. 1996;14(4):1218–23.
3. Eggermont AM, Gore M. Randomized adjuvant therapy trials in melanoma: surgical and systemic. Semin Oncol. 2007;34(6):509–15.
4. Hauschild A. Adjuvant interferon alfa for melanoma: new evidence based treatment recommendations? Curr Oncol. 2009;16(3):3–6.
5. Kirkwood JM, Strawderman MH, Ernstoff MS, et al. Interferon alfa-2b adjuvant therapy of high-risk resected cutaneous melanoma: the Eastern Cooperative Oncology Group Trial EST 1684. J Clin Oncol. 1996;14:7–17.
6. Kirkwood JM, Ibrahim JG, Sondak VK, et al. High- and low-dose interferon alfa-2b in high-risk melanoma: first analysis of inter-group trial E1690/S9111/C9190. J Clin Oncol. 2000;18:2444–58.
7. Kirkwood JM, Ibrahim JG, Sosman JA, et al. High-dose interferon alfa-2b significantly prolongs relapse-free and overall survival compared with the GM2-KLH/QS-21 vaccine in patients with resected stage IIB-III melanoma: results of intergroup trial E1694/S9512/C509801. J Clin Oncol. 2001; 19:2370–80.
8. Eggermont AM, Suciu S, MacKie R, et al. Post-surgery adjuvant therapy with intermediate doses of interferon alfa 2b versus observation in patients with stage IIb/III melanoma (EORTC 18952): randomised controlled trial. Lancet. 2005;366:1189–96.
9. Hancock BW, Wheatley K, Harris S, et al. Adjuvant interferon in high-risk melanoma: the AIM HIGH Study–United Kingdom Coordinating Committee on Cancer Research randomized study of adjuvant low-dose extended- duration interferon alfa-2a in high-risk resected malignant melanoma. J Clin Oncol. 2004;22:53–61.
10. Cascinelli N, Belli F, MacKie RM, et al. Effect of long-term adjuvant therapy with interferon alpha-2a in patients with regional node metastases from cutaneous melanoma: a randomised trial. Lancet. 2001; 358:866–9.
11. Cameron DA, Cornbleet MC, MacKie RM, et al. Adjuvant interferon alpha 2b in high risk melanoma—the Scottish study. Br J Cancer. 2001;84:1146–9.
12. Garbe C, Radny P, Linse R, et al. Adjuvant low-dose interferon_2a with or without dacarbazine compared with surgery alone: a prospective-randomized phase III DeCOG trial in melanoma patients with regional lymph node metastasis. Ann Oncol. 2008; 19:1195–201.
13. Eggermont AM, Suciu S, Santinami M, et al. Adjuvant therapy with pegylated interferon alfa-2b versus observation alone in resected stage III melanoma: final results of EORTC 18991, a randomised phase III trial. Lancet. 2008;372:117–26.
14. Eggermont AM, Suciu S, Santinami M, et al. EORTC 18911 phase III trial: long-term adjuvant pegylated interferon-α2b (PEG-IFN) versus observation in resected stage III melanoma: long-term results at 7.6 years follow-up. Program and abstracts of the 2011 American Society of Clinical Oncology Annual Meeting. 2011. Chicago. Abstract 8506b.
15. Lens MB, Dawes M. Interferon alpha therapy for malignant melanoma: a systematic review of randomized controlled trials. J Clin Oncol. 2002;20:1818–25.

16. Wheatley K, Ives N, Hancock B, et al. Does adjuvant interferon alfa for high-risk melanoma provide a worthwhile benefit? A meta-analysis of the randomized trials. Cancer Treat Rev. 2003;29(4):241–52.

17. Kirkwood JM, Manola J, Ibrahim J, et al. A pooled analysis of eastern cooperative oncology group and intergroup trials of adjuvant high-dose interferon for melanoma. Clin Cancer Res. 2004;10:1670–7.

18. Verma S, Quirt I, McCready D, et al. Systematic review of systemic adjuvant therapy for patients at high risk for recurrent melanoma. Cancer. 2006;106:1431–42.

19. Eggermont AM, Testori A, Marsden J, et al. Utility of adjuvant systemic therapy in melanoma. Ann Oncol. 2009;20 Suppl 6:vi30–4.

20. Mocellin S, Pasquali S, Rocci CR, et al. Interferon alpha adjuvant therapy in patients with high risk melanoma: a systematic review and meta-analysis. J Natl Cancer Inst. 2010;102:493–501.

21. Spitler LE, Grossbard ML, Ernstoff MS. Adjuvant therapy of stage III and IV malignant melanoma using granulocyte-macrophage colony-stimulating factor. J Clin Oncol. 2000;18(8):1614–21.

22. Lawson DH, Lee SJ, Tarhiini AA, et al. Phase III cooperative group study of yeast-derived granulocyte macrophage colony-stimulating factor (GM-CSF) versus placebo as adjuvant treatment of patient with completely resected stage III-IV melanoma. J Clin Oncol (ASCO Annual Meeting Proceedings). 2010;28:abstract 8504.

23. Kruit WH, Suciu S, Dreno B, et al. Immunization with recombinant MAGE-A3 protein combined with adjuvant systems AS15 or AS02B in patients with unresectable and progressive metastatic cutaneous melanoma: a randomized open-label phase II study of the EORTC Melanoma Group (16032–18031). J Clin Oncol (ASCO Annual Meeting Proceedings). 2008;26:abstract 9065.

24. Avril MF, Aamdal S, Grob JJ, et al. Fotemustine compared with dacarbazine in patients with disseminated malignant melanoma: a phase III study. J Clin Oncol. 2004;22:1118–25.

25. Bedikian AY, Millward M, Pehamberger H, et al. Bcl-2 antisense (oblimersen sodium) plus dacarbazine in patients with advanced melanoma: the Oblimersen Melanoma Study Group. J Clin Oncol. 2006; 24:4738–45.

26. Schadendorf D, Ugurel S, Schuler-Thurner B, et al. Dacarbazine (DTIC) versus vaccination with autologous peptide-pulsed dendritic cells (DC) in first-line treatment of patients with metastatic melanoma: a randomized phase III trial of the DC study group of the DeCOG. Ann Oncol. 2006;17:563–70.

27. Middleton MR, Grob JJ, Aaronson N, et al. Randomized phase III study of temozolomide versus dacarbazine in the treatment of patients with advanced metastatic malignant melanoma. J Clin Oncol. 2000;18(1):158–66.

28. Patel PM, Suciu S, Mortier L, et al. Extended schedule, escalated dose temozolomide versus dacarbazine in stage IV malignant melanoma: final results of the randomised phase III study (EORTC 18032). Ann Oncol. 2008;19:viii3, abstract LBA8.

29. Margolin K, Atkins B, Thompson A, et al. Temozolomide and whole brain irradiation in melanoma metastatic to the brain: a phase II trial of the Cytokine Working Group. J Cancer Res Clin Oncol. 2002;128(4):214–8.

30. Atkins MB, Lotze MT, Dutcher JP, et al. High-dose recombinant interleukin 2 therapy for patients with metastatic melanoma: analysis of 270 patients treated between 1985 and 1993. J Clin Oncol. 1999;17:2105–16.

31. Atkins MB. Interleukin-2 in metastatic melanoma: what is the current role? Cancer J Sci Am. 2000;6:S8–10.

32. Atkins MB, Kunkel L, Sznol M, et al. High-dose recombinant interleukin-2 therapy in patients with metastatic melanoma: long term survival update. Cancer J Sci Am. 2000;6:S11–4.

33. Peggs KS, Quezada SA, Korman AJ, et al. Principles and use of anti-CTLA4 antibody in human cancer. Curr Opin Immunol. 2006;18:206–13.

34. Robert C, Ghiringhelli F. What is the role of cytotoxic T lymphocyte-associated antigen 4 blockade in patients with metastatic melanoma? Oncologist. 2009;14:848–61.

35. Read S, Malmstrom V, Powrie F. Cytotoxic T lymphocyte associated antigen 4 plays an essential role in the function of CD25(+)CD4(+) regulatory cells that control intestinal inflammation. J Exp Med. 2000;192:295–302.

36. Tarhini A, Lo E, Monor DR. Releasing the brake on the immune system: ipilimumab in melanoma and other tumor. Cancer Biother Radiopharm. 2010;25:601–13.

37. Hersh EM, O'Day SJ, Powderly J, et al. A phase II multicenter study of ipilimumab with or without dacarbazine in chemotherapy-naïve patients with advanced melanoma. Invest New Drugs. 2010;29:489–98.

38. O'Day SJ, Maio M, Chiarion-Sileni V, et al. Efficacy and safety of ipilimumab monotherapy in patients with pretreated advanced melanoma: a multicenter single-arm phase II study. Ann Oncol. 2010;21:1712–7.

39. Wolchok JD, Neyns B, Linette G, et al. Ipilimumab monotherapy in patients with pretreated advanced melanoma: a randomised, double-blind, multicentre, phase 2, dose-ranging study. Lancet Oncol. 2010;11:155–64.

40. Hersh EM, O'Day SJ, Powderly J, et al. A phase II multicenter study of ipilimumab with or without dacarbazine in chemotherapy-naïve patients with advanced melanoma. Invest New Drugs. 2011;29:489–98.

41. Weber J, Thompson JA, Hamid O, et al. A randomized, double-blind, placebo-controlled, phase II study comparing the tolerability and efficacy of ipilimumab administered with or without prophylactic budesonide in patients with unresectable stage III or IV melanoma. Clin Cancer Res. 2009;15:5591–8.

42. Maio M, Lebbe' C, Sileni VC, et al. Long-term survival in advanced melanoma patients treated with ipilimumab at 10 mg/kg: ongoing analyses from completed phase II trials[abstr]. Eur J Cancer. 2009; 7(suppl):578, abstract P-9307.

43. Wolchok JD, Hoos A, O'Day S, et al. Guidelines for the evaluation of immune therapy activity in solid tumors: immune-related response criteria. Clin Cancer Res. 2009;15:7412–20.

44. Hodi FS, O'Day SJ, McDermott DF, et al. Improved survival with ipilimumab in patients with metastatic melanoma. N Engl J Med. 2010;363:711–23.

45. Robert C, Thomas L, Bondarenko I, et al. Ipilimumab plus dacarbazine for previously untreated metastatic melanoma. N Engl J Med. 2011;364:2517–26.

46. Houben R, Becker JC, Kappel A, et al. Constitutive activation of the Ras-Raf signaling pathway in metastatic melanoma is associated with poor prognosis. J Carcinog. 2004;3:6.

47. Long GV, Menzies AM, Nagrial AM, et al. Clinicopathologic correlates of BRAF mutation status in 207 consecutive patients with metastatic melanoma. J Clin Oncol (ASCO Annual Meeting Proceedings). 2010;28:abstract 8548.

48. Eisen T, Ahmand T, Flaherty KT, et al. Sorafenib in advanced melanoma: a phase II randomized discontinuation trial analysis. Br J Cancer. 2006;95:581–6.

49. Hauschild A, Agarwala SS, Trefzer U, et al. Results of a phase III, randomized, placebo-controlled study of sorafenib in combination with carboplatin and paclitaxel as second-line treatment in patients with unresectable stage III or stage IV melanoma. J Clin Oncol. 2009;27:2823–30.

50. Flaherty KT, Lee SJ, Schuchter LM, et al. Final results of E2603: a double-blind, randomized phase III trial comparing carboplatin/paclitaxel with or without sorafenib in metastatic melanoma. J Clin Oncol (ASCO Annual Meeting Proceedings). 2010;28:abstract 8511.

51. Garnett MJ, Marais R. Guilty as charged: B-RAF is a human oncogene. Cancer Cell. 2004;6:313–9.

52. Flaherty KT, Puzanov I, Kim KB, et al. Inhibition of mutated, activated BRAF in metastatic melanoma. N Engl J Med. 2010;363:809–19.

53. Ribas A, Kim KB, Schuchter LM, et al. BRIM-2: an open-label, multicenter phase II study of vemurafenib in previously treated patients with BRAFV600E mutation positive melanoma. J Clin Oncol (ASCO Annual Meeting Proceedings). 2011;29:abstract 8509.

54. Chapman PB, Hauschild A, Robert C, et al. Improved survival with vemurafenib in melanoma with BRAF V600E mutation. N Engl J Med. 2011;364:2507–16.

55. Kefford RF, Arkenau H, Brown MP, et al. Phase I/II study of GSK 2118436, a selective inhibitor of oncogenic mutant BRAF kinase in patients with metastatic melanoma and other solid tumor. J Clin Oncol (ASCO Annual Meeting Proceedings). 2010;28:abstract 8503.

56. Long GV, Kefford RF, Carr PJA, et al. Phase 1/2 study of GSK2118436, a selective inhibitor of V600 mutant (mut) BRAF kinase: evidence of activity in melanoma brain metastases (mets). Ann Oncol. 2010;21:viii12.

57. Long GV, Trefzer U, Davies MA, Kefford RF, Ascierto PA, Chapman PB, Puzanov I, Hauschild A, Robert C, Algazi A, Mortier L, Tawbi H, Wilhelm T, Zimmer L, Switzky J, Swann S, Martin AM, Guckert M, Goodman V, Streit M, Kirkwood JM, Schadendorf D. Dabrafenib in patients with Val600Glu or Val600Lys BRAF-mutant melanoma metastatic to the brain (BREAK-MB): a multicentre, open-label, phase 2 trial. Lancet Oncol. 2012;13(11):1087–95.

58. Poulikakos PI, Rosen N. Mutant BRAF melanomas: dependence and resistance. Cancer Cell. 2011;19:11–5.

59. Solit DB, Rosen N. Resistance to B-RAF inhibition in melanoma. N Engl J Med. 2011;364:772–4.

60. Hauschild A, Grob JJ, Demidov LV, Jouary T, Gutzmer R, Millward M, Rutkowski P, Blank CU, Miller Jr WH, Kaempgen E, Martín-Algarra S, Karaszewska B, Mauch C, Chiarion-Sileni V, Martin AM, Swann S, Haney P, Mirakhur B, Guckert ME, Goodman V, Chapman PB. Dabrafenib in BRAF-mutated metastatic melanoma: a multicentre, open-label, phase 3 randomised controlled trial. Lancet. 2012;380(9839): 358–65. doi:10.1016/S0140-6736(12)60868-X. Epub 2012 Jun 25.

61. Kirkwood JM, Bastholt L, Robert C, Sosman J, Larkin J, Hersey P, Middleton M, Cantarini M, Zazulina V, Kemsley K, Dummer R. Phase II, open-label, randomized trial of the MEK1/2 inhibitor selumetinib as monotherapy versus temozolomide in patients with advanced melanoma. Clin Cancer Res. 2012;18(2):555–67. doi:10.1158/1078-0432.CCR-11-1491. Epub 2011 Nov 2. PMID:22048237 [PubMed - indexed for MEDLINE].

62. LoRusso PM, Krishnamurthi SS, Rinehart JJ, et al. Phase I pharmacokinetic and pharmacodynamic study of the oral MAPK/ERK kinase inhibitor PD-0325901 in patients with advanced cancers. Clin Cancer Res. 2010;16:1924–37.

63. Haura EB, Ricart AD, Larson TG, et al. A phase II study of PD-0325901, an oral MEK inhibitor, in previously treated patients with advanced non-small cell lung cancer. Clin Cancer Res. 2010;16:2450–7.

64. Flaherty KT, Robert C, Hersey P, Nathan P, Garbe C, Milhem M, Demidov LV, Hassel JC, Rutkowski P, Mohr P, Dummer R, Trefzer U, Larkin JM, Utikal J, Dreno B, Nyakas M, Middleton MR, Becker JC, Casey M, Sherman LJ, Wu FS, Ouellet D, Martin AM, Patel K, Schadendorf D, METRIC Study Group. Improved survival with MEK inhibition in BRAF-mutated melanoma. N Engl J Med. 2012;367(2): 107–14.

65. Flaherty KT, Infante JR, Daud A, Gonzalez R, Kefford RF, Sosman J, Hamid O, Schuchter L, Cebon J, Ibrahim N, Kudchadkar R, Burris 3rd HA, Falchook G, Algazi A, Lewis K, Long GV, Puzanov I, Lebowitz P, Singh A, Little S, Sun P, Allred A, Ouellet D, Kim KB, Patel K, Weber J. Combined BRAF and MEK inhibition in melanoma with BRAF V600 mutations. N Engl J Med. 2012;367(18):1694–703. doi:10.1056/NEJMoa1210093. Epub 2012 Sep 29.

Systemic Therapy for Rare Tumours of the Skin and Soft Tissue Tumour

31

Bruno Vincenzi, Anna Maria Frezza, Daniele Santini, and Giuseppe Tonini

Key Points

- Systemic therapy represents today the mainstay of soft tissue sarcoma, DFSP and MCC treatment in the metastatic setting; its role has also been evaluated in the adjuvant and neoadjuvant settings.
- Doxorubicin and ifosfamide are the principal compounds used in combination or as single agents in the treatment of metastatic soft tissue sarcoma, even if new chemotherapy regimens (i.e. gemcitabine and docetaxel) and target therapies (mTOR inhibitors, TKIs) are under investigation.
- The results regarding the role of adjuvant chemotherapy in the management of sarcoma are contradictory, but it can be proposed to those patients with a high risk of recurrence. The neoadjuvant chemotherapy is a reasonable approach in order to promote a non-demolishing surgery, but no impact on the survival has been proven.
- On the basis of a solid preclinical rational, imatinib mesylate has been tested in

DFSP, and it is today approved in the treatment of locally advanced and metastatic disease; its role in the neoadjuvant setting is under investigation.

- Cis-platinum (or carboplatinum) and etoposide are the most wildly used compounds in the management of metastatic MCC; unfortunately, their use in the adjuvant setting is associated to a detrimental impact on survival, and the evaluation of different agents, such as imatinib, has led to disappointing results.

Introduction and Basic Principles

Soft tissue sarcomas are a group of rare and extremely heterogeneous disease which comprise more than a hundred different histological subtypes, mainly originating from the embryonic mesoderm. Today, they represent less than 1 % of all the tumours in adults and almost 15 % of all paediatric neoplasm. According to SEER programme data, soft tissue sarcomas account for 1.3 % of all deaths for cancer, and the median age at the time of death is 65 years [1].

Among different histological subtypes of soft tissue sarcoma, the relative frequency varies according to age: during childhood, rhabdomyosarcoma is the most frequent kind of sarcoma, Ewing sarcoma and synovial sarcoma

B. Vincenzi • A.M. Frezza • D. Santini • G. Tonini (✉)
Medical Oncology, University Campus Bio-Medico,
200 Via Alvaro del Portillo, Rome 00128, Italy
e-mail: g.tonini@unicampus.it

A. Baldi et al. (eds.), *Skin Cancer*, Current Clinical Pathology,
DOI 10.1007/978-1-4614-7357-2_31, © Springer Science+Business Media New York 2014

in adolescence and in young adults, while in the adult age there is an increased incidence of leiomyosarcoma and liposarcoma.

Even if soft tissue sarcoma can arise anywhere in the body, the most commonly affected sites comprise lower limbs and limb girdle (40 %), upper limbs and limb girdle (20 %) and abdominal cavity (20 %); trunk and head and neck are affected only in 10 % of all cases.

Unfortunately, the symptoms at the time of the diagnosis are not specific and often confusing: the most common presentation finding is a painful progressively enlarging mass, whose dimensions can vary according to the onset site (usually bigger in trunk, thigh and abdominal cavity and smaller in distal limbs and head and neck). The growth of the tumour can determine the compression of surrounding structure, comprising vessels, nerves or cave organs, with site-dependent symptoms of increased pressure, such as paresthesia and pain, distal oedema and organ dysfunction. The diagnosis of soft tissue sarcoma must be confirmed through an appropriate imaging (MRI for limbs and limb girdles and CT scan for the abdomen) and through a core needle or excisional biopsy. Fine needle aspiration is useful to establish the diagnosis of recurrent disease in a previously treated patient. Given the fact that a correct diagnosis is the first step toward the definition of the prognosis and the choice of the best treatment, the biopsy should be analysed by a pathologist with great expertise in the field in order to identify the specific subtype. However, because of the heterogeneity of these diseases, soft tissue sarcoma morphological diagnosis can be still challenging mainly when the findings at the time of the onset are unusual; the availability of molecular techniques, such as the determination of karyotype, the fluorescence in situ hybridisation (FISH), the polymerase chain reaction (PCR) and the reverse transcriptase PCR (RT-PCR), is today an extremely important tool in the diagnostic part of the initial work-up, because it allows to detect those specific translocations which are known to characterise at least one-third of soft tissue sarcoma. Soft tissue sarcoma is an aggressive disease, and almost 80 % of patients will develop distant metastases within

3 years from the diagnosis [2]; on the contrary, only 5 % of patients affected by soft tissue sarcoma show a lymph nodal involvement [3]. Sarcomas of the extremities tend to metastasise mainly to the lung by haematogenous spreading, while abdominal sarcomas are more often associated with liver and peritoneal metastases. Given these data, a CT scan of chest, abdomen and pelvis should be considered for the initial systemic staging in this disease.

Apart from soft tissue sarcoma, we can find rare, non-melanocytic tumours which affect the skin: among this group, the most important and well-defined nosological entities are represented by dermatofibrosarcoma protuberans (DFSP) and by Merkel cell carcinoma. DFSP is a rare sarcoma of the skin with fibroblastic/myofibroblastic origin, which usually affects the dermis and underlying soft tissue. Even if it accounts only for 2–6 % of all sarcomas, it is today the most frequent sarcoma of the skin. From a clinical point of view, DFSP is characterised by a highly irregular plaque-like shape, with frequent fingerlike extensions. The lesion is usually covered by telangiectatic atrophic skin, and it is locally destructive. The most frequent presenting location of the lesions is the skin of the trunk with 42–72 % of cases, followed by proximal extremities (16–30 %) and head and neck, involved in approximately 10–16 % of patients [4]. The biological behaviour of this disease is characterised by a local aggressiveness and tendency to recurrence (the data reported in the literature varies between 10 and 80 %). On the other side, the rate of developing distant metastases is low (4–5 %), and there are only few cases in which a regional lymph node involvement was reported (1 %) [5]. A definitive diagnosis of DFSP requires histology after a core needle or excisional biopsy. Of interest, more than 90 % of DFSP possess supernumerary ring chromosomes or a unique translocation involving chromosomes 17 and 22, which fuses the strongly expressed collagen type 1 alpha 1 (COL1A1) gene on chromosome 17 with the platelet-derived growth factor B-chain gene (PDGFB) on chromosome 22: the detection of the t(17;22) translocation through molecular techniques is today mandatory for the diagnosis of DFSP, even if in about 8 % of cases this fusion transcript is not found [6]. The extent of the tumour must be assessed with a local MRI, and, given the low rate of metastatic disease, a complete stage is not routinely required.

Merkel cell carcinoma (MCC) is a rare and aggressive neuroendocrine tumour of the skin arising from dermoepidermal junction. It occurs most frequently in sun-exposed areas of skin, particularly the head and neck, followed by the extremities and then the trunk. Of interest, MCC incidence increases progressively with age (median age at the time of diagnosis is 65 years), and it is also significantly higher in immunocompromised patients. Moreover, in 2008, a new polyomavirus (Merkel cell polyomavirus (MCPyV)) was identified in a specimen of MCC, and today we know that 43–100 % of MCC are positive for MCPyV [7]: the possible pathogenic and prognostic values of immunosuppression and MCPyV are today still uncertain and under active investigation. MCC usually presents as an asymptomatic and indurated dermal nodule with a slightly erythematous to deeply violaceous colour which infiltrates locally via dermal lymphatics resulting in multiple satellite lesions. Even if the diagnosis can be suspected on the basis of clinical and epidemiological data, a definitive confirmation can only be obtained through histology. Furthermore, given this similarity to a variety of other small round blue cell tumours, such as small cell lung cancer, the morphological diagnosis can still be challenging. Immunohistochemical analysis can be of great help by assessing the positivity of CK20 (a very sensitive marker of MCC) and the negativity of TTF-1 (usually expressed in lung cancer). Even if the role of imaging in the initial work-up of MCC is still to be clarified, a CT scan of chest and abdomen should be perform in order to rule out the presence of a primitive lung cancer and to assess the presence of distant metastasis. As discussed before, MCC is an aggressive disease, with a high rate of both local recurrence (25–30 %) and distant metastatic disease (34–36 %) [8]. MCC prognosis is poorer than that of melanoma, and the 5 years' overall survival ranges from 30 to 64 % [9].

Current Treatment: Practical Considerations and Application

Despite the progresses done in the last years, systemic therapy represents today one of the principal therapeutic approaches in the treatment of soft tissue sarcomas and rare tumour of the skin. Among this heterogeneous group of neoplasm, we can identify subtypes known to be extremely responsive to chemotherapy (such as Ewing sarcoma and MCC), subtypes which are resistant to any compound today available (alveolar soft part sarcoma) and finally subtypes in which the better understanding of the pathogenesis brought to the development of effective target therapy (DFSP).

In the field of soft tissue sarcoma, standard chemotherapy has been investigated with unsatisfactory results in the management of advanced disease and, more recently, in the neoadjuvant and adjuvant setting.

The aim of the neoadjuvant therapy in the management of soft tissue sarcoma is to allow a radical resection of the primary tumour with a more conservative surgery. This is important mainly in the treatment of extremity sarcoma in order to avoid the amputation. According to the data today available in the literature, tumour shrinkage can be obtained in 30–40 % of all cases, but only 20–30 % will reach a more conservative surgery. The only prospective phase II trial is the one from EORTC done in 2001, in which patients affected by high-risk sarcoma (≥8 cm in size; grade II/III <8 cm in size; grade II/III recurrent) were randomised to receive surgery only or surgery preceded by three cycles of doxorubicin (50 mg/m^2/cycle) and ifosfamide (5 g/m^2/cycle). This trial pointed out the feasibility of neoadjuvant chemotherapy but failed in demonstrating a significant impact in terms of DFS (52 % vs 56 % at 5 years) and OS (64 % vs 65 % at 5 years) [10]. Further studies are currently evaluating the relevance of neoadjuvant chemotherapy in modifying the prognosis of locally advanced soft tissue sarcoma. The role of the adjuvant chemotherapy in the treatment of soft tissue sarcoma today is still unclear. One of the first studies conducted in 2001 by Frustaci et al. [11] proved initially a benefit both in DFS and OS for those patients who received an adjuvant chemotherapy with doxorubicin and ifosfamide: unfortunately, a further analysis at 10 years proved a significant reduction of the benefit in OS. A meta-analysis conducted by Peraiz et al. evaluated 18 different randomised clinical trials about adjuvant chemotherapy in locally advanced resectable soft tissue sarcoma. The results proved a marginal efficacy of chemotherapy in adjuvant setting in terms of local recurrence (OR 0.73) and distant and overall recurrence (OR 0.67). In terms of survival, doxorubicin alone had an OR of 0.84, which is not statistically significant. However, the OR for doxorubicin combined with ifosfamide was 0.56 in favour of chemotherapy, but it was associated with a worst tolerability profile (Table 31.1) [12]. The 62771 and the 62931 are two large phase III studies conducted by EORTC which compared surgery versus surgery followed by adjuvant chemotherapy with ifosfamide- and doxorubicin-based regimens (Table 31.2). A pooled analysis of these two studies presented by Le Cesne et al. [13] has shown how adjuvant chemotherapy was an independent favourable prognostic factor for PFS but not for OS. On the basis of these results, an adjuvant treatment can be proposed to those patients with a high risk of recurrence, but the

patient should be informed about the uncertainty of the data today available.

Among the different antineoplastic agents available in the treatment of soft tissue sarcoma in the metastatic setting, doxorubicin- and ifosfamide-based regimens are still the most widely used. Doxorubicin is an anthracycline which was introduced in the management of metastatic soft tissue sarcoma in 1970. The administration of doxorubicin single agent as a first-line treatment ($50-75$ mg/m^2 every 3–4 weeks, given both as bolus and as continuous infusion) is associated to a response rate of almost 20 %, and it is usually well tolerated. Unfortunately, doxorubicin use is however limited by its well-known cardiotoxicity, which is related to cumulative dose (higher than 550 mg/mq) and probably also to the administration manner (lower with continuous infusion and higher with bolus) [14]. A possible alternative could be represented by pegylated liposomal doxorubicin, which seems to share the same efficacy of the non-pegylated formulation with a better tolerability profile: in fact, a phase II trial by EORTC pointed out how the incidence of myelosuppression, alopecia and left ventricle dysfunction is significantly lower in patients treated with pegylated liposomal form [15]. Ifosfamide is an alkylating agent which has been introduced in the treatment of metastatic soft tissue sarcoma in 1980, and its administration, at the dose of 9 g/m^2 every 3 week, is associated with a 20 % response rate; better results are obtained if it is used as a first line. Comparing doxorubicin- and ifosfamide-based treatment, no differences have been identified in terms of PFS and OS, but the tolerability profile seems to be better when doxorubicin is used [10]. A phase III study in adults with advanced soft tissue

Table 31.1 Results from a systematic meta-analysis of 18 studies evaluating the efficacy of adjuvant chemotherapy in the treatment of soft tissue sarcoma

	Odds ratios	P value
Local relapse	0.73	0.02
Distant relapse	0.67	0.0001
Overall survival		
Doxorubicin	0. 84	0.09
Doxorubicin + ifosfamide	0.56	0.01

Table 31.2 Phase III study evaluating the efficacy of adjuvant chemotherapy in the treatment of soft tissue sarcoma

Study	Regimen	Patients (*n*)	Results
Frustaci et al.	Doxorubicin: 120 mg/sqm	104	>DFS
	Ifosfamide: 9 g/sqm + GCSF		>OS
EORTC 62771	Doxorubicin: 50 mg/sqm	468	>DFS
	DTIC: 400 mg/sqm gg 1–3		=OS
	Cyclophosphamide: 500 mg/sqm		
	Vincristine: 1.5 mg/sqm		
EORTC 62931	Doxorubicin: 74 mg/sqm	351	=DFS
	Ifosfamide: 9 g/sqm + GCSF		=OS

sarcomas which aimed to compare the objective regression rates, toxicity and survival of patients receiving doxorubicin alone and ifosfamide plus doxorubicin proved how the combination therapy reduced a significantly higher regression rate than did doxorubicin alone (34 % vs 20 %, $P = 0.03$), but it was also associated to a significantly more intense myelosuppression [16].

Trabectedin (ET743 or Yondelis) is a marine-derived antineoplastic molecule isolated from the Caribbean tunicate *Ecteinascidia turbinata* and currently produced synthetically. In Europe, today, trabectedin given as monotherapy (1.5 mg/mq as a 24-h continuous infusion every 3 weeks) is the only agent approved as a second line in the treatment of advanced soft tissue sarcoma after the failure of anthracycline- and ifosfamide-based regimens and received orphan drug status from the European Commission for the treatment of ovarian cancer in October 2003. The US FDA granted trabectedin orphan drug status both for soft tissue sarcoma and ovarian cancer. Trabectedin mechanism of action is today still not completely understood. What we know today is that, thanks to its structure, trabectedin can bind to DNA minor groove and alkylated guanine at the N2 position, bending DNA toward the major groove. Three nonrandomised phase II studies assessed the efficacy of trabectedin in patients with heavily pretreated, advanced/metastatic soft tissue sarcoma: the results from those studies benefit associated with trabectedin therapy in terms of overall response rate (4–8 %), 6-month progression-free survival (24–29 %) and overall survival (9.2–12.8 months); this benefit was particularly evident in the treatment of liposarcomas and leiomyosarcomas compared to other soft tissue sarcoma subtypes [17–19]. Trabectedin is also associated with an acceptable tolerability profile: the most significant side effects observed were grade 3 or 4 transaminase increase (26–50 %) and neutropenia (34–61 %). As for trabectedin hepatic effects, plasma liver enzyme level (transaminases, bilirubin, alkaline phosphatases and 5′-nucleotidase) should be checked before each course, because patients with any baseline alterations have a significant higher probability of developing a severe liver toxicity. The risk

of developing grade 3–4 toxicities seems to be strongly reduced through the patients' premedication with dexamethasone (4 mg per os bid 24 h before therapy). A study by Grosso et al. showed how elevation of transaminases, neutropenia and thrombocytopenia incidence was significantly lower in patients with prior dexamethasone (2, 2 and 0 %) and then in those who have not been previously premedicated (34, 24 and 25 %, respectively) [20].

Recently, particular attention has been dedicated to the evaluation of the association between gemcitabine and docetaxel in the treatment of soft tissue sarcoma, which seems to be promising. A phase II trial conducted by Maki et al. in 2007 randomised 122 patients to receive gemcitabine alone (1,200 mg/m^2 days 1 and 8) or gemcitabine (900 mg/m^2 days 1 and 8) plus docetaxel (100 mg/m^2 day 8) every 21 days: in those patients who received the combined regimen, the radiological response rate resulted higher than in those treated with gemcitabine alone (16 % vs 10 %), as also PFS (6.2 vs 2.6 months) and OS (18 vs 11.2 months). The toxicity, even if higher in the gemcitabine/docetaxel arm, was acceptable [21]. The association between gemcitabine and docetaxel has been found to be tolerable and highly active especially in leiomyosarcoma, for which a response rate of 57 % has been recorded [22].

In the management of MCC, surgery remains today the primary treatment modality. The role for systemic therapy today is still extremely marginal, and the data today available on the efficacy of standard chemotherapy in the treatment of this extremely aggressive disease are disappointing. The most common regimen used in the treatment of MCC is cis-platinum (or carboplatinum) and etoposide, both in the adjuvant and metastatic settings. While a role for adjuvant radiotherapy is increasingly supported by retrospective data, several recent studies have failed to demonstrate a benefit for MCC from adjuvant chemotherapy, whose use should be on the contrary strictly limited to clinical trials. A phase II study conducted by Allan et al. pointed out how the administration of adjuvant therapy in patients with stage II, nodal-positive MCC was associated with a detrimental effect on survival: in fact, the 4 years' survival in those patients who received an adjuvant treatment was 42 % compared with the 60 % of those who underwent surveillance [9]. Moreover, different studies which assessed the safety of an adjuvant treatment for MCC have proved how chemotherapy is associated with a significant treatment-related mortality (3.4 %) [23] and morbidity (63 % of patients experienced serious skin toxicity and 40 % were admitted for neutropenia) [24]. Data about the use of chemotherapy in the metastatic setting show how, despite the chemosensitive disease, the impact of the treatment on the survival is minimal. In fact, the response rate for MCC metastatic patients treated with standard chemotherapy is 57 %, but the median overall survival was only 9 months and the 3 years overall survival 17 %. Of note, a high rate of toxic death during first-line treatment ($n = 7.7$ %) was reported for these patients. A further trial, which aimed to specifically evaluate the efficacy of the association between cisplatin (or carboplatin) and etoposide, confirmed the previous observations according to which MCC appears to be chemosensitive but can progress rapidly with fatal outcomes [25].

Unlike soft tissue sarcoma and MCC, the identification of a specific pathway which seems to drive the growth of DFSP has led to the development of a target therapy with a well-recognised activity. As discussed before, nearly 90 % of DFSP are characterised by the presence of a rearrangement of chromosomes 17 and 22, which can be represented both by translocation t(17;22) (q22;q13) and by a supernumerary ring chromosome containing several copies of the t(17;22) breakpoint region. This genetic aberration results in the fusion of the COL1A1 and PDGFB genes, with PDGFB passing under the control of COL1A1 promoter which is more transcriptionally active than its own promoter. Upregulated PDGFB acts as a ligand for both PDGFRα and PDGFRβ, and it causes an autocrine/paracrine stimulation which is thought to be a key point in DFSP pathogenesis. It is important to remember that 8–10 % of DFSB do not present the t(11;22) translocation: in this case, other pathways not still recognised probably drive the tumour growth (Fig. 31.1) [26]. This pathogenic mechanism represents the rational according to which imatinib mesylate was tested in the treatment of DFSP. Apart from many case reports today present in the literature, an important experience was published in 2005 by McArthur et al. who analysed the efficacy of imatinib, at the dose of 400 mg twice a day, in the treatment of six patients with locally advanced DFSP and two patients with metastatic disease. Of interest, all the patients with t(11;22) translocation reported a partial response, while one metastatic patient, in whose DFSP the translocation was not present, progressed [27]. These data have led to approval of imatinib by the US Food and Drug Administration for treating locally advanced DFSP. Although

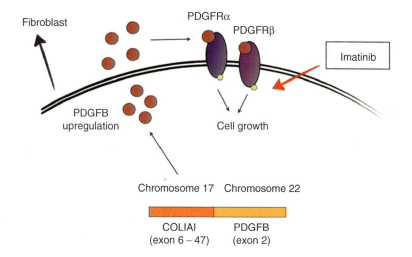

Fig. 31.1 DFSP pathogenesis and imatinib mesylate mechanism of action

wide surgical excision remains standard care, patients with locally advanced disease not suitable for surgical excision can be treated with the PDGFR inhibitor imatinib, which sometimes allows residual DFSP to be surgically excised. Because tumours lacking the t(11;22) translocation may not respond to imatinib treatment, DFSP molecular analyses should be always performed before starting a systemic therapy.

Future Considerations

Given the poor results obtained with standard chemotherapy, currently many ongoing clinical trials are investigating the efficacy of alternative systemic therapy in the treatment of metastatic soft tissue sarcoma. Of interest, promising results have been obtained with the inhibition of the PI3K/Akt/mTOR pathway (Fig. 31.2). The PI3K/Akt/mTOR pathway has been found to be deregulated in many different human sarcomas, including leiomyosarcoma, rhabdomyosarcoma and GIST [28], underlining its importance in the promotion of cancer cell growth and survival. mTOR (mammalian target of rapamycin) appears to be regulated by the insulin-like growth factor (IGF) through the PI3K/Akt pathway, while mTOR downstream targets are mainly represented

by S6K1 (ribosomal kinase) and 4E-BP1 (translational initiation factor) [29]. Rapamycin (or sirolimus), a macrolide antibiotic isolated from a strain of *Streptomyces hygroscopicus*, is an mTOR inhibitor routinely used in immunosuppressive regimen, which has shown efficacy in the treatment of iatrogenic [30, 31] and classic [32, 33] Kaposi's sarcoma. Among the mTOR inhibitors which are currently in clinical development as anticancer agents, AP23573 (deforolimus), developed by ARIAD Pharmaceuticals Inc. both in intravenous and oral formulations, has recently demonstrated a single-agent activity in a broad range of soft tissue sarcoma in a phase II trial: in 212 patients affected by advanced soft tissue and bone sarcoma treated with deforolimus, the clinical benefit response rate (CBR, defined as a complete or partial response or stable disease for at least 16 weeks) was found to be 29 %, and the overall survival (OS) was 67.6 weeks. On the basis of these promising results, a multinational, phase 3 trial (SUCCEED: sarcoma multi-center clinical evaluation of the efficacy of deforolimus) has been conducted in order to investigate the efficacy and safety of oral deforolimus when administered as maintenance therapy to patients with metastatic soft tissue or bone sarcomas who have had a favourable outcome to chemotherapy. The results from the SUCCEED trial showed an

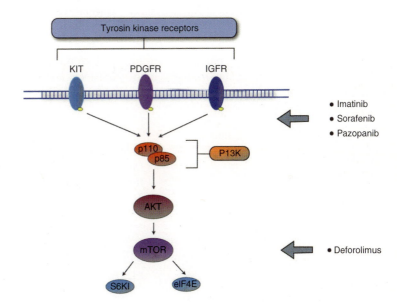

Fig. 31.2 New therapeutic targets in the treatment of soft tissue sarcoma and DFSP

improvement in PFS by 21 % and in terms of overall survival, a trend in favour of deforolimus (88 vs 77.8 weeks) [34]. Among the new therapy under development in the treatment of soft tissue sarcoma, encouraging data have been also obtained through the inhibition of tyrosine kinase receptors (VEGFR, PDGFR, c-Kit, Raf), whose activation is known to be involved in angiogenesis, cell proliferation and apoptosis (Fig. 31.2). Among small molecule tyrosine kinase inhibitors (smTKI), the most promising results in the treatment of soft tissue sarcoma have been obtained with pazopanib and sorafenib. Pazopanib, developed by GlaxoSmithKline Inc., is an oral, second-generation multi-targeted tyrosine kinase inhibitor that targets PDGFR, VEGFR and c-kit, key proteins responsible for tumourigenesis and tumour progression. A recent phase II trial [35], which enrolled 142 patients affected by adipocytic STS, leiomyosarcomas, synovial sarcomas or other soft tissue sarcoma types to be treated with pazopanib, proved an increase of PFS at 12 weeks only in the leiomyosarcoma cohort (44 %), in the synovial sarcomas (49 %) and in the other soft tissue sarcoma types (39 %). On the basis of these results, a phase III trial is ongoing to investigate whether treatment with pazopanib improves the outcome of patients with metastatic soft tissue sarcoma when compared to placebo. Sorafenib is an oral multikinase inhibitor that acts through the inhibition of Raf1 (and additional Raf isoforms) and RTK (VEGFR-1/VEGFR-2/VEGFR-3), involved both in cell proliferation and in angiogenesis [36, 37]. A multiarm phase II study by Maki et al. [38] proved an interesting activity of sorafenib in the treatment of angiosarcoma (RR 13 %; PFS 3.8; OS 14.9) and leiomyosarcoma (RR 2 %; PFS 3.2; OS 22.4), while the activity against other sarcoma subtypes was minimal. On the basis of a strong biological rational and given the encouraging results obtained in the treatment of angiosarcoma, several phase I and phase II trials are now evaluating sorafenib efficacy in the treatment of locally advanced and metastatic soft tissue sarcoma, both as a single agents and in combination with standard chemotherapy, but no phase III trials are available at the moment. Finally, given the good results obtained with trabectedin, two new compounds that act by binding DNA minor groove are under clinical development. The first one, brostallicin (PNU-166196), has been evaluated in a phase II study conducted by EORTC in metastatic or inoperable soft tissue sarcoma, and it has been found to be associated with two confirmed partial responses on 21 patients recruited and with 3 months PFS of 46 % [39]. Given the previous data, three phase II studies are currently evaluating brostallicin efficacy in advanced soft tissue sarcoma in association with doxorubicin as first-line therapy or alone as second line. Eribulin mesylate (E7389, Eisai Research Institute) is a microtubule dynamics inhibitor that is a more stable, synthetic analogue of the marine natural macrolide halichondrin B. In phase I studies, eribulin has shown a manageable tolerability profile, and a phase II study is currently evaluating its impact on 12 months PFS in the treatment of advanced soft tissue sarcoma (Table 31.3).

Unfortunately, disappointing results have been obtained so far in the search for alternative approach for the management of MCC. On the

Table 31.3 Approved and experimental therapies in the treatment of soft tissue sarcoma, DFSP and MCC

Tumours	Standard treatment	Regimens/compounds under investigations	Current study level
Soft tissue sarcoma	Doxorubicin	Gemcitabine and docetaxel	Phase II
	Ifosfamide	Deforolimus	Phase III
	Trabectedin (second line)	Sorafenib	Phase II
		Pazopanib	Phase III
		Brostallicin	Phase II
		Eribulin	Phase I
DFSP	Imatinib	Pazopanib	Phase II
MCC	CDDP/ CBCDA ± etoposide	–	

basis of data in vitro, supporting the hypothesis that KIT receptor activation by autocrine and paracrine stem cell factor could stimulate the growth of MCC [40], the efficacy of imatinib was assessed in the treatment of this aggressive disease. The only phase II trial published so far showed a partial response only in the 4 % of patients and a median overall survival of 5 months [41]. However, a second phase II study is currently ongoing.

As for the treatment of locally advanced and metastatic DFSP, apart for many ongoing trials which are still assessing imatinib efficacy both in the metastatic and neoadjuvant settings, an interesting phase II study is currently evaluating the efficacy of pazopanib. In fact, pazopanib is characterised by a multi-tyrosine kinase inhibitor activity which affects in particular PDGFR and VEGFR, both of which have been shown to be activated in DFSP; moreover, as discussed before, pazopanib has already shown antitumour activity in sarcoma patients with an acceptable safety profile: because of all these reasons, there seems to be a strong rationale to assess its efficacy in the treatment of DFSP, especially in those patients who are not expected to derive a sufficient benefit from imatinib.

Glossary

Adjuvant chemotherapy Additional cancer treatment given after the primary treatment to lower the risk that the cancer will come back.

Neoadjuvant chemotherapy Treatment given as a first step to shrink a tumour before the main treatment, which is usually surgery, is given.

Overall survival The percentage of people in a study or treatment group who are alive for a certain period of time after they were diagnosed with or treated for a disease, such as cancer. The overall survival rate is often stated as a 5-year survival rate, which is the percentage of people in a study or treatment group who are alive 5 years after diagnosis or treatment.

Progression-free survival The length of time during and after treatment in which a patient is living with a disease that does not get worse.

Soft tissues Non-epithelial extraskeletal tissue, including muscle, fat and fibrous supporting structures, arising mainly from embryonic mesoderm, with some neuroectodermal contribution.

References

1. Ries LAG, Melbert D, Krapcho M, Stinchcomb DG, Howlader N, Horner MJ, Mariotto A, Miller BA, Feuer EJ, Altekruse SF, Lewis DR, Clegg L, Eisner MP, Reichman M, Edwards BK (editors). SEER Cancer Statistics Review, 1975–2005. Bethesda: National Cancer Institute; 2008. http://seer.cancer.gov/csr/1975_2005/, based on November 2007 SEER data submission, posted to the SEER web site.
2. Cormier JN, Pollock RE. Soft tissue sarcomas. CA Cancer J Clin. 2004;54(2):94–109.
3. Fong Y, Coit DG, Woodruff JM, Brennan MF. Lymph node metastasis from soft tissue sarcoma in adults. Analysis of data from a prospective database of 1772 sarcoma patients. Ann Surg. 1993;217:72–7.
4. Criscione VD, Weinstock MA. Descriptive epidemiology of dermatofibrosarcoma protuberans in the United States, 1973 to 2002. J Am Acad Dermatol. 2007;56:968–73.
5. Rutgers EJ, Kroon BB, Albus-Lutter CE, Gortzak E. Dermatofibrosarcoma protuberans: treatment and prognosis. Eur J Surg Oncol. 1997;18:241–8.
6. Patel KU, Szabo SS, Hernandez VS, Prieto VG, Abruzzo LV, Lazar AJ, et al. Dermatofibrosarcoma protuberans COL1A1-PDGFB fusion is identified in virtually all dermatofibrosarcoma protuberans cases when investigated by newly developed multiplex reverse transcription polymerase chain reaction and fluorescence in situ hybridization assays, Hum Pathol. 2008;39(2):184–93.
7. Rollison DE, Giuliano AR, Becker JC. New virus associated with Merkel cell carcinoma development. J Natl Compr Canc Netw. 2010;8(8):874–80.
8. Medina-Franco H, Urist MM, Fiveash J, Heslin MJ, Bland KI, Beenken SW. Multimodality treatment of Merkel cell carcinoma: case series and literature review of 1024 cases. Ann Surg Oncol. 2001;8(3):204–8.
9. Allen PJ, Bowne WB, Jaques DP, Brennan MF, Busam K, Coit DG. Merkel cell carcinoma: prognosis and treatment of patients from a single institution. J Clin Oncol. 2005;23(10):2300–9.
10. Lorigan P, Verweij J, Papai Z, Rodenhuis S, Le Cesne A, Leahy MG, et al. Phase III trial of two investigational schedules of ifosfamide compared with standard-dose doxorubicin in advanced or metastatic soft tissue sarcoma: a European Organisation for Research and Treatment of Cancer Soft Tissue and Bone Sarcoma Group Study. J Clin Oncol. 2007;25(21):3144–50.

11. Frustaci S, Gherlinzoni F, De Paoli A, et al. Adjuvant chemotherapy for adult soft tissue sarcomas of the extremities and girdles: results of the Italian randomized cooperative trial. J Clin Oncol. 2001;19:1238–47.

12. Pervaiz N, Colterjohn N, Farrokhyar F, Tozer R, Figueredo A, Ghert M. A systematic meta-analysis of randomized controlled trials of adjuvant chemotherapy for localized resectable soft-tissue sarcoma. Cancer. 2008;113(3):573–81.

13. Le Cesne A, Van Glabbeke M, Woll PJ, Bramwell VH, Casali PG, Hoekstra HJ, Reichardt P, Hogendoorn PC, Hohenberger P, Blay JY. The end of adjuvant chemotherapy (adCT) era with doxorubicin-based regimen in resected high-grade soft tissue sarcoma (STS): Pooled analysis of the two STBSG-EORTC phase III clinical trials. J Clin Oncol (ASCO Annual Meeting). 2008;20(15S):10525.

14. Shapira J, Gotfried M, Lishner M, Ravid M. Reduced cardiotoxicity of doxorubicin by a 6-hour infusion regimen: a prospective randomized evaluation. Cancer. 1990;65:870–3.

15. Judson I, Radford JA, Harris M, Blay JY, van Hoesel Q, le Cesne A, et al. Randomised phase II trial of pegylated liposomal doxorubicin (DOXIL/CAELYX) versus doxorubicin in the treatment of advanced or metastatic soft tissue sarcoma: a study by the EORTC Soft Tissue and Bone Sarcoma Group. Eur J Cancer. 2001;37(7):870–7.

16. Edmonson JH, Ryan LM, Blum RH, Brooks JS, Shiraki M, Frytak S, et al. Randomized comparison of doxorubicin alone versus ifosfamide plus doxorubicin or mitomycin, doxorubicin, and cisplatin against advanced soft tissue sarcomas. J Clin Oncol. 1993;11(7):1269–75.

17. Garcia-Carbonero R, Supko JG, Manola J, et al. Phase II and pharmacokinetic study of ecteinascidin 743 in patients with progressive sarcomas of soft tissues refractory to chemotherapy. J Clin Oncol. 2004;22:1480–90.

18. Le Cesne A, Blay JY, Judson I, et al. Phase II study of ET-743 in advanced soft tissue sarcomas: a European Organisation for the Research and Treatment of Cancer (EORTC) Soft Tissue and Bone Sarcoma Group Trial. J Clin Oncol. 2005;23:576–84.

19. Yovine A, Riofrio M, Blay JY, et al. Phase II study of ecteinascidin-743 in advanced pretreated soft tissue sarcoma patients. J Clin Oncol. 2004;22:890–9.

20. Grosso F, Dileo P, Sanfilippo R, Stacchiotti S, Bertulli R, Piovesan C, et al. Steroid premedication markedly reduces liver and bone marrow toxicity of trabectedin in advanced sarcoma. Eur J Cancer. 2006;42(10):1484–90.

21. Maki RG, Wathen JK, Patel SR, Priebat DA, Okuno SH, Samuels B, et al. Randomized phase II study of gemcitabine and docetaxel compared with gemcitabine alone in patients with metastatic soft tissue sarcomas: results of sarcoma alliance for research through collaboration study 002. J Clin Oncol. 2007;25(19):2755–63.

22. Hensley ML, Maki R, Venkatraman E, Geller G, Lovegren M, Aghajanian C, et al. Gemcitabine and docetaxel in patients with unresectable leiomyosarcoma: results of a phase II trial. J Clin Oncol. 2002;20(12):2824–31.

23. Tai PT, Yu E, Winquist E, Hammond A, Stitt L, Tonita J, et al. Chemotherapy in neuroendocrine/Merkel cell carcinoma of the skin: case series and review of 204 cases. J Clin Oncol. 2000;18(12):2493–9.

24. Poulsen M, Rischin D, Walpole E, Harvey J, Macintosh J, Ainslie J, et al. Analysis of toxicity of Merkel cell carcinoma of the skin treated with synchronous carboplatin/etoposide and radiation: a Trans-Tasman Radiation Oncology Group Study. Int J Radiat Oncol Biol Phys. 2001;51(1):156–63.

25. Pectasides D, Pectasides M, Psyrri A, Koumarianou A, Xiros N, Pectasides E, et al. Cisplatin-based chemotherapy for Merkel cell carcinoma of the skin. Cancer Invest. 2006;24(8):780–5.

26. Labropoulos SV, Razis ED. Imatinib in the treatment of dermatofibrosarcoma protuberans. Biologics. 2007;1(4):347–53.

27. McArthur GA, Demetri GD, van Oosterom A, Heinrich MC, Debiec-Rychter M, Corless CL, et al. Molecular and clinical analysis of locally advanced dermatofibrosarcoma protuberans treated with imatinib: Imatinib Target Exploration Consortium Study B2225. J Clin Oncol. 2005;23(4):866–73.

28. Okuno S. Mammalian target of rapamycin inhibitors in sarcomas. Curr Opin Oncol. 2006;18:360–2.

29. Magenau JM, Schuetze SM. New targets for therapy of sarcoma. Curr Opin Oncol. 2008;20:400–6.

30. Campistol JM, Schena FP. Kaposi's sarcoma in renal transplant recipients—the impact of proliferation signal inhibitors. Nephrol Dial Transplant. 2007;22 Suppl 1:i17–22.

31. Montaner S. Akt/TSC/mTOR activation by the KSHV G protein-coupled receptor: emerging insights into the molecular oncogenesis and treatment of Kaposi's sarcoma. Cell Cycle. 2007;6:438–43.

32. Guenova E, Metzler G, Hoetzenecker W, Berneburg M, Rocken M. Classic Mediterranean Kaposi's sarcoma regression with sirolimus treatment. Arch Dermatol. 2008;144:692–3.

33. Merimsky O, Jiveliouk I, Sagi-Eisenberg R. Targeting mTOR in HIV-negative classic Kaposi's sarcoma. Sarcoma. 2008;2008:825093.

34. Chawla SP. Results of the phase III, placebo-controlled trial (SUCCEED) evaluating the mTOR inhibitor ridaforolimus (R) as maintenance therapy in advanced sarcoma patients (pts) following clinical benefit from prior standard cytotoxic chemotherapy (CT). J Clin Oncol (ASCO Annual Meeting). 2011;29(15 suppl):10005 (abstract).

35. Sleijfer S, Ray-Coquard I, Papai Z, Le Cesne A, Scurr M, Schöffski P, et al. Pazopanib, a multikinase angiogenesis inhibitor, in patients with relapsed or refractory advanced soft tissue sarcoma: a phase II study from the European Organisation for Research and Treatment of Cancer-soft Tissue and Bone

Sarcoma Group (EORTC study 62043). J Clin Oncol. 2009;27(19):3126–32.

36. Wilhelm SM, Carter C, Tang L, et al. BAY43-9006 exhibits broad spectrum oral antitumor activity and targets the RAF/MEK/ERK pathway and receptor tyrosine kinases involved in tumor progression and angiogenesis. Cancer Res. 2004;64:7099–109.

37. Levy AP, Pauloski N, Braun D, et al. Analysis of transcription and protein expression changes in the 786-O human renal cell carcinoma tumor xenograft model in response to treatment with the multi-kinase inhibitor sorafenib (BAY 43–9006). Proc Am Assoc Cancer Res. 2006;47:213–4.

38. Maki RG, D'Adamo DR, Keohan ML, Saulle M, Schuetze SM, Undevia SD, et al. Phase II study of sorafenib in patients with metastatic or recurrent sarcomas. J Clin Oncol. 2009;27(19):3133–40.

39. Leahy M, Ray-Coquard I, Verweij J, Le Cesne A, Duffaud F, Hogendoorn PC, et al. Brostallicin, an agent with potential activity in metastatic soft tissue sarcoma: a phase II study from the European Organisation for Research and Treatment of Cancer Soft Tissue and Bone Sarcoma Group. Eur J Cancer. 2007;43(2):308–15.

40. Krasagakis K, Fragiadaki I, Metaxari M, Krüger-Krasagakis S, Tzanakakis GN, Stathopoulos EN, et al. KIT receptor activation by autocrine and paracrine stem cell factor stimulates growth of Merkel cell carcinoma in vitro. J Cell Physiol. 2011;226(4):1099–109. doi:10.1002/jcp.22431.

41. Samlowski WE, Moon J, Tuthill RJ, Heinrich MC, Balzer-Haas NS, Merl SA, et al. A phase II trial of imatinib mesylate in Merkel cell carcinoma (neuroendocrine carcinoma of the skin): a Southwest Oncology Group Study (S0331). Am J Clin Oncol. 2010;33(5):495–9.

Sentinel Lymph Node

32

Paolo Persichetti, Stefania Tenna,
Beniamino Brunetti, and Stefano Campa

Key Points
- Basic principles
- Knowledge of the microscopic and macroscopic anatomy of the lymphatic system (head and neck, upper extremity and lower extremity, lymph node basins).
- Indications
  - Validated indications: melanoma; breast cancer.
  - Suggested indications: atypical or borderline Spitz tumors; squamous cell carcinoma; Merkel cell carcinoma; eccrine/apocrine carcinoma.
- Equipments and surgical technique
  - Lymphoscintigraphy; blue dye injection; handheld gamma probe.
  - Minimal, atraumatic dissection.
- Postoperative management
  - *Drainage*; extremity elevation; elastic compressive bandages.
  - Prevention of complications (immediate and short-term vs long-term expected side effects).

P. Persichetti • S. Tenna • S. Campa
Plastic and Reconstructive Surgery Unit,
Campus Bio-Medico University of Rome, Rome, Italy

B. Brunetti, MD (✉)
Plastic and Reconstructive Surgery Unit,
Campus Bio-Medico University of Rome,
Via Alvaro del Portillo 200, Rome 00128, Italy
e-mail: b.brunetti@unicampus.it

Introduction

The theory of lymphatic spread of cancer represents a basic chapter in the book of modern oncology. The concept of "anticipatory gland excision," which opened the field to modern elective lymph node dissection, was first introduced by Snow [1] in 1898, but only in 1955 Seaman and Powers [2] introduced radiolabeled colloidal gold to describe the path of lymphatic channels followed by cancer. Then, lymphoscintigraphy evolved with the introduction in the clinical practice of technetium Tc 99m sulfur colloid, albumin colloid, or human serum albumin.

In 1960, Gould and colleagues [3] described the first node to be involved in lymphatic spread, defining it as "sentinel node," but it was Cabanas [4] in 1977 who introduced in the clinical practice the sentinel lymph node dissection (SLND) to stage penile carcinoma.

In the 1990s, sentinel lymph node biopsy became the gold standard in the staging of melanoma patients, thanks to Morton, Alex, and Krag [5, 6], who first used blue dye injected around the primary melanoma to identify the sentinel node and then described radio-guided sentinel lymph node biopsy with gamma-probe localization of sentinel lymph nodes.

These experiences standardized the method, allowing transcutaneous identification of the sentinel lymph node and performing biopsy through a small incision, limiting the extent of the dissection needed to identify it.

Since those early efforts, many studies have clarified SLND crucial role in the staging of ectoderm-derived tumors, particularly in melanoma and breast cancer; anyway, the efficacy of SLN biopsy in the staging or treatment of nonmelanoma skin cancer has still to be proved.

Basic Principles

Anatomy of the Lymphatic System for SLND [7]

The lymphatic system consists of a complex capillary networks which collect the lymph in the various organs and tissues. It is an elaborate system of collecting vessels, lymph glands or nodes, and lymphatic chains. Vessels conduct the lymph from the capillaries to the large veins of the neck at the junction of the internal jugular and subclavian veins, where the lymph is poured into the bloodstream; nodes are interspaced in the pathways of the collecting vessels filtering the lymph as it passes through them and contributing lymphocytes to it.

The lymph glands are small oval- or bean-shaped bodies situated in the course of lymphatic and lacteal vessels so that the lymph and chyle pass through them on their way to the blood. Each generally presents on one side a slight depression (the hilus) through which the blood vessels enter and leave the interior. The efferent lymphatic vessel also emerges from the gland at this spot, while the afferent vessels enter the organ at different parts of the periphery. On section, a lymph gland displays two different structures: an external, of lighter color (the cortical), and an internal, darker (the medullary). The cortical structure does not form a complete investment, but is deficient at the hilus, where the medullary portion reaches the surface of the gland, so that the efferent vessel is derived directly from the medullary structures, while the afferent vessels empty themselves into the cortical substance.

Lymphatic Chains and Their Drainage Areas [7]

The lymphatic chains are anatomically divided according to major districts. Considering skin cancer, the most important areas can be summarized as follows:

Lymph Glands of the Head and Neck

The lymph glands of the head are usually involved by oncologic dissemination from cancers of the scalp, the face, and the auricle. They are divided in the following groups: occipital, facial, posterior auricular, deep facial, anterior auricular, lingual, parotid, and retropharyngeal.

Occipital glands usually drain lymph from the scalp; posterior auricular glands drain the temporoparietal region, the upper part of the cranial surface of the auricular, and the back of the external acoustic meatus; the anterior auricular glands drain the lateral surface of the auricula and the skin of the adjacent part of the temporal region; parotid and facial glands, respectively, drain the root of the nose, the eyelids, the frontotemporal region, the external acoustic meatus and the tympanic cavity and eyelids, the conjunctiva, and the skin and mucous membrane of the nose and cheek.

The lymph glands of the neck are usually involved by oncologic dissemination from cancers of the upper/lower lip and the oral cavity. They are divided in superficial and deep glands.

The superficial cervical glands lie in close relationship with the external jugular vein as it emerges from the parotid gland and, therefore, superficial to the sternocleidomastoideus. Their afferents drain the lower parts of the auricula and parotid region, while their efferents pass around the anterior margin of the sternocleidomastoideus to join the superior deep cervical glands. The deep glands are divided in the following surgical levels according to the Robbins classification [8], originally proposed by the Memorial Sloan-Kettering Cancer Group:

- Ia: Submental nodes—draining the floor of the mouth, anterior tongue, anterior mandibular alveolar ridge, and lower lip.
- Ib: Submandibular nodes—draining the oral cavity, anterior nasal cavity, soft tissue structures of the midface, and submandibular gland.
- II: Upper jugular nodes—draining the oral cavity, nasal cavity, nasopharynx, oropharynx, hypopharynx, larynx, and parotid gland.

- III: Middle jugular nodes—draining the oral cavity, nasopharynx, oropharynx, hypopharynx, and larynx.
- IV: Lower jugular nodes—draining larynx, hypopharynx, thyroid, and cervical esophagus.
- V: Posterior triangle nodes—draining nasopharynx, oropharynx, and skin of the posterior scalp and neck.
- VI: Anterior nodes—they are usually removed during surgery for thyroid, laryngeal, and hypopharyngeal cancer.

Lymph Glands of the Upper Extremity

The lymph glands of the upper extremity are divided into two groups, superficial and deep.

The superficial lymph glands are few and of small size. They are rarely involved in dissemination from skin cancers or melanoma of the hand and forearm.

Supratrochlear glands are placed above the medial epicondyle of the humerus, medial to the basilic vein. Their afferents drain the middle, ring, and little fingers, the medial portion of the hand, and the superficial area over the ulnar side of the forearm; these vessels are, however, in free communication with the other lymphatic vessels of the forearm. Their efferents accompany the basilic vein and join the deeper vessels.

Deltoideopectoral glands, in number of one or two, are found beside the cephalic vein, between the pectoralis major and deltoideus, immediately below the clavicle. They are situated in the course of the external collecting trunks of the arm.

The deep lymph glands are mainly grouped in the axilla, although a few may be found in the forearm, in the course of the radial, ulnar, and interosseous vessels, and in the arm along the medial side of the brachial artery.

The axillary glands are usually involved by oncologic dissemination from skin cancers of the thorax, back, and upper extremity.

They consist of a lateral group, an anterior or pectoral group, a posterior or subscapular group, a central or intermediate group, and a medial or subclavicular group.

By a practical point of view, the axillary glands are usefully divided according to the Fisher classification [9], which recognizes three levels, usually progressively involved in metastatic dissemination:

- Level I: They are located inferior and lateral to the lateral margin of the pectoralis minor muscle.
- Level II: They are located on the undersurface of the pectoralis minor muscle.
- Level III: They are located superior and medial to the medial margin of the pectoralis minor muscle.

Lymph Glands of the Lower Extremity

The lymph glands of the lower extremity consist of the popliteal and inguinal glands.

They are usually involved by oncologic dissemination from skin cancers of the lower extremity, lower back, lower abdomen, and perineum.

The popliteal glands, small in size, six or seven in number, are imbedded in the fat contained in the popliteal fossa. One lies immediately beneath the popliteal fascia, near the terminal part of the small saphenous vein. Another is placed between the popliteal artery and the posterior surface of the knee joint; it receives the lymphatic vessels from the knee joint together with those which accompany the genicular arteries. The others lie at the sides of the popliteal vessels and receive as efferents the trunks which accompany the anterior and posterior tibial vessels. They are rarely involved in metastatic dissemination, usually by skin cancers and melanoma arising in the lateral aspect of the leg and dorsolateral aspect of the foot [10].

The inguinal glands [11] are situated at the upper part of the femoral triangle. They are divided in superficial and deep glands and represent the common site of metastasis of skin cancers and melanoma arising in the lower extremity and genitalia.

The superficial inguinal glands, in number of 22–24, are situated in a surface described by Daseler, near to the saphenous vein, in a superficial plane. They usually drain in the deep inguinal nodes and, sometimes, directly in external iliac nodes.

Five subgroups are identified:
- Central: Located near the saphenous-femoral crosse
- Superolateral: Located near the superficial circumflex vein

- Inferolateral: Located near the accessory saphenous vein
- Superomedial: Located near the superficial epigastric and pudendal vein
- Inferomedial: Located near the great saphenous vein

The deep inguinal glands, in number of 2 or 3, lie deeper to fascia lata of the leg, medially to the femoral vein. The commonest is the Cloquet gland, located between the femoral vein and Gimbernat's ligament.

Indications and Contraindications

Sentinel lymph node biopsy is currently approved for cutaneous melanoma and breast cancer; guidelines for nonmelanoma skin cancer are not available and the use of sentinel lymph node biopsy in these cases represents only a clinical suggestion.

Melanoma

Proper selection of patients for sentinel lymph node biopsy is an important aspect of the procedure. No survival benefit has been proven yet for sentinel lymph node biopsy for patients with clinically node-negative melanoma. In this scenario, sentinel node biopsy assumes a crucial value in the staging of the disease.

Indications

Appropriate candidates include patients with clinically node-negative melanomas thicker than or equal to 1 mm. While general agreement [12–14] exists that sentinel lymph node biopsy is indicated for patients with intermediate-thickness melanomas (1–4 mm thick), debate continues among surgical oncologists regarding the expansion of these indications to patients with thinner or thicker tumors. Many centers expand the inclusion of patients to tumors thicker than 0.75 mm. Patients with high-risk lesions [15, 16] (Clark level IV or V, ulceration, vertical growth phase, angiolymphatic invasion, or a high mitotic rate), even if thinner than 1 mm, should be included in the sentinel lymph node biopsy protocol.

Other patients who may benefit from sentinel lymph node biopsy include patients with tumors thicker than 4 mm [17]. In this group of patients, the procedure can permit to identify individuals with a better prognosis (negative sentinel lymph node biopsy results) or to achieve long-term locoregional control of disease (selective lymphadenectomy). Sentinel lymph node biopsy may also be proposed to patients with isolated local cutaneous recurrence in the absence of clinically evident regional nodal disease.

Contraindications

Patients with clinically palpable lymphadenopathy or suspected lymphadenopathy demonstrated on imaging studies (eventually confirmed by preoperative fine-needle aspiration) should undergo a therapeutic lymph node dissection and are not eligible to sentinel node biopsy. However, in such patients with primary melanomas of the trunk or head and neck, lymphoscintigraphy should be considered to identify other nodal basins at risk, and sentinel lymph node biopsy in these areas may be performed in conjunction with therapeutic lymphadenectomy of the clinically involved nodal basin.

Sentinel lymph node biopsy should be also excluded in case of primary wide local excision (margins equal or more than 2 cm) or when large skin flaps (rotation flaps) or skin grafts are used for closure after primary excision [18]. In these patients, the pattern of lymphatic drainage could theoretically be altered. The situation is similar in patients who have undergone prior surgery involving the regional nodal basin, such as open lymph node biopsy or skin grafting, or prior surgery that disrupts the native lymphatic drainage patterns between the primary site and the at-risk nodal basin. Elective lymph node dissection may be discussed with these patients; nevertheless, further investigation on this group of patients is mandatory.

The presence of satellitosis or in-transit metastasis at the time of initial presentation is a relative contraindication to sentinel lymph node biopsy (the validity of the procedure in this setting is unknown) [19].

Atypical or Borderline Spitz Tumors

Atypical Spitzoid lesions that are difficult to classify as clearly benign or malignant may represent undiagnosed malignant melanoma. Sentinel lymph node biopsy may be offered to patients with atypical or borderline lesions [20] (whose features may include size >1 cm, ulceration, deep dermal mitoses, extension into subcutaneous fat, and cytologic atypia).

Other Skin Cancers (Squamous Cell Carcinoma, Merkel Cell Carcinoma, Eccrine/Apocrine Carcinoma)

Application of the principles of sentinel lymph node biopsy to other cutaneous malignancies with a propensity for regional lymphatic spread has garnered tremendous interest. Unfortunately, no official guidelines can be followed in these cases (further multicenter studies are required), and the indication to sentinel node biopsy, proposed in the presence of high-risk factors for nodal dissemination, needs to be discussed with the single patients.

Sentinel lymph node biopsy has been used to treat high-risk *squamous cell carcinomas* of the skin or mucosa [21–25]. It may be considered for patients with head and neck or urogenital squamous cell carcinomas (lip SCCs; T1–T2, N0 oral and oropharyngeal SCCs; penile or vulvar SCCs) or in case of skin tumors extending into subcutaneous fat or invading deeper structures, for patients with tumors greater than 4–6 mm in depth, for patients with extensive peritumoral lymphatic invasion, for patients with Marjolin ulcer, and for some patients with locally recurrent carcinomas. Contraindications to SLN biopsy are a palpable lymph node, tumors larger than 4–5 cm, disruption of lymphatic drainage, prior extensive surgery, or previous radiation to nodal basins.

The technique has been reported most frequently for *neuroendocrine carcinoma of the skin* (Merkel cell carcinoma or trabecular carcinoma), which frequently is a rapidly progressive and often fatal cutaneous cancer [26].

While only approximately 30 % of patients with neuroendocrine carcinoma of the skin present with clinically apparent regional lymph node metastases, as many as 70 % of the remainder of patients experience relapse in the regional lymph nodes within 2 years of diagnosis if the regional lymph nodes are not treated. Half of the patients with regional failure develop systemic disease. Sentinel lymph node biopsy with selective lymph node dissection is suggested for clinical stage I Merkel cell carcinoma patients.

Other indications reported in the literature (eccrine and apocrine skin carcinomas, porocarcinoma, hidradenocarcinoma, and invasive extramammary Paget disease) have no scientific validity.

Noncutaneous Malignancies

Since its initial description for melanoma patients, the concept and technique of sentinel lymph node biopsy with or without selective lymph node dissection has been applied to a number of noncutaneous malignancies with varying degrees of efficacy. Most widely accepted is sentinel lymph node biopsy for early-stage breast cancer as an alternative to routine levels I and II axillary lymph node dissection.

Sentinel lymph node biopsy has also been applied to the treatment of colon cancer [27], small bowel tumors (e.g., carcinoid tumor), gastric cancer, pancreatic cancer, thyroid cancer, prostate cancer, pediatric soft tissue sarcoma, and clear cell sarcoma (melanoma of the soft parts).

Equipments and Techniques

Lymphoscintigraphy

SNB for clinically localized cutaneous and noncutaneous cancer should be preceded by preoperative lymphoscintigraphy to identify the regional drainage basins and the approximate site of SNs within that basin. Dynamic lymphoscintigraphy can distinguish SNs which receive direct drainage from the primary tumor site from second-echelon

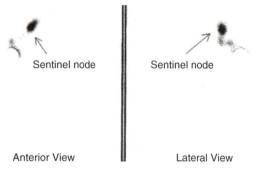

Sentinel node   Sentinel node

Anterior View   Lateral View

Fig. 32.1 Preoperative lymphoscintigraphy allows to identify nodal basins involved in the lymphatic spread of cancer. The *arrows* identify sentinel node in anterior and latenal views

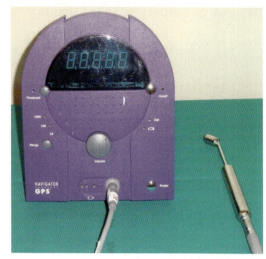

Fig. 32.2 The handheld gamma probe routinely used in our operative rooms

non-SNs, which may be near SNs but do not receive direct drainage from tumor site (Fig. 32.1).

Vital Blue Dye

Vital blue dyes complement lymphoscintigraphy by helping to visualize the SNs during dissection. Isosulfan blue (Lymphazurin) and patent blue V are both effective. Methylene blue has also been used because of its greater availability; however, it is less effective at highlighting lymphatic channels and has been associated with soft tissue necrosis. Vital blue dye is injected intradermally using a tuberculin syringe (27 G) around the primary lesion or biopsy scar. The volume of dye depends on the anatomic site: 1–2 ml for sites on the trunk, extremity, and scalp, but only 0.5–0.75 ml on the face because of wider diffusion, particularly around the eye. Injection into the subcutaneous tissue should be avoided because lymphatic density is lower and the dye may not migrate. Also, subcutaneous tissues have separate and distinct lymphatic channels and therefore may lead to incorrect SN identification. The time interval from injection of blue dye to surgical dissection depends on the distance from the primary lesion to the regional nodal basin that will be explored. Lymphatic flow is fastest for the distal limbs and slowest for the head-neck region. Typically within 5–15 min, the blue dye has entered the SN and washout from the node is evident after approximately 45 min [28].

A contraindication to blue dye injection is known as allergic reaction to blue dye; anaphylaxis is rare but has been reported. As mentioned above, pregnancy is a relative contraindication because the long-term toxicity to the fetus is unknown. Adverse side effects to blue dye include allergic reactions ("blue hives"), which are seen in up to 2 % of cases and may be influenced by blue dye volume. Other side effects are blue-colored urine for up to 24 h following administration and a factitious drop in intraoperative oxygen saturation measured by pulse oximetry.

Handheld Gamma Probe

The handheld gamma probe is a radiation detector that provides a count rate from gamma rays. It is an effective tool that facilitates the intraoperative identification of radioactive lymph nodes that may or may not be blue stained (Fig. 32.2). If SN biopsy is performed shortly after preoperative lymphoscintigraphy, the handheld gamma probe can be used to identify residual radiotracer in the SN. After a few hours, radioactivity decreases in the SN but can be measured in second-tier nodes. Because the radioisotope has a half-life of approximately 5–6 h, SN biopsy can also be performed the day after lymphoscintigraphy. In this case, radioactive counts will be lower

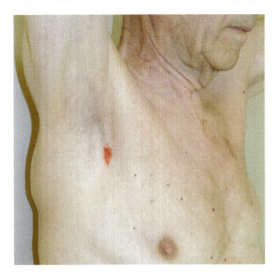

Fig. 32.3 The marked skin site (right axillary sentinel node biopsy) needs to be confirmed in the chosen operative position before skin incision

and the SN sometimes may be more difficult to identify.

Before the skin is incised, the gamma probe should be moved systematically over the lymphatic basin to confirm the accuracy of the marked skin site (Fig. 32.3); if the patient's position during surgery differs from that during lymphoscintigraphy, then the skin marks may no longer approximate the location of the SN. Because the preoperative lymphoscintigraphic image given to the surgeon represents only a snapshot of a dynamic process, potential drainage basins (including ectopic locations such as the intermuscular triangle of the back) should be checked with the probe to confirm the absence of radioactivity.

The general function of the probe can be crudely checked by pointing the probe at the injection site to test for a response. The nuclear medicine report and the skin mark act as reference point for the SN search. First, set initial count range to the lowest setting and volume to a clearly audible setting. Correct range is important because an insufficient pitch variation can prevent identification of some radioactive nodes. Record the count activity at the injection site and the background count activity around the basin. Start at the position in the basin closest to the injection site, place the probe perpendicular to

the skin surface, and scan in a back and forth pattern moving away from the injection site. When count activity increases, localize the hot spot by scanning perpendicular to the initial scan line. The speed of scanning should be approximately 1–5 cm/s [29].

The distance between the injection site and the drainage basin can affect hot spot identification: the closer the injection site is to the drainage basin, the more likely that background counts will be constant because radioactivity "shines through" from the primary injection site. If the injection site is within the probe's field, counts will be falsely elevated. As a practical rule, we suggest to always perform radicalization of the primary site, with excision margins indicated by official guidelines, prior to identifying the SN.

Surgical Technique

After lymphoscintigraphy, the patient is transported to the operative room; anesthesia is induced at the discretion of the anesthesiologist in consultation with the surgeon. Many surgeons still prefer adjunctive intradermal injection of blue dye (approximately 1 ml) at the site of the lesion. A handheld gamma probe is used to identify "hot spots," which will indicate areas where SLNs are and to place the skin incision.

The key principle of the procedure is to remove all SNs avoiding unnecessary tissue trauma, with minimal dissection (which is facilitated either by the blue dye trace or by the count rate of the gamma probe). The probe is in fact usually placed on the tissue and pointed in different directions to ensure the radioactivity pathway. Meticulous, gentle dissection should avoid transecting the lymphatics, because disruption of these vessels leads to contamination of radiotracer and dye and to an increased risk of seroma. Electrocautery is used to dissect through the subcutaneous tissue and fascia. Blunt dissection towards the hot node is preferred using a tonsil clamp. Afferent and efferent lymphatic and blood vessels are ligated with clips and/or suture. Care is taken to neither crush nor cauterize the specimen.

After a node is dissected free, the radioactivity of this node is checked by placing it on a surface away from the patient to avoid interference. The operative site is finally tested for remaining activity. The decision to remove eventual further nodes will depend on the persistence of radioactivity in the operative field. Lymphatic vessels and lymph nodes may be replaced by tumor and fail to take up mapping agents; therefore, the operative site should be inspected and palpated for clinically suspicious lymph nodes. All such lymph nodes should be removed.

Lymphatic mapping in the groin and axilla is associated with high rates of SN identification and low rates of false-negative SNs (1 % for the groin and 5 % for the axilla). There is no consensus on whether to excise external iliac or obturator SNs identified by lymphoscintigraphy; we recommend removing them through a retroperitoneal approach if the lymphoscintigram demonstrates direct drainage to these nodes from the primary site on the skin.

Lymphatic mapping in the head and neck region requires much more experience for comparable success, because this area has a dense and complex pattern of communicating lymphatic channels, often with multiple SNs. Though the lymphoscintigram may indicate only one hot node, there may actually be multiple hot nodes in a cluster that appear as one due to the limited resolution of the gamma camera. Reported false-negative rates for the head-neck region have been as high as 15 %. For these reasons, we agree with many authors that the head-neck region is the most difficult site to map.

Failure rate to identify a sentinel lymph node is <5 %. If no SN can be found, a complete lymph node dissection should be considered for high-risk primary lesions.

Frozen Section

Sentinel nodes are fixed in 10 % neutral, buffered formalin, and, after fixation, they are bisected through the hilum (if identifiable) or through the long axis of the node. If the halves are thicker than 2 mm, the slices are further trimmed to provide additional blocks of 2 mm. If sentinel nodes are found to be free from tumor after the initial histologic examination, step-serial sections are prepared at an additional six levels in the block at intervals of approximately 150 μm.

For permanent sectioning, it's possible to perform hematoxylin and eosin (H&E) staining followed by staining with immunohistochemical (IHC) markers S-100, MART-1, and HMB-45. In addition to IHC evaluation, National Comprehensive Cancer Network (NCCN) guidelines also recommend that multiple sectioning of each node be performed to pick up potential micrometastatic deposits. Consideration can also be given in performing polymerase chain reaction (PCR) evaluation of the SLN.

Postoperative Care

In general, patients undergoing sentinel lymph node biopsy are discharged the same day of the procedure or on postoperative day 1, depending on the treatment of the primary neoplasm and the reconstructive strategy chosen. Drainage in axillary or inguinal cavity after lymph node sentinel biopsy is not mandatory. Sutures are usually removed within 2 weeks postoperative. Extremity elevation and elastic compressive bandage wraps help to prevent lymphedema. These patients are usually advised to wear compression stockings 4–6 weeks postoperatively.

Expected Side Effects and Complications

Although sentinel lymph node dissection with selective lymphadenectomy is less morbid than elective lymph node dissection, as with any invasive procedure, complications do occur. In the Sunbelt Melanoma Trial [30], the overall complication rate was less than 5 % for sentinel lymph node biopsy. The mortality rate was 0 %.

Complications occur more frequently in patients with cardiac disease, obesity, diabetes mellitus, and cigarette smoking. The complication rate has also been reported to increase with the number of sentinel nodes removed.

Immediate and Short-Term Expected Side Effects

Immediate complications of the procedure include anaphylaxis or other allergic reactions to the intradermal injection of blue dye (<1 %) and bleeding. Short-term postoperative complications of the procedure include hematoma, wound infection, seroma, and flap necrosis. Seroma and wound infection are the most common but the incidence rate is under 2 %.

Long-Term Expected Side Effects

Long-term postoperative sequelae may include persistent blue discoloration of the skin at the injection site, lymphatic fistulae, lymphocele, lymphedema (generally <2 %), and neurologic complications, including transient or persistent neurapraxia, cutaneous anesthesia, paresthesias, and neuropathy. Sentinel lymph node biopsy does not increase the risk of in-transit metastases. The risk of locoregional recurrence after lymph node sentinel dissection, with follow-up ranging from 13 to 60 months, is 1–6 %, while the locoregional relapse rate ranges from 5 to 10 % [31].

Potential technical reasons for failure include errors in surgical technique; failure of nuclear medicine mapping; alterations in lymphatic drainage due to inflammation, infection, or previous surgery; and errors in the pathologic examination of a correctly identified true sentinel node. Most (30–60 %) clinical relapses in sentinel node-negative patients are distant metastasis without any evidence of local, in-transit, or regional disease.

Future Considerations

New agents for lymphatic mapping are currently being developed. One agent with exciting potential is ^{99m}Tc-diethylenetriamine pentaacetic acid (DPTA)-mannosyl-dextran, a radiocolloid that binds mannose receptors on antigen-presenting cells of lymph nodes. Studies have shown that this agent has rapid clearance from the primary injection site and accumulates in the SN for at least 24 h [32]. Other interesting studies [33] have recently introduced in the clinical practice the use of indocyanine green fluorescence for lymphatic mapping and sentinel node biopsy in breast cancer: the advantage of the technique is represented by transcutaneous visualization of lymphatic vessels and intraoperative lymph node detection without the use of the radioisotope.

Despite advances in pathologic assessment of the SN, nodal micrometastasis may be missed if the wrong section of the node is examined or if the node is non-sentinel. A carbon dye mapping has been developed, as a way to permanently label a node as the SN and to help the pathologist identify the intranodal site of lymphatic drainage. Carbon particles (sterile India ink) are mixed with the blue dye prior to injection. The SN uptakes the blue dye and carbon particles; these carbon particles are seen in the SN and correlate with the intranodal location of tumor cells. As a result, the location of carbon particles in the SN may assist the pathologist in identifying metastasis. Currently there are no commercial preparations available and use of carbon particles is restricted to research studies [34].

Glossary

Handheld gamma probe Radiation detector that provides a count rate from gamma rays and facilitates the intraoperative identification of radioactive lymph nodes.

Lymphoscintigraphy Preoperative exam that allows to identify, by injecting a radioactive tracer in the site of primary neoplasm, nodal basins involved in the metastatic process.

Sentinel lymph node biopsy Surgical identification of the first node involved in lymphatic spread of cancer through a small incision and a limited extent dissection.

Vital blue dye Injection of a colored tracer in the site of primary neoplasm that complements lymphoscintigraphy and helps visualize the sentinel node during dissection.

References

1. Snow H. Twenty two years' experience in the treatment of cancerous and other tumours. London: Bailliere, Tindall and Cox; 1898.
2. Seaman WB, Powers WE. Studies on the distribution of radioactive colloidal gold in regional lymph nodes containing cancer. Cancer. 1955;8(5):1044–6.
3. Gould EA, Winship T, Philbin PH, Kerr HH. Observations on a "sentinel node" in cancer of the parotid. Cancer. 1960;13:77–8.
4. Cabanas RM. An approach for the treatment of penile carcinoma. Cancer. 1977;39(2):456–66.
5. Morton DL, Wen DR, Wong JH, Economou JS, Cagle LA, Storm FK, et al. Technical details of intraoperative lymphatic mapping for early stage melanoma. Arch Surg. 1992;127(4):392–9.
6. Alex JC, Weaver DL, Fairbank JT, Rankin BS, Krag DN. Gamma-probe-guided lymph node localization in malignant melanoma. Surg Oncol. 1993;2(5):303–8.
7. Lewis WH. Gray's Anatomy of the human body. 20th ed. Philadelphia: Lea & Febiger; 1918.
8. Robbins TK, Clayman G, Levine PA, et al. Neck dissection classification update: revisions proposed by the American Head and Neck Society and the American Academy of Otolaryngology-Head and Neck Surgery. Arch Otolaryngol Head Neck Surg. 2002;128(7):751–8.
9. Townsend CM. Jr, Daniel Beauchamp R, Mark Evers B, Mattox KL. Sabiston textbook of surgery: the biological basis of modern surgical practice. Elsevier, 13th Edition, 2012.
10. Thompson JF, Hunt JA, Culjak G, Uren RF, Howman-Giles R, Harman CR. Popliteal lymph node metastasis from primary cutaneous melanoma. Eur J Surg Oncol. 2000;26:172–6.
11. Lengelé B, Scalliet P. Anatomical bases for the radiological delineation of lymph node areas. Part III: pelvis and lower limbs. Radiother Oncol. 2009;92(1):22–33.
12. Essner R, Conforti A, Kelley MC, et al. Efficacy of lymphatic mapping, sentinel lymphadenectomy, and selective complete lymph node dissection as a therapeutic procedure for early-stage melanoma. Ann Surg Oncol. 1999;6(5):442–9.
13. Gershenwald JE, Thompson W, Mansfield PF, et al. Multi-institutional melanoma lymphatic mapping experience: the prognostic value of sentinel lymph node status in 612 stage I or II melanoma patients. J Clin Oncol. 1999;17(3):976–83.
14. Cascinelli N, Belli F, Santinami M, et al. Sentinel lymph node biopsy in cutaneous melanoma: the WHO Melanoma Program experience. Ann Surg Oncol. 2000;7(6):469–74.
15. Jacobs IA, Chang CK, DasGupta TK, Salti GI. Role of sentinel lymph node biopsy in patients with thin (< 1 mm) primary melanoma. Ann Surg Oncol. 2003;10(5):558–61.
16. Puleo CA, Messina JL, Riker AI, et al. Sentinel node biopsy for thin melanomas: which patients should be considered? Cancer Control. 2005;12(4):230–5.
17. Gershenwald JE, Mansfield PF, Lee JE, Ross MI. Role for lymphatic mapping and sentinel lymph node biopsy in patients with thick (> or = 4 mm) primary melanoma. Ann Surg Oncol. 2000;7(2):160–5.
18. Gannon CJ, Rousseau Jr DL, Ross MI, Johnson MM, Lee JE, Mansfield PF. Accuracy of lymphatic mapping and sentinel lymph node biopsy after previous wide local excision in patients with primary melanoma. Cancer. 2006;107(11):2647–52.
19. Yao KA, Hsueh EC, Essner R, Foshag LJ, Wanek LA, Morton DL. Is sentinel lymph node mapping indicated for isolated local and in-transit recurrent melanoma? Ann Surg. 2003;238(5):743–7.
20. Su LD, Fullen DR, Sondak VK, Johnson TM, Lowe L. Sentinel lymph node biopsy for patients with problematic Spitzoid melanocytic lesions: a report on 18 patients. Cancer. 2003;97(2):499–507.
21. Broglie MA, Haile SR, Stoeckli SJ. Long-term experience in sentinel node biopsy for early oral and oropharyngeal squamous cell carcinoma. Ann Surg Oncol. 2011;18(10):2732–8. Epub 2011 May 19.
22. Sloan P. Head and neck sentinel lymph node biopsy: current state of the art. Head Neck Pathol. 2009;3(3):231–7. Epub 2009 Aug 21. Review.
23. Neto AS, Tobias-Machado M, Ficarra V, Wroclawski ML, Amarante RD, Pompeo AC, et al. Dynamic sentinel node biopsy for inguinal lymph node staging in patients with penile cancer: a systematic review and cumulative analysis of the literature. Ann Surg Oncol. 2011;18(7):2026–34.
24. Kwon S, Dong ZM, Wu PC. Sentinel lymph node biopsy for high-risk cutaneous squamous cell carcinoma: clinical experience and review of literature. World J Surg Oncol. 2011;9:80.
25. Crosbie EJ, Winter-Roach B, Sengupta P, Sikand KA, Carrington B, Murby B, et al. The accuracy of the sentinel node procedure after excision biopsy in squamous cell carcinoma of the vulva. Surg Oncol. 2010;19(4):e150–4.
26. Mehrany K, Otley CC, Weenig RH, Phillips PK, Roenigk RK, Nguyen TH. A meta-analysis of the prognostic significance of sentinel lymph node status in Merkel cell carcinoma. Dermatol Surg. 2002;28(2):113–7.
27. De Jong JS, Beukema JC, van Dam GM, Slart R, Lemstra C, Wiggers T. Limited value of staging squamous cell carcinoma of the anal margin and canal using the sentinel lymph node procedure: a prospective study with long-term follow-up. Ann Surg Oncol. 2010;17(10):2656–62.
28. Amersi F, Morton DL. The role of sentinel lymph node biopsy in the management of melanoma. Adv Surg. 2007;41:241–56.
29. Bagaria SP, Faries MB, Morton DL. Sentinel node biopsy in melanoma: technical considerations of the procedure as performed at the John Wayne Cancer Institute. J Surg Oncol. 2010;101(8):669–76.

30. McMasters KM, Noyes RD, Reintgen DS, Goydos JS, Beitsch PD, Davidson BS, et al. Lessons learned from the Sunbelt Melanoma Trial. J Surg Oncol. 2004; 86(4):212–23.

31. Morton DL, Cochran AJ, Thompson JF, Elashoff R, Essner R, Glass EC, et al. Sentinel node biopsy for early-stage melanoma: accuracy and morbidity in MSLT-I, an international multicenter trial. Ann Surg. 2005;242(3):302–11; discussion 311–3.

32. Leung K. 99mTc-Diethylenetriamine pentaacetic acid superparamagnetic iron oxide nanoparticles conjugated with lactobionic acid. Molecular Imaging and Contrast Agent Database (MICAD) [INTERNET].

Bethesda, MD: National Cemer for biotechnology information US; 2004–2013. 2010 Apr 28.

33. Hirche C, Lehnhardt M, Hunerbein M. Real-time lymphography and sentinel lymph node biopsy for breast cancer guided by indocyanine green fluorescence: clinical experience. In: Acta of twenty second Euraps annual meeting, Mykonos, 2–4 June 2011.

34. Pramanik M, Song KH, Swierczewska M, Green D, Sitharaman B, Wang LV. In vivo carbon nanotube-enhanced non-invasive photoacoustic mapping of the sentinel lymph node. Phys Med Biol. 2009;54(11): 3291–301.

Sunlight-Induced Skin Cancer in Companion Animals

33

Paulo Vilar-Saavedra and Barbara E. Kitchell

Key Points

- Animals with pale skin and thin hair coats are at increased risk of suffering solar injury.
- The two most prevalent neoplastic lesions induced by ultraviolet irradiation are cutaneous squamous cell carcinomas (cSCC), in dogs and cats, and cutaneous hemangiosarcoma (cHSA), primarily seen in dogs.
- Squamous cell carcinomas account for 1.25–15 % of all cutaneous tumors in dogs and for approximately 15–50 % of all cutaneous tumors in cats.
- The classic multistep colorectal carcinogenesis model is useful for understanding the progression of sunlight-induced skin lesions from the premalignant actinic keratosis (AK) stage to fully manifested cSCC.
- Alterations in the *p53* gene product comprise the most common genetic abnormalities found in actinic keratosis (AK), in situ SCC (ISSCC) and cSCC. In addition, immunocompromised status and viral pathogenesis may play a contributory role in cSCC development.
- Prognostic factors for cSCC in veterinary medicine related to recurrence and metastasis are unknown. Cutaneous SCC lesions in dogs and cats are considered to be slow to metastasize. In humans, prognostic factors include size and location of the primary tumor, tumor differentiation, and histologic features such as involvement of the reticular dermis or underlying tissues.
- Most veterinary patients with primary sunlight-induced cSCC have a good-to-excellent prognosis when lesions are detected and addressed early in the course of disease.
- Squamous cell carcinoma lesions occurring on sun-exposed skin have better prognosis than those occurring in unexposed skin.
- Local modalities of treatment include complete surgical excision as the most cost-effective and successful means of local control for cSCC.
- Molecular understanding of the pathogenesis of HSA is primarily focused on visceral disease and seems to be consistent with the biology of human angiosarcoma lesions.

P. Vilar-Saavedra, DVM, MS
Center for Comparative Oncology, D 208,
Veterinary Medicine Center, Michigan State University,
East Lansing, MI 48824, USA

B.E. Kitchell, DVM, PhD, DACVIM (✉)
Department of Small Animal Clinical Sciences, Center
for Comparative Oncology, D 208, Veterinary Medicine
Center, Michigan State University,
East Lansing, MI 48824, USA
e-mail: kitchell@cvm.msu.edu

A. Baldi et al. (eds.), *Skin Cancer*, Current Clinical Pathology,
DOI 10.1007/978-1-4614-7357-2_33, © Springer Science+Business Media New York 2014

- Heterozygosity of chromosome 22, chromosomal deletions of the tumor suppressor gene PTEN, and amplifications or rearrangements of various genes are genomic abnormalities frequently found in cHSA in humans.
- Cutaneous HSA is commonly observed in predisposed breeds such as American Staffordshire terriers, pit bulls, beagles, Dalmatians, Italian greyhounds, whippets, and bull terriers.
- Identified prognostic factors included breed, tumor location, and the presence of solar actinic changes.
- Locoregional recurrence is very common in predisposed thin-coated breeds with the solar-induced form of this disease.
- Metastasis was documented or suspected in 34 % of dogs with cHSA and occurred at a median of 326 days from diagnosis. Progression to the visceral form of HSA was observed in 62 % of dogs with metastatic disease.
- Overall, the median survival for dogs treated by surgical excision with no adjuvant chemotherapy was reported to range from 780 to 987 days, with 1-, 2-, and 3-year survival rates of 79, 60, and 44, respectively. Median survival was 1,095 days in surgically treated cats with cHSA.
- Cutaneous HSA lesions are most often treated with curative-intent surgical excision.
- Biopsy margin status documenting complete surgical excision, absence of metastasis, and no subcutaneous invasion were surprisingly unassociated with incidence of local recurrence.
- The dearth of prospective studies defining the clinical behavior of cHSA results in uncertainty and controversy regarding the role of complete surgical excision of the lesion as a predictor of clinical outcome in dogs and cats.

- Use of chemotherapy in management of dogs and cats affected by cHSA is largely recommended only if there is evidence of invasion of the subcutaneous tissue or of distant metastasis.
- Doxorubicin-based protocols provide several more months of survival time for these cats, when compared to no therapy.
- Metronomic therapy may be feasible as a first-line therapy option for patients with cHSA that cannot undergo surgery protocols.

Background and Pathogenesis of Dermal Injury by UV Light

As the skin is the largest organ in the body, it is perhaps unsurprising that skin tumors represent one third of the tumors diagnosed in dogs [1]. The incidence rate of skin tumors has been increasing throughout the past decades (1960–2000), representing 1.9–3.6 % of tumors diagnosed in dogs examined at veterinary teaching hospitals in North America, as compiled by the Veterinary Medical Database [2].

Companion animals are largely protected from the carcinogenic effects of ultraviolet light by having adequate pelage and dermal pigmentation. However, animals with pale skin and thin hair coats are at increased risk of suffering solar injury. The two most prevalent neoplastic lesions induced by ultraviolet irradiation are cutaneous squamous cell carcinomas (cSCC), in dogs and cats, and cutaneous hemangiosarcoma (cHSA), primarily seen in dogs.

Squamous cell carcinoma arises from epidermal stem cells that have the potential for self-renewal and multi-lineage differentiation. These stem precursors are located in the hair follicle bulge and the basal layer of the interfollicular epidermis. There is also evidence that bone marrow-derived cells may home to the bulge region of the epidermis in response to skin wounding and there differentiate into keratinocyte stem cells [3]. The classic multistep colorectal carcinogenesis model described by Fearon and Vogelstein et al., in 1990, is useful for understanding the progression of sunlight-induced skin lesions from the premalignant actinic keratosis (AK) stage to fully manifested cSCC [4].

The spectrum of electromagnetic solar radiation interfacing the Earth's atmosphere is comprised of five regions based upon light wavelengths. Light in the ultraviolet spectrum (UV-A, UV-B, and UV-C) is in an invisible wavelength form that comprises 3 of the 5 spectra. The UV spectrum of radiation is of medical interest because these wavelengths have both carcinogenic and germicidal properties [5]. In fact, the high incidence of cSCC is caused by the mutagenic effects of ultraviolet light (UV) which is intensified by geographic latitude [6, 7]. The mechanism leading to genomic instability in keratinocytes likely results from ultraviolet-β (UV-B)-induced inactivation of the p53 gene product, which acts as a tumor suppressor gene in skin cancer. In humans, it is estimated that approximately 58 % of cSCCs harbor UV-B signature mutations such as CC:GG to TT:AA and C:G to T:A transitions [8]. The precise mutational events in cutaneous carcinogenesis in dogs and cats are less well established, although missense mutations in highly conserved regions of the p53 gene have been reported in the veterinary literature [9, 10]. Alterations in the *p53* gene product comprise the most common genetic abnormalities found in actinic keratosis (AK), in situ SCC (ISSCC) and cSCC, demonstrating that dysplastic lesions have acquired an initiating genetic mutation prior to becoming cSCC. This is evidenced by the fact that p53 dysfunction generally occurs prior to tumor invasion [11]. Additionally, aberrant activation of epidermal growth factor receptor (EGFR) and Fyn, a Src-family tyrosine kinase, is seen in human cSCCs. These kinases downregulate p53 mRNA and protein levels, revealing another mechanism for controlling p53 function [12].

Loss of heterozygosity has also been observed in human cSCCs at chromosome 9p21. This region contains several tumor suppressor genes, including p16INK4A (CDKN2A), p15INK4B,

and MTAP. These genes are hypothesized to be associated with progression from AKs to cSCCs [13, 14].

Activating mutations of the Ras oncogene have been found in cSCCs and AKs [15]. Ras family members are proto-oncogenes that transduce cellular growth and proliferation signals downstream of cell-membrane-bound receptor tyrosine kinases (RTKs). Ras can be activated by gene amplification, activating mutations, or overexpression of upstream RTKs [16].

Epigenetic effects refer to the molecular mechanisms that regulate gene expression in the absence of changes in the DNA sequence itself. Epigenetic alterations include DNA promoter methylation and histone protein modifications, which consist among others of methylation, acetylation, or phosphorylation of histone cores [17]. Epigenetic dysregulation is thought to be involved in tumor biology and cancer progression. In fact, a higher level of expression of FOXE1, a promoter of hypermethylation, was found in cSCC compared to normal skin, indicating that FOXE1 may be a direct target for the aberrant methylation noted in cSCC lesions [18]. In a similar manner, it has been shown that a distinct microRNA profile is modulated by UV radiation [19].

Cutaneous HSA has been also associated with ultraviolet light exposure in dogs [20, 21]. Molecular understanding of the pathogenesis of cHSA is primarily focused on visceral disease and seems to be consistent with the biology of human angiosarcoma lesions. In human dermatology, cHSA lesions are predominantly seen in older men who work in outdoor occupations that result in excessive sunlight exposure to the scalp, face, and ears [22]. Tumor-derived HSA cell lines express hematopoietic stem cell markers, suggesting that they arise from bone marrow-derived pluripotent stem cells [23, 24]. Genomic abnormalities have been noted in cHSA lesions in people. These include large chromosomal abnormalities such as loss of heterozygosity of chromosome 22, chromosomal deletions such as at the C-terminal domain of the tumor suppressor gene PTEN, and amplifications or rearrangements of various genes. However, the importance of these mutations or gene amplifications for tumorigenesis in canine and feline cHSA is still unknown [25].

Loss of vascular endothelial cadherin (VE-cadherin) may be involved in cancer gene regulation, facilitating angiogenesis, tumor cell invasion, and metastasis [26]. Mutations of tumor suppressor gene p53, Kras, VEGFR2, and VEGFR3 have been associated with angiosarcoma pathogenesis in humans [27–29]. A progression from cutaneous hemangioma to cHSA may occur, reflecting phenotypic development of more malignant tumor as a result of repeated genetic damage. Subcutaneous hemangiomas do not seem to have this progression [20].

Viral pathogenesis may play a contributory role in cSCC development. Viruses associated with SCC lesions include papillomavirus (PV) and retroviruses such as FIV which cause immunosuppression in cats. Papillomavirus is commonly present in normal skin, and it is possible that this virus is an innocent bystander. Papillomavirus DNA has been detected within cutaneous in situ SCCs of cats and dogs, but evidence that PVs increase the development and progression of these lesions is less conclusive in animals [30–32]. However, the frequent and rapid progression of endophytic papillomas to in situ SCCs observed in severe combined immunodeficiency (SCID) dogs suggests that CfPV-2 infection can cause neoplastic transformation [33, 34]. Three theories have been suggested for the mechanism of human PV (HPV) carcinogenesis. First, UV radiation-induced immunosuppression may explain enhanced interaction between HPV and UV radiation [35]. Second, viral expression of E6 and E7 oncoproteins can inactivate p53 and Rb tumor suppressor genes, leading to an unregulated system of cell proliferation and apoptosis [36]. Finally, integration of HPV DNA may disrupt genomic stability [37].

An immunocompromised status is associated with marked escalation of cSCC, with up to 64–250 times greater incidence noted than that seen in the general human population. Immunosuppression significantly impacts the biology of cSCC. In solid organ transplant patients, cSCC tumors, mostly associated with papillomaviruses, tend to be numerous, exhibit a strong propensity to recur, and metastasize at a high rate regardless of lesion size [38].

Feline immunodeficiency virus (FIV) causes immune dysfunction, and it is also associated with an increased incidence of cancers [39–41]. Reported incidence of FIV-associated tumors, predominantly lymphomas, ranges from 1 to 21 % of FIV-positive cats. Infection with this chronic retrovirus has also been described in cats with cutaneous tumors [42].

The general epidemiologic information referenced here reflects the geographic diversity of the reported studies cited (Australia, Greece, the United Kingdom, the United States of America, and Zimbabwe). Also, the diagnostic methodology employed in these studies was varied. Therefore, epidemiologic information must always be interpreted cautiously rather than as broadly applicable discrete facts.

Squamous Cell Carcinoma of the Skin

Incidence and Risk Factors

Squamous cell carcinomas account for 1.25–15 % of all cutaneous tumors in dogs. Squamous cell carcinomas reportedly range between the second and the sixteenth most common canine skin tumor type, depending on the referenced study [2, 43]. In cats, SCC accounts for approximately 15–50 % of all cutaneous tumors, making this among the four most common feline skin tumors, along with basal cell tumors, mast cell tumors, and fibrosarcomas [44, 45]. Common locations for SCC in dogs are the oral cavity, nasal planum, and nail bed (Fig. 33.1). This is as opposed to locations associated with ultraviolet sunlight exposure, such as on the flank, medial thighs, or abdomen in the skin of short-coated, lightly pigmented dogs [46, 47]. The most common location of cSCC in cats is the head, where 57–65 % may be observed on the ear pinna. Other common sites of feline cSCC include the nasal planum, eyelids, preauricular area, and lips (Fig. 33.2) [44, 45]. Cutaneous SCC commonly affects older dogs and cats, with a mean of 8 and 12 years of age, respectively, and there appears to be no gender predilection [47]. Overall, cSCC is most common in

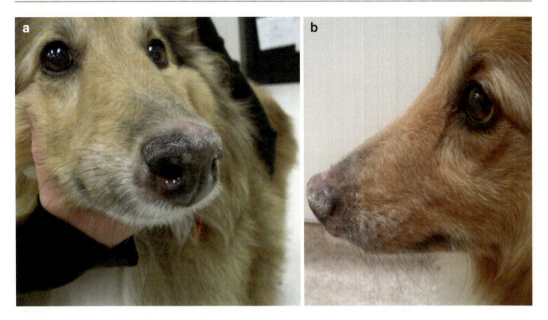

Fig. 33.1 Frontal (**a**) and lateral (**b**) view in a dog with diffuse and infiltrative SCC of the nasal planum. Please note marked depigmentation and asymmetry associated with the lesions

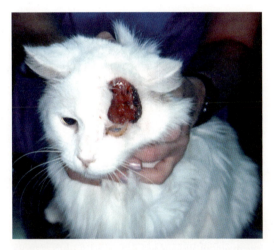

Fig. 33.2 White-coated cat with advanced, aggressive cutaneous SCC lesion and progressing to the periorbital area

Biologic Behavior

Canine SCC of the oral cavity has site-associated metastatic behavior, with tumors of the rostral aspect of the mouth less prone to metastasis than those of the caudal tongue, oropharynx, and tonsil [49]. However, this site-associated metastatic behavior has not been reported for cSCC. Prognostic factors for cSCC in veterinary medicine related to recurrence and metastasis are unknown. In humans, the most important factors affecting risk of recurrence and metastasis are the size and location of the primary tumor. Large lesions, considered to be those greater than 2 cm in diameter, recur at a rate of 15 %, which is twice that of smaller lesions. These larger lesions also metastasize at a rate of 30 %, three times that of smaller lesions [50]. Squamous cell carcinomas of the human lip and ear are also aggressive lesions, with rates of recurrence and metastasis ranging from 10 to 25 % [50, 51]. Other sites associated with a high risk of recurrence and metastasis in humans are eyelid, nose, and mucous membranes [52, 53]. Locally recurrent squamous cell carcinomas metastasize at rates that range from 25 % for most cutaneous lesions to 30–45 % for ear and lip tumors [50, 52]. Squamous cell carcinomas arising in injured,

animals without pigmentation in areas of sparse hair coat, and there is a reported 5–13 times higher incidence in white-coated than in pigmented cats [47, 48]. Similarly, cSCC are overrepresented in Dalmatian dogs (6.94 odds ratio compared to dogs with no cutaneous neoplasias) and Basset hounds (3.97 odds ratio vs. dogs with no cutaneous neoplasias). Not surprisingly, cSCC lesions are underrepresented in colorpoint breeds, such as Siamese cats [2, 45].

chronically diseased or chronically inflamed skin can also demonstrate more aggressive clinical behavior and a greater propensity to metastasize, with an overall metastatic rate of 40 % [50, 54]. Clinical features associated with recurrence and metastases include rapid growth and local recurrence of the tumor as well as immunosuppression [52]. Histologic features that are predictive of recurrence or metastasis include a depth of more than 4 mm, involvement of the reticular dermis or underlying tissues. Poorly differentiated cSCC in humans recurred at a rate of 28.6 %; in contrast, well-differentiated tumors had a local recurrence rate of 13.6 % [50].

However, despite the fact that the majority of these tumors present at early stages, cSCC accounts for the majority of non-melanotic skin cancer deaths and 20 % of all skin-cancer-related deaths in humans [50, 55]. For those with metastatic disease, however, the long-term prognosis is extremely poor [56]. In humans, if metastasis does occur, regional lymph nodes are involved in approximately 85 % of cases; approximately 15 % of cases involve distant sites, including the lungs, liver, brain, skin, and bone [56, 57].

Most veterinary patients with primary sunlight-induced cSCC have a good-to-excellent prognosis when lesions are detected and addressed early in the course of disease. Lesions occurring on sun-exposed skin have better prognosis than those occurring in unexposed skin. In North America, dogs and cats affected by sunlight-induced cSCC are often kept outdoors, and lesions may not be detected in early stages. Also, owners may be less willing or financially unable to seek veterinary care for their outdoor pets, when the lesions are most manageable. Fortunately, cSCC lesions in dogs and cats are slow to metastasize. Small and superficial lesions may never progress, whereas more deeply invasive lesions can become metastatic by the lymphatic route primarily. Ultimate visceral metastasis can be seen in end-stage cases [47].

Diagnosis

Cytology may allow differentiation of neoplastic from inflammatory lesions and of epithelial from spindle cell tumors. Cytologic diagnosis of ulcerative lesions may be problematic, as inflammation can induce secondary proliferative changes in epithelial cells even in benign lesions. Moreover, ulcerative lesions may be associated with lymphadenopathy, which may be reactive or may represent metastasis to regional nodes in cases with cSCC. Cytologic examination of enlarged regional lymph nodes should be performed before definitive therapy. Histologic examination of the tumor is important for further treatment planning and identifies possible prognostic factors associated with the suspected malignancy such as grade or level of cellular differentiation. In addition, histopathology allows determination of invasion and whether surgical excision was adequate. Cutaneous lesions are rarely metastatic to visceral organs; however, systemic staging for pulmonary metastasis is indicated for patients with advanced local disease or nodal metastasis. Advance local staging with CT scanning may be helpful for surgical and radiation therapy planning [47].

Treatment

Cutaneous SCC lesions may be locally aggressive but are slow to metastasize. Thus, adequate local control may be curative for these tumors, particularly when they are addressed early in the clinical course of disease. Local modalities of treatment include complete surgical excision as the most cost-effective and successful means of local control. Complete excision with 1–3 cm surgical margins may be curative for most lesions. This might necessitate ear pinna amputation in cats, or nasal planum resection, which owners may consider unacceptably disfiguring. For lesions not amenable to resection due to size or location, radiation therapy, cryosurgery, electrochemotherapy, photodynamic therapy, or intralesional chemotherapy may be helpful.

Cryosurgery

Cryosurgery is a minimally invasive procedure that destroys malignant tissue through inducing cell death by formation of intracellular and extracellular ice crystals. Liquid nitrogen, argon, and dimethyl ether-propane are frequently used as cryotherapy agents. The agent is directly applied to the skin or introduced by cryoneedles for delivery. Most canine and feline cSCC treated with cryosurgery achieve good-to-excellent overall remission rates (80 %), although many required multiple treatments and development of recurrence is observed in up to 73 % of cases. Recurrence of the malignancy is mostly associated with degree of infiltration (deep vs. superficial) and volume size (>0.5 cm in diameter) of the mass [48, 58, 59].

Most of the adverse effects associated with this low-cost therapy, including erythema, bleeding, blisters, and minimal pain, are localized and well tolerated by the patient.

Electrochemotherapy

Electrochemotherapy is a form of localized treatment for tumors that involves administration of a chemotherapeutic agent combined with delivery of appropriate energy waveforms. The ultimate goal of those waveforms is to induce an increased uptake of the drug by cancer cells. One published manuscript for treatment of cSCC describes the local administration of bleomycin ($1-1.5$ mg/cm^3 of lesion) followed in 5 min by permeabilizing biphasic electric pulses. Eight pulses of $50+50$ μ (microns) at 1,300 V/cm^3 are delivered by a pair of electrodes. Total treatment consists of two sessions of electrochemotherapy 1 week apart. Toxicity reported was described as mild erythema localized to tumor lesion and was transient and well tolerated by cats. Almost 80 % (7/9 cases) of the patients had a complete response (CR), and 55 % (5/9) had durable control lasting more than 1 year [60, 61].

Intralesional Chemotherapy

This treatment modality involves the direct intratumoral delivery of chemotherapeutic agents. Site-directed administration of the drug is intended to achieve local control of malignancy by providing a higher tumor-to-plasma ratio of the drug over a prolonged period of time. An additional advantage of this therapy is reduced to absent systemic adverse effects.

Cisplatin (1 mg/cm^3 of tissue target in oily emulsion) and bleomycin (1 mg/cm^3 of tissue)

four times a week on a 2-week interval has proven efficacious in treatment of cSCC in horses. The local control rate at 1 year for lesions treated with cisplatin was approximately 93 % and with bleomycin was approximately 78 % [62, 63]. Cisplatin in cats at standard IV doses (50–70 mg/m^2) is lethal through induction of severe pulmonary edema. However, local injection as repositol implants, consisting of purified cosmetic-grade bovine collagen matrix (20 mg/ml), epinephrine (0.1 mg/ml), and the chemotherapy agent (cisplatin 3.3 mg/ml), resulted in 86 % CR and 4 % partial response (PR) after 2 weekly treatments on average for a study population of 17 cats with a total of 51 cSCC lesions. Average disease-free interval (DFI) was 10.5 months with a local recurrence rate of 30 % in these cats (B. Kitchell 1994, personal communication).

The antimetabolite chemotherapeutic agent fluorouracil (5-FU) inhibits both RNA and DNA synthesis and targets dividing cells. Fluorouracil in cats at standard IV human doses (400–600 mg/m^2) induces rapidly lethal neurotoxicity. In fact, it is possible to see fatal neurotoxicosis in cats with the use of 5 % topical fluorouracil cream to the ear tips [64].

One study described the use of collagen implants as described above, substituting fluorouracil (5-FU 30 mg/ml) for cisplatin in the formulation. Using a regimen of 3 weekly implants, 58 % CR and 17 % PR were noted for a study population of six cats with a total of 16 lesions. Average DFI was 5 months with local recurrence rate of 14 %. Mild-to-moderate local adverse effects such as erythema and desquamation were noticed (B. Kitchell 1994, personal communication).

Intralesional delivery of chemotherapy in purified bovine collagen with fluorouracil as described above was applied to 13 dogs with sunlight-induced cSCC with 100 % overall response rate (54 % CR, 46 % PR). Cisplatin (3.3 mg/ml) in the collagen gel implant was given sequentially when CR was not achieved with fluorouracil, and no further reduction in area of the tumor was apparent after 2 weekly injections of fluorouracil implants. Cisplatin implants achieved CR that provided DFI of 44 months in two cases that achieved initial PR after treatment with fluorouracil implants. Partial remission allowed complete surgical excision to achieve cure in 3/6 dogs. The average DFI was almost 50 months. Further, weekly fluorouracil or cisplatin collagen implant treatments were well tolerated with minimal local erythema and no systemic adverse effects [65, 66].

Photodynamic Therapy (PDT)

This treatment modality consists of intravenous injection of an inert photosensitizer that is activated by light at the appropriate wavelength (600–900 nm "therapeutic windows"). Upon activation, the photosensitizer can undergo type I reaction, reacting directly with substrates such as DNA. Alternately, the photosensitizer can undergo type II reaction, directly producing free radicals or interacting with molecular oxygen to generate cytotoxic reactive oxygen species.

In a previous study, six feline cSCC were treated, resulting in two partial responses and four long-term complete responses with DFI that ranged from 276 to 576 days. Toxicity was described as tolerable and mostly localized to the skin. Erythema was noted and ulceration was occasionally observed, especially when PDT was applied for lesions of the eyelid. Systemic toxicity included nausea associated with the photosensitizer injection and elevated body temperatures 2 days after PDT. In one cat, anorexia and peripheral neuropathy of undetermined cause noted 2 weeks after PDT resolved without treatment [67]. Another study described the use of a novel liposomal photosensitizer for PDT in 18 cats. Local toxicity consisting of erythema and edema was reported in 15 % of the patients, and the CR rate was 100 %. The overall 1-year control rate was 75 %. The tumor recurrence rate in this cohort of patients was 20 % with a median time to recurrence of 172 days [68]. Similar response rates (overall response rate 96 %; CR 84 % and PR 11 %) to a single treatment with topical photosensitizer (5-ALA) were observed by Bexfield et al. [69] in a population of 56 cats with nasal planum cSCC. Recurrence was noticed in 51 % of the cases, with a median time to recurrence of 157 days. At a median follow-up of 1,146 days, 45 % of cats were alive and disease-free but 33 %

had to be euthanized due to local tumor recurrence. In this study, erythema and edema were observed in all cats after treatment, but these adverse effects were localized, mild, and transient. The lesions appeared to cause some discomfort, as manifested by occasional rubbing of the nasal planum [69].

Topical Therapy

Imiquimod is an antiproliferative agent and immune system stimulator. Imiquimod acts as a Toll-like receptor 7 agonist. Activation of this receptor protein plays a fundamental role in pathogen recognition and activation of innate immunity. Imiquimod is available as a topical cream and has been used to treat in situ cSCC presented as multiple lesions not invading the basal layer of the skin [70]. Imiquimod 5 %, used once daily on an alternate-day dosing regimen was associated with 100 % (40 % CR, 60 % PR) response rate in 12 cats affected by in ISSSC. Because of multifocal nature of the disease, appearance of new masses was observed in 75 % of the cats included in the study, and treatment duration extended to approximately 300 days on average. New lesions also responded to treatment in all cats. Toxicity was reported in 40 % of the cats. The toxicity observed included local erythema, mildly increased liver enzymes, mild neutropenia, anorexia, and vomiting [71–73].

Radiation Therapy

Most of the published data is focused on radiation therapy for cSCC of the nasal planum in cats. The volume of cSCC lesion treated was inversely associated with DFI and survival time [74]. Orthovoltage fractionated radiotherapy given as a total dose of 40 Gy provided a 1-year progression-free survival rate of 60 % in 90 cats with nasal planum SCC [74]. Proton therapy achieved similar control rates to orthovoltage radiotherapy with an overall response rate of 93 % in 15 cats with nasal planum SCC [75]. Plesiotherapy is a direct application of a strontium-90 radiation source to superficial cutaneous lesions. In this therapy, 50 Gy of radiation is delivered to a depth of 2 mm and administered in five fractions over a 10-day period to small (2–5 cm diameter) superficial lesions. This treatment achieved 87 % complete remission with no local recurrence noted for 2 years in 15 cats with cSCC [76]. Radiotherapy was not as effective in controlling residual cSCC in seven dogs that failed surgical curative-intent resection. Radiation therapy alone in three dogs only provided control of the disease for no longer than 8 weeks as an average [77].

The retinoic acid drugs called retinoids are derivatives of vitamin A, which is an essential factor for epithelial cell differentiation. Retinoids have been demonstrated to induce growth inhibition of premalignant lesions such as actinic keratoses, by induction of terminal differentiation, apoptosis, and cell cycle arrest [78]. Administration of etretinate to ten dogs at 1 mg/kg twice daily for a minimum of 90 days induced complete resolution of preneoplastic lesions in two dogs and partial responses in three dogs. Treatment toxicity included reversible hypertriglyceridemia and transient serum liver enzyme elevations in three dogs [79].

Systemic chemotherapy is not typically used to treat cSCC, as these lesions are rarely systemically disseminated. Agents such as carboplatin, bleomycin, fluorouracil, and doxorubicin have been administered with limited effect. The use of nonsteroidal anti-inflammatory agents such as piroxicam has been used in adjunctive protocols, as there is some evidence of tumor regression in oral SCC in the dog. Pain control afforded by NSAIDS may have a palliative effect for the patients, even if direct anticancer effect is not noted [80].

Future Treatment Strategies

The signal transducing G-coupled peptide Hras upregulates *Fyn* mRNA, and this suggests the potential for an interesting biologic relationship between Ras and Fyn in cutaneous neoplasms such as cSCC. Ratushny et al. [4] proposed the topical application of small-molecule kinase inhibitors (SMKIs) that have the physical properties required to penetrate the skin. The ideal SMKIs would target Fyn and related tyrosine kinases or would target kinases in the Ras path-

way. The tyrosine kinase inhibitor dasatinib is smaller than 500 Da in molecular size and targets multiple tyrosine kinase receptors, including Fyn. Topical dasatinib has been proposed as a possible therapeutic agent in this context [81]. Metronomic chemotherapy protocols involving the use of the oral receptor tyrosine kinase inhibitors toceranib and masitinib have some modest evidence of efficacy against oral SCC lesions, which might prove helpful in cSCC management as well [82].

Cutaneous Hemangiosarcoma

Incidence and Risk Factors

Hemangiosarcoma is a malignancy of vascular- or vessel-forming cells. The median of age range of dogs at the time of diagnosis of hemangiosarcomas affecting the cutis (cHSA) is approximately 10 years; in cats the median age at diagnosis is approximately 12 years [20, 83–85]. There is no known sex predilection, but most cutaneous vascular tumors (hemangiomas and hemangiosarcomas) in cats have been reported in males [20, 45, 83–85]. Hemangiosarcomas of the skin have predilection for cutaneous over subcutaneous tissue and for glabrous, lightly pigmented skin when compared with haired skin. Dogs with short hair coats and lightly pigmented skin have more hemangiomas and hemangiosarcomas of the cutis than do dogs with variable length hair coats and pigmentation [20]. Cutaneous HSA is commonly observed in predisposed breeds such as American Staffordshire terriers, pit bulls, beagles, Dalmatians, Italian greyhounds, whippets, and bull terriers [20, 83, 85]. Outdoor cats with unpigmented skin may be predisposed to cutaneous tumor development in areas without adequate pelage, particularly on the pinna and head [84].

Cutaneous HSA usually presents as solitary or multiple small cutaneous lesions, often less than 1 cm in diameter. In a recent report of 94 dogs with suspected or confirmed diagnosis of cHSA, 71 % of the cases at initial diagnosis had one solitary dermal lesion, and 29 % had multiple cutaneous lesions [20, 83]. Whether the presence of multiple sites of cHSA is a result of metastasis or whether the lesions arise de novo as multiple primary tumors is unclear.

Biologic Behavior

Recently, Szivek et al. [83] were able to identify prognostic factors that predict outcome for cHSA in dogs. Identified prognostic factors included breed, tumor location, and the presence of solar actinic changes. Predisposed breeds were found to have a median survival of 1,570 days compared with 593 days in non-predisposed or atypical breeds. Predisposed breeds had a lower metastatic relative risk of 0.45 when compared with non-predisposed breeds. Tumor location predicted survival of dogs with cHSA. Dogs with lesions arising in typical sun-exposed ventral abdominal locations had a median survival of 1,085 days compared with 539 days for dogs with tumors seen in other body locations. Tumor location also predicted locoregional recurrence. The solar-induced form associated with actinic changes has a reported median survival of 1,549 days compared with 545 days in dogs without actinic lesions [83]. The prognostic significance of association of solar elastosis or actinic changes with outcome of cHSA is controversial in the literature, however [83, 85]. Dogs of non-predisposed breeds with tumors in areas other than the ventrum, and that also lack actinic changes, or those with subcutaneous involvement appear to have a more aggressive form of HSA with higher risk of developing visceral HSA. Dogs with subcutaneous invasion have an associated metastatic relative risk of 2.04 when compared to dogs with only cutaneous involvement [83].

Lesions confined to the dermis are correlated with better prognostic outcome and lower recurrence rates, possibly because of ease of surgical excision [85]. Cutaneous HSA lesions may be easier to excise completely, and recurrence is much less frequent than for tumors involving deeper tissues. Locoregional recurrence is very common in predisposed thin-coated breeds with the solar-induced form of this disease. The incidence of metastasis is considered to be low in

cHSA in dogs and cats, but some patients may ultimately develop metastatic disease. Metastasis was documented or suspected in 34 % of dogs with cHSA and occurred at a median of 326 days from diagnosis. Progression to the visceral form of HSA was observed in 62 % of dogs with metastatic disease. These dogs are frequently diagnosed by the presence of hemoabdomen that occurs in more than the 95 % of the cases with visceral metastasis. Overall, the median survival for dogs treated by surgical excision with no adjuvant chemotherapy was reported to range from 780 to 987 days, with 1-, 2-, and 3-year survival rates of 79, 60, and 44 %, respectively. Median survival was 1,095 days in surgically treated cats with cHSA [20, 83, 84].

Diagnosis

Cutaneous HSA lesions closely resemble benign hemangiomas of the dermis, in both gross and cytologic appearance. Therefore, a cytologic approach may not be adequate for accurate diagnosis. Histologic examination allows determination of invasion and whether surgical excision was adequate. Systemic staging for pulmonary and visceral metastasis is indicated based on potential for spread to distant organs. Advanced local staging with computed tomography scanning may be helpful for surgical and radiation therapy planning.

Treatment

Surgery

Cutaneous HSA lesions are most often treated with curative-intent surgical excision. When patients have cHSA present in multiple sites, multiple surgeries are required. Locoregional recurrence was documented in 77 % of the cases at a median time of 211 days after initial diagnosis. Locoregional recurrence only occurred in skin anatomically close to the previously resected tumor. Predisposed breeds were found to be more affected by the development of locoregional recurrence, particularly when

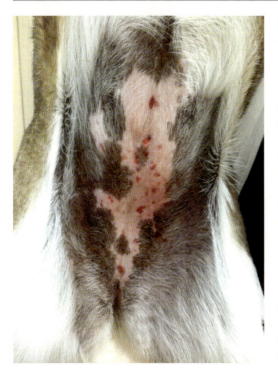

Fig. 33.3 Multiple small cutaneous HSA lesions located in the unpigmented skin of the ventral abdomen of a dog

masses were located on the ventrum, and also for dogs with multiple masses at initial presentation (Fig. 33.3). Biopsy margin status documenting complete surgical excision, absence of metastasis, and no subcutaneous invasion were surprisingly unassociated with incidence of local recurrence [83]. This may represent the effect of solar field cancerization, in which case all cells in the solar-exposed field have increased risk of carcinogenesis [86]. The dearth of prospective studies defining the clinical behavior of cHSA results in uncertainty and controversy regarding the role of complete surgical excision of the lesion as a predictor of clinical outcome in dogs and cats [83, 85].

Chemotherapy

Use of chemotherapy in the management of dogs and cats affected by cHSA is largely recommended only if there is an evidence of invasion of the subcutaneous tissue or of distant metastasis. Recent studies have documented a

possibly higher metastatic potential than previously believed in cats with cHSA [20, 83, 87]. Doxorubicin-based protocols provide several more months of survival time for these cats, when compared to no therapy. The most common chemotherapeutic agent used to treat systemic HSA is doxorubicin. Doxorubicin may be administered as a single agent every 2 or 3 weeks at 30 mg/m^2 for dogs, and 20–25 mg/m^2 or 1 mg/kg for dog <10 kg or for cats affected by cHSA with poor prognostic features. Doxorubicin may be used as described above in combination with cyclophosphamide 200–250 mg/m^2 IV, or 50 mg/m^2 PO for 4 days during week 1, and vincristine 0.5–0.7 mg/m^2 on days 8 and 15 of a 21-day cycle (VAC protocol). The DAV protocol substitutes the alkylating agent dacarbazine (DTIC) for cyclophosphamide in the VAC protocol. In the DAV protocol, dacarbazine is delivered at 800 mg/m^2 as an 8-h infusion diluted in 0.9 % NaCl at maintenance rate on day 1, with doxorubicin and vincristine delivered as scheduled for the VAC protocol. The DAV protocol has been used for treatment of visceral HSA. However, no chemotherapy protocol has been proven superior when compared to single-agent doxorubicin. More intense protocols such as VAC and DAV are associated with more toxicity [88–90].

Other therapies used to treat visceral HSA include ifosfamide delivered at a dose of 350–375 mg/m^2 IV every 3 weeks as a single agent. Complete response with tolerable toxicity was observed in a dog with metastatic cHSA [91].

Targeting tumor-associated neovasculature is the object of many anticancer therapeutics strategies. These investigations have been conducted in dogs with HSA and include studies of the efficacy of doxorubicin nanoconjugates that target transmembrane proteins expressed in the neovasculature of cHSA and other solid tumors. In vitro and in vivo studies using nanoconjugates showed measurable anticancer activity in cHSA cell lines and in xenograft mouse models implanted with canine cancer cells. These promising preliminary results warrant further investigation on macroscopic solid tumors [92].

Radiation Therapy

The use of radiation therapy for treatment of cHSA has not been extensively explored in dogs and cats. Palliative radiation therapy has been reported to have relative success in controlling nonsurgical cutaneous bleeding masses. The treatment protocol consisted of 3–4 Gy fractions to achieve a 24 Gy total radiation dose [90]. Other investigators have suggested the use of radiation therapy for control of cutaneous cHSAs with incomplete surgical resection. These studies reported poor responses in two cats with large, unresectable cHSA lesions [93].

Future Treatment Strategies

A newer concept in chemotherapy drug delivery is referred to as metronomic chemotherapy. Metronomic therapy is based on continuous drug exposure to susceptible cancer cells that results in direct inhibition of tumor cell replication, as well as inhibition of angiogenesis and alteration of immune function. The metronomic strategy is attractive as a cost-effective and well-tolerated treatment alternative for veterinary patients with malignancy.

Most of the metronomic treatment protocols in common veterinary use consist of combinations of NSAIDS and oral alkylating agents. Oral alkylating agents such as cyclophosphamide at 15–25 mg/m^2 or chlorambucil at 4 mg/m^2 may be given daily or on alternate days in combination with the oral administration of an NSAID such as piroxicam at the dose of 0.3 mg/kg daily. Increased benefit also appears to occur when metronomic chemotherapy is used in combination tyrosine kinase inhibitor drugs, such as toceranib and masitinib [94].

In human medicine, metronomic therapy has been used to treat patients with cutaneous angiosarcomas using a similar protocol to those employed for veterinary patients. This metronomic protocol consisted of low-dose trofosfamide in combination with the peroxisome proliferator-activated receptor gamma agonist pioglitazone and the selective cyclooxygenase-2 inhibitor rofecoxib. Response was observed in four out of the six patients and stabilization of the disease in the other two cases for a period of almost 8 months on average. This treatment protocol was well tolerated with minimal adverse effects [95]. Similarly in veterinary medicine, canine splenic hemangiosarcoma was treated with metronomic therapy using daily cyclophosphamide at 12.5–25 mg/m^2 on an alternating 3-week schedule with orally administered etoposide at 50 mg/m^2. The protocol's performance was similar to that seen in historical controls treated with conventional intravenous biweekly doxorubicin at 30 mg/m^2 IV for 5 doses [96, 97]. Metronomic therapy may be feasible as a first-line therapy option for patients with cHSA that cannot undergo surgery. However, further study is needed to determine the ultimate value of metronomic chemotherapy for treatment of canine and feline cHSA.

Glossary

Actinic keratosis Solar-induced premalignant condition of the skin characterized by abnormal maturation of keratinocytes, thickening of the epidermis, and inflammatory infiltrate of the dermis.

Cryosurgery Treatment modality for localized tumors that induces cell death by formation of intracellular and extracellular ice crystals.

Electrochemotherapy Treatment modality for localized tumors that involves administration of a chemotherapeutic agent combined with delivery of appropriate energy waveforms that induces increased cell drug uptake.

Epigenetic effects Molecular mechanisms that regulate gene expression in the absence of changes in the DNA sequence itself.

Hemangiosarcoma Malignant neoplastic condition of vascular- or vessel-forming cells.

Intralesional chemotherapy Treatment modality for localized tumors that involves the direct intratumoral delivery of chemotherapeutic agents.

Metronomic therapy Treatment modality based on continuous drug exposure that results in direct inhibition of tumor cell replication, as well as inhibition of angiogenesis and stimulation of immune function.

MicroRNAs (miRNA) Small RNA fragments of no more than 25–50 nucleotides that act as post-transcriptional regulators by hybridizing complementary bases in strands of messenger RNA.

Missense mutation Single-point nucleotide change, mutation that results in substituted amino acids or mRNA chain termination.

Nanoconjugates Nano-sized particles compounded to incorporate a polymer and an anticancer drug.

Oncogene Altered or mutated gene associated with unregulated cell replication that results in cancer.

Peroxisome proliferator-activated receptor Nuclear receptors that modulate expression of growth regulatory genes and enzymes involved in oxidative stress leading to DNA damage.

Photodynamic therapy Treatment modality for localized tumors that consists of intravenous injection of an inert photosensitizer that is activated by light at the appropriate wavelength, resulting in a reactive agent that ultimately induces DNA damage.

Retrovirus Single-strain RNA viruses that require the host transcriptase enzyme to create the DNA-viral genome.

Solar elastosis Elastic fiber proliferation in the dermis of chronically sun-exposed skin.

Squamous cell carcinoma Epithelial tumor that arises from epidermal stem cells located in the hair follicle bulge and the basal layer of the interfollicular epidermis.

Stem cells Cell lineage precursors with the potential for self-renewal and multi-lineage differentiation.

Topical therapy Treatment modality that consists in the delivery of drug in target site lesion of the skin.

Tyrosine kinases Enzymes that induce changes in cell communication pathways that regulate cellular activity by phosphorylation of other proteins.

Ultraviolet light Invisible wavelength forms of the electromagnetic solar radiation spectrum with carcinogenic, germicidal, and other multiple properties.

References

1. Finnie JW, Bostock DE. Skin neoplasia in dogs. Aust Vet J. 1979;55(12):602–4.
2. Villamil JA, Henry CJ, Bryan JN, et al. Identification of the most common cutaneous neoplasms in dogs and evaluation of breed and age distributions for selected neoplasms. J Am Vet Med Assoc. 2011; 239(7):960–5.
3. Brittan M, Braun KM, Reynolds LE, et al. Bone marrow cells engraft within the epidermis and proliferate in vivo with no evidence of cell fusion. J Pathol. 2005;205(1):1–13.
4. Ratushny V, Gober MD, Hick R, Ridky TW, Seykora JT. From keratinocyte to cancer: the pathogenesis and modeling of cutaneous squamous cell carcinoma. J Clin Invest. 2012;122(2):464–72.
5. Sung B, Prasad S, Yadav VR, Aggarwal BB. Cancer cell signaling pathways targeted by spice-derived nutraceuticals. Nutr Cancer. 2012;64(2):173–97.
6. Ramos J, Villa J, Ruiz A, Armstrong R, Matta J. UV dose determines key characteristics of nonmelanoma skin cancer. Cancer Epidemiol Biomarkers Prev. 2004;13(12):2006–11.
7. Tufaro AP, Chuang JC, Prasad N, Chuang A, Chuang TC, Fischer AC. Molecular markers in cutaneous squamous cell carcinoma. Int J Surg Oncol. 2011; 2011:231475.
8. Brash DE, Rudolph JA, Simon JA, et al. A role for sunlight in skin cancer: UV-induced p53 mutations in squamous cell carcinoma. Proc Natl Acad Sci U S A. 1991;88(22):10124–8.
9. Mayr B, Blauensteiner J, Edlinger A, et al. Presence of p53 mutations in feline neoplasms. Res Vet Sci. 2000;68(1):63–70.
10. Jasik A, Reichert M. New p53 mutations in canine skin tumours. Vet Rec. 2011;169(26):684.
11. Ortonne JP. From actinic keratosis to squamous cell carcinoma. Br J Dermatol. 2002;146 Suppl 61: 20–3.
12. Kolev V, Mandinova A, Guinea-Viniegra J, et al. EGFR signalling as a negative regulator of Notch1 gene transcription and function in proliferating keratinocytes and cancer. Nat Cell Biol. 2008;10(8): 902–11.
13. Mortier L, Marchetti P, Delaporte E, et al. Progression of actinic keratosis to squamous cell carcinoma of the skin correlates with deletion of the 9p21 region encoding the p16(INK4a) tumor suppressor. Cancer Lett. 2002;176(2):205–14.

14. Burnworth B, Arendt S, Muffler S, et al. The multistep process of human skin carcinogenesis: a role for p53, cyclin D1, hTERT, p16, and TSP-1. Eur J Cell Biol. 2007;86(11–12):763–80.
15. Pierceall WE, Goldberg LH, Tainsky MA, Mukhopadhyay T, Ananthaswamy HN. Ras gene mutation and amplification in human nonmelanoma skin cancers. Mol Carcinog. 1991;4(3):196–202.
16. Khavari PA. Modelling cancer in human skin tissue. Nat Rev Cancer. 2006;6(4):270–80.
17. Gibbons RJ. Histone modifying and chromatin remodelling enzymes in cancer and dysplastic syndromes. Hum Mol Genet. 2005;14 Spec No 1:R85–92.
18. Venza I, Visalli M, Tripodo B, et al. FOXE1 is a target for aberrant methylation in cutaneous squamous cell carcinoma. Br J Dermatol. 2010;162(5):1093–7.
19. Dziunycz P, Iotzova-Weiss G, Eloranta JJ, et al. Squamous cell carcinoma of the skin shows a distinct microRNA profile modulated by UV radiation. J Invest Dermatol. 2010;130(11):2686–9.
20. Hargis AMIP, Spangler WL, Stannard AA. A retrospective clinicopathologic study of 212 dogs with cutaneous hemangiomas and hemangiosarcomas. Vet Pathol. 1992;4(29):316–28.
21. Nikula KJ, Benjamin SA, Angleton GM, Saunders WJ, Lee AC. Ultraviolet radiation, solar dermatosis, and cutaneous neoplasia in beagle dogs. Radiat Res. 1992;129(1):11–8.
22. Glickstein J, Sebelik ME, Lu Q. Cutaneous angiosarcoma of the head and neck: a case presentation and review of the literature. Ear Nose Throat J. 2006;85(10):672–4.
23. Tamburini BA, Phang TL, Fosmire SP, et al. Gene expression profiling identifies inflammation and angiogenesis as distinguishing features of canine hemangiosarcoma. BMC Cancer. 2010;10:619.
24. Thamm DH, Dickerson EB, Akhtar N, et al. Biological and molecular characterization of a canine hemangiosarcoma-derived cell line. Res Vet Sci. 2006;81(1):76–86.
25. Zu Y, Perle MA, Yan Z, Liu J, Kumar A, Waisman J. Chromosomal abnormalities and p53 gene mutation in a cardiac angiosarcoma. Appl Immunohistochem Mol Morphol. 2001;9(1):24–8.
26. Zanetta L, Corada M, Grazia Lampugnani M, et al. Downregulation of vascular endothelial-cadherin expression is associated with an increase in vascular tumor growth and hemorrhagic complications. Thromb Haemost. 2005;93(6):1041–6.
27. Yonemaru K, Sakai H, Murakami M, et al. The significance of p53 and retinoblastoma pathways in canine hemangiosarcoma. J Vet Med Sci. 2007;69(3):271–8.
28. Antonescu CR, Yoshida A, Guo T, et al. KDR activating mutations in human angiosarcomas are sensitive to specific kinase inhibitors. Cancer Res. 2009;69(18):7175–9.
29. Marion MJ, Froment O, Trepo C. Activation of Ki-ras gene by point mutation in human liver angiosarcoma associated with vinyl chloride exposure. Mol Carcinog. 1991;4(6):450–4.
30. Zaugg N, Nespeca G, Hauser B, Ackermann M, Favrot C. Detection of novel papillomaviruses in canine mucosal, cutaneous and in situ squamous cell carcinomas. Vet Dermatol. 2005;16(5):290–8.
31. Munday JS, Kiupel M, French AF, Howe L. Amplification of papillomaviral DNA sequences from a high proportion of feline cutaneous in situ and invasive squamous cell carcinomas using a nested polymerase chain reaction. Vet Dermatol. 2008;19(5):259–63.
32. Munday JS, O'Connor KI, Smits B. Development of multiple pigmented viral plaques and squamous cell carcinomas in a dog infected by a novel papillomavirus. Vet Dermatol. 2011;22(1):104–10.
33. Goldschmidt MH, Kennedy JS, Kennedy DR, et al. Severe papillomavirus infection progressing to metastatic squamous cell carcinoma in bone marrowtransplanted X-linked SCID dogs. J Virol. 2006;80(13):6621–8.
34. Munday JS, Kiupel M. Papillomavirus-associated cutaneous neoplasia in mammals. Vet Pathol. 2010;47(2):254–64.
35. Asgari MM, Kiviat NB, Critchlow CW, et al. Detection of human papillomavirus DNA in cutaneous squamous cell carcinoma among immunocompetent individuals. J Invest Dermatol. 2008;128(6):1409–17.
36. zur Hausen H. Papillomaviruses and cancer: from basic studies to clinical application. Nat Rev Cancer. 2002;2(5):342–50.
37. Dubina M, Goldenberg G. Viral-associated nonmelanoma skin cancers: a review. Am J Dermatopathol. 2009;31(6):561–73.
38. Moloney FJ, Comber H, O'Lorcain P, O'Kelly P, Conlon PJ, Murphy GM. A population-based study of skin cancer incidence and prevalence in renal transplant recipients. Br J Dermatol. 2006;154(3):498–504.
39. Pedersen NC, Yamamoto JK, Ishida T, Hansen H. Feline immunodeficiency virus infection. Vet Immunol Immunopathol. 1989;21(1):111–29.
40. Gabor LJ, Love DN, Malik R, Canfield PJ. Feline immunodeficiency virus status of Australian cats with lymphosarcoma. Aust Vet J. 2001;79(8):540–5.
41. Magden E, Quackenbush SL, VandeWoude S. FIV associated neoplasms – a mini-review. Vet Immunol Immunopathol. 2011;143(3–4):227–34.
42. Hutson CA, Rideout BA, Pedersen NC. Neoplasia associated with feline immunodeficiency virus infection in cats of southern California. J Am Vet Med Assoc. 1991;199(10):1357–62.
43. Mukaratirwa S, Chipunza J, Chitanga S, Chimonyo M, Bhebhe E. Canine cutaneous neoplasms: prevalence and influence of age, sex and site on the presence and potential malignancy of cutaneous neoplasms in dogs from Zimbabwe. J S Afr Vet Assoc. 2005;76(2):59–62.
44. Sabattini S, Marconato L, Zoff A, et al. Epidermal growth factor receptor expression is predictive of poor prognosis in feline cutaneous squamous cell carcinoma. J Feline Med Surg. 2010;12(10):760–8.
45. Miller MA, Nelson SL, Turk JR, et al. Cutaneous neoplasia in 340 cats. Vet Pathol. 1991;28(5):389–95.

46. Henry CJ, Brewer Jr WG, Whitley EM, et al. Canine digital tumors: a veterinary cooperative oncology group retrospective study of 64 dogs. J Vet Intern Med. 2005;19(5):720–4.

47. Vail D, Withrow S. Tumors of the skin and subcutaneous tissues. In: Vail D, Withrow S, editors. Small animal clinical oncology. 4th ed. St. Louis: Saunders/Elsiever; 2007. p. 375–99.

48. Lana SE, Ogilvie GK, Withrow SJ, Straw RC, Rogers KS. Feline cutaneous squamous cell carcinoma of the nasal planum and the pinnae: 61 cases. J Am Anim Hosp Assoc. 1997;33(4):329–32.

49. Vail D, Withrow S. Cancer of the gastrointestinal tract. In: Vail D, Withrow S, editors. Small animal clinical oncology. St. Louis: Saunders/Elsiever; 2007. p. 455–510.

50. Rowe DE, Carroll RJ, Day Jr CL. Prognostic factors for local recurrence, metastasis, and survival rates in squamous cell carcinoma of the skin, ear, and lip. Implications for treatment modality selection. J Am Acad Dermatol. 1992;26(6):976–90.

51. Molnar L, Ronay P, Tapolcsanyi L. Carcinoma of the lip. Analysis of the material of 25 years. Oncology. 1974;29(2):101–21.

52. Conley J. Cancer of the skin of the nose. Ann Otol Rhinol Laryngol. 1974;83(1):2–8.

53. Chernosky ME. Squamous cell and basal cell carcinomas: preliminary study of 3,817 primary skin cancers. South Med J. 1978;71(7):802–3, 806.

54. Pocholle E, Reyes-Gomez E, Giacomo A, Delaunay P, Hasseine L, Marty P. [A case of feline leishmaniasis in the south of France]. Parasite. 2012;19(1): 77–80.

55. Reszko AAS, Wilson L, Leffell D. Cancer of the skin. In: DeVita VLT, Rosenberg S, editors. Cancer: principles and practice of oncology. Philadelphia: Lippincott Williams & Wilkins; 2011. p. 1620–3.

56. Kwa RE, Campana K, Moy RL. Biology of cutaneous squamous cell carcinoma. J Am Acad Dermatol. 1992;26(1):1–26.

57. Dinehart SM, Pollack SV. Metastases from squamous cell carcinoma of the skin and lip. An analysis of twenty-seven cases. J Am Acad Dermatol. 1989;21(2 Pt 1):241–8.

58. Thomson M. Squamous cell carcinoma of the nasal planum in cats and dogs. Clin Tech Small Anim Pract. 2007;22(2):42–5.

59. Clarke R. Cryosurgical treatment of feline cutaneous squamous cell carcinoma. Aust Vet Pract. 1991;21: 148–53.

60. Spugnini EP, Vincenzi B, Citro G, et al. Electrochemotherapy for the treatment of squamous cell carcinoma in cats: a preliminary report. Vet J. 2009;179(1): 117–20.

61. Cemazar M, Tamzali Y, Sersa G, et al. Electrochemotherapy in veterinary oncology. J Vet Intern Med. 2008;22(4):826–31.

62. Theon AP, Pascoe JR, Galuppo LD, Fisher PE, Griffey SM, Madigan JE. Comparison of perioperative versus postoperative intratumoral administration of cisplatin for treatment of cutaneous sarcoids and squamous cell

carcinomas in horses. J Am Vet Med Assoc. 1999;215(11):1655–60.

63. Theon AP, Pascoe JR, Carlson GP, Krag DN. Intratumoral chemotherapy with cisplatin in oily emulsion in horses. J Am Vet Med Assoc. 1993;202(2): 261–7.

64. Theilen GH. Adverse effect from use of 5% fluorouracil. J Am Vet Med Assoc. 1987;191:216.

65. Kitchell BK, Orenberg EK, Brown DM, et al. Intralesional sustained-release chemotherapy with therapeutic implants for treatment of canine sun-induced squamous cell carcinoma. Eur J Cancer. 1995;31A(12):2093–8.

66. Orenberg EK, Luck EE, Brown DM, Kitchell BE. Implant delivery system: intralesional delivery of chemotherapeutic agents for treatment of spontaneous skin tumors in veterinary patients. Clin Dermatol. 1991;9(4):561–8.

67. Frimberger AE, Moore AS, Cincotta L, Cotter SM, Foley JW. Photodynamic therapy of naturally occurring tumors in animals using a novel benzophenothiazine photosensitizer. Clin Cancer Res. 1998;4(9): 2207–18.

68. Buchholz J, Wergin M, Walt H, Grafe S, Bley CR, Kaser-Hotz B. Photodynamic therapy of feline cutaneous squamous cell carcinoma using a newly developed liposomal photosensitizer: preliminary results concerning drug safety and efficacy. J Vet Intern Med. 2007;21(4):770–5.

69. Bexfield NH, Stell AJ, Gear RN, Dobson JM. Photodynamic therapy of superficial nasal planum squamous cell carcinomas in cats: 55 cases. J Vet Intern Med. 2008;22(6):1385–9.

70. Zagon IS, Donahue RN, Rogosnitzky M, McLaughlin PJ. Imiquimod upregulates the opioid growth factor receptor to inhibit cell proliferation independent of immune function. Exp Biol Med (Maywood). 2008;233(8):968–79.

71. Gill VL, Bergman PJ, Baer KE, Craft D, Leung C. Use of imiquimod 5% cream (Aldara) in cats with multicentric squamous cell carcinoma in situ: 12 cases (2002–2005). Vet Comp Oncol. 2008;6(1): 55–64.

72. Patel U, Mark NM, Machler BC, Levine VJ. Imiquimod 5% cream induced psoriasis: a case report, summary of the literature and mechanism. Br J Dermatol. 2011;164(3):670–2.

73. van der Fits L, Mourits S, Voerman JS, et al. Imiquimod-induced psoriasis-like skin inflammation in mice is mediated via the IL-23/IL-17 axis. J Immunol. 2009;182(9):5836–45.

74. Theon AP, Madewell BR, Shearn VI, Moulton JE. Prognostic factors associated with radiotherapy of squamous cell carcinoma of the nasal plane in cats. J Am Vet Med Assoc. 1995;206(7):991–6.

75. Fidel JL, Egger E, Blattmann H, Oberhansli F, Kaser-Hotz B. Proton irradiation of feline nasal planum squamous cell carcinomas using an accelerated protocol. Vet Radiol Ultrasound. 2001;42(6):569–75.

76. Goodfellow M, Hayes A, Murphy S, Brearley M. A retrospective study of 90Strontium plesiotherapy

for feline squamous cell carcinoma of the nasal planum. J Feline Med Surg. 2006;8(3):169–76.

77. Lascelles BD, Parry AT, Stidworthy MF, Dobson JM, White RA. Squamous cell carcinoma of the nasal planum in 17 dogs. Vet Rec. 2000;147(17):473–6.

78. de Mello Souza CH, Valli VE, Selting KA, Kiupel M, Kitchell BE. Immunohistochemical detection of retinoid receptors in tumors from 30 dogs diagnosed with cutaneous lymphoma. J Vet Intern Med. 2010;24(5): 1112–7.

79. Marks SL, Song MD, Stannard AA, Power HT. Clinical evaluation of etretinate for the treatment of canine solar-induced squamous cell carcinoma and preneoplastic lesions. J Am Acad Dermatol. 1992;27(1): 11–6.

80. Schmidt BR, Glickman NW, DeNicola DB, de Gortari AE, Knapp DW. Evaluation of piroxicam for the treatment of oral squamous cell carcinoma in dogs. J Am Vet Med Assoc. 2001;218(11):1783–6.

81. Muller BA. Imatinib and its successors – how modern chemistry has changed drug development. Curr Pharm Des. 2009;15(2):120–33.

82. Kitchell B. Review of U.S cases treated with Masivet. In: VCS proceedings, Alburquerque, 2011, p. 66.

83. Szivek A, Burns RE, Gericota B, et al. Clinical outcome in 94 cases of dermal haemangiosarcoma in dogs treated with surgical excision: 1993-2007*. Vet Comp Oncol. 2012;10(1):65–73.

84. Miller MA, Ramos JA, Kreeger JM. Cutaneous vascular neoplasia in 15 cats: clinical, morphologic, and immunohistochemical studies. Vet Pathol. 1992;29(4): 329–36.

85. Schultheiss PC. A retrospective study of visceral and nonvisceral hemangiosarcoma and hemangiomas in domestic animals. J Vet Diagn Invest. 2004;16(6): 522–6.

86. Dakubo GD, Jakupciak JP, Birch-Machin MA, Parr RL. Clinical implications and utility of field cancerization. Cancer Cell Int. 2007;7:2.

87. Kraje AC, Mears EA, Hahn KA, McEntee MF, Mitchell SK. Unusual metastatic behavior and clinicopathologic findings in eight cats with cutaneous or visceral hemangiosarcoma. J Am Vet Med Assoc. 1999;214(5):670–2.

88. Dervisis NG, Dominguez PA, Newman RG, Cadile CD, Kitchell BE. Treatment with DAV for advanced-stage hemangiosarcoma in dogs. J Am Anim Hosp Assoc. 2011;47(3):170–8.

89. Hammer AS, Couto CG, Filppi J, Getzy D, Shank K. Efficacy and toxicity of VAC chemotherapy (vincristine, doxorubicin, and cyclophosphamide) in dogs with hemangiosarcoma. J Vet Intern Med. 1991;5(3): 160–6.

90. Smith AN. Hemangiosarcoma in dogs and cats. Vet Clin North Am Small Anim Pract. 2003;33(3): 533–52, vi.

91. Rassnick KM, Frimberger AE, Wood CA, Williams LE, Cotter SM, Moore AS. Evaluation of ifosfamide for treatment of various canine neoplasms. J Vet Intern Med. 2000;14(3):271–6.

92. Fan T. Preclinical evaluation of vascular targeting doxorubicin nanoconjugates using a canine hemangiosarcoma xenograft model. In: VCS 2011 Proceedings, Alburquerque, 2001.

93. Meleo KA. Tumors of the skin and associated structures. Vet Clin North Am Small Anim Pract. 1997; 27(1):73–94.

94. London CA, Hannah AL, Zadovoskaya R, et al. Phase I dose-escalating study of SU11654, a small molecule receptor tyrosine kinase inhibitor, in dogs with spontaneous malignancies. Clin Cancer Res. 2003;9(7): 2755–68.

95. Vogt T, Hafner C, Bross K, et al. Antiangiogenetic therapy with pioglitazone, rofecoxib, and metronomic trofosfamide in patients with advanced malignant vascular tumors. Cancer. 2003;98(10):2251–6.

96. Lana S, U'Ren L, Plaza S, et al. Continuous low-dose oral chemotherapy for adjuvant therapy of splenic hemangiosarcoma in dogs. J Vet Intern Med. 2007;21(4):764–9.

97. Mutsaers AJ. Metronomic chemotherapy. Top Companion Anim Med. 2009;24(3):137–43.

Job Paul van der Heijden and Leonard Witkamp

Key Points

- Teledermatology is the delivery of dermatologic care through information and communication technology.
- Over the last 5 years Teledermatology services have fully matured in countries such as USA and The Netherlands.
- Teledermoscopy is the result of combining digitalized dermoscopic images with the technology provided by teledermatology.
- Teledermoscopy is mostly used for the purpose of triage in skin cancer screening programs.
- Accuracy and reliability of teledermatology and teledermoscopy are comparable to in vivo consultation, but are highly dependent on image quality.

J.P. van der Heijden, MSc (✉)
Department of Dermatology,
Academic Medical Center,
University of Amsterdam,
22700, 1100 DE Amsterdam,
The Netherlands

KSYOS TeleMedical Center,
Amsterdamseweg 206, 1182 HL
Amstelveen, The Netherlands
e-mail: j.vanderheijden@ksyos.org

L. Witkamp, MD, PhD
KSYOS TeleMedical Center,
Amsterdamseweg 206, 1182 HL
Amstelveen, The Netherlands

Introduction

Telemedicine is the delivery of healthcare and sharing of medical knowledge by use of information and communication technology (ICT), enabling caregivers and caretakers to work together independent of place and time for the purpose of consultation, remote medical procedures or examinations, and education [1].

Currently many countries are experiencing a high demand on their healthcare, either due to a scarcity of healthcare workers in rural areas where access to healthcare is difficult and costly or due to overpopulation resulting in ever-growing waiting times and pressured, stressful work environments. This demand will only continue to rise, as Europe is facing population aging across the board. For example, take a look at the situation in the Netherlands. Forty-seven percent (47 %) of the Dutch population (16,725,902 inhabitants on 13,082 m^2 of land in 2011) will be nonworking in 2030 as compared to 39 % in 2008, and 25 % of the population will be over 65 years old [2]. This last group will count for 37.5 % of the total costs of care [3]. These figures show that considerable increased demand for care, leading to higher costs in the next 20 years, will not be followed by an increase in healthcare workers.

Telemedicine has been thought as an organizational answer to keep healthcare accessible for the general population [4]. Its benefits may be vital for the restructuring of healthcare systems in the Anglo-Saxon world and the progression towards better healthcare in developing countries

A. Baldi et al. (eds.), *Skin Cancer*, Current Clinical Pathology,
DOI 10.1007/978-1-4614-7357-2_34, © Springer Science+Business Media New York 2014

in the coming decades. This chapter describes teledermatology (TD), the adaptation of telemedicine on the field of dermatology, the various TD implementations, the growing participation of TD in skin cancer care, and how not the technology but the whole telemedicine concept can be adopted as the advocate for change.

Teledermatology

Teledermatology is the delivery of dermatologic care through information and communication technology. It has evolved rapidly in the last decade [4, 5]. MEDLINE has indexed 336 papers (search term: "teledermatology," March 2012) presenting studies on TD in over 30 countries. Over the years various actors, modes of delivery, capturing technologies, and purposes have been developed and studied in TD research [6, 7].

Actors

There are various actors (e.g., patient, general practitioner (GP), dermatologist) who play a role in the TD process. A categorization of TD processes can be made dependent on the actors involved (Fig. 34.1).

Primary (or patient-initiated or patient-supplied) TD encompasses communication between the patient and the GP or dermatologist. Primary TD has scarcely been researched thus far. Self-monitoring and patient empowerment are mentioned as important reasons for primary TD in acne or psoriasis patients [8–11]. Primary TD may be used to improve outpatient clinic triage for patients that the GP has already referred to the dermatologist for a face-to-face consultation [12].

In secondary TD, the GP or the homecare nurse communicates with the dermatologist. Secondary TD may be one of the most evolved telemedicine services so far, having been subject of research since 1995 [13, 14]. Research has shown secondary TD to be diagnostically accurate and reliable in many implementations [15, 16]. Recent studies showed that secondary TD is implemented in regular healthcare systems with reimbursement for the actors, is more efficient compared to conventional care, and is more cost-effective [17, 18].

Tertiary TD facilitates communication among dermatologists. Tertiary TD cases with a more specialized character are presented to get an

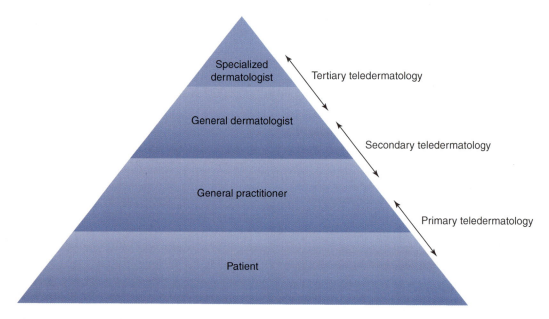

Fig. 34.1 Teledermatology actors

expert opinion from a specialized (often academic) dermatologist; also tertiary TD often has an educational character [19].

Mode of Delivery

Two main technologies are used for the delivery of information and care in TD. The most common is store-and-forward (SAF), asynchronous data transfer in which photos and videos are created, sent, and assessed at the actors' time of convenience independent of the actors' location. Another less popular mode is real-time (RT), synchronous data transfer in which photos but more often video streams are created, sent, and assessed at a time all actors are available independent of the actors' location. Lastly there is a hybrid mode where SAF and RT are used simultaneous.

Capturing Technology

Teledermatology has been made possible through the introduction of consumer digital (video) cameras. As store-and-forward is the main delivery mode of choice, video camera equipment is not discussed in this chapter [20]. In the late 1990s and early 2000s, the costs of digital camera equipment posed a barrier for the use of TD, and the quality of different cameras continued to be a critical topic of discussion. With the current hardware, these issues are off the table. Any off-the-shelf digital camera can produce an image of more than sufficient quality for TD. This day, the quality of the image is highly dependent, not on the camera but on the skills of the photographer. It is recommended, when practicing TD, to take an introductory course in taking (clinical) pictures.

High-quality dermoscopic images can be acquired when a dermoscope is attached to a digital camera. The assessment of dermoscopic images through TD is called teledermoscopy and is used for screening and management of skin cancer. Its advantages and risks are described in the next section.

The development of digital cameras in mobile phones brought a new capturing device to TD.

Pilot studies show mobile phone TD to be feasible [21–25] and to contribute to mobility and self-management [8, 26]. Recently, mobile phone TD used as a skin cancer screening tool has shown promising results in a number of pilot studies [27–30].

Purpose

The most common purpose for TD is consultation: to get an advice from an expert on diagnosis, management, or both, with the underlying goal to avoid physical referral, or to obtain a second opinion.

Triage is the second use of TD and overlaps with consultation, as the result of a consultation improves a patient's triage by either avoiding physical referral or accelerating referral. When used to prevent a referral, TD can reduce physical referrals up to 74 %. When a second opinion is obtained, 16% of these patients will have an accelerated physical referral, hence improving quality of care [18]. TD is also used as a triage tool in skin cancer screening [31, 32] and in outpatient clinic triage [12].

Monitoring, a third purpose of TD, is used for and by patients with chronic disorders such as psoriasis patients on systemic treatment and patients with open wounds. Pilot studies show that monitoring can optimize treatment, improve compliance, and improve empowerment of the patient's responsibility [11, 33, 34]. Monitoring of patients with chronic wounds via TD can offer a better quality of life and gives potential to cost-effective long-term wound care [35, 36].

Teledermatology is also used in education programs. Online discussion groups and Internet fora are used as a stage to present interesting cases as continuing medical education for colleagues [19]. There are resident training programs developed that incorporate TD in their courses [37]. Lastly, there is a huge passive learning experience found in GPs practicing TD and gaining knowledge from the answers provided by the dermatologists [18].

Finally there is the purpose of cost reduction that has so far been subordinate to aforementioned purposes, as availability and quality of care are the first priority. Nevertheless, cost reduction is a very important motivator of all telemedicine implementations. Only after cost-effectiveness has been proven in TD, it can grow into a fully implemented practice of care delivery. Due to the many variables and different perspectives, it has proven difficult to design complete cost analysis in telemedicine [38]. Recent studies however indicate that teledermatology is cost-effective under the right conditions and can save healthcare costs up to 18 % [17, 18, 39].

Satisfaction and Acceptance

Although reliable validated methods to assess satisfaction of patients and referring and consulting clinicians do not yet exist in telemedicine research, there are still a number of publications with, be it mostly anecdotal, results on the subject.

Main positive results on patient satisfaction display high rates of acceptance, confidence, and favoritism of TD (76–93 %) [40–45]. Concerns with TD were mainly expressed as "not seeing a dermatologist in-person" but were post by a lower percentage of the population (30–40 %) [40, 41, 45].

Clinicians are generally satisfied with TD and acceptance is high, but express concerns on time consumption and complex or faulty software [40, 43, 46]. As one would expect, most clinicians who are using teledermatology are frontrunners who embrace innovative techniques and tend to be more positive. Indeed, studies by Collins et al. and Bowns et al., in which participation for dermatologists was not voluntary, showed not all clinicians embrace this new method as easily with satisfaction rates as low as 20 % [40, 46].

Teledermoscopy

Teledermoscopy is the obvious result of combining digitalized dermoscopic images with the technology provided by teledermatology (Fig. 34.2). The concept of teledermoscopy had already been developed as early as 1999 [47]. A major

concern with teledermoscopy has always been its diagnostic accuracy and reliability, even more so than with regular teledermatology. The main reason, the relative high mortality risk found in melanoma skin cancer, warrants this caution. Still, the use of dermoscopy by trained dermoscopists increases diagnostic accuracy for pigmented and nonpigmented skin lesions, especially in melanoma [48, 49]. Many papers have been published reporting on the diagnostic accuracy [27, 28, 31, 32, 47, 50–56] and diagnostic reliability [32, 57–60] of teledermoscopy for (non) pigmented skin lesions. Several recent studies have reported high diagnostic accuracy of teledermoscopy (Cohen's kappa 0.74–0.95), comparable with diagnostic accuracy found in face-to-face dermoscopic examination. Diagnostic reliability studies reported moderate to good concordance between observers (Cohen's kappa 0.44–0.93). The diagnostic accuracy of teledermoscopy is mostly dependent on the observer's level of experience [55] and the quality of the provided images.

As teledermoscopy is mostly used for the purpose of triage in skin cancer screening programs, it is perhaps of more importance to look at the management plan accuracy. Several studies have showed that, although agreement on a diagnostic level is sometimes moderate (possibly due to differences in terminology and classification), management plan agreement is high and equal to face-to-face consultation [31, 32, 56]. A recent study by Lim et al. reported on the first completely implemented and reimbursed teledermoscopy triage service [61]. Instead of a live visit, patients could be referred to a commercially run virtual lesion clinic (VLC). Results showed 88% prevented referrals to the dermatologist and faster detection and treatment of skin cancer patients in the patient group that was treated through the VLC.

Two risk factors must be addressed when practicing teledermoscopy. Its accuracy can be significantly lowered when diagnosis is performed by inexperienced teledermoscopists or when the dermoscopic photography is of a nongradable quality. A study by Piccolo et al. showed an accuracy of kappa 0.69–0.87 with experienced

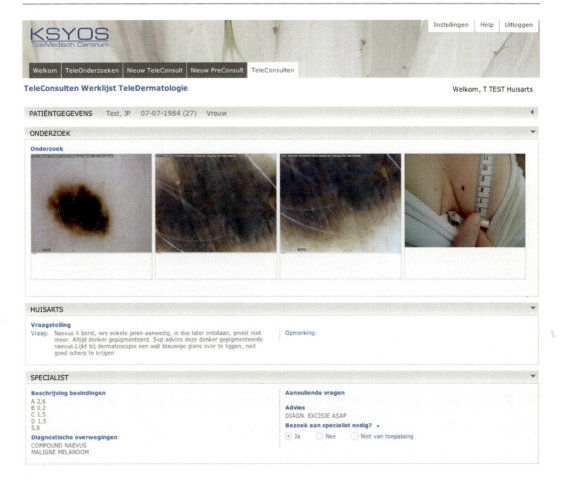

Fig. 34.2 A teledermoscopy consultation

dermatologists and an accuracy of kappa 0.40–0.56 with less experienced dermatologists [55]. Preliminary results from a study performed by the authors in the Netherlands showed a diagnostic accuracy of 29 % compared to in vivo diagnosis where the photographs were classified as non-gradable by two independent dermatologists ($n=7$ patients) and an accuracy of 79 % where the photographs were classified as gradable ($n=24$ patients). Photographs were taken by general practitioners during regular practice with a DermLite II Pro (3Gen, USA) attached to a Cybershot DSC-W560 digital camera (SONY, Japan).

Training is of vital importance for the referring and consulting actors in TD and even more so in teledermoscopy, both on how to capture a (dermoscopic) photo that is gradable and on the grading methods. Repetition and experience is key in obtaining and maintaining these skills.

From Pilot to Practice

Teledermatology services have started up all over the world, in most cases as part of a research program. Results are positive more often than not, but TD services have predominantly remained in the pilot setting [20]. Over the last 5 years however, in several countries, TD services have fully matured. In the USA, 36 active services have been identified with an annual median consult volume per service of 309 (range, 5–6,500) and all with a sustainable method of reimbursement [62]. In the Netherlands TD is practiced by the majority of Dutch GPs and dermatologists [18].

The consult volume is still increasing yearly, with over 30,000 teleconsultations performed in 2011 and its reimbursement integrated in the national health insurance plan. New Zealand has a successful melanoma screening service with clinics for dermoscopic photography across the country receiving over 20,000 patients per year [61].

The common factor in many of these success stories is the cooperation of both scientific institutes and commercial companies. This combination proves to be a driving force in the evolution of TD. The authors have described this route in a model called Health Management Practice, in which private and public parties and independent knowledge institutes jointly develop and study telemedicine tools and their outcomes and drive introduction in regular care [63].

Health Management Practice Model
Telemedicine Development
Technology and new healthcare processes lead to an integrated telemedicine service including software, hardware, infrastructure, hosting, education, and management meeting (national) requirements of safety, security, connectivity, and user-friendliness.

Health Management Research
Independent research aims to collect evidence that the use of telemedicine services increases efficiency leading to increased production volume and better quality of care at equal or lower costs.

Health Management Implementation
Telemedicine stakeholders – manufacturers, users, policy makers, and health insurers – should all be actively involved in the design of practice and reimbursement models. When significant reductions in costs on a macro-level have been proven, the next step is to create a healthy business case to support the complete telemedicine service. In order to assure successful implementation in regular care, active support and marketing from all stakeholders should take place.

Conclusion

Telemedicine is a potentially strong instrument to keep healthcare accessible and affordable in the future. Since its introduction in 1995, teledermatology has proven itself a highly successful healthcare delivery method in rural as well as in overpopulated areas for a number of different purposes, resulting in healthcare that can be more efficient and has higher quality and lower costs. Teledermoscopy is an exciting new method that can greatly improve triage of patients with skin cancer when implemented under the right conditions. Several mature teledermatology services with sustainable reimbursement models have developed in the last 5 years and more are on the way. Still, the success of teledermatology highly depends on the people who choose to adopt, use, and promote it and their determination to change the way healthcare is delivered.

Glossary

Teledermatology delivery of dermatologic care through information and communication technology.

Teledermoscopy digital dermoscopic lesion images (with or without clinical images) are transmitted electronically to a specialist for examination.

Telemedicine delivery of healthcare and sharing of medical knowledge by use of information and communication technology.

References

1. Strode SW, Gustke S, Allen A. Technical and clinical progress in telemedicine. JAMA. 1999;281:1066–8.
2. Central Bureau for Statistics. Centraal Bureau voor de Statistiek. Den Haag/Heerlen. http://www.cbs.nl. Accessed 17 Sept 2010.
3. National Institute for Public Health and the Environment. RIVM. Bilthoven: Kosten van Ziekten in Nederland; 2003, versie 1.1. http://www.kostenvan-ziekten.nl. Accessed 22 Sept 2010.
4. Wurm EM, Hofmann-Wellenhof R, Wurm R, et al. Telemedicine and teledermatology: past, present and future. J Dtsch Dermatol Ges. 2008;6:106–12.

5. Massone C, Wurm EM, Hofmann-Wellenhof R, et al. Teledermatology: an update. Semin Cutan Med Surg. 2008;27:101–5.

6. Kanthraj GR. Newer insights in teledermatology practice. Indian J Dermatol Venereol Leprol. 2011;77: 276–87.

7. Pathipati AS, Lee L, Armstrong AW. Health-care delivery methods in teledermatology: consultative, triage and direct-care models. J Telemed Telecare. 2011;17:214–6.

8. Schreier G, Hayn D, Kastner P, et al. A mobile-phone based teledermatology system to support self-management of patients suffering from psoriasis. Conf Proc IEEE Eng Med Biol Soc. 2008;2008:5338–41.

9. Watson AJ, Bergman H, Williams CM, et al. A randomized trial to evaluate the efficacy of online follow-up visits in the management of acne. Arch Dermatol. 2010;146:406–11.

10. Hayn D, Koller S, Hofmann-Wellenhof R, et al. Mobile phone-based teledermatologic compliance management – preliminary results of the TELECOMP study. Stud Health Technol Inform. 2009;150:468–72.

11. Fruhauf J, Schwantzer G, Ambros-Rudolph CM, et al. Pilot study on the acceptance of mobile teledermatology for the home monitoring of high-need patients with psoriasis. Australas J Dermatol. 2012;53:41–6.

12. Eminovic N, Witkamp L, Ravelli AC, et al. Potential effect of patient-assisted teledermatology on outpatient referral rates. J Telemed Telecare. 2003;9:321–7.

13. Perednia DA, Brown NA. Teledermatology: one application of telemedicine. Bull Med Libr Assoc. 1995;83:42–7.

14. Perednia DA, Allen A. Telemedicine technology and clinical applications. JAMA. 1995;273:483–8.

15. Levin YS, Warshaw EM. Teledermatology: a review of reliability and accuracy of diagnosis and management. Dermatol Clin. 2009;27:163–76, vii.

16. Warshaw EM, Hillman YJ, Greer NL, et al. Teledermatology for diagnosis and management of skin conditions: a systematic review. J Am Acad Dermatol. 2011;64:759–72.

17. Eminovic N, Dijkgraaf MG, Berghout RM, et al. A cost minimisation analysis in teledermatology: model-based approach. BMC Health Serv Res. 2010;10:251.

18. van der Heijden JP, de Keizer NF, Bos JD, et al. Teledermatology applied following patient selection by general practitioners in daily practice improves efficiency and quality of care at lower cost. Br J Dermatol. 2011;165:1058–65.

19. van der Heijden JP, Spuls PI, Voorbraak FP, et al. Tertiary teledermatology: a systematic review. Telemed J E Health. 2010;16:56–62.

20. Eminovic N, de Keizer NF, Bindels PJ, et al. Maturity of teledermatology evaluation research: a systematic literature review. Br J Dermatol. 2007;156:412–9.

21. Chung P, Yu T, Scheinfeld N. Using cellphones for teledermatology, a preliminary study. Dermatol Online J. 2007;13:2.

22. Ebner C, Wurm EM, Binder B, et al. Mobile teledermatology: a feasibility study of 58 subjects using mobile phones. J Telemed Telecare. 2008;14:2–7.

23. Lamel SA, Haldeman KM, Ely H, et al. Application of mobile teledermatology for skin cancer screening. J Am Acad Dermatol. 2012;67:576–81.

24. Massone C, Lozzi GP, Wurm E, et al. Cellular phones in clinical teledermatology. Arch Dermatol. 2005;141: 1319–20.

25. Tran K, Ayad M, Weinberg J, et al. Mobile teledermatology in the developing world: implications of a feasibility study on 30 Egyptian patients with common skin diseases. J Am Acad Dermatol. 2011;64:302–9.

26. Farshidi D, Craft N, Ochoa MT. Mobile teledermatology: as doctors and patients are increasingly mobile, technology keeps us connected. Skinmed. 2011;9: 231–8.

27. Kroemer S, Fruhauf J, Campbell TM, et al. Mobile teledermatology for skin tumour screening: diagnostic accuracy of clinical and dermoscopic image tele-evaluation using cellular phones. Br J Dermatol. 2011;164:973–9.

28. Massone C, Hofmann-Wellenhof R, Ahlgrimm-Siess V, et al. Melanoma screening with cellular phones. PLoS One. 2007;2:e483.

29. Massone C, Brunasso AM, Campbell TM, et al. Mobile teledermoscopy – melanoma diagnosis by one click? Semin Cutan Med Surg. 2009;28:203–5.

30. Varma S. Mobile teledermatology for skin tumour screening. Br J Dermatol. 2011;164:939–40.

31. Moreno-Ramirez D, Ferrandiz L, Galdeano R, et al. Teledermatoscopy as a triage system for pigmented lesions: a pilot study. Clin Exp Dermatol. 2006;31:13–8.

32. Tan E, Yung A, Jameson M, et al. Successful triage of patients referred to a skin lesion clinic using teledermoscopy (IMAGE IT trial). Br J Dermatol. 2010; 162:803–11.

33. Koller S, Hofmann-Wellenhof R, Hayn D, et al. Teledermatological monitoring of psoriasis patients on biologic therapy. Acta Derm Venereol. 2011;91:680–5.

34. Fruhauf J, Schwantzer G, Ambros-Rudolph CM, et al. Pilot study using teledermatology to manage high-need patients with psoriasis. Arch Dermatol. 2010;146: 200–1.

35. Binder B, Hofmann-Wellenhof R, Salmhofer W, et al. Teledermatological monitoring of leg ulcers in cooperation with home care nurses. Arch Dermatol. 2007;143:1511–4.

36. Salmhofer W, Hofmann-Wellenhof R, Gabler G, et al. Wound teleconsultation in patients with chronic leg ulcers. Dermatology. 2005;210:211–7.

37. Scheinfeld N. The use of teledermatology to supervise dermatology residents. J Am Acad Dermatol. 2005;52:378–80.

38. Whited JD. Economic analysis of telemedicine and the teledermatology paradigm. Telemed J E Health. 2010;16:223–8.

39. Pak HS, Datta SK, Triplett CA, et al. Cost minimization analysis of a store-and-forward teledermatology consult system. Telemed J E Health. 2009;15:160–5.

40. Bowns IR, Collins K, Walters SJ, et al. Telemedicine in dermatology: a randomised controlled trial. Health Technol Assess. 2006;10:iii–xi, 1.

41. Collins K, Walters S, Bowns I. Patient satisfaction with teledermatology: quantitative and qualitative results from a randomized controlled trial. J Telemed Telecare. 2004;10:29–33.

42. Hsueh MT, Eastman K, McFarland LV, et al. Teledermatology patient satisfaction in the Pacific Northwest. Telemed J E Health. 2012;18:377–81.

43. Kvedar JC, Menn ER, Baradagunta S, et al. Teledermatology in a capitated delivery system using distributed information architecture: design and development. Telemed J. 1999;5:357–66.

44. Whited JD, Hall RP, Foy ME, et al. Patient and clinician satisfaction with a store-and-forward teledermatology consult system. Telemed J E Health. 2004;10: 422–31.

45. Williams TL, Esmail A, May CR, et al. Patient satisfaction with teledermatology is related to perceived quality of life. Br J Dermatol. 2001;145:911–7.

46. Collins K, Nicolson P, Bowns I, et al. General practitioners' perceptions of store-and-forward teledermatology. J Telemed Telecare. 2000;6:50–3.

47. Piccolo D, Smolle J, Wolf IH, et al. Face-to-face diagnosis vs telediagnosis of pigmented skin tumors: a teledermoscopic study. Arch Dermatol. 1999;135: 1467–71.

48. Argenziano G, Soyer HP. Dermoscopy of pigmented skin lesions – a valuable tool for early diagnosis of melanoma. Lancet Oncol. 2001;2:443–9.

49. Kittler H, Pehamberger H, Wolff K, et al. Diagnostic accuracy of dermoscopy. Lancet Oncol. 2002;3:159–65.

50. Braun RP, Meier M, Pelloni F, et al. Teledermatoscopy in Switzerland: a preliminary evaluation. J Am Acad Dermatol. 2000;42:770–5.

51. Coras B, Glaessl A, Kinateder J, et al. Teledermatoscopy in daily routine – results of the first 100 cases. Curr Probl Dermatol. 2003;32:207–12.

52. Fabbrocini G, Balato A, Rescigno O, et al. Telediagnosis and face-to-face diagnosis reliability for melanocytic and non-melanocytic 'pink' lesions. J Eur Acad Dermatol Venereol. 2008;22:229–34.

53. Ferrara G, Argenziano G, Cerroni L, et al. A pilot study of a combined dermoscopic-pathological approach to the telediagnosis of melanocytic skin neoplasms. J Telemed Telecare. 2004;10:34–8.

54. Ishioka P, Tenorio JM, Lopes PR, et al. A comparative study of teledermatoscopy and face-to-face examination of pigmented skin lesions. J Telemed Telecare. 2009;15:221–5.

55. Piccolo D, Smolle J, Argenziano G, et al. Teledermoscopy – results of a multicentre study on 43 pigmented skin lesions. J Telemed Telecare. 2000;6: 132–7.

56. Warshaw EM, Lederle FA, Grill JP, et al. Accuracy of teledermatology for pigmented neoplasms. J Am Acad Dermatol. 2009;61:753–65.

57. Argenziano G, Soyer HP, Chimenti S, et al. Dermoscopy of pigmented skin lesions: results of a consensus meeting via the Internet. J Am Acad Dermatol. 2003;48:679–93.

58. Di Stefani A, Zalaudek I, Argenziano G, et al. Feasibility of a two-step teledermatologic approach for the management of patients with multiple pigmented skin lesions. Dermatol Surg. 2007;33: 686–92.

59. Piccolo D, Soyer HP, Chimenti S, et al. Diagnosis and categorization of acral melanocytic lesions using teledermoscopy. J Telemed Telecare. 2004;10:346–50.

60. Tan E, Oakley A, Soyer HP, et al. Interobserver variability of teledermoscopy: an international study. Br J Dermatol. 2010;163:1276–81.

61. Lim D, Oakley AM, Rademaker M. Better, sooner, more convenient: a successful teledermoscopy service. Australas J Dermatol. 2012;53:22–5.

62. Armstrong AW, Wu J, Kovarik CL, et al. State of teledermatology programs in the United States. J Am Acad Dermatol. 2012;67:939–44.

63. Witkamp L, van der Heijden JP. Health management practice as a method to introduce teledermatology: experiences from the Netherlands. In: Telemedicine in dermatology. Berlin/Heidelberg: Springer; 2012.

Automated Content-Based Image Retrieval: Application on Dermoscopic Images of Pigmented Skin Lesions

Alfonso Baldi, Raffaele Murace, Emanuele Dragonetti, Mario Manganaro, and Stefano Bizzi

---

Key Points

- Dermoscopy is a noninvasive diagnostic technique for the in vivo observation of PSLs, allowing a better visualization of surface and subsurface structures.
- The results of dermoscopic examination have limitations especially for the inexperienced, and they are effective only if the users are trained formally.
- In order to reduce the learning curve of nonexpert clinicians and to mitigate problems inherent in the reliability and reproducibility of the diagnostic criteria used in pattern analysis, several indicative methods based on diagnostic algorithms have been introduced in the last few years.
- Automatic image-based diagnosis attempts have been the subject of active research in biomedical image analysis since a number of years.
- FIDE is a CBIR system effective in retrieving PSL images with known pathology visually similar to the image under evaluation giving a valuable and intuitive aid to the clinician in the decision-making process.

A. Baldi (✉)
Department of Environmental, Biological and Pharmaceutical Sciences and Technologies, Second University of Naples,
Via L. Armanni 5, Naples 80138, Italy

Futura-onlus, Via Pordenone 2,
Rome 00182, Italy
e-mail: alfonsobaldi@tiscali.it

R. Murace • E. Dragonetti
Futura-onlus, Via Pordenone 2,
Rome 00182, Italy

M. Manganaro • S. Bizzi
Advanced Computer Systems (ACS),
Via della Bufalotta 378, Rome 00139, Italy

Introduction

Human cutaneous melanoma is a highly aggressive neoplasm, characterized by rapidly growing incidence and elevated mortality rate. Precocious diagnosis is very important, since early melanomas are locally controlled with surgical excision [1]. Nevertheless, about 20 % of patients will develop metastatic tumors due to its high malignancy [2]. In fact, when this tumor reaches the metastatic stage, it establishes powerful mechanisms of resistance to chemotherapy, radiation, and biological intervention, thus affecting the efficacy of current medical therapies [3, 4]. Melanoma incidence has significantly increased in the last decade, reaching currently 18 new cases per 100,000 population per year in the USA [5, 6]. Early detection and surgical excision still remain the only tactics to reduce mortality.

A. Baldi et al. (eds.), *Skin Cancer*, Current Clinical Pathology,
DOI 10.1007/978-1-4614-7357-2_35, © Springer Science+Business Media New York 2014

The traditional screening tests require a skin naked-eye examination by an experienced clinician, generally based on the ABCD rule [7]. However, this system may fail to detect many difficult or borderline pigmented skin lesions (PSLs) which are small or/and regular in shape or color.

Dermatoscopy and Computer-Aided Analysis of Digital Images

Dermoscopy (dermatoscopy, epiluminescence microscopy, incident light microscopy, skin surface microscopy) is a noninvasive diagnostic technique for the in vivo observation of PSLs. Dermoscopy allows the identification of dozens of morphological features such as pigment networks, dot/globules, streaks, blue-white areas, and blotches. Several studies [7] have shown that this method may significantly improve diagnostic sensitivity compared with clinical diagnosis by naked eye. However, it must be underlined that great limitations exist if this technique is used by inexperienced people, due to the complexity of patterns and their interpretation. In fact, it has been demonstrated that dermoscopy may actually lower the diagnostic accuracy in the hands of inexperienced dermatologists [8]. To overcome this problem, several methods based on diagnostic algorithms have been developed in the last years. The ABCD rule, the 3-point checklist, the 7-point checklist, the Menzies' method, and the CASH algorithm are the most relevant ones [7–11]. Recently, it has been proposed that the transfer of the ABCD attributes, as well as of other features based on texture, into automatically computed quantities, could be the basis for the development of systems designed to provide computer-aided analysis of digital images obtained by dermoscopy [12]. The proposed computer-assisted methods have different set of features extracted, digitized dermoscopic images, feature selection, and classification methods. Logically, the effectiveness of these systems depends largely on the dataset used [13, 14]. Interestingly, some recent works have investigated the possibility to set up automated analysis of dermoscopic images in melanoma diagnosis, using different strategies based on machine learning algorithms [15–19].

Unfortunately, all these studies have shown that at this stage, all the proposed image analysis systems are effective in the identification of melanomas that are also clinically obvious, but they have significant limited capabilities to discriminate between borderline lesions and early malignant melanoma [20]. Therefore, so far, these computer-assisted diagnostic imaging tools fail to provide a diagnostic advantage to the experienced clinicians.

Content-Based Image Retrieval (CBIR) Systems

Today, medical images represent the major amount of information collected for medical data. In hospitals, medical images are normally processed and saved digitally on picture archiving and communication systems (PACS) along with some text description. An image retrieval system is part of a digital asset management system for browsing, searching, and retrieving images from a large database. Content-based image retrieval (CBIR) technology exploits the visual content in image data. It has been proposed to benefit the management of increasingly large biomedical image collections as well as to aid clinical medicine, research, and education [21–23]. CBIR intends overcoming the limitations inherent in metadata-based systems. Actually, the search of textual information about images is really simple, but it is impossible to retrieve data based on the characteristics of the images, using existing technology. In fact, all the searches on figures must be carried on metadata, such as captions or keywords, since there is not the possibility to examine image content. Indeed, CBIR is the application of computer vision to the image retrieval problem. "Content based" means that the search will be based on the actual contents of the image. The term "content" could refer to colors, shapes, textures, or any other information that can be derived from the image itself.

A workshop in Redwood, California, organized in 1992 by the US National Science

Foundation can be considered the first step of a large volume of scientific research of the last 20 years about CBIR development in different fields, including medicine [24]. This scientific activity has developed techniques, tools, and algorithms that have originated from fields such as statistics, pattern recognition, signal processing, and computer vision.

Among the others, CBIR of medical images has achieved a significant improvement [21, 24–26]. However, medical CBIR is still not usable in clinical practice. Principal cause of this situation is the gap that is still very important, between people involved in the generation of the mathematical applications and the medical community. As a logical consequence of this situation, the large volume of scientific research produced on the topic of CBIR is still not paralleled by an equally significant availability of operational tools available in the clinical setting.

Dermoscopic CBIR: The FIDE System

Automatic image-based diagnosis attempts have been the subject of active research in biomedical image analysis in the recent years [27–30]. The process of describing picture content in textual terms takes on a specific meaning in the case of image-based diagnostic activities, e.g., in dermatological settings. Abstract features and machine learning methodologies or problem-oriented model-based systems have been employed. Yet, the main problem with automated diagnostic analysis is their real effectiveness in the clinical practice with a disproportionate cost of false negatives. Specifically for the diagnosis of melanomas, it has been already underlined the fact that these automatic image-based tools are real effective only when applied on clinical obvious melanomas. Indeed, the role of the expert interpreter and the related responsibilities should not be abdicated.

Our research group has recently proposed an original CBIR system for dermoscopic image analysis; we have named it FIDE [31]. The original approach is to documenting the image analysis side of the diagnostic process, focusing on

accompanying and aiding it and on providing efficient digital atlas navigation. The aim of this system is to provide precision (cases most similar to the one under analysis) and to clarify context (similar cases in different categories). In Fig. 35.1 a scheme of the FIDE system is depicted. FIDE does not give indications on a possible diagnosis by an automated interpretation system. On the contrary, the system presents a number of similar cases from a large atlas. Therefore, this CBIR system can be used to retrieve and display cases that are objectively similar by image content to the one under analysis, together with medical records for the analyst to consider in order to document and assist the interpretation and diagnosis procedures. Furthermore, the diagnostic procedure can be documented by logging the acquired images.

The statistical analysis performed in order to assess the similarity among image items is based on a hierarchical Bayesian model-based data analysis approach. The RGB signal level model $p(D)$ is linked to a high-dimensional primitive descriptor level $p(P)$ taking into account the color as well as geometric information extracted from the data and in turn to a secondary, lower-dimensionality, independent synthetic descriptor level $p(S)$ by conditional probabilistic links $p(P|S)$, $p(S|P)$. Inference is conducted in order to obtain the posterior density $p(S|P)\ p(P|D)\ p(D)$. The obtained densities are compared with each other taking into account a bank of distance and divergence measures to carry out an association level search procedure. Category search is employed to limit search results discriminating among retrieval outcomes of different natures. Standard measures of retrieval performance are considered in the development and evaluation of the system performance. Clusters are defined by the available supervised diagnoses attached to each of the items. The centers of mass of each of the clusters can be calculated, as the relative distances of the different centers of mass provide a further measure of the quality of the ranking output by the retrieval system. The methodological strategies used for images retrieving and archive access have been described in detail in a previous publication [31].

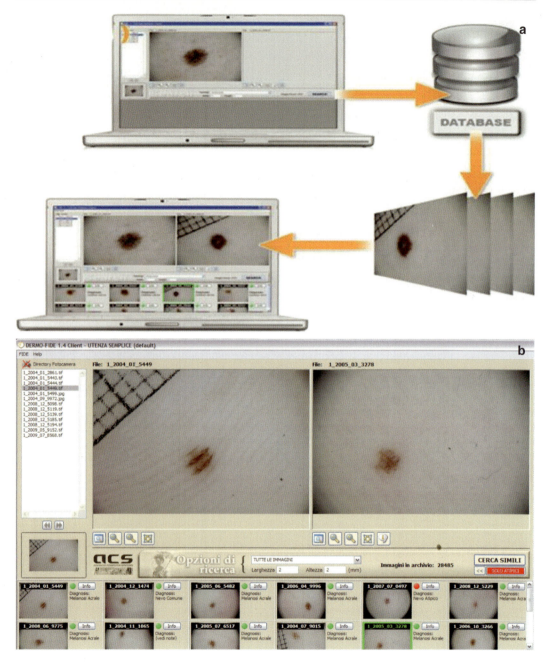

Fig. 35.1 (**a**) Scheme of the FIDE system. (**b**) An exemplificative outcome of the search for similar pigmented skin lesions

The FIDE system, indeed, is effective in retrieving PSL images with known pathology visually similar to the image under evaluation. This performance gives a helpful and valuable aid to the clinician in the decision-making process. Indeed, we argue that a system, able to retrieve

and present cases with known pathology similar in appearance to the lesion under evaluation, may provide an intuitive and effective support to clinicians which potentially can improve their diagnostic accuracy. Nevertheless, based on its ability to retrieve images similar to the one chosen as query, FIDE can be useful as a training tool for medical students and inexpert practitioners. In fact, by using it would be possible to browse large collections of PSL images using their visual attributes. The system will allow the user to mark retrieved images as positive and negative relevance feedback. Finally, the proposed system can be used to create appropriate CBIR Web Services that can be used remotely to perform query by example in various PSL image databases around the world and can be a very good complement to text-based retrieval methods [32].

Conclusion

Dermoscopy, actually, is one of the major imaging modalities used in the diagnosis of melanoma, having significant higher discrimination power than naked-eye examination. Computer-assisted automated diagnosis of PSL by means of CBIR systems is a promising research field that probably will greatly increase the early diagnosis of melanomas in the near future. FIDE represents, indeed, the first CBIR system successfully applied to dermoscopic images. In order to assess the real clinical impact of this system, it will be necessary to greatly increase the number of cases analyzed and the medical groups using it. Finally, a similar search engine finds possible usage in all other sectors of imaging diagnostic or digital signals (NMR, video, radiography, endoscopy, TAC, etc.), which could be supported by the huge amount of information available in medical archives.

Acknowledgments This work was supported by a grant from FUTURA-onlus to A.B. and by a grant from Regione Lazio (Legge 598/94 grant MCC-1792) to Advanced Computer System. A.B., R.M., and E.D. are scientific advisers of Advanced Computer System.

Glossary

Content-based image retrieval (CBIR) also known as *query by image content* (*QBIC*) and *content-based visual information retrieval* (*CBVIR*) is the application of computer vision techniques to the image retrieval problem, that is, the problem of searching for digital images in large databases.

Dermoscopy A noninvasive diagnostic technique for the early diagnosis of melanoma and the evaluation of other pigmented and nonpigmented lesions on the skin that are not as well seen with the unaided eye.

References

1. Nathan FE, Mastrangelo MJ. Systemic therapy in melanoma. Semin Surg Oncol. 1998;14:319–27.
2. Soengas MS, Lowe SW. Apoptosis and melanoma chemoresistance. Oncogene. 2003;22:3138–51.
3. Campioni M, Santini D, Tonini G, Murace R, Dragonetti E, Spugnini EP, Baldi A. Role of Apaf-1, a key regulator of apoptosis, in melanoma progression and chemoresistance. Exp Dermatol. 2005;14:811–8.
4. Helmbach H, Rossmann E, Kern MA, Schadendorf D. Drug-resistance in human melanoma. Int J Cancer. 2001;93:617–22.
5. Lens MB, Dawes M. Global perspectives of contemporary epidemiological trends of cutaneous malignant melanoma. Br J Dermatol. 2004;150:179–85.
6. Schaffer JV, Rigel DS, Kopf AW, Bolognia JL. Cutaneous melanoma: past, present, and future. J Am Acad Dermatol. 2004;51:S65–9.
7. Soyer HP, Argenziano G, Zalaudek I, Corona R, Sera F, Talamini R, Barbato F, Baroni A, Cicale L, Di Stefani A, Farro P, Rossiello L, Ruocco E, Chimenti S. Three-point checklist of dermoscopy. A new screening method for early detection of melanoma. Dermatology. 2004;208:27–31.
8. Binder M, Schwarz M, Winkler A, et al. A useful tool for the diagnosis of pigmented skin lesions for formally trained dermatologists. Arch Dermatol. 1995;131:286–91.
9. Argenziano G, Fabbrocini G, Carli P, De Giorgi V, Sammarco E, Delfino M. Epiluminescence micros copy for the diagnosis of doubtful melanocytic skin lesions. Comparison of the ABCD rule of dermatoscopy and a new 7-point checklist based on pattern analysis. Arch Dermatol. 1998;134:1563–70.
10. Scott Henning MJ, Dusza SW, Wang SQ, Marghoob AA, Rabinovitz HS, Polsky D, Kopf AW. The CASH (color, architecture, symmetry, and homogeneity) algorithm for dermoscopy. J Am Acad Dermatol. 2007;56:45–52.
11. Massone C, Di Stefani A, Soyer HP. Dermoscopy for skin cancer detection. Curr Opin Oncol. 2005;17: 147–53.
12. Perrinaud A, Gaide O, French LE, Saurat JH, Marghoob AA, Braun RP. Can automated dermoscopy image analysis instruments provide added

benefit for the dermatologist? A study comparing the results of three systems. Br J Dermatol. 2007;157: 926–33.

13. Boldrick JC, Layton CJ, Nquyen J, Swetter SM. Evaluation of digital dermoscopy in a pigmented lesion clinic: clinician versus computer assessment of malignancy risk. J Am Acad Dermatol. 2007;56: 417–21.

14. Burroni M, Sbano P, Cevenini G. Dysplastic naevus vs. in situ melanoma: digital dermoscopy analysis. Br J Dermatol. 2005;152:679–84.

15. Hoffmann K, Gambichler T, Rick A, Kreutz M, Anschuetz M, Grünendick T, Orlikov A, Gehlen S, Perotti R, Andreassi L, Newton Bishop J, Césarini JP, Fischer T, Frosch PJ, Lindskov R, Mackie R, Nashan D, Sommer A, Neumann M, Ortonne JP, Bahadoran P, Penas PF, Zoras U, Altmeyer P. Diagnostic and neural analysis of skin cancer (DANAOS). A multicentre study for collection and computer-aided analysis of data from pigmented skin lesions using digital dermoscopy. Br J Dermatol. 2003;149:801–9.

16. Burroni M, Corona R, Dell'Eva G, Sera F, Bono R, Puddu P, Perotti R, Nobile F, Andreassi L, Rubegni P. Melanoma computer-aided diagnosis: reliability and feasibility study. Clin Cancer Res. 2004;10:1881–6.

17. Gerger A, Pompl R, Smolle J. Automated epiluminescence microscopy: tissue computer analysis using CART and 1-NN in the diagnosis of melanoma. Skin Res Technol. 2003;9:105–10.

18. Oka H, Hashimoto M, Iyatomi H, Argenziano G, Soyer HP, Tanaka M. Internet-based program for automatic discrimination of dermoscopic images between melanomas and Clark naevi. Br J Dermatol. 2004;150:1041.

19. Seidenari S, Pellacani G, Grana C. Computer description of colours in dermoscopic melanocytic lesion images reproducing clinical assessment. Br J Dermatol. 2003;149:523–9.

20. Emre Celebi M, Iyatomi H, Schaefer G, Stoecker WV. Lesion border detection in dermoscopy images. Comput Med Imaging Graph. 2009;33:148–53.

21. Long LR, Antani S, Deserno TM, Thoma GR. Content-based image retrieval in medicine: retrospective assessment, state of the art, and future directions. Int J Health Inf Syst Inform. 2009;4:1–16.

22. Zhu Y, Huang X, Wang W, Lopresti D, Long R, Antani S, Xue Z, Thoma G. Balancing the role of priors in multi-observer segmentation evaluation. J Signal Process Syst. 2008;55:185–207.

23. Uwimana E, Ruiz ME. Integrating an automatic classification method into the medical image retrieval process. AMIA Annu Symp Proc. 2008;6:747–51.

24. Jain R. NSF workshop on visual information management systems. NSF workshop report, Redwood, 24–25 Feb 1992.

25. Smeulders AWM, Worring M, Santini S, Gupta A, Jain R. Content-based image retrieval at the end of the early years. IEEE Trans Pattern Anal Mach Intell. 2000;22:1349–58.

26. Müller H, Michoux N, Bandon D, Geissbuhler A. A review of content-based image retrieval systems in medical applications-clinical benefits and future directions. Int J Med Inform. 2004;73:1–23.

27. Schmid-Saugeons P, Guillod J, Thiran JP. Towards a computer-aided diagnosis system for pigmented skin lesions. Comput Med Imaging Graph. 2003;27:65–78.

28. Dorileo EAG, Frade MAC, Roselino AMF, Rangayyan RM, Azevedo-Marques PM. Color image processing and content-based image retrieval techniques for the analysis of dermatological lesions. In: 30th annual international conference of the IEEE Engineering in Medicine and Biology Society (EMBS 2008), Aug 2008. p. 1230–3.

29. Wollina U, Burroni M, Torricelli R, Gilardi S, Dell'Eva G, Helm C, Bardey W. Digital dermoscopy in clinical practise: a three-centre analysis. Skin Res Technol. 2007;13:133–42 (10).

30. Rahman MM, Desai BC, Bhattacharya P. Image retrieval-based decision support system for dermatoscopic images. In: IEEE symposium on computer-based medical systems, Los Alamitos, IEEE Computer Society, 2006, p. 285–90.

31. Baldi A, Murace R, Dragonetti E, Manganaro M, Guerra O, Bizzi S, Galli L. Definition of an automated Content-based Image Retrieval (CBIR) system for the comparison of dermoscopic images of pigmented skin lesions. Biomed Eng Online. 2009;8:18.

32. Baldi A, Quartulli M, Murace R, Dragonetti E, Manganaro M, Guerra O, Bizzi S. Cancers. 2010;2: 262–73.

Gene Expression Profiling in Melanoma

36

Stefania Crispi and Emilia Caputo

Key Points
- Microarray for transcriptome analysis and identification of melanoma deregulated genes.
- Next-generation sequencing (NGS) for analysis of structural genome variants and methylation patterns in melanoma.
- Molecular profiling in melanoma for development of diagnostic tools and of targeted therapy.

Introduction

Melanoma is the most aggressive skin cancer, accounting 75 % of all skin tumour deaths. In the recent years, its incidence has rapidly increased, especially in the USA and in Australia, where more frequently fair-skinned people are found [1]. The number of new melanoma estimated cases in 2009 reached 70,000 that, in turn, correspond to a total of about 8,000 estimated deaths [2]. Surgical

S. Crispi, PhD (✉)
Institute of Genetics and Biophysics,
I.G.B., A.Buzzati-Traverso, CNR,
Via Pierto Castellino, 111, Naples, Italy
e-mail: stefania.crispi@igb.cnr.it

E. Caputo
Department of Genetics and Biophysics,
Institute of Genetics and Biophysics,
Naples, Italy

resection is curative at early stage of melanoma diagnosis, while chemotherapy, biotherapy and immunotherapy remain ineffective for more advanced melanomas, with a median survival rate of only 6–9 months [3].

To date the molecular basis responsible for melanoma carcinogenesis and progression is still unknown [4].

In the last years, the advent of new high-throughput technologies, such as microarrays and next-generation sequencing (NGS), has made it possible to molecularly dissect complex diseases as cancer and has contributed to shed some light also in melanoma. Microarray technology allows to analyse simultaneously the expression of thousands of genes and to classify human tumours into homogeneous groups [5]. It also permits to realise genome-wide association (GWA) studies, examining up to two million markers in a single assay. GWAs are critical in melanoma research, where the association between mutations and patients is not well defined.

NGS technology is able to produce millions of DNA sequence reads in a single run, generating giga base pairs (Gbp) of data [6]. It is based on massive parallel sequencing in short reads (25–70 bases) of preamplified and tagged DNA/RNA template molecules, representing the whole genetic content of selected samples. The short reads are aligned to a known genome sequence as reference: the higher is the number of reads, the "deeper" sequence analysis is obtained, and more robust is the final outcome. The different applications related to this technology all provide a definitive and whole genome coverage, at both a quantitative

A. Baldi et al. (eds.), *Skin Cancer*, Current Clinical Pathology,
DOI 10.1007/978-1-4614-7357-2_36, © Springer Science+Business Media New York 2014

and a qualitative level, providing a digital transition from the analogical array-based assay.

The biggest challenge of NGS technology is to catalogue human genetic variations (http://www.genome.gov) with the aim to associate them with diseases, including cancer. The huge amount of data coming out from these applications needs to use specific bioinformatic tools in order to make the results helpful in translational medicine.

Here we describe new high-throughput analysis and, after a brief illustration on melanoma biology, we report the main microarray findings in the field of melanoma research.

High-Throughput Gene Expression Analysis Methods

Microarray Technology

Cell biology studies were widely transformed after the sequencing of human genome, giving rise to the birth of novel -*omics* disciplines. Thus, new high-throughput methods were applied to study specific cellular compartments or complements like proteins (*proteome*) and metabolites (*metabolome*).

Transcriptomics, usually referred as microarray analysis, measures thousands of genes in a single RNA sample. Transcriptomic analyses have greatly improved the understanding of genotypic-phenotypic correlation and of gene function in normal and disease states. Transcriptomic analysis also allows to associate specific combination of genes, proteins and metabolites with healthy or pathological conditions (biomarker profile), an important issue to clinically translate the microarray data and to perform better diagnosis and design the right therapeutic intervention [7].

Microarray technology was initially developed measuring differential expression of 45 Arabidopsis genes simultaneously [8]. A microarray is an ordered arrangement of samples where it is possible to pair known and unknown RNA samples based on base pairing rules. Thousands of spotted samples – with known identity – are immobilised on a solid support. The spots contain single-stranded DNA, cDNA or oligonucleotides (probes),

and their position is used for genes identification. The sequences in each spot bind unknown sequences in the sample (target) by means of base pairing, thus allowing parallel analysis for gene expression and gene discovery. The hybridisation is performed using as starting material total RNA extracted from biological samples of interest. The RNA is then converted into either single-stranded cDNA or cRNA, before hybridisation to the microarray surface. After washing procedures and laser scansion, it is possible to detect the probe-target interactions (Fig. 36.1).

Microarray is classified into double-channel and single-channel array, according to the labelling methods. Double-channel array [9] uses cDNA or oligonucleotides spotted on a solid surface. Two different samples, each labelled with a different fluorescent dye (usually Cye3 and Cye5), can be hybridised at the same time on a single array. After laser scansion, it is possible to visualise upregulated and downregulated genes at once (Fig. 36.1).

The surface of a single-channel array is coated by spotted- or "in situ" synthesised oligonucleotides, and one sample is hybridised on a single array (Fig. 36.1). One of the most used single-channel arrays, Affymetrix GeneChip® (www.Affymetrix.com), uses a photolithographic process for a high-density oligonucleotide synthesis, where over 1.4 million probe set are accommodated on a very small surface (11 μm^2 features on glass slides). In GeneChip®, multiple short oligonucleotides, perfectly matching to the 3′ ends of transcripts, are used to detect the whole expression level and multiple probe pairs (11–16 probe pairs or probe set) interrogate each transcript. Among the commercial single-channel microarray platforms, Affymetrix has the highest panel of microarray designed for a variety of different organisms and the highest public available datasets (www.ncbi.nlm.nih.gov/geo/). Another single-channel commercial platform is provided by Illumina (www.illumina.com) and is characterised by two interesting features: long oligonucleotides and probe replication. These arrays (Bead Array) are based on randomly arranged beads [10]. A specific oligonucleotide sequence, represented at about 30-fold redundancy, is assigned to each bead type. A series

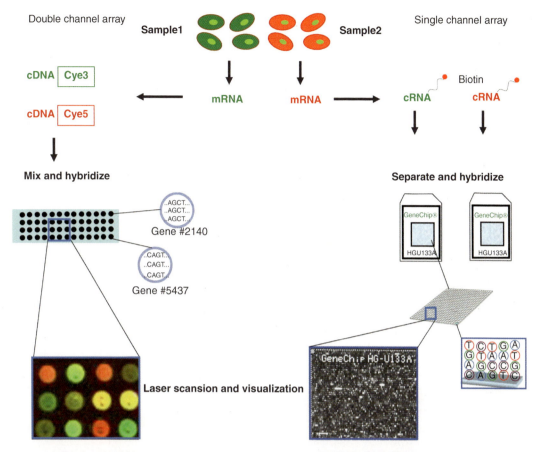

Fig. 36.1 Schematic representation of the double- and single-channel array technologies. The two methods differ in the sample preparation and labelling procedures. A typical microarray experiment consists in the expression profile comparison of at least two experimental conditions. In the double-channel technology, mRNA extracted from samples is converted in cDNA labelled using a different fluorescent. These molecules are then mixed and used to hybridise a single array. After laser scansion it is possible to associate differentially expressed genes with a starting sample. In the single-channel technology, mRNA from each sample is converted in cRNA (RNA copy) labelled with biotin. Each cRNA is separately hybridised to a single array. After laser scansion it is possible to visualise the hybridisation

of decoding hybridisations is used to identify each bead, and the high degree of replication makes robust measurements for each bead type.

Microarray Data Analysis

Microarray data analysis is a multistep process in which any step can be performed combining different computational tools. The advantage is that all the necessary tools are implemented in Bioconductor (www.bioconductor.org), an open source and open development project, based on the R statistical programming language.

The main steps in microarray data process are:

1. Quality control
2. Data analysis
3. Differential expression and data annotation

Each step described below can be applied to the different microarray platforms, downloading from the Bioconductor web page all the specific packages. Furthermore, for users with limited experience, it is possible to analyse data by using a graphical interface (OneChannelGUI) [11]. For simplicity, here we refer to GeneChip® 3′IVT array analysis.

1. Quality controls include (a) hybridisation/ construction artefact identification, (b) probe intensity distribution and (c) replicate quality

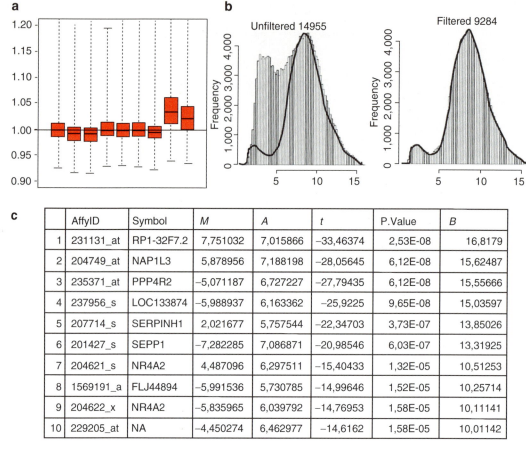

Fig. 36.2 Microarray data analysis, an example of output for the different steps: quality control (**a**), filtering (**b**) and annotation (**c**). (**a**) The NUSE box plot visualises a standard error from the probe-level model. NUSE plot allows to identify the divergent arrays that usually are not centred at 1.0 and appear spread out in comparison to the other arrays (as the last two box plots). (**b**) The IQR filtering output allows to filter out nonsignificant transcripts and select transcripts that will subsequently be analysed to detect the differential expression. In this example only genes with an intensity of at least 100 in at least half (50 %) of the arrays were selected. (**c**) Annotation of differentially expressed genes (top table). The table for each transcript returns different information associated to each probe ID and relative gene symbol. M log 2-fold change, A average intensity, $P.$ $Value$ p-value, T t-statistics, B log-odd statistics

evaluation. This step allows excluding the presence of array artefacts and dishomogeneity of different experimental groups. A function that can be used to identify hybridisation/washing artefacts is the "affyPLM". It produces probe-level models (PLM) by fitting a linear model to the probe data and enables a model to be fitted with probe-level and chip-level parameters for each probe set. The function generates array pseudo-images very useful for detecting artefacts on arrays. Another PLM method is based on plot of Normalized Unscaled Standard Errors (NUSE) (Fig. 36.2).

2. Data analysis allows to eliminate nonsignificant transcript. It includes (a) background subtraction, (b) data normalisation, (c) transcript intensity summary and (d) filtering of nonsignificant transcripts.

Normalisation and background correction procedures ensure that differences in intensities are really due to differential expression. The "affy" Bioconductor package uses intensities scaled so that each array has the same average value used for constant normalisation. If a non-linear relationship between arrays exists, it is more accurate to apply the quantile normalisation method [12] that makes the distribution of probe intensities for each set of arrays the same. This method is based on the concept that a quantile-quantile plot will show the same distribution of two data vectors if the plot is a straight diagonal line, but not if it is other than diagonal. Of course it is possible to have up to "n" dimensions if more than two arrays are available.

Genes estimated to be not expressed, according to user-defined specific parameters, are removed from the dataset by filtering (Fig. 36.2). IQR (interquartile range) is a filtering approach [13] implemented in the "genefilter" package which eliminates genes with no sufficient variation in expression across all samples, because of their weak discriminatory power.

Statistical validation methods are finally applied to identify differentially expressed genes and to obtain biological information from microarray data (data annotation). However, microarray experiments are conducted on a very limited number of biological replicates that is the exact opposite for an ideal statistical test. So many efforts have been made to optimise the statistical tests for microarray data. Furthermore, due to the reduced number of samples, the resulting differential expressed genes must be biologically validated using different approaches, such as real-time PCR or TMA assays. Several well-known statistical tests (e.g. t-test, ANOVA, linear model analysis) have been subjected to sophisticated optimisation to secure a good estimate of inter-/intra-sample variance despite the limited number of replicates. All methods assume that the transcription expression level of one gene is independent from that of the others. Best results are obtained with multiple statistical methods sharing a core of very robust differentially expressed genes that are always identified. The central issue is to find the best condition to obtain the highest number of only true signals [14].

In performing multiple statistical tests, two errors are possible: Type I error or false positive (a gene is identified as differentially expressed when it is not) and Type II error or false negative (a failure to identify a real differentially expressed gene). The Bioconductor package "multtest" implements widely applicable resampling-based single-step and stepwise Multiple Testing Procedures (MTP) that control a broad class of Type I error rates, null hypotheses and test statistics.

3. The ultimate goal in gene expression analyses is to identify differentially expressed genes and to understand their biological significance in the specific context.

An important issue is the specific association of probe set identifiers with genome-annotated transcripts (Fig. 36.2). A critical point is how the annotation has been produced. Generally, commercial arrays define probes retrieving transcript sequences from the last release Unigene (www.ncbi.nlm.nih.gov/entrez/query.fcgi?db=unigene), the major repository of sequences belonging to transcriptomes for all known organisms. To associate a probe set with a specific gene, Bioconductor uses a specific annotation library (AnnBuilder) which creates Bioconductor annotation libraries or XML annotation files starting from the association "probe set identifier"/"GenBank accession number" (i.e. the primary target for probes design).

The biological knowledge extraction from the candidate gene list represents the last step of the data analysis procedure. The assignment of functional categories to a gene list is the main challenge in understanding the biological question. Furthermore, it is generally accepted that genes sharing a similar expression profile might have similar biological functions.

Different public databases, as Gene Ontology (http://www.geneontology.org/), KEGG (http://www.genome.ad.jp/kegg/) and GSEA (www.broadinstitute.org/gsea/index.jsp), allow performing a functional analysis.

Gene Ontology (GO) contains a controlled vocabulary of terms (ontologies) describing gene product characteristics and gene product annotation. Three structured ontologies describe gene products in terms of their associated molecular functions, the biological processes they act and the cellular components they belong to. GO is organised as a graph, where each term is a node and the relationships between the terms are arcs between the nodes.

KEGG is another database based on hierarchal graphs representing the various KEGG objects, from the molecular level to the more complex levels. The structure contains graphs (each graph is a set of nodes or KEGG objects) and edges (that are the biological relationships).

GSEA is a tool that functionally associates pathways and differential expression by performing a "per-gene" statistics across genes. In this way, it is possible to determine if a priori defined set of genes shows statistically significant differences between two biological states and to identify either small changes in many genes or large changes in few genes [15].

Different commercial tools are also available to extract biological meaning from a candidate gene list, as IPA (www.ingenuity.com) and Pathway Studio (www.ariadnegenomics.com/products/databases/). IPA is a web-based software application, which enables to analyse and integrates gene expression data in which information is manually curated by experts in order to ensure accurate and detailed content.

Pathway Studio bases its core technology on MedScan® technology, a software able to extract biological information from multiple sources of public information (text, journals) and from different datasets.

Both software use databases derived from primary literature sources and the users can always link back to the original findings in the original source article.

NGS Technology

The completion of human genome sequence has represented the first step for the development of new sequencing methods to rapidly assemble and sequence whole genomes. NGS represents the latest methods that allow to studying structural genome variants and methylation patterns over gene expressions.

Three main platforms are used in NGS application: the 454 Genome Sequencer (Roche, www.454.com), the Genome Analyzer (Illumina, www.illumina.com) and the SOLiD (Life Technologies, www.appliedbiosystems.com). The other two available platforms, the Polonator G.007 and the HeliScope (Helicosbio), will not be described here.

NGS technologies are based on the clonal amplification of the sample to analyse, followed by sequencing and imaging procedures. The template preparation consists in a random fragmentation of DNA needed to obtain a library of fragments to amplify. These fragments are then ligated to adaptors that can bind universal primers in the amplification reaction.

454 and SOLiD realise the template amplification in a cell-free system, through an emulsion PCR (ePCR). Single-stranded DNA binding beads are encapsulated in micro-reactors by vigorous vortexing of the aqueous micelles containing PCR reactants and PCR oil. The amplified beads are purified and then deposited in the micro-wells of the slide (Roche) or onto the glass slide surface (Applied) where the sequencing reaction takes place (Fig. 36.3).

Illumina amplifies the DNA, by a solid amplification. The glass slides contain forward and reverse primers covalently attached to the surface. The fragmented DNA is linked to the adaptors that can bind the primers on the glass slide. Then clonally amplified clusters from each fragment are produced (Fig. 36.4).

The sequencing reactions in the Roche GS FLX 454 Genome Sequencer is based on sequencing-by-synthesis method, or pyrosequencing developed by Ronaghi [16], in which a chemiluminescent signal is produced when a nucleotide complementary to the template is inserted. The nucleotide incorporation is connected to inorganic pyrophosphate release that is measured by converting it into a light signal through the ATP that converts luciferin in oxyluciferin and light (Fig. 36.3). The 454 Sequencer produces an average read length of 400 bp, and its more powerful application is in the de novo genome assembly. The latest model (GS FLX+) can produce up to 750 bp per read with Sanger-like read length generating 500 Mbp (mega base pairs) of mappable sequences per run.

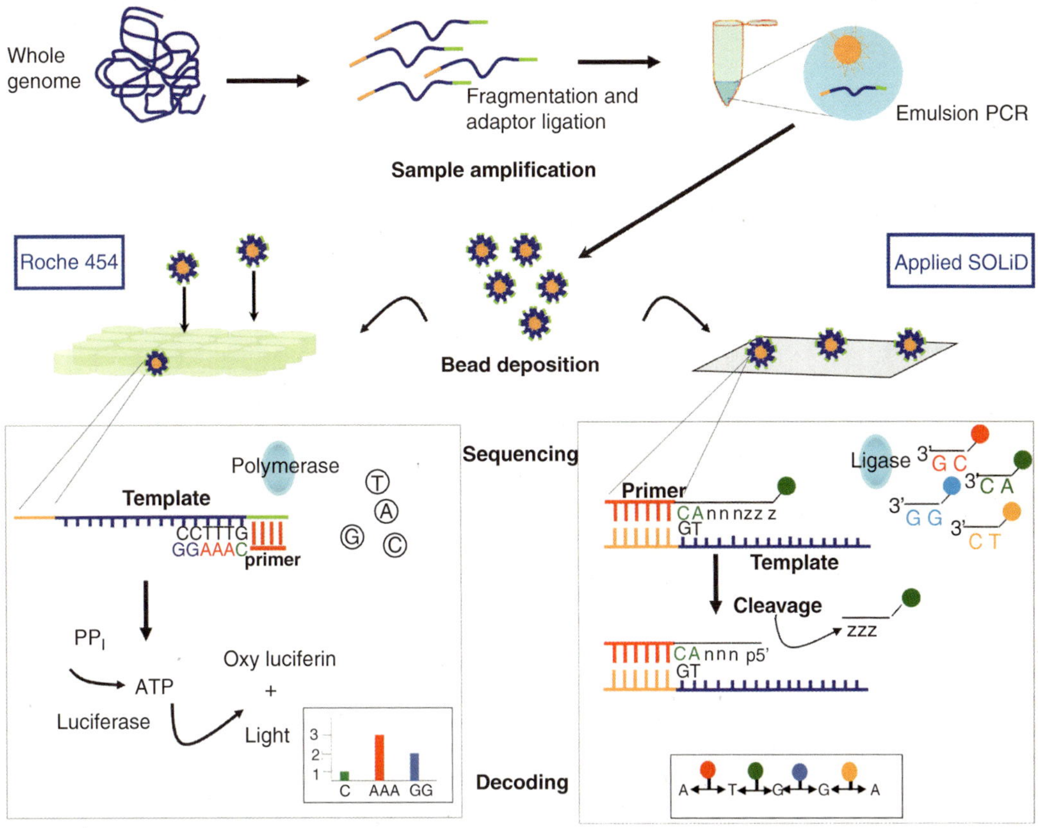

Fig. 36.3 NGS sample amplification and sequencing procedures for 454 and SOLiD platform. Samples to sequence are clonally amplified by emulsion PCR after fragmentation and ligation of adapter to the fragments. After amplification the bead-containing fragments deposited into picotiter-plate wells with sequencing enzymes (454) or onto a glass slide (SOLiD). Sequencing in 454 platforms is based on pyrosequencing. A nucleotide incorporation results in pyrophosphate (PPi) release that is then converted into light. The order and the intensity of the light peaks are recorded as a fluorogram revealing the DNA sequence. The light signal generated by complementary nucleotides will be proportional to the number of nucleotides incorporated. The SOLiD system uses sequencing-by-ligation method and a colour-space decoding. Sixteen different dinucleotides, corresponding to all possible 2-base combinations, are linked to six degenerate bases (nnnzzz) and to four different fluorescent labels at 5′ end. The template binds the complementary dinucleotide, and after ligation the degenerated nucleotides are cleaved and the fluorescence is recorded. The cycle is then repeated and completed after ten ligases and five different primers. The colour-base reads are converted into base-space reads based on a two-colour method, in which each base corresponds to different and fixed colour combination

The sequencing method in SOLiD platform is based on sequencing by ligation, with two-base encoding probes and four colours. The beads containing the template fragments are deposited on the slide and are ligated to specific 8-mer primers, fluorescently labelled in the 4 and 5 positions. The reads produced are in colour space and each ligation step is followed by fluorescence detection. A specific two-base encoding scheme permits to associate the four dinucleotides with one colour (Fig. 36.3). The sequence is then retrieved through the alignment with a colour-space reference sequence. The advantage of this method is that each template is interrogated twice. A complete round of ten ligations and five different primers sequence 50 base fragments and produce 80–100 Gbp of mappable sequences per run. A new recent model (5500xl) is able to generate over 2.4 billion reads per run and 200 Gbp.

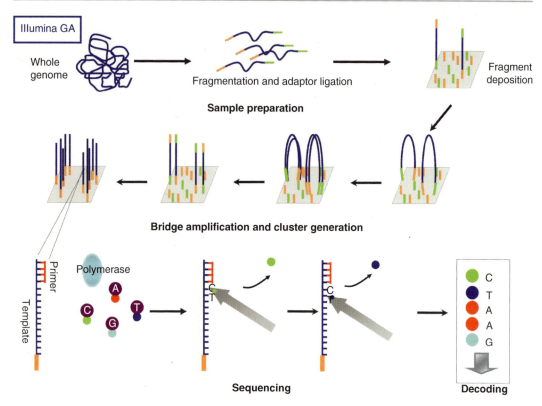

Fig. 36.4 Illumina Genome Analyzer sequencing with reversible terminators. Samples to sequence are fragmented and ligated to adapters. Single-stranded DNA fragments are added to glass surface where they bind complementary primers. Fragments are clonally amplified by bridge amplification generating clusters. Clusters are then denatured and sequencing starts with the addition of primer, polymerase and 4-colour reversible dye terminators. Fluorescence is recorded at each nucleotide incorporation. After imaging fluorescent dye is removed and the cycle restarts until the template is sequenced

The Illumina Genome Analyzer uses a sequencing method based on the use of reversible terminators in a cyclic three-step way: nucleotide incorporation, fluorescence imaging and cleavage. The clonally amplified molecules located on the slide are detected using a bridge amplification that extends cluster strands with all four nucleotides, each labelled with a different fluorescent dye. Each nucleotide is identified after the incorporation (Fig. 36.4). The cycle is repeated until the imaging reveals the sequence corresponding to each amplified template (50–75 bp). The latest Illumina sequencer (HiSeq 2000 Genome Analyzer) generates about 200 Gbp of short sequences per run.

Illumina and SOLiD platforms both represent the ideal solution for genome resequencing or for exomes and transcriptome assays, where reference sequences are available.

NGS Data Analysis

NGS assay produces large datasets of sequence reads in a massively parallel format. The reads must be aligned to reference data in order to obtain quantitative information about any parameter (position, variation or frequency) and relative to read differences from the reference sequence.

There are three main steps in NGS data management and analysis:
- Primary analysis or alignment
- Secondary analysis or assembly
- Tertiary analysis

The first two steps allow mapping the reads to the right genomic location before assembling them into longer contiguous sequences. The primary analysis is the transformation of image data in sequence data. The reads obtained can be in

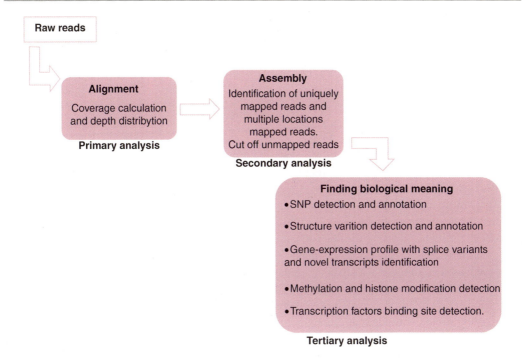

Fig. 36.5 NGS data analysis. Pipeline for NGS data analysis

sequence or in colour space depending on the platform used to generate data. This step also ranks the quality value of each nucleotide. Sequences obtained from the primary analysis are aligned to reference sequence in the secondary analysis. The reference is specifically selected based on the application. We can select a complete genome or a genome subset if we are analysing only the expressed genes. The tertiary analysis is a multistep procedure used for the extraction of biological information from the obtained data (Fig. 36.5).

1. The alignment to a reference sequence is fundamental to establish the failure or the success of an NGS experiment. Different algorithms can be used for alignment and assembly depending on the sequencing platform used. The two fundamental alignment algorithms are the hash-based method [17] and the Burrows-Wheeler transform method [18].

   The hash-based methods generate a lookup table that is designed to efficiently store noncontiguous keys (account numbers, part numbers, etc.) that may have wide gaps in their alphabetic and numeric sequences. In order to map a sequence, the program identifies in the reference sequence small strings where it is probable to find the best mapping. This step is then followed by a more accurate alignment algorithm, such as the Smith-Waterman [19]; it is used to determine the exact position of the reads on the genome reference sequence. This approach is used by different tools that can build the hash table either from input reads (MAQ, ZOOM, SHRiMP or ELAND that is part of the Illumina Suite) or from reference genome (SOAP, BFAST and MOSAIK).

   The Burrows-Wheeler transform method is an algorithm originally created for text compression (zip), which uses suffix arrays for rapid exact subsequence search. The method first generates an index of the reference genome, which is used for a rapid positioning of the reads on the genome. This method can be easily improved resulting in a faster processivity without loss in sensitivity. BOWTIE, BWA and SOAP2 are examples of tools that use BWT method.

2. Assembly has a more important role in analysing organisms for which a reference genome is not available. It is a procedure that allows having large continuous regions of

DNA sequence. The algorithms used to read the long sequences (800 bp) obtained from gel-capillary technologies were based on the assembly of overlapping sequences. Because of the short read lengths (25–50 bp) and large volumes of data generated by NGS assays, it is complex to assemble short reads using the classical shotgun method [20]. In fact it is difficult to distinguish repetitive sequences derived from adjacent genomic regions or from highly polymorphic loci. The NGS technology overcomes this limitation by oversampling the target genome with short reads from random positions, by using specific software.

Assembly methods are based on "graphs", a concept used in computer science composed by sets of nodes connected by sets of edges. The graph can be visualised as balls in space connected by arrows, with edges directionally connected from a node to another. Different paths can be viewed from different edges and it is possible to have intersecting paths. So an overlap graph might represent the reads and their overlaps [21]. Furthermore, the graph is able to discriminate in the 5′ and 3′ ends' reads, their length and the overlap length and type. Finally, paths between graphs represent contiguous parts and they can be converted in sequence.

The "de Bruijn graph" is a compact representation based on short words (k-mers). In the graph (k-mer graph), the nodes are all possible fixed-strength sequences (of symbols from the DNA alphabet) and the edges indicate the potentially overlapping sequences. The structure is based on very small sequences of fixed length k (k-mers), not reads; thus, high redundancy is naturally handled by the graph without affecting the number of nodes. Nonrepetitive sequences induce formation of a single path, while repeats induce convergent and divergent paths [22]. Many assembler tools are based on the "de Bruijn graph" (SHARCGS, VCAKE, VELVET, EULER-SR, EDENA, AbySS and ALLPATHS).

3. The complexity of the tertiary analysis is tightly linked to the assay. While pattern variation analysis is easy, digital gene expression assays are very complex. In fact expression measurements need to be normalised between datasets and statistical comparisons are critical in order to assess differences. Various bioinformatic approaches are available according to the application, as de novo sequencing, resequencing, and transcriptome (RNA-seq) or chromatin immunoprecipitation (ChIP-seq) sequencing analyses. Given the complexity of the final step in NGS data analysis, we will not further discuss in detail the methods available.

Tertiary analysis can be done using different packages from Bioconductor (www.bioconductor.org) and several commercial tools such as Golden Helix (www.goldenhelix.com) software and SeqSolve (www.integromics.com/ngs) that provide a global analysis starting from mapped reads. Golden Helix was specifically designed for genotype analysis, while SeqSolve performs RNA-seq or ChIP-seq analyses on any annotated genome.

Applications in Melanoma

Melanoma Biology

Melanoma originates from the pigment-producing melanocytes that are positioned at the epidermal-dermal junction and are interspersed among every five to ten basal keratinocytes. Despite the dynamic nature of epidermal shedding, involving constant growth, differentiation and vertical migration of keratinocytes, proliferation of melanocytes is strictly controlled and rarely observed under physiologic conditions, albeit melanocytes maintain a lifelong proliferation potential.

The developmental process of melanoma is characterised by a dramatic change of the cellular homeostasis due to the deregulated expression of many genes [4, 23].

The Clark model of melanoma genesis and progression has provided a basic and relatively straightforward platform for the hypothesised stepwise transformation of normal human epidermal melanocytes (NHEM) to melanoma, describing five distinct stages of progression based on histological criteria (Fig. 36.6) [24]. According to this model, melanocytes can proliferate and

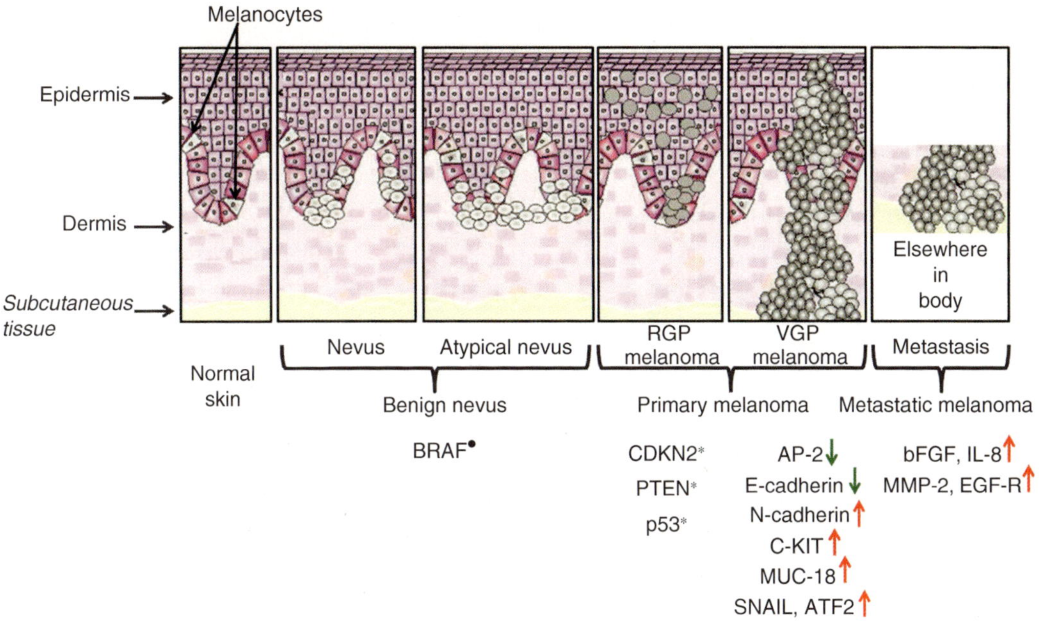

Fig. 36.6 Stepwise changes involved in melanoma genesis. Five distinct stages associated with the evolution of melanoma, from naevus to metastatic melanoma, are represented. Molecular events associated with melanoma progression are also reported. Constitutive activation was indicated with the symbol (•), while inactivation by mutation, deletion or epigenetic alterations was indicated with the symbol (*). Upregulated (↑) and downregulated (↓) genes were reported

spread, leading to a formation of a naevus or common mole. Based on the localisation of proliferating melanocytes, naevi can be classified as junctional, dermal or compound. Some naevi are dysplastic with morphologically atypical melanocytes. In the most cases, naevi are benign but can progress to the radial growth phase (RGP) melanoma, which consists of an intra-epidermal lesion, which could involve some local invasion of dermis. RGP cells can progress to vertical growth phase (VGP) primary cutaneous melanoma (PCM). This represents a more dangerous stage, in which the cells have potential metastatic properties, with nodules or nests of cells invading the dermis. Not all melanomas pass through each of these individual phases. RGP or VGP primary melanoma can develop directly from both isolated melanocytes and naevi, and both can progress directly to metastatic melanoma (MM).

There are four main clinical subtypes of melanoma [25]: superficial spreading melanoma (SSM), nodular melanoma, acral lentiginous melanoma (ALM) and lentigo maligna melanoma.

SSM is by far the most common form of melanoma, comprising approximately 70 % of all cases. It is usually flat with an intra-epidermal component, particularly at the edges, and it is linked to episodes of severe sunburn, especially at early age.

Nodular melanomas account for 15–30 % of all melanomas. It consists of raised nodules without a significant flat portion.

ALM accounts for 5 % of melanomas and is the most common subtype found in dark-skinned individuals. ALM tends to be found on the palms of the hands, the soles of the feet and in the nail bed and so is not associated with UV exposure.

Another 5 % of melanomas are lentigo maligna melanomas, which are typically located on the head and neck that seems associated with lifetime chronic sun exposure.

However, some lesions cannot be unequivocally classified as naevus or melanoma by histological evaluation of the primary tumour. These lesions are reported as borderline or melanocytic tumours of uncertain malignant potential.

Recently, a naevus/melanocytoma/melanoma paradigm for classification and clinical management of borderline melanocytic tumours has been reported [26], and the term *melanocytoma* has been introduced to indicate a group of melanocytic lesions with intermediate malignant potential, capable of metastasis to regional lymph nodes but showing limited potential for distant spread.

Microarray and NGS Output in Melanoma

The molecular basis of melanoma genesis and progression has not been fully elucidated [27]. Several validated genetic mutations have been described as responsible for melanocytic transformation. They include the deletion of the 9p21 CDKN2A familial melanoma locus, encoding the tumour suppressor INK4A and ARF, as well as the amplification of MITF as a lineage-specific oncogene [28]. Although naevi and melanomas at a very early stage share genetic alterations, such as oncogenic mutations in BRAF and NRAS [29–33], melanomas show recurrent pattern of chromosomal aberrations such as losses of chromosome 6q, 8p,9p and 10q along with gains of chromosomes 1q, 6p, 7, 8q, 17q and 20q, while naevi do not show detectable chromosomal aberrations by comparative genomic hybridisation (CGH) or karyotyping [34–36].

A wide variety of DNA and tissue microarray studies have been applied to identify potential candidate genes involved in the transition from melanocytes to metastatic melanomas [37–45]. A brief summary of these data is reported in Table 36.1, of which only few central ones will be discussed below in more details.

DeRisi and colleagues were one of the first group able to demonstrate the potentiality of high-density DNA microarray [46]. This work confirmed several candidate genes and putative melanoma-associated antigens, such as TRP-1, gp75, MCP-1 and WAF1 (p21) [47–49], by using a spotted microarray containing sequences corresponding to about 1,100 genes.

A comprehensive subsequent study examined the gene expression profiles of 31 cutaneous melanoma samples with the aim to identify a molecular

Table 36.1 Metastatic melanoma and differential gene expression

Study	Gene names	Expression in the metastatic phenotype
DeRisi et al. [46]	TRP-1/melanoma antigen gp75	Up
	MCP-1	Down
	P21 (WAF-1)	Down
Bittner et al. [50]	WNT-5	Up
Carr et al. [37]	Fibronectin	Up
	MART-1	Down
	CD63	Down
Haqq et al. [38]	REH	Up
	IGFBP1	Down
	S100A2	Down
	RBP1	Down
	PDGFRA	Down
	LUM	Down
	HLA-DQ	Down
	HLA-B1/2	Down
	ALOX5	Down
	TMP21	Down
Jaeger et al. [40]	AQP3*	Up
	DSC1	Up
	LGALS7*	Down
	SFN*	Down
	FGFBP1	Down
	KRT10/14	Down
	TACSTD2	Down
Riker et al. [41]	MAGEA1/2	Up
	MMP14	Up
	CSAG2	Up
	SPRR1A/B	Down
	AQP3*	Down
	CD24	Down
	FLG	Down
	KLK7	Down
	LGALS7*	Down
	RAB25	Down
	SFN*	Down
	ICEBERG	Down
	HAS3	Down
	ASAH3	Down
Karim et al. [44]	Cyclin D1	Down
	pRb	Down
Mehnert et al. [45]	VEGF-R2	Up

*Same genes identified in different studies

classification helpful to discriminate between a metastatic and non-metastatic phenotype in melanoma [50]. To this end 7,000 genes were studied using a cDNA microarray. Samples analysed were derived either by primary melanoma biopsy or by melanoma lymph node metastases. Hierarchical clustering analysis revealed a major cluster containing 19 samples distinct from the remaining samples. This cluster was further analysed to obtain a weighted gene list subsequently used for re-analysing all the samples. This analysis identified specific genes with reduced expression within the major cluster as integrin b1, integrin b3, integrin a1, syndecan 4 and vinculin 21. On the other hand, an enhanced expression outside this cluster was found for fibronectin, a pro-migratory molecule, which plays an important role for focal contacts in modulating cell motility.

Biological validation on samples belonging to the major cluster showed that they had reduced motility, invasive ability and vasculogenic mimicry compared to the cells deriving from tissues of the rest of specimens. To this respect, the molecular signature obtained from this study could be regarded as a marker for less aggressive phenotype. This study has been successively reviewed and discussed with additional experiments demonstrating that WNT-5 represents another good discriminator between the two clusters, being correlated with increased motility and invasiveness of melanoma cells. Moreover, high WNT-5 protein expression in melanoma specimens has been associated with bad prognosis of melanoma patients [37].

Several recent expression-profiling studies have been made to compare differential gene expression levels from benign or non-metastatic cells/tissues versus clinically aggressive tumours. These studies evidenced a complex molecular pattern in melanoma transcriptome, resulting in a not well-defined gene set whose expression changes are tightly linked to the phenotype [39–41].

A more recent study examined a larger number of tumours and compared a wide variety of specimens, including a well-documented gradation from thin to thick primary melanomas to metastatic melanomas [41]. In particular, GeneChip® array measuring transcript levels of the entire human genome (HG U133Plus 2.0) was used to investigate gene expression profiles of 40 MM and 42 PCM samples. However, considering that thin melanomas are the most difficult specimens

to acquire in a research setting where it is crucial to preserve RNA integrity, the analysis following hybridisation was limited to only few samples of thin melanomas. Nevertheless, some genes potentially involved in metastasis development were identified: MAGE, TRAG3 and PRAME; three genes known as melanoma tumour antigens showed an increased expression in advanced disease. These genes resulted highly expressed in thicker tumours, suggesting that melanoma phenotype becomes more metastatic-like as it gets thicker. The data were also integrated to GO database, showing a reduction or loss in the expression for genes involved in keratinocyte differentiation, epidermal development, cell adhesion and cell-to-cell signalling. All these pathways reflect a migratory potential gain that is typical of metastatic cell type. In addition, the homogeneity of expression shared by genes belonging to the same pathway, and the similar relative expression level, suggested a developmental change, rather than a regulation of cellular metabolism, thus supporting an epithelial-mesenchymal transition as the metastatic signature emerges [42].

Metastasis-relevant genes have been recently described in a genome-wide characterisation study [51] of primary and metastatic melanoma samples. Thirty genes significantly altered in metastatic relative to primary melanomas were identified by a statistical approach. A subset of these genes, including MET, ASPM, AKAP9, IMP3, PRKC9, RPA3 and SCAP2, were functionally validated and provided another tool for patient stratification.

A critical issue in melanoma research is the number of misdiagnoses that constitutes 13 % of total medical malpractice lawsuits. In this respect gene expression analysis has been helpful in discovering potential genes able to discriminate melanomas from naevi. Distinction of a melanoma from a benign naevus by standard histological criteria can be very difficult and/or impossible. Introduction of the sentinel lymph nodes technique [52] has increased the sensitivity of melanoma micro-metastasis detection compared to haematoxylin and eosin staining (H&E) method alone [53, 54]. Furthermore, histological analysis is limited by the ability of light microscopy to recognise the tumour cells, even enhanced by immunohistochemistry. Recently, 36 differentially expressed genes have been identified in melanomas and naevi [55]. The most statistically significant genes (PTN, L1CAM, GPX3, FABP7, RPL12, PHACTR1, DLC1, HLA-B, PRAME, NACA, Stat1, LCP2, GSTM2, HLA-A) might be used as a supplement to standard histology in melanoma.

Gene expression analysis has also been used to decipher the potential epigenetic mechanisms involved in melanoma development and progression. Several studies have also aimed to identify alterations in epigenetic of NHEM leading to an aggressive melanoma-like cell phenotype [56–60]. Muthusamy et al. used a strategy based on the combined treatment of cancer cells with a DNA methyltransferase and a histone deacetylase (HDAC) inhibitor. The treated cells were then analysed for their gene expression, and 17 epigenetically modulated genes were identified [61]. Among these genes QPCT, CYP1B1 and LXN resulted to be densely methylated in more than 95 % of melanoma samples, suggesting their potential use as therapeutic targets in melanoma clinical trials. These genes could be induced and reactivated via demethylation. Other putative gene targets with a differential methylation status in melanoma could be the suspected tumour suppressor genes (TSG) that are critical for the progression of melanoma, although they are not yet demonstrated [59, 60].

NGS has been recently applied to discover and quantify small, no-coding RNAs called miRNAs, in melanoma [62]. Little is known about the repertoire and the function of miRNAs in melanoma. In particular, three-pigment cell-specific miRNAs have been reported (MELmiRNA_197, MELmiRNA_434 and MELmiRNA_677), which could represent novel potential therapeutic modulators.

Finally, high-throughput gene expression analysis has also been used in melanoma research as a powerful diagnostic tool for clinical applications. A comprehensive DNA microarray study by the EORTC Melanoma group was aimed to investigate the correlation between gene expression profiles and clinical outcome in primary melanomas. A signature consisting of 254 genes

Table 36.2 An example of gene signature for good-prognosis melanomas

Gene names	Expression in the good-prognosis melanoma
PLXNB2	Up
ARFRP1	Up
IGKC	Up
Similar to tubulin a6	Up
OSIL; A170; p62B	Up
KCNIP2	Up
MHC, class I, E	Up
HLA-E	Up
GTPBP2	Up
MFGE8	Up
kiaa0353; dmn	Up
TXNDC5	Up
PILRA	Up
kiaa1067; kiaa1067	Up
Partial n-myc exon 3	Down
NFKBIB	Down
MTCH2	Down
CHST4	Down
MRPS5	Down
IDH1	Down
ITPA	Down

was described as an accurate indicator for patients at risk of developing distant metastasis. In particular, a novel gene signature, including karyopherin alpha 2, minichromosome maintenance proteins (MCMs), geminin and PCNA, was reported to discriminate patients with a poor clinical outcome [63].

Another recent study [43] used molecular profiling as a tool to predict the clinical outcome in patients suffering from stage III melanoma. To this end, RNA samples were collected from lymph node sections of melanoma patients and analysed for gene expression. A predictive algorithm based on the expression of a subset of 21 genes (Table 36.2) was specifically developed and could be applied to distinguish good-prognosis patients from those with bad prognosis.

The information obtained from gene expression profiling has been helpful for defining some molecular pathways associated to melanoma development. To date several molecules have been explored as targets for biological therapeutic design. In particular, several drugs have been developed for targets such as VEGFR, PDGFR, Raf kinases [64], MEK, Bcl-2 [65] and NF-kB [66] (Ras, HSP90,mTOR, PTEN, PI(3)K/Akt pathway) [67, 68]. However, more work needs to be made since these drugs are not very specific and show dangerous side effects. Several efforts are now going towards to the development of drugs targeting multiple pathways.

Conclusions

Although high-throughput gene analysis provides a plethora of genes, with many more genes being discovered every month, the mechanism of human melanoma progression and metastasis is still not fully understood. The development of advanced bioinformatics is becoming a critical step in order to analyse all these genes and pathways with overall function in cancer cells. Only a complete integration of gene microarray data to bioinformatic analysis will provide a more complete picture of the genesis and progression of melanoma, which will be helpful in designing novel diagnostic tools and tailored therapeutic strategies.

Acknowledgement   We are grateful to Anna Maria Aliperti for her assistance in the editing of the manuscript.

Glossary

ALM   Acral lentiginous melanoma, a melanoma subtype not associated with UV exposure

Cye3 and Cy5   Fluorescent dyes belonging to the cyanine dye family

Gbp   Giga base pairs, one billion pairs of DNA nucleotide bases

GWA   Genome-wide association

LMM   Lentigo maligna melanoma, a melanoma subtype associated with chronic sun exposure

MM   Metastatic melanoma

NGS   Next-generation sequencing

NHEM   Normal human epidermal melanocytes

PCM   Primary cutaneous melanoma

RGP   Radial growth phase melanoma

SSM   Superficial spreading melanoma, a melanoma subtype linked to severe sunburns

TMA   Tissue microarray

VGP   Vertical growth phase melanoma

References

1. Tsao H, Atkins MB, Sober AJ. Management of cutaneous melanoma. N Engl J Med. 2004;351(10):998–1012.
2. Jemal A, Siegel R, Ward E, Hao Y, Xu J, Thun MJ. Cancer statistics, 2009. CA Cancer J Clin. 2009;59(4):225–49.
3. Korn EL, Liu PY, Lee SJ, et al. Meta-analysis of phase II cooperative group trials in metastatic stage IV melanoma to determine progression-free and overall survival benchmarks for future phase II trials. J Clin Oncol. 2008;26(4):527–34.
4. Herlyn M, Ferrone S, Ronai Z, Finerty J, Pelroy R, Mohla S. Melanoma biology and progression. Cancer Res. 2001;61(11):4642–3.
5. Van't Veer LJ, Dai H, van de Vijver MJ, et al. Gene expression profiling predicts clinical outcome of breast cancer. Nature. 2002;415(6871):530–6.
6. Venter JC, Adams MD, Myers EW, et al. The sequence of the human genome. Science. 2001;291(5507):1304–51.
7. West M, Ginsburg GS, Huang AT, Nevins JR. Embracing the complexity of genomic data for personalized medicine. Genome Res. 2006;16(5):559–66.
8. Schena M, Shalon D, Davis RW, Brown PO. Quantitative monitoring of gene expression patterns with a complementary DNA microarray. Science. 1995;270(5235):467–70.
9. Shalon D, Smith SJ, Brown PO. A DNA microarray system for analyzing complex DNA samples using two-color fluorescent probe hybridization. Genome Res. 1996;6(7):639–45.
10. Gunderson KL, Kruglyak S, Graige MS, et al. Decoding randomly ordered DNA arrays. Genome Res. 2004;14(5):870–7.
11. Sanges R, Cordero F, Calogero RA. oneChannelGUI: a graphical interface to Bioconductor tools, designed for life scientists who are not familiar with R language. Bioinformatics. 2007;23(24):3406–8.
12. Bolstad BM, Irizarry RA, Astrand M, Speed TP. A comparison of normalization methods for high density oligonucleotide array data based on variance and bias. Bioinformatics. 2003;19(2):185–93.
13. von Heydebreck A, Huber W, Gentleman RC. Differential expression of the Bioconductor Project. Bioconductor Project Working Papers. 2004;Working Paper 7.
14. Jeffery IB, Higgins DG, Culhane AC. Comparison and evaluation of methods for generating differentially expressed gene lists from microarray data. BMC Bioinformatics. 2006;7:359.
15. Subramanian A, Tamayo P, Mootha VK, et al. Gene set enrichment analysis: a knowledge-based approach for interpreting genome-wide expression profiles. Proc Natl Acad Sci U S A. 2005;102(43):15545–50.
16. Ronaghi M. Pyrosequencing sheds light on DNA sequencing. Genome Res. 2001;11(1):3–11.
17. Hash Functions. Dr. Dobb's Web site. http://drdobbs.com/database/184410284. Accessed 4 Sept 1997.

18. Burrows M, Wheeler D. A block sorting lossless data compression algorithm. Technical Report 124, Digital Equipment Corporation. 1994.

19. Smith TF, Waterman MS. Identification of common molecular subsequences. J Mol Biol. 1981;147(1): 195–7.

20. Sanger F, Coulson AR, Barrell BG, Smith AJ, Roe BA. Cloning in single-stranded bacteriophage as an aid to rapid DNA sequencing. J Mol Biol. 1980; 143(2):161–78.

21. Myers EW. Toward simplifying and accurately formulating fragment assembly. J Comput Biol. 1995;2(2): 275–90.

22. Zhi D, Raphael BJ, Price AL, Tang H, Pevzner PA. Identifying repeat domains in large genomes. Genome Biol. 2006;7(1):R7.

23. Perlis C, Herlyn M. Recent advances in melanoma biology. Oncologist. 2004;9(2):182–7.

24. Miller AJ, Mihm Jr MC. Melanoma. N Engl J Med. 2006;355(1):51–65.

25. Clark Jr WH, Elder DE, Guerry DT, Epstein MN, Greene MH, Van Horn M. A study of tumor progression: the precursor lesions of superficial spreading and nodular melanoma. Hum Pathol. 1984;15(12): 1147–65.

26. Zembowicz A, Scolyer RA. Nevus/melanocytoma/melanoma: an emerging paradigm for classification of melanocytic neoplasms? Arch Pathol Lab Med. 2011;135(3):300–6.

27. Uong A, Zon LI. Melanocytes in development and cancer. J Cell Physiol. 2010;222(1):38–41.

28. Chin L, Garraway LA, Fisher DE. Malignant melanoma: genetics and therapeutics in the genomic era. Genes Dev. 2006;20(16):2149–82.

29. Satyamoorthy K, Li G, Gerrero MR, et al. Constitutive mitogen-activated protein kinase activation in melanoma is mediated by both BRAF mutations and autocrine growth factor stimulation. Cancer Res. 2003; 63(4):756–9.

30. Willmore-Payne C, Holden JA, Tripp S, Layfield LJ. Human malignant melanoma: detection of BRAF- and c-kit-activating mutations by high-resolution amplicon melting analysis. Hum Pathol. 2005;36(5): 486–93.

31. Ackermann J, Frutschi M, Kaloulis K, McKee T, Trumpp A, Beermann F. Metastasizing melanoma formation caused by expression of activated N-RasQ61K on an INK4a-deficient background. Cancer Res. 2005;65(10):4005–11.

32. Gray-Schopfer VC, da Rocha Dias S, Marais R. The role of B-RAF in melanoma. Cancer Metastasis Rev. 2005;24(1):165–83.

33. Spittle C, Ward MR, Nathanson KL, et al. Application of a BRAF pyrosequencing assay for mutation detection and copy number analysis in malignant melanoma. J Mol Diagn. 2007;9(4):464–71.

34. Greulich KM, Utikal J, Peter RU, Krahn G. c-MYC and nodular malignant melanoma. A case report. Cancer. 2000;89(1):97–103.

35. Bastian BC, Olshen AB, LeBoit PE, Pinkel D. Classifying melanocytic tumors based on DNA copy number changes. Am J Pathol. 2003;163(5):1765–70.

36. Cowan JM, Halaban R, Francke U. Cytogenetic analysis of melanocytes from premalignant nevi and melanomas. J Natl Cancer Inst. 1988;80(14):1159–64.

37. Carr KM, Bittner M, Trent JM. Gene-expression profiling in human cutaneous melanoma. Oncogene. 2003;22(20):3076–80.

38. Haqq C, Nosrati M, Sudilovsky D, et al. The gene expression signatures of melanoma progression. Proc Natl Acad Sci U S A. 2005;102(17):6092–7.

39. Smith AP, Hoek K, Becker D. Whole-genome expression profiling of the melanoma progression pathway reveals marked molecular differences between nevi/melanoma in situ and advanced-stage melanomas. Cancer Biol Ther. 2005;4(9):1018–29.

40. Jaeger J, Koczan D, Thiesen HJ, et al. Gene expression signatures for tumor progression, tumor subtype, and tumor thickness in laser-microdissected melanoma tissues. Clin Cancer Res. 2007;13(3):806–15.

41. Riker AI, Enkemann SA, Fodstad O, et al. The gene expression profiles of primary and metastatic melanoma yields a transition point of tumor progression and metastasis. BMC Med Genomics. 2008;1:13.

42. Alonso SR, Tracey L, Ortiz P, et al. A high-throughput study in melanoma identifies epithelial-mesenchymal transition as a major determinant of metastasis. Cancer Res. 2007;67(7):3450–60.

43. John T, Black MA, Toro TT, et al. Predicting clinical outcome through molecular profiling in stage III melanoma. Clin Cancer Res. 2008;14(16):5173–80.

44. Karim RZ, Li W, Sanki A, et al. Reduced p16 and increased cyclin D1 and pRb expression are correlated with progression in cutaneous melanocytic tumors. Int J Surg Pathol. 2009;17(5):361–7.

45. Mehnert JM, McCarthy MM, Jilaveanu L, et al. Quantitative expression of VEGF, VEGF-R1, VEGF-R2, and VEGF-R3 in melanoma tissue microarrays. Hum Pathol. 2010;41(3):375–84.

46. DeRisi J, Penland L, Brown PO, et al. Use of a cDNA microarray to analyse gene expression patterns in human cancer. Nat Genet. 1996;14(4):457–60.

47. el-Deiry WS, Tokino T, Velculescu VE, et al. WAF1, a potential mediator of p53 tumor suppression. Cell. 1993;75(4):817–25.

48. Graves DT, Barnhill R, Galanopoulos T, Antoniades HN. Expression of monocyte chemotactic protein-1 in human melanoma in vivo. Am J Pathol. 1992;140(1): 9–14.

49. Vijayasaradhi S, Doskoch PM, Wolchok J, Houghton AN. Melanocyte differentiation marker gp75, the brown locus protein, can be regulated independently of tyrosinase and pigmentation. J Invest Dermatol. 1995;105(1):113–9.

50. Bittner M, Meltzer P, Chen Y, et al. Molecular classification of cutaneous malignant melanoma by gene expression profiling. Nature. 2000;406(6795): 536–40.

51. Kabbarah O, Nogueira C, Feng B, et al. Integrative genome comparison of primary and metastatic melanomas. PLoS One. 2010;5(5):e10770.

52. Morton DL, Wen DR, Wong JH, et al. Technical details of intraoperative lymphatic mapping for early stage melanoma. Arch Surg. 1992;127(4):392–9.

53. Yu LL, Flotte TJ, Tanabe KK, et al. Detection of microscopic melanoma metastases in sentinel lymph nodes. Cancer. 1999;86(4):617–27.

54. Messina JL, Glass LF, Cruse CW, Berman C, Ku NK, Reintgen DS. Pathologic examination of the sentinel lymph node in malignant melanoma. Am J Surg Pathol. 1999;23(6):686–90.

55. Koh SS, Opel ML, Wei JP, et al. Molecular classification of melanomas and nevi using gene expression microarray signatures and formalin-fixed and paraffin-embedded tissue. Mod Pathol. 2009;22(4):538–46.

56. Seftor EA, Brown KM, Chin L, et al. Epigenetic transdifferentiation of normal melanocytes by a metastatic melanoma microenvironment. Cancer Res. 2005;65(22):10164–9.

57. Hoon DS, Spugnardi M, Kuo C, Huang SK, Morton DL, Taback B. Profiling epigenetic inactivation of tumor suppressor genes in tumors and plasma from cutaneous melanoma patients. Oncogene. 2004;23(22): 4014–22.

58. Furuta J, Nobeyama Y, Umebayashi Y, Otsuka F, Kikuchi K, Ushijima T. Silencing of Peroxiredoxin 2 and aberrant methylation of 33 CpG islands in putative promoter regions in human malignant melanomas. Cancer Res. 2006;66(12):6080–6.

59. Liu S, Ren S, Howell P, Fodstad O, Riker AI. Identification of novel epigenetically modified genes in human melanoma via promoter methylation gene profiling. Pigment Cell Melanoma Res. 2008;21(5):545–58.

60. Rothhammer T, Bosserhoff AK. Epigenetic events in malignant melanoma. Pigment Cell Res. 2007;20(2): 92–111.

61. Muthusamy V, Duraisamy S, Bradbury CM, et al. Epigenetic silencing of novel tumor suppressors in malignant melanoma. Cancer Res. 2006;66(23): 11187–93.

62. Stark MS, Tyagi S, Nancarrow DJ, et al. Characterization of the melanoma miRNAome by deep sequencing. PLoS One. 2010;5(3):e9685.

63. Winnepenninckx V, Lazar V, Michiels S, et al. Gene expression profiling of primary cutaneous melanoma and clinical outcome. J Natl Cancer Inst. 2006;98(7): 472–82.

64. Eisen T, Ahmad T, Flaherty KT, et al. Sorafenib in advanced melanoma: a phase II randomised discontinuation trial analysis. Br J Cancer. 2006;95(5):581–6.

65. Bedikian AY, Millward M, Pehamberger H, et al. Bcl-2 antisense (oblimersen sodium) plus dacarbazine in patients with advanced melanoma: the Oblimersen Melanoma Study Group. J Clin Oncol. 2006;24(29): 4738–45.

66. Markovic SN, Geyer SM, Dawkins F, et al. A phase II study of bortezomib in the treatment of metastatic malignant melanoma. Cancer. 2005;103(12):2584–9.

67. End DW, Smets G, Todd AV, et al. Characterization of the antitumor effects of the selective farnesyl protein transferase inhibitor R115777 in vivo and in vitro. Cancer Res. 2001;61(1):131–7.

68. O'Donnell A, Faivre S, Burris 3rd HA, et al. Phase I pharmacokinetic and pharmacodynamic study of the oral mammalian target of rapamycin inhibitor everolimus in patients with advanced solid tumors. J Clin Oncol. 2008;26(10):1588–95.*same genes identified in different studies

Index

A. Baldi et al. (eds.), *Skin Cancer*, Current Clinical Pathology,
DOI 10.1007/978-1-4614-7357-2, © Springer Science+Business Media New York 2014

Printed by Printforce, the Netherlands